D0189453

THE PILL BOOK, 8th REVISED EDITION:
THE ILLUSTRATED GUIDE TO THE MOST
PRESCRIBED DRUGS IN THE UNITED STATES
Illustrated with 32 pages of actual-size color photographs

With more than 10 million copies in print, THE PILL BOOK is the bestselling consumer drug reference ever, offering the most up-to-date, comprehensive information, now in a revised format designed for ease of use.

This new 8th edition of THE PILL BOOK is bigger than ever and contains more profiles of commonly prescribed drugs than any other consumer reference. Compiled by a team of eminent pharmacologists, it is based on official, FDA-approved information usually available only to doctors and pharmacists, plus the latest information gathered from computer databases and on-line resources. It synthesizes the most important facts about each drug in a concise, readable, easy-to-understand entry.

Here are complete profiles of more than 1,500 of the most commonly prescribed drugs, including:

- Generic and brand names
- What the drug is for and how it works
- Usual dosages, and what to do if a dose is skipped
- Side effects and possible adverse reactions, highlighted for quick reference
- Interactions with other drugs and foods
- Overdose and addiction potential
- Alcohol-free and sugar-free medications
- Information for seniors, pregnant and breast-feeding women, and others with special needs
- Cautions and warnings, and when to call your doctor

This completely revised and updated 8th edition contains dozens of new brand names and more than 50 important new drugs approved by the FDA in late 1997 that will go on sale for the first time in 1998. A 32-page insert provides actual-size full color photographs of the most-prescribed pills.

THE PILL BOOK

8th EDITION

Editor-in-Chief
HAROLD M. SILVERMAN, Pharm. D.

Production
CMD PUBLISHING
A DIVISION OF
CURRENT MEDICAL DIRECTIONS

Consultants
MARIA WASILIK, R.Ph.
JUDITH I. BROWN

Digital Photography and Color Separations
WACE, NEW YORK
SIGLER AND FLANDERS

Original Creators of THE PILL BOOK
LAWRENCE D. CHILNICK
BERT STERN
HAROLD M. SILVERMAN, Pharm. D.
GILBERT I. SIMON, Sc.D.

BANTAM BOOKS
NEW YORK • TORONTO • LONDON • SYDNEY • AUCKLAND

THE PILL BOOK

A Bantam Book

PUBLISHING HISTORY

*Bantam edition published June 1979
Bantam revised edition / October 1982
Bantam 3rd revised edition / March 1986
Bantam 4th revised edition / February 1990
Bantam 5th revised edition / May 1992
Bantam 6th revised edition / June 1994
Bantam 7th revised edition / June 1996
Bantam 8th revised edition / May 1998
This revised edition was published simultaneously in
trade paperback and mass market paperback.*

ISBN: 0-553-57971-1

*Bantam Books are published by Bantam Books, a division of Bantam
Doubleday Dell Publishing Group, Inc. Its trademark, consisting of the
words "Bantam Books" and the portrayal of a rooster, is Registered in U.S.
Patent and Trademark Office and in other countries. Marca Registrada.
Bantam Books, 1540 Broadway, New York, New York 10036.*

PRINTED IN THE UNITED STATES OF AMERICA

OPM   17   16   15   14

Contents

How to Use This Book

How to Find Your Medication in *The Pill Book*

- *The Pill Book* lists most medications in alphabetic order by generic name because a medication may have many brand names but has only 1 generic name. Most generic medications produce the same therapeutic effects as their brand-name equivalents but are much less expensive. Drugs that are available generically are indicated by the [G] symbol.

- When a medication has 2 or more active ingredients, it is listed by the most widely known brand name. In a few cases, pill profiles are listed by drug type (e.g., antidiabetes drugs).

- *The Pill Book* includes brand names of the top 100 drugs, with the page numbers they appear on, in alphabetic order with the pill profiles.

- Most over-the-counter (OTC) medications are not included in *The Pill Book*. For complete information on OTC medications, refer to *The Pill Book Guide to Over-the-Counter Medications*.

- All brand and generic names are listed in the Index. Brand names are indicated by boldface.

- Sugar-free and alcohol-free brand-name drugs are indicated by the [S] and [A] symbols in the beginning of each pill profile.

The Pill Book, like pills themselves, should be taken with caution. Used properly, this book may save you money and, perhaps, your life. It contains life-size pictures of the most prescribed brand-name drugs in the U.S. *The Pill Book*'s product identification system is designed to help you check that the medication you are about to take is the one your doctor prescribed. Although many dosage forms are included, not all available forms and strengths of every medication have been shown. While every effort has been made to create accurate photographic reproductions of the products, some variations in size or color may be expected as a result of the printing process. Do not rely solely on the photographic images to identify your pills; check with your pharmacist if you have any product identification questions.

Each pill profile in *The Pill Book* contains the following information:

Generic and Brand Name: The generic name is the common name of the drug approved by the Food and Drug Administration (FDA). It is listed along with the current brand names available for each generic drug. Medications that are available in a generic form are indicated by the Ⓖ symbol.

Most prescription drugs are sold in more than one strength. Some drugs, such as oral contraceptives, come in packages containing different numbers of pills. A few manufacturers reflect this fact by adding letters and/or numbers to the basic drug name; others do not. An example: Loestrin 21 1.5/30 and Loestrin 21 1/20. (The numbers here refer to the number of tablets in each monthly packet, 21, and the amount of medication found in the tablets.) Other drugs come in different strengths: This is often indicated by a notation such as "DS" (double strength) or "Forte" (stronger).

The Pill Book lists generic and brand names together only where there are no differences in basic ingredients (e.g., Loestrin). However, the amount of the ingredient (strength) may vary from product to product. In most cases, the brand names and generic versions listed for each medication are interchangeable; you can use any version of the drug and expect that it will work for you. *The Pill Book* identifies those medications for which generic versions are not considered equivalent and which should not be interchanged with a brand-name product or another generic version of the same drug.

Type of Drug: Describes the general pharmacologic class of each drug: "antidepressant," "tranquilizer," "decongestant," "expectorant," and so on.

Prescribed for: All drugs are approved for some symptoms or conditions by federal authorities, but doctors also commonly prescribe drugs for other, as yet unapproved, reasons; these are also listed in *The Pill Book*. Check with your doctor if you are not sure why you have been given a certain pill.

General Information: Information on how the drug works, how long it takes for you to feel its effects, or a description of how this drug is similar to or different from other drugs.

Cautions and Warnings: This information alerts you to important and more dangerous reactions and to physical conditions, such as heart disease, that can have serious consequences if the medication is prescribed for you.

Possible Side Effects: Side effects are generally divided into 4 categories—those that are most common, common, less common, and rare—to help you better understand what to expect from your pills. If you are not sure whether you are experiencing a drug side effect, ask your doctor.

Drug Interactions: Describes what happens when you combine your medication with other drugs and lists what should not be taken at the same time as your medication. Some interactions may be deadly. At every visit, be sure to inform your doctor of any medication you are already taking. Your pharmacist should also keep a record of all your prescription and OTC medications. This listing, called a *Patient Drug Profile*, is used to check for potential problems. You may want to keep your own drug profile and take it to your pharmacist for review whenever a new medication is added. You would be surprised at how many drug interaction problems may develop.

Food Interactions: Provides information on foods to avoid while taking your medication, whether to take your medication with meals, and other important facts.

Usual Dose: Tells you the largest and smallest doses usually prescribed. You may be given different dosage instructions by your doctor. Do not change the dosage of ANY medication you take without first calling your doctor.

Overdosage: Describes overdose symptoms and what to do.

Special Information: Includes symptoms to watch for, when to call your doctor, what to do if you forget a dose of your medication, and any special instructions.

Special Populations: *Pregnancy/Breast-feeding:* For women who are or might be pregnant, and what to do if you must take a medication during the time you are nursing your baby. *Seniors:* This section presents the special facts an older adult needs to know about every drug and explains how reactions may differ from those of a younger person.

In an Emergency!

Each year over 70,000 people experience drug-related poisoning in the U.S., and about 10% of those cases result in death. In fact, drug overdose is a leading cause of fatal poisoning in the U.S.

Although each of the pill profiles in *The Pill Book* has specific information on drug overdose, there are a few general rules to remember if you are faced with an accidental poisoning.

1. Make sure the victim is breathing, and call for medical help immediately.
2. Learn the phone number for your local poison control center and post it near the phone. Call the center in an emergency. When you call, be prepared to explain:

   - What drug was taken and how much.
   - Status of the victim (e.g., conscious, sleeping, vomiting, or having convulsions).
   - The approximate age and weight of the victim.
   - Any chronic medical problems of the victim (e.g., diabetes, epilepsy, or high blood pressure), if you know them.
   - What medications, if any, the victim takes regularly.

3. Remove anything that might interfere with breathing. A person who is not getting enough oxygen will turn blue

(the fingernails or tongue change color first). If this happens, lay the victim on his or her back, open the collar, place one hand under the neck, and lift, pull, or push the victim's jaw so that it juts outward. This will open the airway between the mouth and lungs as wide as possible. Begin mouth-to-mouth resuscitation ONLY if the victim is not breathing.

4. If the victim is unconscious or having convulsions, call for medical help immediately. While waiting for the ambulance, lay the victim on his or her stomach and turn the head to one side. Should the victim throw up, this will prevent inhalation of vomit. DO NOT give an unconscious victim anything by mouth. Keep the victim warm.

5. If the victim is conscious, call for medical help and give the victim an 8-oz. glass of water to drink. This will dilute the poison.

Only a small number of poisoning victims require hospitalization. Most may be treated with simple actions or need no treatment at all.

The poison control center may tell you to make the patient vomit. The best way to do this is to use ipecac syrup, which is available over-the-counter at any pharmacy. Specific instructions on how much to give infants, children, or adults are printed on the label and will also be given by your poison control center. Remember, DO NOT make the victim vomit unless you have been instructed to do so. Never make the victim vomit if the victim is unconscious, is having a convulsion, or has a painful, burning feeling in the mouth or throat.

Be Prepared

The best way to deal with a poisoning is to be prepared for it. Do the following now:

1. Write the telephone number of your local poison control center next to your other emergency phone numbers.
2. Decide which hospital you will go to, if necessary, and how you will get there.
3. Buy 1 oz. of ipecac syrup from your pharmacy. The pharmacist will tell you how to use it. Remember, this is a potent drug to be used only if directed.
4. Learn to give mouth-to-mouth resuscitation.

Reduce the Risk of Drug Related Poisoning

1. Keep all medication in a locked place out of the reach of young children.
2. Do not store medications in containers that once held food.
3. Do not remove the labels from bottles so that the contents are unknown.
4. Discard all medications when you no longer need them.

The Most Commonly Prescribed Drugs in the United States, Generic and Brand Names, with Complete Descriptions of Drugs and Their Effects

Generic Name

Acarbose (uh-CAR-bose)

Brand Name

Precose

Type of Drug

Antidiabetic.

Prescribed for

Non-insulin-dependent diabetes mellitus.

General Information

Acarbose works in a different way than many other antidiabetes drugs, such as the sulfonylureas and metformin. Acarbose interferes with enzymes in the intestine responsible for
breaking down the complex carbohydrates found in starchy
foods into simple sugars, including glucose. Acarbose lowers
blood sugar by delaying the absorption of glucose into the
blood after eating. Because it works against diabetes in this
way, the blood-sugar-lowering effect of acarbose is additive
to that of other antidiabetes drugs. Acarbose may also be
used by people who are unable to control their blood sugar
by diet alone. Half of each dose of acarbose remains unchanged in the intestines, passing out of the body in the stool;
about 2% is absorbed into the blood, and the rest is broken
down in the intestines. Most of acarbose's side effects are
related directly to the fact that it leaves undigested carbohydrates in the lower intestines. In studies of acarbose, black
and white patients responded similarly, but a better response
was seen in Hispanic patients.

Cautions and Warnings

Acarbose should not be used if you are **allergic** or sensitive to
it. People should not use acarbose if they have **diabetic
ketoacidosis, cirrhosis, severe kidney disease, inflammatory
bowel disease, ulcers of the colon, intestinal obstruction,
severe digestive disease** or **absorption diseases,** or if **intestinal gas** will be a severe problem. Acarbose may lead to liver
inflammation.

Possible Side Effects

▼ Most common: stomach gas (in ¾ of people who take it), abdominal pains, and diarrhea. These side effects tend to improve or go away after a few weeks.

▼ Rare: liver irritation and minor abnormalities in blood tests.

Drug Interactions

• Acarbose adds to the blood-sugar-lowering effect of sulfonylureas and other antidiabetes drugs.

• Activated charcoal and antacids—and other drugs intended to absorb stomach contents—and digestive enzyme preparations may reduce the effectiveness of acarbose. Separate these drugs from acarbose by at least 2 hours.

Food Interactions

Acarbose must be taken with the first bite of each meal.

Usual Dose

Adult: 25–50 mg (up to 100 mg) 3 times a day.
Child: not recommended.

Overdosage

Acarbose overdose does not cause low blood sugar, but diarrhea, abdominal pains and intestinal gas can be expected. Call your local poison control center for more information.

Special Information

It is essential to take each dose of acarbose at the beginning of each meal. Since the drug works in the intestines, it has to be there at the same time as the food you are digesting.

As with all antidiabetes medicines, people taking acarbose must follow their doctors' instructions for diet, exercise, and blood sugar testing.

Read product labels carefully or check with your pharmacist before buying any nonprescription drug to be sure it is safe for diabetics to take with acarbose.

If you forget a dose of acarbose, skip it and continue with your regular schedule. Taking a missed dose between meals will not provide any benefit.

Special Populations

Pregnancy/Breast-feeding
Animal studies of acarbose showed no effects on the fetus, but there is no information available on its effect in humans. Blood sugar control is considered essential during pregnancy and insulin is usually prescribed for that purpose. When acarbose is considered crucial by your doctor, its potential benefits must be weighed against its risks.

It is not known if acarbose passes into human breast milk. Nursing mothers who must take this medicine should consider bottle-feeding their babies.

Seniors
Blood levels of acarbose are higher in older adults, but this is not considered important. Seniors with severe kidney disease should avoid this medicine.

Accupril

see *Quinapril*, page 951

Generic Name

Acebutolol (ah-seh-BUTE-uh-lol) Ⓖ

Brand Name
Sectral

Type of Drug
Beta-adrenergic blocking agent.

Prescribed for
High blood pressure and abnormal heart rhythms.

General Information
Acebutolol hydrochloride is one of 15 beta-adrenergic blocking drugs, or beta blockers, that interfere with the action of a specific part of the nervous system. Beta receptors are found all over the body and affect many body functions. This accounts for the usefulness of beta blockers against a wide

variety of conditions. The oldest of these drugs, propranolol, affects the entire beta-adrenergic range of the nervous system. Newer, more refined beta blockers affect only a portion of that system, making them more useful in the treatment of cardiovascular disorders and less useful for other purposes. Other of the newer beta blockers act as mild stimulants to the heart or have particular characteristics that make them adapted to specific purposes or certain people.

Cautions and Warnings

You should be cautious about taking acebutolol if you have **asthma**, **severe heart failure**, a **very slow heart rate**, or **heart block** (disruption of the electrical impulses that control heart rate) because the drug may aggravate these conditions. Compared with other beta blockers, acebutolol has less of an effect on pulse and bronchial muscles—which affect asthma—and less of a rebound effect when discontinued; it also produces less tiredness, depression, and intolerance to exercise.

People with **angina** taking acebutolol for high blood pressure risk aggravating their angina if they suddenly stop taking the drug. These patients should have their acebutolol dosage reduced gradually over 1 to 2 weeks.

Acebutolol should be used with caution if you have **liver or kidney disease** because your ability to eliminate this drug from your body may be impaired.

Acebutolol reduces the amount of blood pumped by the heart with each beat. This reduction in blood flow may aggravate the condition of people with **poor circulation** or **circulatory disease**.

If you are undergoing **major surgery**, your doctor may want you to stop taking acebutolol at least 2 days before surgery to permit the heart to respond more acutely to stresses that can occur during the procedure. This practice is still controversial and may not be appropriate for all surgeries.

Possible Side Effects

Side effects are relatively uncommon and usually mild; normally they develop early in the course of treatment and are rarely a reason to stop taking acebutolol.

▼ Most common: impotence.
▼ Less common: unusual tiredness or weakness, slow

Possible Side Effects *(continued)*

heartbeat, heart failure (symptoms include swelling of the legs, ankles, or feet), dizziness, breathing difficulties, bronchospasm, depression, confusion, anxiety, nervousness, sleeplessness, disorientation, short-term memory loss, emotional instability, cold hands and feet, constipation, diarrhea, nausea, vomiting, upset stomach, increased sweating, urinary difficulties, cramps, blurred vision, skin rash, hair loss, stuffy nose, facial swelling, aggravation of lupus erythematosus (chronic condition affecting the body's connective tissue), itching, chest pain, back or joint pain, colitis, drug allergy (symptoms include fever and sore throat), and liver toxicity.

Drug Interactions

• Acebutolol may interact with surgical anesthetics to increase the risk of heart problems during surgery. Some anesthesiologists recommend having gradually stopped the drug by 2 days before surgery.

• Acebutolol may interfere with the normal signs of low blood sugar and with the action of oral antidiabetes drugs.

• Acebutolol increases the blood-pressure-lowering effects of other blood-pressure-reducing agents, including clonidine, guanabenz, and reserpine; and calcium-channel blockers, such as nifedipine.

• Aspirin-containing drugs, indomethacin, sulfinpyrazone, and estrogen drugs may interfere with the blood-pressure-lowering effect of acebutolol.

• Cocaine may reduce the effectiveness of all beta-blockers.

• Acebutolol may worsen the problem of cold hands and feet associated with ergot alkaloids, used to treat for migraine headaches. Gangrene is a possibility in people taking both an ergot and acebutolol.

• Acebutolol will counteract thyroid hormone replacements.

• Calcium channel blockers, flecainide, hydralazine, oral contraceptives, propafenone, haloperidol, phenothiazine tranquilizers—molindone and others—quinolone antibacterials, and quinidine may increase the amount of acebutolol in the bloodstream and lead to increased acebutolol effects.

• Acebutolol should not be taken within 2 weeks of taking a monoamine oxidase inhibitor (MAOI) antidepressant.

• Cimetidine increases the amount of acebutolol absorbed into the bloodstream from oral tablets.

• Acebutolol may interfere with the effects of some anti-asthma drugs including theophylline and aminophylline, and especially ephedrine and isoproterenol.

• Combining acebutolol with phenytoin or digitalis drugs may result in excessive slowing of the heart, possibly causing heart block.

• If you stop smoking while taking acebutolol, your dose may have to be reduced because your liver will break down the drug more slowly afterward.

Food Interactions

None known.

Usual Dose

Adult: starting dose—400 mg a day, taken all at once or in 2 divided doses. The daily dose may be gradually increased. Maintenance dose—400–1200 mg a day.

Senior: Older adults may respond to lower doses and should be treated more cautiously, beginning with 200 mg a day, increasing gradually to a maximum of 800 mg a day.

Overdosage

Symptoms of overdose include changes in heartbeat—unusually slow, unusually fast, or irregular—severe dizziness or fainting, breathing difficulties, bluish-colored fingernails or palms, and seizures. The victim should be taken to a hospital emergency room. ALWAYS bring the prescription bottle or container with you.

Special Information

Acebutolol is meant to be taken continuously. When ending acebutolol treatment, dosage should be reduced gradually over a period of about 2 weeks. Do not stop taking this drug unless directed to do so by your doctor: Abrupt withdrawal may cause chest pain, breathing difficulties, increased sweating, and unusually fast or irregular heartbeat.

Call your doctor at once if you develop back or joint pain, breathing difficulties, cold hands or feet, depression, skin rash, or changes in heartbeat. Acebutolol may produce an undesirable lowering of blood pressure, leading to dizziness or fainting; call your doctor if this happens to you. Call your doctor if you experience persistent or bothersome anxiety, diarrhea, constipation, impotence, headache, itching, nausea or vomiting, nightmares or vivid dreams, upset stomach, trouble sleeping, stuffy nose, frequent urination, unusual tiredness, or weakness.

Acebutolol may cause drowsiness, dizziness, light-headedness, or blurred vision. Be careful when driving or performing complex tasks.

It is best to take acebutolol at the same time each day. If you forget a dose, take it as soon as you remember. If you take acebutolol once a day and it is within 8 hours of your next dose, skip the dose you forgot and continue with your regular schedule. If you take acebutolol twice a day and it is within 4 hours of your next dose, skip the missed dose and continue with your regular schedule. Never take a double dose.

Special Populations

Pregnancy/Breast-feeding

Infants born to women who took a beta blocker while pregnant had lower birth weights, low blood pressure, and reduced heart rates. Acebutolol should be avoided by pregnant women and women who might become pregnant while taking it. When the drug is considered crucial by your doctor, its potential benefits must be carefully weighed against its risks.

Large amounts of acebutolol pass into breast milk. Nursing mothers taking acebutelol should bottle-feed their babies.

Seniors

Seniors may absorb and retain more acebutolol and may require less of the drug to achieve results. Your doctor should adjust your dosage to meet your individual needs. Seniors taking acebutolol may be more likely to suffer from cold hands and feet, reduced body temperature, chest pain, general feelings of ill health, sudden breathing difficulties, increased sweating, or changes in heartbeat.

Generic Name

Acetazolamide (uh-sete-uh-ZOLE-uh-mide)

Brand Names

Dazamide   Diamox Sequels
Diamox

Type of Drug

Carbonic-anhydrase inhibitor.

Prescribed for

Glaucoma and prevention or treatment of mountain sickness; also prescribed for epilepsy, including absence seizures, petit mal and grand mal epilepsy, tonic-clonic seizures, mixed seizures, and partial seizures.

General Information

Acetazolamide inhibits an enzyme in the body called carbonic anhydrase. This effect allows the drug to be used as a weak diuretic; as part of the treatment of glaucoma it helps to reduce pressure inside the eye. The same effect on carbonic anhydrase makes acetazolamide a useful drug in treating certain epileptic seizure disorders. The exact way in which the effect is produced is not understood.

Cautions and Warnings

Do not take acetazolamide if you have serious **kidney, liver, or Addison's disease**. This drug should not be used by people with **low blood sodium or potassium**.

Possible Side Effects

Side effects of short-term acetazolamide therapy are usually minimal.

▼ Most common: nausea or vomiting; tingling feeling in the arms, legs, lips, mouth, or anus; appetite and weight loss; a metallic taste; increased frequency in urination (to be expected, since this drug has a weak diuretic effect); diarrhea; not feeling well; occasional drowsiness, and weakness. Since this drug is chemically a sulfa drug, it can have sulfa side effects, including rash, drug crystals in the urine, painful urination, low back pain, urinary difficulty, and low urine volumes.

▼ Rare: breathing difficulties, fever, sore throat, unusual bleeding or bruising, hives, itching, rash or sores, black or tarry stools, darkened urine, yellow skin or eyes, transient nearsightedness, clumsiness or unsteadiness, confusion, convulsions, ringing or buzzing in the ears, headache, sensitivity to bright light, increased blood

---

Possible Side Effects *(continued)*

sugar, weakness and trembling, nervousness, depression, dizziness, dry mouth, excessive thirst, abnormal heart rhythms, muscle cramps or pains, weak pulse, disorientation, muscle spasms, and loss of taste or smell.

Drug Interactions

• Avoid nonprescription drug products that contain stimulants or anticholinergics, which tend to aggravate glaucoma or cardiac disease. Ask your pharmacist about ingredients contained in over-the-counter drugs.

• Acetazolamide may increase blood concentrations of cyclosporine, used to prevent the rejection of transplanted organs and for other purposes.

• Acetazolamide may inhibit or delay the absorption of primidone—prescribed for seizure—into the bloodstream.

• Avoid aspirin while taking acetazolamide, since acetazolamide side effects can be enhanced by this combination.

• The combination of diflunisal and acetazolamide can result in an unusual lowering of eye pressure.

Food Interactions

Acetazolamide may be taken with food if it upsets your stomach. Because acetazolamide can increase potassium loss, take this drug with foods that are rich in potassium, like apricots, bananas, orange juice, or raisins.

Usual Dose

250–1000 mg a day, according to disease and patient's condition.

Overdosage

Symptoms of overdose may include drowsiness, loss of appetite, nausea, vomiting, dizziness, tingling in the hands or feet, weakness, tremors, or ringing or buzzing in the ears. Overdose victims should be made to vomit as soon as possible with ipecac syrup—available at any pharmacy—and taken to a hospital emergency room. ALWAYS bring the prescription bottle or container with you.

Special Information

Acetazolamide may cause minor drowsiness and confusion,

particularly during the first 2 weeks of therapy. Take care while performing tasks that require concentration, such as driving or operating appliances or machinery.

Call your doctor if you develop sore throat, fever, unusual bleeding or bruises, tingling in the hands or feet, rash, or unusual pains. These can be signs of side effects.

Acetazolamide can make you unusually sensitive to the sun. Avoid prolonged sun exposure and protect your eyes while taking this medicine.

If you forget a dose of acetazolamide, take it as soon as you remember. If it is almost time for your next dose, skip the dose you forgot and continue with your regular schedule. Do not take a double dose.

Special Populations

Pregnancy/Breast-feeding
High doses of this drug may cause birth defects or interfere with fetal development. Check with your doctor before taking it if you are or might be pregnant.

Small amounts of acetazolamide may pass into breast milk, but the drug has not caused problems in breast-fed infants.

Seniors
Seniors are more likely to have problems with acetazolamide. Take this medication according to your doctor's prescription.

Generic Name

Acitretin (ah-sih-TREH-tin)

Brand Name
Soriatane

Type of Drug
Antipsoriatic.

Prescribed for
Severe psoriasis; also prescribed for a variety of other skin conditions.

General Information
Acitretin is related to vitamin A and prescription drugs such

as etretinate and isotretinoin. It is produced when etretinate is broken down in the body and its effects are very similar to those of etretinate. The way that acitretin works is not known. Its effects are not likely to be seen until you have taken it for 2 or 3 months. Because of the risks associated with acitretin, your doctor is urged to use this medication only in cases of severe psoriasis that have not responded to other treatments.

Cautions and Warnings

Women who take acitretin must not be pregnant during the treatment or become pregnant for 3 years following the completion of treatment.

A small number of people taking this drug have developed **liver damage** including jaundice (symptoms include yellowing of the skin and whites of the eyes). People with **kidney failure** have much less acitretin in their blood than people with normal kidneys. Caution is advised for people with liver or kidney damage.

Blood fat levels rise in 25% to 50% of people·taking acitretin. Very large increases in triglycerides are uncommon but a few cases of **pancreatitis (pancreas inflammation)** have occurred. Your doctor should measure your blood fat levels before you start taking acitretin and monitor them weekly or biweekly until your response to the medication has been determined. People with **diabetes**, who are **obese**, or who have a **history of these conditions** are at increased risk for high blood fat levels as are people who **drink alcohol excessively**.

Drugs similar to acitretin have been associated with **pseudotumor cerebri (increased pressure in the brain)**. Symptoms of pseudotumor cerebri include **visual disturbances, headache, nausea, and vomiting**. Report these or any unusual symptoms to your doctor at once.

People taking acitretin who had **spine or bone—including knee or ankle—problems** before starting the drug may find that their problems worsen while on the drug.

People with **diabetes** may find it more difficult to control their blood sugar while on acitretin.

Possible Side Effects

▼ Most common: hair loss, peeling skin, and inflammation of the lips.

Possible Side Effects *(continued)*

▼ Common: dry eyes, chills or stiffness, dry skin, fingernail problems, itching, rash, tingling in the hands or feet, increased sensory awareness, loss of some sections of skin, sticky skin, and runny nose.

▼ Less common: drying and thickening of eye tissue, eye irritation, eyebrow or eye lash loss, changes in appetite, swelling, fatigue, hot flashes, flushing, sinus irritation, headache, pain, Bell's palsy, crusting of the eyelids, blurred vision, conjunctivitis (pinkeye), double vision, itchy eyes or eyelids, cataracts, swelling inside the eye, unusual sensitivity to bright light, dry mouth, nosebleeds, joint pain, and worsening of existing spinal problems.

▼ Rare: unusual skin odor, changes in hair texture, sweating, large blisters erupting on the skin, cold or clammy skin, skin irritation, skin infection, bleeding or clotting under the skin, cracks in the skin, seborrhea, sunburn, blurred or abnormal vision, poor night vision, eye pain, sensitivity to bright light, abdominal pain, diarrhea, nausea, tongue problems, gum irritation or bleeding, increased salivation, mouth sores, thirst, arthritis, back pain, bone pain, muscle stiffness, muscle ache, bone spurs in arm or leg joints, depression, sleeplessness, tiredness, earache, changes in sense of taste, and ringing or buzzing in the ears.

Drug Interactions

• People combining acitretin and glyburide (an antidiabetic) may have unusually low blood-sugar levels. Your doctor may have to adjust your diabetic treatment program while you are taking acitretin.

• Combining acitretin with methotrexate increases the risk of liver damage.

• Acitretin reduces the effectiveness of low-progestin oral contraceptives (the "mini-pill"). If you are taking one of these contraceptives, switch to another type of birth control and use at least one other contraceptive method for at least 3 years after treatment is completed.

• Combining alcohol with acitretin produces acitretin's parent compound, etretinate. Etretinate stays in the body much longer than acitretin and may therefore affect the fetus for an even longer period of time than might acitretin. Avoid alcoholic beverages.

• Acitretin is related to vitamin A. Do not take a vitamin A supplement that has more than the standard minimum daily requirement. Taking excess vitamin A with acitretin exposes you to the possibility of vitamin A toxicity.

Food Interactions

Acitretin is best absorbed when taken with food or meals.

Usual Dose

Adult: 25–50 mg a day with your main meal. Dosage must be individualized to your specific needs.

Child: not recommended.

Overdosage

One case of overdose is known and that person vomited several hours after taking the drug. Call your local hospital emergency room or local poison control center for more information.

Special Information

Contact your doctor at once if you become pregnant while taking acitretin or in the 3 years following treatment. The risk of birth defects persists as long as the drug is in your body. A case is known in which small amounts of etretinate were found in blood plasma and fatty tissue more than 5 years after treatment.

Report visual disturbances, headache, nausea, vomiting, or anything unusual to your doctor at once.

Do not drink any alcoholic beverages during acitretin treatment and for at least 2 months after treatment has been completed.

Avoid excess vitamin A.

Some birth control methods, including low-dose progestin contraceptives and tubal ligation may fail while taking this drug. Be sure to use at least one additional form of contraception while taking acitretin to avoid pregnancy.

You may have problems tolerating contact lenses while you are taking acitretin.

Do not donate blood while taking acitretin or for 3 years afterwards because of the possibility that your blood will be given to a pregnant woman.

Avoid exposure to excessive sunlight or to sunlamps because of unusual sensitivity caused by acitretin.

If you forget to take a dose of acitretin, take it with food as soon as you remember. If it is almost time for your next dose, skip the one you forgot and continue with your regular schedule. Do not take a double dose.

Special Populations

Pregnancy/Breast-feeding
Acitretin causes birth defects and may damage the fetus.

Women who take acitretin must be sure that they are not pregnant before starting therapy by using a reliable contraceptive method for at least 1 month before starting the drug and taking a pregnancy test within one week of starting treatment. You must use 2 reliable contraceptive methods during treatment and for 3 years following the completion of treatment. Be cautious. Some birth control pills may lose their effectiveness if you are taking acitretin. It is not known if men taking acitretin also pose a risk to the fetus, though several healthy babies have been born to fathers who took acitretin during conception.

Acitretin may pass into breast milk. Nursing mothers who must take this drug should bottle-feed their infants.

Seniors
Seniors have twice as much acitretin in their blood as do younger adults but may take acitretin without special precaution.

Generic Name

Acyclovir (ae-SYE-kloe-vir)

Brand Name
Zovirax

Type of Drug
Antiviral.

Prescribed for
Serious, frequently recurring herpes simplex infections of the genitals, mucous membrane tissue, and central nervous

system; herpes zoster (shingles); varicella (chickenpox); and viral infections including nongenital herpes simplex, herpes simplex and cytomegalovirus (CMV) in immunocompromised patients, and varicella pneumonia.

General Information

Acyclovir is the only oral drug that reduces growth rates of the herpes virus and the related viruses, Epstein-Barr, varicella, and CMV; both oral acyclovir and oral ganciclovir work against CMV. Other intravenous drugs, including acyclovir injection, may be used for these viral infections; however, intravenous antiviral drugs are usually reserved for patients with AIDS, cancer, or otherwise compromised immune systems.

Acyclovir is selectively absorbed into cells that are infected with the herpes simplex virus, where it is converted into its active form. Acyclovir works by interfering with the reproduction of viral DNA, slowing the growth of existing viruses. It has little effect on recurrent infections. To treat both local and systemic (whole-body) symptoms acyclovir must be given by intravenous injection in a hospital or doctor's office or taken by mouth. Local symptoms may be treated with the ointment alone. Oral acyclovir may be taken every day to reduce the number and severity of herpes attacks in people who suffer 10 or more attacks a year; it may also be used to treat intermittent attacks as they occur, but treatment must be started as soon as possible to have the greatest effect.

Cautions and Warnings

Do not use acyclovir ointment if you have had an **allergic** reaction to it or to the major component of the ointment base, polyethylene glycol. Do not apply acyclovir ointment inside the vagina because the polyethylene glycol base may cause irritation and swelling of sensitive vaginal tissue. Acyclovir ointment is not intended for use in the eye and should not be used to treat a herpes infection of the eye.

Some people develop **tenderness, swelling, or bleeding of the gums** while taking acyclovir. Regular brushing, flossing, and gum massage may help prevent these conditions.

Long-term high doses of acyclovir have caused reduced sperm counts in animals, but this effect has not been reported in men.

Possible Side Effects

Ointment
▼ Most common: mild burning, irritation, rash, and itching. These effects are more likely to occur when treating an initial herpes attack than a recurrent attack. Women are 4 times more likely to experience burning than men.

Capsules/Suspension/Tablets
▼ Most common: dizziness, headache, diarrhea, nausea, and vomiting.
▼ Less common: appetite loss, stomach gas, constipation, fatigue, rash, not feeling well, leg pains, sore throat, a bad taste in the mouth, sleeplessness, and fever.
▼ Rare: aching joints, weakness, and tingling in the hands or feet.

Intravenous
▼ Rare: pain or inflammation at the injection site, liver inflammation, confusion, hallucinations, tremors, agitation, seizures, coma, anemia, kidney damage, blood in the urine, pain or pressure when urinating, loss of bladder control, abdominal pain, fluid in the lungs, and bluish-colored fingertips.

Drug Interactions

• Do not apply acyclovir together with any other ointment or topical medication.
• Oral probenecid may decrease elimination of acyclovir from the body, which increases blood levels of oral or injected acyclovir, increasing the chance of side effects.
• Combining acyclovir and zidovudine (an AIDS drug— also known as AZT) may lead to severe drowsiness and lethargy.

Food Interactions

Acyclovir may be taken with food if it upsets your stomach.

Usual Dose

Capsules/Suspension/Tablets: For maximum benefit, treatment should be started as soon as possible. If you have kidney disease, your doctor should adjust your dose according to the degree of functional loss.

Adult: genital herpes attack—200 mg every 4 hours, 5 times a day for 10 days. Recurrent infections—400 mg twice a day or 200 mg 2–5 times a day. Suppressive therapy for chronic herpes—400–800 mg a day, every day. Herpes zoster—800 mg 5 times a day for 7–10 days.

Child (age 2 and over): Acyclovir has been given to children in daily doses as high as 36 mg per lb. of body weight without any unusual side effects.

Child (under age 2): not recommended.

Ointment: Apply every 3 hours, 6 times a day for 7 days. Apply enough medication to cover all visible skin lesions. About ½ in. of ointment should cover about 4 sq. in. of lesions. Your doctor may prescribe a longer course of treatment to prevent the delayed formation of new lesions over the duration of an attack.

Overdosage

Divided oral doses of up to 4.8 g a day for 5 days have been taken without serious adverse effects; however, acyclovir overdose would likely lead to kidney damage due to deposits of acyclovir crystals in the kidneys. The chance of experiencing toxic side effects from swallowing acyclovir ointment is quite small because there are only 50 mg of drug per gram of ointment. Observe the overdose victim for side effects and call your poison control center for more detailed information.

Special Information

Use a finger cot or rubber glove when applying acyclovir ointment to protect against inadvertently spreading the virus. Be sure to apply the medication exactly as directed and to completely cover all lesions. Keep affected areas clean and dry. Loose-fitting clothing will reduce possible irritation of a healing lesion. If you skip several doses, or a day or more of treatment, the drug will not exert its maximum effect.

Herpes may be transmitted even if you do not have symptoms of active disease. To avoid giving the condition to a sexual partner, do not have intercourse while visible herpes lesions are present. A condom offers some protection against transmission of the herpes virus, but spermicidal products and diaphragms do not. Acyclovir alone will not prevent herpes transmission.

Women with genital herpes have an increased risk of cervical cancer. Speak with your doctor about the need for an annual Pap smear. Call your doctor if acyclovir does not relieve your symptoms, if side effects become severe or intolerable, or if you become pregnant or want to begin breast-feeding. Check with your dentist if you notice swelling or tenderness of the gums.

Special Populations

Pregnancy/Breast-feeding

Acyclovir crosses into the circulation of the fetus. Animal studies have shown that large doses—up to 125 times the human dose—cause damage to both mother and fetus. While there is no information to indicate that acyclovir affects a human fetus, do not use it during pregnancy unless it is specifically prescribed by your doctor and the possible benefit outweighs the risk.

Acyclovir passes into breast milk in concentrations up to 4 times the concentration in blood, and it has been found in the urine of a nursing infant. Although no side effects have been found in nursing babies, mothers who must take acyclovir should consider bottle-feeding their infants.

Seniors

Shingles attacks in people over age 50 tend to be more severe and respond best to acyclovir treatment if the drug is started within 48 to 72 hours of the appearance of the first rash. Seniors with reduced kidney function should be given a lower dose of oral acyclovir than younger adults.

Adalat CC

see **Nifedipine**, page 781

Generic Name

Adapelene (uh-DAP-uh-lene)

Brand Name

Differin

Type of Drug

Anti-acne.

Prescribed for

Acne.

General Information

Adapelene is similar to a retinoid. Retinoids are compounds related to vitamin A and are used in acne treatment. When adapelene is applied to an acne lesion, it modifies several of the processes involved in skin cell function. It reduces inflammation in the acne lesion and slows the formation of the material that fills the lesion. Very little adapelene is absorbed through the skin. It passes out of the body via the bile and feces.

Cautions and Warnings

Do not use adapelene if you are **sensitive** or **allergic** to it. If you are **sunburned**, wait until your sunburn clears before applying adapelene to your skin. **Avoid sun or sunlamp exposure** while using adapelene. If you must be in the sun, be sure to apply sunscreen or wear protective clothing over areas where you have applied adapelene. Extreme wind or cold can also be irritating to skin where adapelene has been applied.

Adapelene can be **highly irritating** if it gets into your eyes or if it is applied to your lips, the angles of your nose, mucous membranes, cuts, abrasions, or sunburned or damaged skin.

Possible Side Effects

▼ Most common: redness, irritation, dryness, scaling, itching, and burning are common after applying adapelene to your skin. These effects usually occur during the first 2 to 4 weeks of adapelene use and may be severe enough to cause you to stop using adapelene; call your doctor if this happens to you.

▼ Rare: skin irritation, stinging sunburn, and worsening acne.

Food and Drug Interactions

None known.

Usual Dose

Adult and Child (age 12 and over): Wash affected areas and apply a thin layer of adapelene at bedtime.

Child (under age 12): not recommended.

Overdosage

Using more than a thin film of adapelene does not produce better results and may be more irritating to the skin. Swallowing adapelene can cause liver toxicity and other side effects associated with swallowing large amounts of vitamin A. Ingesting adapelene is like taking vitamin A and can be extremely dangerous for pregnant women, who should not take more vitamin A than is contained in their prenatal vitamins. Infants who swallow adapelene should be taken to a hospital emergency room for treatment. Symptoms of overdose include headache, facial flushing, abdominal pain, dizziness, and weakness.

Special Information

Stop using adapelene and call your doctor if you develop a severe skin reaction or any sign of drug allergy or reaction (symptoms include skin rash, hives, itching, changes in complexion, and breathing difficulties or irregularities).

If you must be in the sun, be sure to apply sunscreen or wear protective clothing over areas to which you have applied adapelene.

If you forget to apply a dose of adapelene, apply it as soon as you remember. If it is almost time for your next application of adapelene, skip the dose you forgot and continue with your regular schedule.

Special Populations

Pregnancy/Breast-feeding

Animal studies of adapelene have shown no effects on the fetus. Since the effect of adapelene on pregnant women is not known, the drug should be used only when the possible benefits outweigh the risks.

Seniors

Seniors may use this medicine without special precautions.

Generic Name

Albendazole (al-BEN-duh-zole)

Brand Name

Albenza

Type of Drug

Anthelmintic.

Prescribed for

Nervous system infections caused by forms of the pork tapeworm, and cysts in the liver, lung, and belly caused by a form of the dog tapeworm. Surgery is the preferred treatment for these kinds of cysts; however, albendazole may be used in place of or in addition to surgery.

General Information

Albendazole fights certain worm infections by interfering with routine functions of the infecting organisms. It is poorly absorbed into the bloodstream, but absorption improves when you take albendazole together with a high-fat meal. The drug circulates widely throughout the body. Albendazole is rapidly broken down in the liver. It passes out of the body through the intestines, which it reaches through liver bile. Your doctor will monitor your liver function and blood count while you are taking albendazole.

Few children younger than age 6 have taken albendazole, but those who have taken it have not had special problems.

Cautions and Warnings

Albendazole can cause **liver inflammation**, but liver function usually returns to normal once the drug is stopped. People with **liver obstruction** may have much more albendazole in their blood than those with normal liver function. Kidney disease is not a problem for people taking this drug.

Women should have a **pregnancy test** to be sure they are not pregnant before they start taking albendazole.

Possible Side Effects

▼ Most common: liver inflammation and headache.

▼ Common: abdominal pain, nausea, and vomiting.

▼ Less common: dizziness, fainting, increased pressure in the head, and hair loss—which reverses when the medicine is stopped.

▼ Rare: fever, decreases in blood-cell counts, itching, skin rash, drug allergy, and kidney failure.

Drug Interactions

• Mixing albendazole with dexamethasone, praziquantal—

another anthelmintic—or cimetidine increases the amount of albendazole in the blood.

Food Interactions

Eating a high-fat meal—about 40 g of fat—with your dose of albendazole improves the absorption of the drug into the blood.

Usual Dose

Adult and Child (130 lbs. and over): 400 mg twice a day with meals.

Adult and Child (under 130 lbs.): about 7 mg per lb. of body weight a day, divided into 2 doses, up to 800 mg total dose.

Dog Tapeworm Disease: Take the prescribed dose for 28 days and stop for 2 weeks. Repeat this cycle 3 times in a row.

Pork Tapeworm Disease: Take the prescribed dose for 8–30 days.

Overdosage

In the one reported case of albendazole overdose there were no serious effects. Overdose victims should be taken to a hospital emergency room for treatment. ALWAYS bring the prescription bottle or container with you.

Special Information

Women must have a pregnancy test with a negative result before starting albendazole treatment. Women who are not pregnant must take special care to avoid becoming pregnant while taking albendazole and for 1 month after finishing the drug. Women who become pregnant while taking albendazole must stop taking it at once to avoid possible birth defects.

Take this medicine exactly as prescribed. If you forget a dose, take it as soon as you remember. If it is almost time for your next dose, skip the dose you forgot and continue with your regular schedule. Do not take a double dose.

Special Populations

Pregnancy/Breast-feeding

Albendazole causes birth defects in animals. Pregnant women should not take albendazole unless no other treatments are available.

Women who are not pregnant must take special care to avoid becoming pregnant while taking albendazole and for 1 month after finishing the medicine. Women who become pregnant while taking albendazole must stop taking it at once to avoid possible birth defects.

It is not known if albendazole passes into breast milk.

Seniors
Seniors may take this medicine without special precaution.

Generic Name

Albuterol (al-BUE-tuh-rawl) Ⓖ

Brand Names

Proventil*   Volmax
Ventolin*

*Some products in this brand-name group are alcohol or sugar free. Consult your pharmacist.

Type of Drug
Bronchodilator.

Prescribed for
Asthma and bronchospasm.

General Information
Albuterol is similar to other bronchodilator drugs, such as metaproterenol and isoetharine, but it has a weaker effect on nerve receptors in the heart and blood vessels; therefore, it is somewhat safer for people with heart conditions.

Albuterol tablets and syrup begin to work within 30 minutes and continue working for up to 8 hours. The long-acting tablet preparation continues to work for up to 12 hours. Albuterol inhalation begins working within 5 minutes and continues for 3 to 8 hours.

Cautions and Warnings
Albuterol should be used with caution by people with a history of **angina pectoris** (condition characterized by brief attacks of chest pain), **heart disease, high blood pressure,**

stroke or **seizure, diabetes, thyroid disease, prostate disease,** or **glaucoma**. Excessive use of albuterol inhalants may lead to worsening **asthma** or other respiratory conditions, and may increase breathing difficulties rather than relieve them. In the most extreme cases, people have had heart attacks after using excessive amounts of inhalant.

Animal studies with albuterol have revealed a significant increase in certain kinds of tumors.

Possible Side Effects

▼ Albuterol's side effects are similar to those of other bronchodilators, except that its effects on the heart and blood vessels are not as pronounced.

▼ Most common: restlessness, weakness, anxiety, fear, tension, sleeplessness, tremors, convulsions, dizziness, headache, flushing, appetite changes, pallor, sweating, nausea, vomiting, and muscle cramps.

▼ Less common: angina, abnormal heart rhythms, rapid heartbeat and heart palpitations, high blood pressure, not feeling well, irritability and emotional instability, nightmares, aggressive behavior, bronchitis, stuffy nose, nosebleeds, increased sputum, conjunctivitis (pinkeye), tooth discoloration, voice changes, hoarseness, and urinary difficulty.

Drug Interactions

• Albuterol's effects may be increased by monoamine oxidase inhibitors (MAOIs), tricyclic antidepressants, thyroid drugs, other bronchodilator drugs, and some antihistamines.

• The chance of cardiotoxicity may be increased in people taking both albuterol and theophylline.

• Albuterol is antagonized by beta-blocking drugs such as propranolol.

• Albuterol may antagonize the effects of blood-pressure-lowering drugs, especially reserpine, methyldopa, and guanethidine.

• Albuterol may reduce the amount of digoxin in the blood of people taking both drugs. Digoxin dose adjustment may be required.

Food Interactions

Albuterol tablets are more effective when taken on an empty

stomach—1 hour before or 2 hours after meals—but can be taken with food if they upset your stomach. Do not inhale albuterol if you have food or anything else in your mouth.

Usual Dose

Inhalation Aerosol
   Adult and Child (age 12 and over): 1–2 puffs every 4–6 hours. Each puff delivers 90 mcg of albuterol. Asthma triggered by exercise may be prevented by taking 2 puffs 15 minutes before exercising.

Inhalation Solution
   Adult and Child (age 12 and over): 2.5 mg 3 or 4 times a day. Dilute 0.5 ml of the 0.5% solution with 2.5 ml of sterile saline. Deliver over 5–15 minutes by nebulizer.

Inhalation Capsules
   Adult and Child (age 4 and over): 200–400 mcg inhaled every 4–6 hours using a special Rotahaler device. Adults and adolescents (age 12 and over) may prevent asthma brought on by exercise by inhaling a single 200-mcg dose 15 minutes before exercising.

Tablets
   Adult and Child (age 12 and over): starting dose—6–16 mg a day in divided doses. The dosage may slowly be increased to a maximum of 32 mg a day until the asthma is controlled.
   Child (age 6–11): starting dose—6–8 mg a day in divided doses. Increase to a maximum daily dose of 24 mg.
   Child (age 2–5): up to 4 mg, 3 times a day.
   Senior: starting dose—6–8 mg a day in divided doses. Increase to the maximum daily adult dosage, if tolerated.

Extended-Release Tablets
   Adult and Child (age 12 and over): 4–8 mg every 12 hours. Dosage may be cautiously increased to a maximum of 32 mg a day. People being switched from regular to extended-release tablets generally take the same dosage per day, in fewer tablets: for example, a 4-mg tablet every 12 hours (1 dose) instead of a 2-mg tablet every 6 hours (2 doses).

Overdosage

Overdose of albuterol inhalation usually results in exaggerated side effects, including heart pain and high blood pressure, although the pressure may drop to a low level after a short period of elevation. People who inhale too much albuterol should see a doctor, who may prescribe a beta-blocking drug such as metoprolol or atenolol to counteract the overdose effect.

Overdose of albuterol tablets is more likely to lead to side effects: changes in heart rate, palpitations, unusual heart rhythm, heart pain, high blood pressure, fever, chills, cold sweats, nausea, vomiting, and dilation of the pupils. Convulsions, sleeplessness, anxiety, and tremors may also develop, and the victim may collapse.

If the overdose was taken within the past half hour, give the victim ipecac syrup to induce vomiting. DO NOT GIVE IPECAC SYRUP IF THE VICTIM IS UNCONSCIOUS OR CONVULSING. If symptoms have already begun to develop, the victim may need to be taken to a hospital emergency room. Call for instructions, and ALWAYS bring the prescription bottle or container with you.

Special Information

If you are inhaling albuterol, be sure to follow the inhalation instructions that come with the product. The drug should be inhaled during the second half of your inward breath, since this will allow it to reach deeper into your lungs. If you use more than 1 puff per dose, wait about 5 minutes between puffs.

Do not take more albuterol than your doctor prescribes. Taking more than you need could actually worsen your symptoms. If your condition worsens rather than improves after taking your dose, stop taking it and call your doctor at once.

Call your doctor immediately if you develop chest pain, palpitations, rapid heartbeat, muscle tremors, dizziness, headache, facial flushing, or urinary difficulty, or if you continue having breathing difficulties after taking the medicine.

If you forget to take a dose of albuterol, take it as soon as you remember. If it is almost time for your next dose, skip the one you forgot. Do not take a double dose.

Special Populations

Pregnancy/Breast-feeding

When used during childbirth, albuterol can slow or delay natural labor. It can cause rapid heartbeat and high blood sugar in the mother and rapid heartbeat and low blood sugar in the baby.

It is not known if albuterol causes birth defects in humans, but it has caused birth defects in animal studies. When your doctor considers this drug crucial, its benefits must be cautiously weighed against its risks.

It is not known if albuterol passes into breast milk. Nursing mothers who must take it should look for any possible side effects in their infants. You may want to consider bottle-feeding your infant.

Seniors

Seniors are more sensitive to the effects of albuterol. Closely follow your doctor's directions and report any side effects at once.

Generic Name

Alendronate (uh-LEN-droe-nate)

Brand Name

Fosamax

The information in this profile also applies to the following drug:

Generic Ingredient: Tiludronate
Skelid

Type of Drug

Bisphosphonate.

Prescribed for

Osteoporosis (condition characterized by loss of bone mass due to depletion of minerals, especially calcium) in women who have gone through menopause; also prescribed for Paget's disease of bone and for cancer that has spread to the bones.

General Information

Alendronate sodium is a bisphosphonate, a group of drugs that has been used for many years to treat a variety of conditions in which bone mass—mostly calcium—is reabsorbed by the body. Alendronate is the first to be reviewed and approved specifically for osteoporosis, although etidro-

nate, another bisphosphonate, has been used for this purpose for some time. Osteoporosis leads to weak and brittle
bones in people. After menopause, women lose their natural
supply of estrogen, which provides a number of important
benefits, including protection against osteoporosis. Bisphosphonate drugs interfere with both normal and abnormal
processes of bone resorption by a mechanism that is not well
understood.

Cautions and Warnings

Do not use alendronate if you are **sensitive** or **allergic** to it.
People with **severe kidney disease** should not take alendronate. People with active gastrointestinal diseases such as
difficulty swallowing, ulcers, and **stomach irritation** should
use this drug with caution because of the chance that it could
worsen the condition. It is not known if **men with osteoporosis** would benefit from taking alendronate.

Possible Side Effects

Alendronate's side effects are generally mild and rarely
serious enough to force people to stop taking the drug.
▼ Most common: abdominal pain and discomfort, upset stomach, nausea, breathing difficulties, constipation,
diarrhea, stomach gas, and ulcers.
▼ Less common: difficulty swallowing, muscle pain,
and headache.
▼ Rare: changes in sense of taste and vomiting.

Drug Interactions

• Other oral medications may interfere with the absorption
of alendronate into the blood. Do not take alendronate within
at least 30 minutes of any other medication.

• Combining aspirin, nonsteroidal anti-inflammatory drugs
(NSAIDs), or other anti-inflammatory drugs with alendronate
may increase your chances of developing stomach or intestinal side effects.

• Do not take calcium, mineral supplements, antacids, or
indomethacin within 2 hours of taking tiludronate.

Food Interactions

Food and drink—even mineral water, orange juice, and
coffee—interfere with the absorption of alendronate into the

blood. Take this medication with plain water at least 30 minutes before eating or drinking. If you have already eaten, wait at least 2 hours before taking your medication.

Usual Dose

Alendronate
    Adult: 10–40 mg a day.
    Child: not recommended.

Tiludronate
    Adult: 400 mg taken with 6–8 oz. of plain water daily for 3 months. Each tablet is equal to 200 mg of tiludronate.
    Child: not recommended.

Overdosage

Very large doses of alendronate are lethal to lab animals, but there is no experience with human overdose. The likely symptoms of alendronate overdose are upset stomach, heartburn, irritation of the esophagus, ulcer, and very low blood-calcium and blood-phosphate levels. Taking milk or antacids will bind any alendronate remaining in the stomach. Overdose victims should be taken to a hospital emergency room. ALWAYS bring the prescription bottle or container with you.

Special Information

Take alendronate with plain water in the morning before any food, drink, or other medicine, and avoid lying down afterward. You must wait at least 30 minutes between taking alendronate and anything else for the drug to be absorbed, but the longer you wait the more drug will be absorbed into the blood.

Exercise, calcium, and vitamin D contribute to the health of your bones. Your doctor will provide a treatment plan, but remember to take any other medications at least 30 minutes after taking alendronate.

If you forget a dose of alendronate, take it as soon as you remember. If it is almost time for your next dose, skip the dose you forgot and continue with your regular schedule. If you forget your morning dose and take one later in the day, remember that you must have an empty stomach: Wait at least 2 hours after eating anything before taking your dose and then wait at least 30 minutes before taking any food or other medications.

Special Populations

Pregnancy/Breast-feeding

Alendronate is not likely to be used by women who are pregnant or nursing, because osteoporosis is common only after menopause. Alendronate affected bone formation in animal fetuses and was toxic to pregnant animals in laboratory studies. Pregnant women should take alendronate only if the possible benefits outweigh the risks.

It is not known if alendronate passes into breast milk. However, because alendronate affects bone formation, nursing mothers who must take this drug should bottle-feed their babies.

Seniors

Alendronate has been studied extensively in seniors without revealing any unusual adverse effect in older adults.

Generic Name

Allopurinol (al-oe-PURE-in-nol) Ⓖ

Brand Name

Zyloprim

Type of Drug

Antigout medication.

Prescribed for

Gout or gouty arthritis; also prescribed for cancer and conditions that may be associated with too much uric acid in the body. In mouthwash form, it helps to prevent mouth, stomach, and intestinal ulcers caused by fluorouracil, an antineoplastic drug. Allopurinol may be given before heart bypass surgery to reduce abnormal rhythms and other surgical complications. It can be used to reduce the relapse rates of duodenal ulcers associated with *Heliobacter pylori* infection and to reduce the vomiting of blood from stomach irritation caused by nonsteroidal anti-inflammatory drugs (NSAIDs). Allopurinol has also been used to control seizures in people for whom standard treatments are not effective.

General Information

Unlike other antigout drugs, which affect the elimination of uric acid from the body, allopurinol acts on the system that manufactures uric acid in your body.

A high level of uric acid can mean that you have gout, psoriasis, or any of a number of other diseases, including various cancers and malignancies. High levels of uric acid can be caused by taking certain drugs, including diuretic medicines. However, a high blood level of uric acid does not point to a specific disease.

Cautions and Warnings

Do not take this medication if you have ever developed a **severe reaction** to it. Stop taking the medication immediately and contact your doctor if you develop a **rash** or any other adverse effects while taking allopurinol. Do not start taking allopurinol again if you have stopped it because of a severe reaction.

Allopurinol should be used by children only if they have high uric acid levels due to neoplastic disease or to very rare metabolic conditions.

A few cases of **liver toxicity** have been associated with allopurinol; they improved when the drug was stopped. People taking allopurinol should periodically be tested for liver and kidney function. People with severely **compromised kidney function** should take a reduced dose of allopurinol.

Possible Side Effects

▼ Most common: rash associated with severe, allergic, or sensitivity reaction to allopurinol. If you develop an unusual rash or other sign of drug toxicity, stop taking this medication and contact your doctor.

▼ Less common: nausea, vomiting, diarrhea, intermittent stomach pain, effects on blood components, and drowsiness or lack of ability to concentrate.

▼ Rare: effects on the eyes, hair loss, fever, chills, breathing difficulties or asthma-like symptoms, arthritis-like symptoms, itching, loosening of the fingernails, pain in the lower back, unexplained nosebleeds, cataracts, conjunctivitis and other eye conditions, numbness, tingling or pain in the hands or feet, confusion, dizziness, fainting, depression, memory loss, ringing or buzzing in the ears, weakness, sleeplessness, and not feeling well.

Drug Interactions

• Large doses of drugs that make your urine more acid, like megadoses of vitamin C, may increase the possibility of kidney stone formation.

• Alcohol, diazoxide, mecamylamine or pyrazinamide can increase the amount of uric acid in your blood; an increase in your allopurinol dose may be required.

• Allopurinol may increase the action of azathioprine, mercaptopurine, or cyclophosphamide and other anticancer medicines, leading to possible bleeding or infection.

• Taking allopurinol with dacarbazine, probenecid, or sulfinpyrazone may cause excessive reduction of uric acid.

• Allopurinol may interact with anticoagulant (blood-thinning) medications, reducing the rate at which the anticoagulant is broken down in the body. Dosage reduction is necessary.

• People who are susceptible to ampicillin, amoxicillin, bacampicillin or hetacillin rash are more likely to develop such a reaction while also taking allopurinol.

• Combining a thiazide diuretic or an ACE-inhibitor (for high blood pressure or heart failure) with allopurinol increases the chances of a drug-sensitivity reaction.

• Combining vidarabine with allopurinol may increase the risk of neurotoxic effects and anemia, nausea, pain, and itching.

• Large doses of allopurinol—more than 600 mg a day—may increase the effects of and chance of toxic reactions to theophylline by interfering with its clearance from the body.

Food Interactions

Take each dose with food or a full glass of water. Drink 10 to 12 glasses of water, juices, soda, or other liquids each day to avoid the formation of crystals in your urine and/or kidneys.

Usual Dose

Adult and Child (age 11 and over): 100–800 mg a day, depending on disease and response.

Child (age 6–10): 300–600 mg a day.

Child (under age 6): 150 mg a day.

The dose should be reviewed periodically by your doctor to be sure that it is producing the desired therapeutic effect.

Overdosage

The expected symptoms of overdose are exaggerated side

effects. Allopurinol overdose victims should be taken to a hospital. ALWAYS bring the prescription bottle or container with you.

Special Information

Allopurinol can make you drowsy or make it difficult to concentrate: Take care while driving a car or operating hazardous equipment.

Call your doctor at once if you develop rash, hives, itching, chills, fever, nausea, muscle aches, unusual tiredness, fever, yellowing of the whites of the eyes or skin, painful urination, blood in the urine, irritation of the eyes, or swelling of the lips and/or mouth.

Avoid large doses of vitamin C, which can cause the formation of kidney stones during allopurinol treatment. Be sure to drink 10 to 12 8-oz. glasses of water a day while taking this medication.

If you forget to take a dose of allopurinol, take the dose you forgot as soon as possible. If it is time for your next regular dose, double this dose. For example, if your regular dose is 100 mg and you miss a dose, take 200 mg at the next usual dose time.

Special Populations

Pregnancy/Breast-feeding

Allopurinol may cause birth defects or interfere with fetal development. Check with your doctor before taking it if you are or might be pregnant.

Allopurinol passes into breast milk. Nursing mothers who must take allopurinol should consider bottle-feeding their baby.

Seniors

No special precautions are required. Follow your doctor's directions and report any side effects at once.

Generic Name

Alprazolam (al-PRAY-zoe-lam) G

Brand Name

Xanax

Type of Drug

Benzodiazepine tranquilizer.

Prescribed for

Anxiety, tension, fatigue, and agitation; also prescribed for irritable bowel syndrome, panic attacks, depression, and premenstrual syndrome (PMS).

General Information

Alprazolam is a member of a group of drugs known as benzodiazepines, which work as antianxiety agents, as anticonvulsants, or as sedatives. Benzodiazepines directly affect the brain. They can relax you and make you more tranquil or sleepier, or they can slow nervous system transmissions in such a way as to act as an anticonvulsant: The exact effect varies according to drug and dosage. Many doctors prefer benzodiazepines to other drugs that can be used to similar effect because they tend to be safer, have fewer side effects, and are usually as effective, if not more so.

Cautions and Warnings

Do not take alprazolam if you know you are **sensitive** or **allergic** to it or to another benzodiazepine drug, including clonazepam.

Alprazolam can aggravate narrow-angle **glaucoma**, but you may take it if you have open-angle glaucoma. Check with your doctor.

Other conditions where alprazolam should be avoided are: severe **depression**, severe **lung disease**, **sleep apnea** (intermittent cessation of breathing during sleep), **liver disease**, **drunkenness**, and **kidney disease**. In each of these conditions, the depressive effects of alprazolam may be enhanced and/or could be detrimental to your overall condition.

Alprazolam should not be taken by **psychotic patients** because it is not effective for them and can trigger unusual excitement, stimulation, and rage.

Alprazolam is meant to be used for no more than 3 to 4 months in a row. Your condition should be reassessed before continuing your medicine beyond that time.

Alprazolam may be **addictive**: You can experience drug withdrawal symptoms if you suddenly stop taking alprazolam after as little as 4 to 6 weeks of treatment. Withdrawal symptoms are more likely if alprazolam is taken for long periods. Withdrawal generally begins with increased feelings of anxiety; it continues with tingling in the extremities, sensitivity to bright lights or the sun, long periods of sleep or sleeplessness, a metallic taste, flulike illness, fatigue, difficulty concentrating, restlessness, appetite loss, nausea, irritability, headache, dizziness, sweating, muscle tension or cramps, tremors, and feeling uncomfortable or ill at ease. Other major withdrawal symptoms include confusion, abnormal perception of movement, depersonalization, paranoid delusions, hallucinations, psychotic reactions, muscle twitching, seizures, and memory loss.

Possible Side Effects

▼ Most common: mild drowsiness during the first few days of therapy. Weakness and confusion may occur, especially in seniors and in those who are sickly. If these effects persist, contact your doctor.

▼ Less common: depression, lethargy, disorientation, headache, inactivity, slurred speech, stupor, dizziness, tremors, constipation, dry mouth, nausea, inability to control urination, sexual difficulties, irregular menstrual cycle, changes in heart rhythm, low blood pressure, fluid retention, blurred or double vision, itching, rash, hiccups, nervousness, inability to fall asleep, and occasional liver dysfunction. If you experience any of these symptoms, stop taking the medicine and contact your doctor immediately.

▼ Rare: diarrhea, coated tongue, sore gums, vomiting, changes in appetite, difficulty swallowing, increased salivation, upset stomach, incontinence, changes in sex drive, urinary difficulties, changes in heart rate, palpitations, swelling, stuffy nose, difficulty hearing, hair loss or gain, sweating, fever, tingling in the hands or feet, breast pain, muscle disturbances, breathing difficulties, changes in blood components, and joint pain.

Drug Interactions

• Alprazolam is a central-nervous-system depressant. Avoid alcohol, other tranquilizers, narcotics, barbiturates, monoamine oxidase inhibitors (MAOIs), antihistamines, and antidepressants. Taking alprazolam with these drugs may result in excessive depression, tiredness, sleepiness, breathing difficulties, or related symptoms.

• Smoking may reduce the effectiveness of alprazolam by increasing the rate at which it is broken down by the body.

• The effects of alprazolam may be prolonged when taken together with cimetidine, oral contraceptives, disulfiram, fluoxetine, isoniazid, itraconazole, ketoconazole, metoprolol, probenecid, propoxyphene, propranolol, rifampin, and valproic acid.

• Theophylline may reduce alprazolam's sedative effects.

• If you take antacids, separate them from your alprazolam dose by at least 1 hour to prevent them from interfering with the absorption of alprazolam into the bloodstream.

• Alprazolam may raise digoxin blood levels and the chances of digoxin toxicity.

• The effect of levodopa may be decreased if it is taken together with alprazolam.

• Combining alprazolam with phenytoin may increase phenytoin blood concentrations and the chances of phenytoin toxicity.

Food Interactions

Alprazolam is best taken on an empty stomach but may be taken with food if it upsets your stomach.

Usual Dose

Adult: 0.75–4 mg a day. Dosage must be tailored to your individual needs. Some people will need less medicine to control anxiety or tension.

Child (under age 18): not recommended.

Overdosage

Symptoms of overdose are confusion, sleepiness, poor coordination, lack of response to pain such as a pinprick, loss of reflexes, shallow breathing, low blood pressure, and coma. The victim should be taken to a hospital emergency room. ALWAYS bring the prescription bottle or container with you.

Special Information

Alprazolam can cause tiredness, drowsiness, inability to concentrate, or related symptoms. Be careful if you are driving, operating machinery, or performing other activities that require concentration.

Anyone taking alprazolam for more than 3 or 4 months at a time may have a drug withdrawal reaction if the medicine is stopped suddenly (see "Cautions and Warnings").

If you forget a dose of alprazolam, take it as soon as you remember. If it is almost time for your next dose, skip the dose you forgot and return to your regular schedule. Do not take a double dose.

Special Populations

Pregnancy/Breast-feeding

Alprazolam may cross into fetal circulation and may cause birth defects if taken during the first 3 months of pregnancy. You should avoid alprazolam while pregnant.

Alprazolam may pass into breast milk. Since infants break down the drug more slowly than do adults, they may accumulate enough alprazolam in their systems to produce undesirable effects. Nursing mothers who must take alprazolam should bottle-feed their babies.

Seniors

Seniors, especially those with liver or kidney disease, are more sensitive to the effects of alprazolam and generally require smaller doses to achieve the same effect. Follow your doctor's directions and report any side effects at once.

Generic Name

Alprostadil (al-PROS-tuh-dil)

Brand Names

Caverject   Muse

Type of Drug

Anti-impotence agent.

Prescribed for

Male sexual dysfunction; also prescribed for a variety of other conditions, including atherosclerosis (hardening of the arteries), gangrene, and pain due to blood vessel disease.

Alprostadil is not usually prescribed for children, although a form of the drug is used to correct a heart birth defect in newborns.

General Information

Male erection happens when blood flows into blood vessels

and holding areas inside the penis. Problems occur when blood cannot move into the penis as it normally should. Men who have problems getting and keeping an erection are usually victims of atherosclerosis, nerve dysfunction—often associated with diabetes, spinal cord injury, or psychological problems. Alprostadil helps men get and keep an erection by dilating blood vessels that supply the penis and by relaxing muscles to help expand holding areas for blood in the penis. Also known as prostaglandin E_1 or PGE_1, alprostadil has a wide variety of actions in the body. It dilates (widens) blood vessels, reduces platelet stickiness—which slows blood-clotting rates—and relaxes some muscle groups. Alprostadil must be injected directly into the cavernosa tissue of the penis (the holding area for blood during an erection) or inserted into the urethra (the tube through which urine flows out of the body) where it is absorbed into the penis.

Cautions and Warnings

Do not take alprostadil if you are **allergic** to it or to other prostaglandin drugs. Alprostadil can cause a **priapism** (painful erection lasting more than 6 hours). People with diseases where priapism is a possibility—**sickle cell anemia** or **trait, multiple myeloma, leukemia**—those with penile deformities, penile implants, women, children, or those for whom **sexual activity could be dangerous** should not use alprostadil.

Penile pain is common after using either form of alprostadil, although it is usually mild or moderate. .

Possible Side Effects

Injection

▼ Most common: penile pain.

▼ Less common: prolonged erection; penile fibrosis (deformity); blood blister or black-and-blue marks at the injection site, usually caused by poor injection technique; penis disorders, including yeast infection, numbness, irritation, sensitivity, itching, redness, and torn skin; penile rash or swelling; headache; dizziness; fainting; respiratory infection; flu symptoms; sinus inflammation; runny or stuffed nose; cough; blood pressure changes; local pain; prostate problems; back pain; and general pain.

▼ Rare: urethral burning, testicular pain, priapism (see "Cautions and Warnings"), penile inflammation or

---

Possible Side Effects *(continued)*

warmth, pain on erection, abnormal ejaculation, pelvic pain, scrotal swelling or other problems, blood in the urine, urinary difficulties, flushing, blood vessel disorders, abnormal heart rhythms, weakness, sweating, reduced sensation, rash, itching, skin cancer, nausea, dry mouth, leg cramps, dilated pupils, and kidney problems.

Pellets

▼ Most common: penile pain.

▼ Common: urethral pain, burning or bleeding, and testicular pain.

▼ Less common: headache, dizziness, respiratory infection, flu symptoms, runny nose, sinus inflammation, low blood pressure, back pain, pelvic pain, and general pain.

▼ Rare: fainting, scrotal swelling or other problems, blood in the urine, urinary difficulties, flushing, blood vessel disorders, abnormal heart rhythms, weakness, sweating, reduced sensation, rash, itching, skin cancer, nausea, dry mouth, leg cramps, dilated pupils, and kidney problems.

Drug Interactions

• Alprostadil can increase the effect of anticoagulant (blood-thinning) drugs. Your doctor may have to adjust the dose of your anticoagulant.

• Alprostadil may decrease the amount of cyclosporine in your blood.

• The safety of combining alprostadil with other drugs that affect blood vessels is not known. These combinations should be used with caution.

Food Interactions

None known.

Usual Dose

Dosage must be individualized to your need and response.

Overdosage

Alprostadil overdose can lead to an extended and painful

erection, as well as other side effects. Overdose victims should seek medical attention.

Special Information

Patient information leaflets are included with each alprostadil prescription. Read this information before you use your prescription.

You must be trained in proper injection technique by your doctor. Self-injection should be permitted only after your doctor has made sure you know how to do it properly.

Alprostadil begins working within 5 to 10 minutes after taking it. Dosage should be set so that your erection lasts for about 30 to 60 minutes. Use the lowest dose that works.

Special Populations

Pregnancy/Breast-feeding

This product should not be used by women. Men using alprostadil must use a condom if they have intercourse with a pregnant woman. Alprostadil passes into semen and will affect the development of a fetal heart if a condom is not worn.

Seniors

Seniors may use alprostadil without special precaution.

Generic Name

Amantadine (uh-MAN-tuh-dene) G

Brand Name

Symmetrel

Type of Drug

Antiviral and antiparkinsonian.

Prescribed for

Certain flu viruses, all varieties of Parkinson's disease, and uncontrolled muscle movements caused by phenothiazines and other psychoactive drugs; also used for fatigue associated with multiple sclerosis.

General Information

Although its action is not entirely understood, amantadine

hydrochloride appears to prevent the release of the infectious part of some flu viruses into body cells; it may also interfere with the penetration of the virus into body cells. Amantadine is used for both prevention and treatment of flu. It is 70% to 90% effective in preventing type A flu and will reduce symptoms of type A flu when taken within 2 days after they begin. Amantadine does not work for type B flu.

In the treatment of Parkinson's disease, amantadine has been shown to increase the amount of stored dopamine that is released in the brain.

Cautions and Warnings

Do not take amantadine if you are **sensitive** or **allergic** to it. People with a history of **epilepsy** may experience increased seizure activity. People have developed **heart failure** while taking amantadine; those who already have heart failure should be carefully monitored for signs that the disease might be worsening. Amantadine is released unmetabolized from the body through the kidneys. People with **kidney disease** must receive reduced doses.

Amantadine should be used with caution by people with **liver disease**, a history of recurrent **eczema**, or **psychosis or severe psychoneurosis** that is not controlled by drug treatment.

Possible Side Effects

▼ Most common: nausea, dizziness, light-headedness, and sleeplessness.

▼ Common: depression; anxiety; irritability; hallucinations; confusion; appetite loss; dry mouth; constipation; weakness; blue or purple discoloration of the skin, which goes away 2–12 weeks after treatment is stopped; swelling in the arms, legs, or ankles; dizziness when rising suddenly from a sitting or lying position; low blood pressure; and headache.

▼ Less common: heart failure, psychotic reactions, urinary difficulties, breathing difficulties, fatigue, skin rash, vomiting, weakness, slurred speech, and visual disturbances.

▼ Rare: convulsions, increased white-blood-cell counts, eczema-type rash, and spasms of the eye muscles leading to uncontrollable eye movement and rolling.

Drug Interactions

• Combining amantadine with anticholinergic drugs like benztropine produces increased side effects. Altering the dose of either drug can solve this problem.

• Hydrochlorothiazide-triamterene (a diuretic combination) interferes with amantadine elimination through the kidneys.

• Alcohol may worsen some of the side effects of amantadine, interfering with your ability to drive or concentrate.

Food Interactions

None known.

Usual Dose

Adult and Child (age 10 and over): 100–300 mg daily.
Senior (age 65 and over): 100 mg a day.
Child (age 1–9): 2–4 mg per lb. a day, up to 150 mg.

Overdosage

Symptoms of overdose include nausea, vomiting, appetite loss, and nervous system side effects—excitability, tremors, weakness, tiredness, blurred vision, slurred speech, and convulsions. Potentially fatal abnormal heart rhythms may also occur with large doses. One person died after taking 2500 mg of amantadine. Overdose victims should be taken to a hospital emergency room for treatment at once. ALWAYS bring the prescription bottle or container with you.

Special Information

Be careful while driving or operating any complex or hazardous equipment; avoid alcoholic beverages while taking amantadine.

Call your doctor immediately if you experience fainting; dizziness or light-headedness; visual difficulties; mood changes; swelling of the arms, legs, or ankles; or any other unusual or intolerable side effect.

A stool softener—for example, docusate—will usually relieve constipation. Dry mouth, nose, or throat can be easily relieved with candy or gum. Dry mouth also leads to tooth and gum disease. Maintain good oral hygiene to prevent cavities and gum disease while taking amantadine.

People taking amantadine for Parkinson's disease may not see any effect for at least 2 weeks.

It is important to take amantadine as your doctor has

prescribed. If you are taking amantadine syrup, be sure to use the measuring spoon supplied with your prescription.

If you forget to take a dose of amantadine, take it as soon as possible. If it is almost time for your next dose, skip the dose you forgot and continue with your regular schedule. Do not take a double dose.

Special Populations

Pregnancy/Breast-feeding

In high doses, amantadine can be toxic and may cause malformations in animal fetuses. A cardiovascular malformation was reported in one infant exposed to amantadine in the first 3 months of pregnancy. Pregnant women should take this drug only if it is absolutely necessary and only after reviewing all of the possible risks with their doctors.

Amantadine passes into breast milk. Amantadine may cause side effects in infants; nursing mothers should bottle-feed their babies.

Seniors

Seniors require reduced doses of amantadine because of normal losses of kidney function. Healthy people age 65 and older should receive half the dose prescribed for younger adults.

Ambien

see *Zolpidem*, page 1188

Generic Name

Amiodarone (ah-mee-OE-duh-rone)

Brand Name

Cordarone

Type of Drug

Antiarrhythmic.

Prescribed for

Abnormal heart rhythms.

General Information·

Amiodarone should be prescribed only in situations where the abnormal rhythm is so severe as to be life-threatening and does not respond to other drug treatments. Amiodarone works by decreasing the sensitivity of heart tissue to nervous impulses within the heart. It has not been proven that people taking this drug will live longer than those with similar conditions who do not take it.

Amiodarone may exert its effects 2 to 5 days after you start taking it, but often takes 1 to 3 weeks to affect your heart. Since amiodarone therapy is often started while you are in the hospital, especially if you are being switched from another antiarrhythmic drug to amiodarone, your doctor will be able to closely monitor how well the drug is working for you. Amiodarone's antiarrhythmic effects can last for weeks or months after you stop taking it.

Cautions and Warnings

Do not take amiodarone if you are **allergic** or **sensitive** to it or if you have **heart block**.

Amiodarone can cause potentially fatal drug side effects. At high doses, 10% or more of people taking this drug can develop potentially fatal **lung and respiratory effects**, beginning with cough and progressive breathing difficulties. **Liver damage** caused by amiodarone is usually mild. In rare cases, amiodarone has been associated with liver failure that resulted in death.

Amiodarone can cause **heart block**, a drastic slowing of electrical impulse movement between major areas of the heart, or extreme slowing of the heart rate. Amiodarone heart block occurs about as often as heart block caused by some other antiarrhythmic drugs, but its effects may last longer than those of the other drugs. Amiodarone can also worsen existing **abnormal heart rhythms** in 2% to 5% of people who take the drug. These effects can be fatal.

People taking amiodarone may develop optic nerve irritation, leading to **partial or complete loss of vision**. Most adults who take amiodarone for 6 months or more develop tiny deposits in the corneas of their eyes. These deposits may cause **blurred vision** or **halos** in up to 10% of people taking amiodarone. Some people develop dry eyes and sensitivity to bright light.

One in ten people taking amiodarone can experience **un-

usual sensitivity to the effects of the sun. Use an appropriate sunscreen product and reapply it frequently.

Amiodarone can cause **thyroid abnormalities** because it interferes with normal thyroid hormone processing in your body. It may worsen an already sluggish thyroid gland in 2% to 10% of people taking the drug, and increase thyroid activity in 2% of people taking it.

Antiarrhythmic drugs are less effective and cause abnormal rhythms if blood potassium is low. Check with your doctor to see if you need extra potassium.

Possible Side Effects

About 75% of people taking 400 mg or more of amiodarone a day develop some drug side effects. As many as 18% have to stop taking the drug because of a side effect. Side effects are more common in people taking amiodarone for 6 months or more, but level off after 1 year.

▼ Common: fatigue, not feeling well, tremors, unusual involuntary movements, loss of coordination, an unusual walk, muscle weakness, dizziness, tingling in the hands or feet, reduced sex drive, sleeplessness, headache, nervous system problems, nausea, vomiting, constipation, appetite loss, abdominal pain, dry eyes, unusual sensitivity to bright light, and seeing halos around bright lights. Unusual sun sensitivity is the most common skin reaction to amiodarone, but people taking this drug can develop a blue skin discoloration that may not go away completely when the drug is stopped. Other skin reactions are sun rashes, hair loss, and black-and-blue spots.

▼ Rare: inflammation of the lung or fibrous deposits in the lungs, changes in thyroid function, changes in taste or smell, bloating, unusual salivation, and changes in blood clotting. Amiodarone can cause heart failure, reduced heart rate, and abnormal rhythms. Up to 9% of people taking amiodarone develop abnormalities in liver function.

Drug Interactions

• Amiodarone increases the effects of metoprolol and other beta blockers, digoxin, flecainide, procainamide, quinidine, theophylline, and warfarin and other anticoagulants. These interactions, which result from the interference of amiodarone with the breakdown of these drugs in the liver, can take from 2 or 3 days to several weeks to develop. The dosage of these drugs must be drastically reduced to take the interaction into account.

• When amiodarone and phenytoin are taken together, both drugs can be affected. Amiodarone can be antagonized by phenytoin and other hydantoin anticonvulsants, and the effect of phenytoin can be increased by amiodarone, which interferes with its breakdown in the liver.

• Cholestyramine interferes with the absorption of amiodarone into the bloodstream.

• Cimetidine and ritonavir interfere with the breakdown of amiodarone, leading to high drug blood levels and the increased possibility of side effects.

Food Interactions

Amiodarone is poorly absorbed into the blood and should be taken on an empty stomach, as food delays its absorption into your bloodstream. If amiodarone upsets your stomach, however, you may take it with food.

Usual Dose

Starting dose—800–1600 mg a day, taken in 1 or 2 doses. Maintenance dose—400 mg a day. You should take the lowest effective dose in order to minimize side effects.

Overdosage

There have been a few reports of amiodarone overdose; no fatalities have occurred, since the drug usually takes several days or weeks to exert an effect on the body. Overdose victims should be taken to a hospital emergency room for treatment. ALWAYS bring the prescription bottle or container with you.

Special Information

Side effects are very common with amiodarone; ¾ of people taking the drug will experience some drug-related problem.

Call your doctor if you develop chest pain, breathing difficulties or any other sign of changes in lung function, abnormal heartbeat, bloating in your feet or legs, tremors, fever, chills, sore throat, unusual bleeding or bruising, changes in skin color, unusual sunburn, or any other unusual side effect. See your doctor for an eye exam if your vision changes at all while taking amiodarone.

Amiodarone can make you dizzy or light-headed. Take care while driving a car or performing any complex tasks.

If you take amiodarone once a day and forget to take a dose, but remember within 12 hours, take it as soon as possible. If you do not remember until later, skip the dose you forgot and continue with your regular schedule.

If you take amiodarone twice a day and remember within 6 hours of your regular dose, take it as soon as you remember. Call your doctor if you forget to take 2 or more doses in a row. Do not take a double dose.

Special Populations

Pregnancy/Breast-feeding

In animal studies, amiodarone has been found to be toxic to a fetus when given at a dose 18 times the maximum adult human dose. Women of childbearing age should use an effective contraceptive while taking amiodarone. If you are or might be pregnant and this drug is considered crucial by your doctor, its potential benefits must be weighed against its risks.

Amiodarone passes into breast milk. Nursing mothers who must take this drug should bottle-feed their babies.

Seniors

Amiodarone must be used with caution, regardless of your age. It is broken down in the liver, and dosage reduction may be needed if you have poor liver function.

Generic Name

Amlexanox (am-LEX-an-ox)

Brand Name

Aphthasol

Type of Drug

Skin-ulcer treatment.

Prescribed for

Mouth ulcers in people with normal immune systems.

General Information

Amlexanox slows the production or release of factors involved in the body's inflammatory response. It aids in the healing of mouth ulcers, but the exact way that it accelerates the healing process is not known. A very small amount of amlexanox is absorbed into the bloodstream after it has been applied to mouth ulcers, but this has not been linked to any effect in the body.

Cautions and Warnings

Do not use amlexanox if you are **sensitive** or **allergic** to it or to any ingredient in the paste.

Possible Side Effects

▼ Less common: pain, stinging, or burning after application.
▼ Rare: mouth irritation, diarrhea, and nausea.

Drug Interactions

None known.

Food Interactions

Do not apply amlexanox while you have any food in your mouth.

Usual Dose

Apply a small amount (¼ in.) to each mouth ulcer after breakfast, lunch, and dinner, and at bedtime.

Overdosage

Swallowing even a whole tube of amlexanox would probably cause only upset stomach, nausea, diarrhea, and vomiting. Call your local poison control center or hospital emergency room for more information.

Special Information

Begin using amlexanox as soon as possible after noticing a mouth ulcer and use it until your ulcers heal. Call your doctor if the pain does not get better or the sores do not heal after 10 days of using amlexanox.

　　Make sure your teeth and mouth are clean before applying amlexanox paste. Squeeze ¼ in. of the paste onto your finger and apply it to each mouth ulcer using gentle pressure.

　　Wash your hands immediately after using amlexanox. If

you get the paste into your eyes, wash it out at once using cool water.

If you forget a dose of amlexanox, use it as soon as you remember. If it is almost time for your next dose, skip the dose you forgot and continue with your regular schedule. Do not apply more than the recommended amount at any time.

Special Populations

Pregnancy/Breast-feeding

The effect of amlexanox on pregnancy is not known; use it only after discussing the possible risks and benefits with your doctor.

Amlexanox passes into the milk of nursing animals, but its effect in humans is not known. Nursing mothers should use this drug with caution.

Seniors

Seniors may use amlexanox without special precaution.

Generic Name

Amlodipine (am-LOE-dih-pene) Ⓖ

Brand Name

Norvasc

Type of Drug

Calcium channel blocker.

Prescribed for

Angina pectoris, Prinzmetal's angina, and high blood pressure; has also been studied for heart failure.

General Information

Amplodipine is one of many calcium channel blockers available in the United States. These drugs block the passage of calcium, an essential factor in muscle contraction, into the heart and smooth muscles. Such blockage interferes with the contraction of these muscles, which in turn dilates (widens) the veins and vessels that supply blood to them. This action has several beneficial effects. Because arteries are dilated, they are less likely to spasm. In addition, because blood vessels are dilated, both blood pressure and the amount of oxygen used by the heart muscles are reduced. Amlodipine is therefore useful in treating not only high blood pressure but also angina pectoris (brief attacks of chest pain), a condition related to poor oxygen supply to the heart muscles.

Amlodipine affects the movement of calcium only into muscle cells; it has no effect on calcium in the blood.

Cautions and Warnings

Amlodipine may, in rare instances, cause unwanted **low blood pressure** in some people taking it for reasons other than hypertension. This is more of a problem with other calcium channel blockers.

Amlodipine may worsen **heart failure** in some people and should be used with caution if heart failure is present.

Calcium channel blockers, alone and with aspirin, have caused **bruises,** black-and-blue marks, and bleeding due to an anticoagulant effect. This is mostly a problem with nifedipine but should be considered for all members of the group.

Amlodipine may cause **angina** when treatment is first started, when dosage is increased, or if the drug is rapidly withdrawn. This can be avoided by gradually reducing dosage.

Studies have shown that people taking calcium channel blockers—usually those taken several times a day, not those taken only once daily—have a greater chance of having a **heart attack** than do people taking beta blockers or other medication for the same purposes. Discuss this with your doctor to be sure you are receiving the best possible treatment.

Do not take this drug if you have had an **allergic** reaction to it in the past.

People with severe **liver disease** break down amlodipine much more slowly than do people with mildly diseased or normal livers. Your doctor should take this into account when determining your amlodipine dosage.

Possible Side Effects

▼ Most common: headache, dizziness or light-headedness, anxiety, nausea, swelling in the arms or legs, heart palpitations, and flushing.

▼ Less common: sleepiness, muscle weakness, cramps

Possible Side Effects *(continued)*

or abdominal discomfort, itching, rash, sexual difficulties, wheezing or shortness of breath, muscle cramps, pain, and inflammation.

▼ Rare: nervousness, depression, memory loss, paranoia, psychosis, hallucination, tingling in the hands or feet, sleeplessness, unusual dreams, anxiety, not feeling well, ringing or buzzing in the ears, hand or other muscle tremors, diarrhea, constipation, vomiting, dry mouth, excessive thirst, stomach gas, low blood pressure, slow heartbeat, abnormal heart rhythm, hair loss, bruising, black-and-blue marks, bleeding, stuffed nose, sinus inflammation, chest congestion, frequent or painful urination, joint stiffness or pain, weight gain, nosebleeds, cough, appetite loss, chest pain, blue discoloration of fingers or toes, difficulty swallowing, double vision, eye pain, abnormal vision, conjunctivitis (pinkeye), heart failure, irregular pulse, apathy, agitation, dry skin, skin discoloration, twitching, migraines, cold and clammy skin, loose stools, changes in sense of taste.

Drug Interactions

• Amlodipine may interact with beta-blocking drugs to cause heart failure, very low blood pressure, or an increased incidence of angina.

• Amlodipine may cause unexpected blood-pressure reduction when combined with other antihypertensive drugs; however, this interaction is more likely with other calcium channel blockers.

• The combination of quinidine (prescribed for abnormal heart rhythm) and amlodipine must be used with caution because it can produce low blood pressure, very slow heart rate, abnormal heart rhythms, and swelling in the arms or legs.

• Amlodipine can increase the effects of theophylline— prescribed for asthma and other respiratory problems—and related drugs.

• Patients taking amlodipine who are given fentanyl as a short-term surgical anesthetic may experience very low blood pressure.

Food Interactions

None known.

Usual Dose

5–10 mg once a day.

Do not stop taking amlodipine abruptly. The dosage should be gradually reduced over a period of time.

Overdosage

Overdose of amlodipine can cause nausea, weakness, dizziness, confusion, and slurred speech. Take overdose victims to a hospital emergency room, or call your local poison control center for directions. You may be asked to make the patient vomit to remove the medication from his or her stomach. If you go to the emergency room, ALWAYS bring the prescription bottle or container with you.

Special Information

Call your doctor if you develop constipation, nausea, weakness or dizziness, swelling in the hands or feet, breathing difficulties, or increased heart pains, or if other side effects are particularly bothersome or persistent.

If you are taking amlodipine for high blood pressure, be sure to continue taking your medication and follow any instructions for diet restriction or other treatments. High blood pressure is a condition with few recognizable symptoms; it may seem to you that you are taking the drug for no good reason. Call your doctor or pharmacist if you have any questions.

It is important to maintain good dental hygiene while taking amlodipine and to use extra care when using your toothbrush or dental floss because of the chance that the drug will make you more susceptible to certain infections.

If you forget a dose of amlodipine, take it as soon as you remember. If it is almost time for your next dose, skip the dose you forgot and continue with your regular schedule. Do not take a double dose.

Special Populations

Pregnancy/Breast-feeding

Animal studies of amlodipine show that it may damage a fetus. Other calcium channel blockers can be used to treat severe high blood pressure associated with pregnancy, so there is no reason for women who are or might become pregnant to take amlodipine.

It is not known if amlodipine passes into breast milk. Nursing mothers who take amlodipine should consider bottle-feeding their babies.

Seniors

Seniors, especially those with liver disease, are more sensitive to the effects of this drug because it takes longer to pass out of their bodies. They should be given somewhat lower starting doses. Follow your doctor's directions and report any side effects at once.

Amoxil

see **Penicillin Antibiotics**, page 846

Generic Name

Anagrelide (ah-NAG-rel-ide)

Brand Name

Agrylin

Type of Drug

Antiplatelet.

Prescribed for

Essential thrombocytopenia (ET), to reduce blood-platelet count and the risk of excess blood clotting associated with high blood-platelet levels.

General Information

Blood platelets play a very important role in the body; they are among the body's first lines of defense. They can quickly initiate the formation of a tiny blood clot to help prevent the loss of blood through a cut or other minor wound. However, when the blood-platelet count is too high, clotting becomes too easy and clots may form when and where they are not wanted. For example, heart attacks and some kinds of strokes

may develop because a small blood clot has blocked circulation to the heart or brain. In persons with ET, there is a risk
that the large numbers of excess platelets may cause an
unwanted clot to form almost anywhere in the body. The
exact way in which anagrelide reduces blood-platelet count is
not known. It is thought to interrupt the formation of new
blood platelets. Anagrelide is not approved for general use by
children age 16 and under, but it has been used without harm
by 8 children between the ages of 8 and 17, who took it in
doses up to 4 mg a day.

Cautions and Warnings

This medicine should be used with caution by people who
have **heart disease**. Anagrelide stimulates the force of each
heartbeat and can cause blood vessels to dilate (widen). Both
of these reactions can be risky for people with heart disease.

Unusually **low blood-platelet counts** can develop in people
treated with anagrelide. Platelet counts should be periodically
checked while you are taking this medicine; they usually rise
soon after the drug is stopped.

Anagrelide can cause **liver or kidney toxicity** and may
worsen the condition of people with liver or kidney disease
who start taking it.

Possible Side Effects

▼ Most common: heart palpitations, diarrhea, abdominal pain, nausea, stomach gas, headache, weakness,
swelling, pain, dizziness, and difficulty breathing.

▼ Common: chest pain, rapid heartbeat, vomiting,
upset stomach, appetite loss, rash and/or itching, tingling
in the hands or feet, back pain, and not feeling well.

▼ Less common: fever, flu symptoms, chills, neck
pains, sensitivity to bright light, abnormal heart rhythms,
bleeding, heart disease, strokes, angina pains, heart failure, dizziness when rising from a sitting or lying position,
flushing, migraines, fainting, depression, confusion,
tiredness, high blood pressure, nervousness, memory
loss, itching, skin disease, hair loss, stomach bleeding,
blood in the stool, stomach irritation, vomiting, anemia,
thrombocytopenia (low blood-platelet count), black-and-
blue marks, swollen lymph glands, painful urination,
blood in the urine, muscle and joint ache, leg cramps,

> **Possible Side Effects** *(continued)*
>
> runny nose, nose bleeds, lung disease, sinus inflamma-
> tion, pneumonia, bronchitis, asthma, double vision, other
> visual difficulties, ringing or buzzing in the ears, liver
> inflammation, and dehydration.

Drug Interactions

• Sucralfate may interfere with the absorption of anagrelide into the blood. Do not combine these two drugs.

Food Interactions

Taking anagrelide with food modestly reduces the amount of
drug absorbed into the blood. In addition, the maximum
blood level of the drug is substantially reduced by food.
Anagrelide is best taken on an empty stomach.

Usual Dose

Adult: 0.5–4 mg a day, or 1 mg twice a day, to start. After at
least a week on the starting dose, the dose should be adjusted
by your doctor to the lowest effective dose.

Child (under age 17): not recommended.

Overdosage

In animals, single doses of anagrelide up to 1250 mg per lb. of
body weight were not toxic, but did cause symptoms including soft stool and decreased appetite. There have been no
reports of human anagrelide overdose, but symptoms can be
expected to be related to a sudden, drastic drop in blood-
platelet count and might affect the heart or nervous system.
Overdose victims should be taken to a hospital emergency
room at once. ALWAYS bring the prescription bottle or
container with you.

Special Information

If you forget to take a dose of anagrelide, take it as soon as
possible. If it is almost time for your next dose, skip the dose
you forgot and continue with your regular schedule. Call your
doctor if you forget 2 or more anagrelide doses in a row. Do
not take a double dose.

Special Populations

Pregnancy/Breast-feeding

Animal studies at doses 49 times the maximum dose recommended for humans resulted in birth defects and other serious problems. Five women became pregnant while taking anagrelide; the drug was stopped as soon as possible and all 5 gave birth to healthy babies. However, pregnant women should not take anagrelide without first discussing its possible risks and benefits with their doctor.

It is not known if this drug passes into breast milk. Because of the possibility of serious effects on nursing infants, mothers who must take anagrelide should bottle-feed their babies.

Seniors

Seniors may take anagrelide without special precaution.

Generic Name

Anastrozole (ah-NAS-troe-zole)

Brand Name

Arimidex

The information in this profile also applies to the following drug:

Generic Ingredient: Letrozole
Femara

Type of Drug

Aromatase inhibitor.

Prescribed for

Advanced breast cancer in postmenopausal women.

General Information

Anastrozole is recommended for use in breast cancer that has advanced despite treatment with tamoxifen. Women with estrogen-receptor negative disease and those who did not respond at all to tamoxifen are not likely to respond to anastrozole. Anastrozole reduces the amount of estradiol, an estrogenic hormone, in the blood. It does this by interfering with the action of the aromatase enzyme, which is an element in the manufacture of estradiol. Most of anastrozole is broken down in the liver; the rest is eliminated through the kidneys.

About 1 in 10 women who took anastrozole in pre-approval studies responded completely or partially to drug treatment.

Cautions and Warnings

Anastrozole **increases blood-cholesterol** levels.

Animal studies of anastrozole have shown that it can affect **fertility**, but this effect has not yet been seen in women.

Possible Side Effects

▼ Most common: weakness, nausea, headache, flushing, pain, and back pain.

▼ Less common: breathing difficulties; vomiting; cough; diarrhea; constipation; abdominal pain; appetite loss; bone pain; sore throat; dizziness; rash; dry mouth; swelling in the arms, legs, or feet; pelvic pain; depression; chest pain; and tingling in the hands or feet.

▼ Rare: vaginal bleeding, weight gain, sweating, increased appetite, flu symptoms, fever, neck pain, feeling sick, infection, weight loss, high blood pressure, blood clots (symptoms include severe leg pain), confusion, sleeplessness, anxiety, nervousness, hair loss, itching, urinary infection, breast pain, anemia, low white blood-cell count, muscle ache, broken bones, runny nose, bronchitis, and sinus irritation.

Drug Interactions

• Usual doses of anastrozole do not affect other medications; however, high doses of anastrozole can reduce the ability of the liver to break down certain drugs.

Food Interactions

Food can reduce the amount of anastrozole absorbed into the blood. Take this drug either 1 hour before or 2 hours after a meal.

Usual Dose

Anastrozole
  Adult: 1 mg once a day.

Letrozole
  Adult: 2.5 mg once a day.

Overdosage

Symptoms of overdose can be exaggerated side effects. Overdose victims should be taken to a hospital emergency room where, in addition to other treatment, they can be made to vomit in order to remove any remaining drug from their systems. ALWAYS bring the prescription bottle or container with you.

Special Information

Call your doctor if your side effects become severe or intolerable.

Use a condom, diaphragm, or other non-hormonal contraceptive while taking anastrozole.

If you forget a dose of anastrozole, take it as soon as you remember. If it is almost time for your next dose, skip the dose you forgot and continue with your regular schedule. Call your doctor if you forget more than two doses in a row.

Special Populations

Pregnancy/Breast-feeding

Animal studies have shown that anastrozole can harm the fetus. Pregnant women who take anastrozole have a good chance of losing the pregnancy or harming the fetus. Conception should be prevented in women taking this drug by the use of a condom, diaphragm, or other non-hormonal contraceptive.

It is not known if anastrozole passes into breast milk. Nursing mothers who must take this drug should consider bottle-feeding their babies.

Seniors

Seniors may take this drug without special precaution.

Type of Drug

Antidiabetes Drugs (Oral Sulfonylureas)

Brand Names

Generic Ingredient: Acetohexamide
Dymelar

Generic Ingredient: Chlorpropamide
Diabinese

Generic Ingredient: Glimepiride
Amaryl

Generic Ingredient: Glipizide
Glucotrol   Glucotrol XL

Generic Ingredient: Glyburide
DiaBeta   Micronase
Glynase PresTab

Generic Ingredient: Repaglinide
Prandin

Generic Ingredient: Tolazamide
Tolinase

Generic Ingredient: Tolbutamide
Orinase

Prescribed for

Diabetes mellitus (sugar in the urine). Chlorpropamide, in doses of 200 to 500 mg a day, may also be used to treat diabetes insipidus (a hormonal condition unrelated to body sugar).

General Information

These medicines work by stimulating the production and release of insulin from the pancreas. They differ from each other in how long they take to start working, the duration of their effectiveness, and the amount of each required to produce a roughly equivalent antidiabetic effect (see table). These drugs do not lower blood sugar directly; they require some working pancreas cells. So-called "second-generation" antidiabetes drugs, glimepiride, glipizide, and glyburide, belong to the same chemical class as the older "first generation" ones, but lower doses of the second-generation agents are required to accomplish the same effect. Other minor differences between the two groups are considered clinically unimportant, and the second-generation drugs offer few advantages over the first-generation agents.

Drug	Equivalent Dose (mg)	Hours to Start Working	Hours of Effectiveness
Acetohexamide	500	1	12 to 24
Chlorpropamide	250	1	up to 60
Glipimepiride	4	1	24
Glipizide	10	1 to 1½	10 to 16
Glyburide (DiaBeta, Micronase)	5	2 to 4	24
Glyburide (Glynase PresTab)	3	1	12 to 24
Tolazamide	250	4 to 6	12 to 24
Tolbutamide	1000	1	6 to 12

Cautions and Warnings

Mild stress, such as infection, minor surgery, or emotional upset, reduces the effectiveness of oral sulfonylurea antidiabetes drugs. Remember that while you are taking these drugs you must be under your doctor's continuous care.

Oral sulfonylurea antidiabetes drugs are **not a form of oral insulin,** nor are they a substitute for insulin. They do not lower blood sugar by themselves. Studies conducted years ago found that people taking an oral sulfonylurea antidiabetic are more likely to have **fatal heart trouble** than those who can control their diabetes with diet alone or diet plus insulin.

Treating diabetes is your responsibility. Follow your doctor's instructions about diet, body weight, exercise, personal hygiene, and all measures to avoid infection.

Oral sulfonylurea antidiabetics are broken down in the liver. They should be used with caution if you have **serious liver, kidney, or endocrine disease;** monitor your blood sugar very closely.

Possible Side Effects

▼ Most common: loss of appetite, nausea, vomiting, and stomach upset. At times you may experience weakness or tingling in the hands and feet. To eliminate these effects, ask your doctor to reduce your daily dosage or,

Possible Side Effects *(continued)*

if necessary, switch you to another oral sulfonylurea antidiabetes drug. The most common side effects of repaglinide are flu-like symptoms, runny nose, and respiratory problems.

▼ Less common: oral sulfonylurea antidiabetics may produce abnormally low blood sugar levels when too much is taken for your immediate requirements. (Other factors which may cause lowering of blood sugar are liver or kidney disease, diseases of the glands, malnutrition, old age, and drinking alcohol.)

▼ Rare: yellowing of the eyes or skin, itching, and rash. Usually these reactions will disappear in time. If they persist, contact your doctor.

Drug Interactions

• The following drugs may increase your need for oral sulfonylurea antidiabetes drugs: beta blockers, cholestyramine, diazoxide, phenytoin and other hydantoin drugs, rifampin, thiazide diuretics, charcoal tablets, and anything that makes your urine less acidic.

• The following drugs may decrease your need for oral sulfonylurea antidiabetes drugs: androgens (male hormones), sulfa drugs, aspirin and other salicylates, chloramphenicol, clofibrate, gemfibrozil, cimetidine, ranitidine, famotidine, nizatidine, oxyphenbutazone, magnesium, methyldopa, phenylbutazone, probenecid, dicumarol, bishydroxycoumarin, warfarin, phenyramidol, sulfinpyrazone, tricyclic antidepressants, large doses of vitamin C, citrus fruits and other foods that make your urine more acidic, and monoamine oxidase inhibitor (MAOI) drugs. These drugs tend to prolong and enhance the action of oral sulfonylurea antidiabetes drugs. Insulin may be used together with an oral sulfonylurea antidiabetes drug, but only under the strict control of a physician. If used indiscriminately, this combination can cause severely low blood sugar.

• Combining these drugs with alcoholic beverages causes flushing of the face and body, as well as breathlessness. Other possible adverse effects are throbbing pain in the head and neck, breathing difficulties, nausea, vomiting, increased sweating, excessive thirst, chest pains, palpitations, lowered blood pressure, weakness, dizziness, blurred vision, and confusion. If you experience any of these reactions, contact your doctor immediately.

• Oral sulfonylurea antidiabetics may increase blood levels of the digitalis drugs, increasing their effects on your body.

• The stimulant ingredients in many nonprescription cough, cold, and allergy remedies may affect your blood sugar; avoid them unless your doctor advises otherwise.

Food Interactions

All oral sulfonylurea antidiabetes drugs except glipizide may be taken with food. Glipizide should be taken 30 minutes before a meal for best results. Repaglinide should be taken about 15 minutes only before eating a meal. You do not need to take the medicine if you skip a meal.

Dietary management is an important part of controlling your diabetes. Be sure to follow your doctor's directions about which foods you should avoid.

Usual Dose

Acetohexamide: 250–1500 mg a day.

Chlorpropamide: starting dose—1–2 g a day. Your doctor will then raise or lower your dose according to your response. Maintenance dose—0.25–2 g a day; rarely, 3 g a day may be prescribed.

Glimepiride: 4–8 mg once a day.

Glipizide: 5 mg once a day. Seniors may be started on 2.5 mg a day. Doses up to 40 mg a day divided into 2 doses may be needed to control more severe diabetes. Single daily doses should not exceed 15 mg.

Glyburide: DiaBeta/Micronase—2.5–20 mg once a day, usually with breakfast or the first main meal. Seniors may start with 1.25 mg a day. Glynase PresTab—1.5–12 mg a day, usually with breakfast or the first main meal. Seniors may start with 0.75 mg a day. Glynase PresTab is not equivalent to DiaBeta or Micronase and may not be substituted for either of them. DiaBeta and Micronase are interchangeable.

Repaglinide: One tablet 15 minutes before each meal. Do not take the medicine if you skip a meal.

Tolazamide: moderate diabetes—100–250 mg a day. Severe diabetes—500–1000 mg a day.

Tolbutamide: starting dose—1–2 g a day. Your doctor will then raise or lower your dosage based on your response. Maintenance dose—0.25–2 g a day; rarely, 3 g a day may be prescribed.

Overdosage

A mild overdose causes low blood sugar (symptoms include tingling of the lips and tongue, nausea, lethargy, yawning, confusion, agitation, nervousness, rapid heartbeat, increased sweating, tremors, and hunger). This can be treated by consuming sugar in such forms as candy, orange juice, or glucose tablets. Ultimately, low blood sugar may lead to convulsions, stupor, and coma. Call your doctor, local poison control center, or hospital emergency room to find out if the overdose victim should be taken to a hospital emergency room. Always bring the prescription bottle or container with you.

Special Information

Diet is essential to the treatment of diabetes. Follow the diet plan your doctor has prescribed and avoid alcoholic beverages.

Call your doctor if you develop low blood sugar (see "Overdosage") or high blood sugar (symptoms include excessive thirst or urination and sugar or ketones in the urine), if you are not feeling well, or if you have symptoms such as itching, rash, yellow skin or eyes, abnormally light-colored stools, a low-grade fever, sore throat, diarrhea, and unusual bruising or bleeding.

Do not stop taking these drugs, except under your doctor's supervision. If you forget a dose of an oral sulfonylurea antidiabetes drug, take it as soon as you remember. If it is almost time for your next dose, skip the one you forgot and continue with your regular schedule. Do not take a double dose.

Special Populations

Pregnancy/Breast-feeding

Animal studies have shown that all oral sulfonylurea antidiabetes drugs except glyburide cause birth defects or interfere with fetal development. Check with your doctor before taking an oral sulfonylurea antidiabetes drug if you are, or might be, pregnant. Blood sugar control is essential in pregnant diabetics since high blood sugar is also associated with an increased chance of birth defects. Pregnant women are best treated with insulin, because oral sulfonylurea antidiabetes drugs generally will not control their blood sugar. Birth defects and other problems are 3 to 4 times more common in diabetic mothers than in nondiabetics.

If you take oral sulfonylurea antidiabetics while nursing, the baby's blood-sugar level may be lowered; nursing mothers taking one of these medications should bottle-feed their babies.

Seniors
Seniors, especially those with reduced kidney function, are very sensitive to the blood-sugar-lowering effects and side effects of these drugs; older adults do not eliminate them from the body as efficiently as do younger people. Low blood sugar, the major sign of drug overdose, may be more difficult to identify in seniors. Also, low blood sugar is more likely to cause nervous-system side effects in seniors.

Seniors taking oral sulfonylurea antidiabetes drugs must keep in close contact with their doctors and follow their directions.

Type of Drug

Antihistamine-Decongestant Combination Products

Brand Names

Generic Ingredients: Acrivastine + Pseudoephedrine
Semprex-D

Generic Ingredients: Azatadine + Pseudoephedrine
Trinalin Repetabs

Generic Ingredients: Brompheniramine + Phenylpropanolamine
E.N.T.

Generic Ingredients: Brompheniramine + Phenylephrine + Phenylpropanolamine
Bromophen T.D.   Tamine S.R.

Generic Ingredients: Brompheniramine + Pseudoephedrine

Allent
Bromfed
Dallergy-JR
Disobrom
Dexaphen-SA
Endafed

Lodrane LD
Respahist
Rondec
Touro A & H
ULTRAbrom

Generic Ingredients: Carbinoxamine + Pseudoephedrine

Carbiset
Carbiset TR
Carbodec

Carbodec TR
Cardec-S
Rondec-TR

Generic Ingredients: Chlorpheniramine + Pseudoephedrine

Anamine
Anamine T.D.
Anaplex S A
Atrohist Pediatric
Brexin L.A.
Chlordrine SR
Chlorphedrine SR
Codimal L.A.
Colfed-A
Cophene No.2
Deconamine*
Deconomed SR
Duralex

Dura-Tap/PD
Fedahist Gyrocaps
Fedahist Timecaps
Histalet A
Klerist-D
Kronofed-A
Kronofed-A Jr.
ND Clear
Novafed A
Rinade B.I.D.
Tanafed
Time-Hist

Generic Ingredients: Chlorpheniramine + Phenylephrine

Dallergy-D A
Ed A-Hist
Histor-D
Novahistine S

Prehist
Rolatuss Plain
Ru-Tuss

Generic Ingredients: Chlorpheniramine + Phenylpropanolamine

A.R.M.
Drize
Dura-Vent/A
Ornade Spansules

Resaid
Rescon ED
Rescon JR
Rhinolar-EX

Generic Ingredients: Chlorpheniramine + Phenylephrine + Phenylpropanolamine

Hista-Vadrin

Generic Ingredients: Chlorpheniramine + Phenindamine + Phenylpropanolamine
Nolamine

Generic Ingredients: Chlorpheniramine + Phenyltoloxamine + Phenylephrine
Comhist

Generic Ingredients: Chlorpheniramine + Phenyltoloxamine + Phenylephrine + Phenylpropanolamine

Naldecon*	Tri-Phen-Chlor
Naldecon Pediatric	Tri-Phen-Mine*
Naldelate	Tri-Phen-Mine SR
Naldelate Pediatric	Tri-Phen-Mine Pediatric
Nalgest*	Uni-Decon

Generic Ingredients: Chlorpheniramine + Pyrilamine + Phenylephrine

Atrohist Pediatric	
Rhinatate	Tanoral
R-Tannate	Triotann
R-Tannamine	Tritan
Rynatan	Tri-Tannate

Generic Ingredients: Chlorpheniramine + Pyrilamine + Phenylephrine + Phenylpropanolamine

Histalet Forte	Vanex Forte

Generic Ingredients: Loratadine + Pseudoephedrine

Claritin-D	Claritin-D 24 Hour

Generic Ingredients: Pheniramine + Pyrilamine + Phenylpropanolamine Ⓖ
Only available generically.

Generic Ingredients: Pheniramine + Phenyltoloxamine + Pyrilamine + Phenylpropanolamine

Liqui-Histine-D	Poly-Histine-D Ped Caps
Poly-Histine-D	

Generic Ingredients: Promethazine + Phenylephrine

Phenergan VC	Prometh VC Plain
Promethazine VC	

*Some products in this brand-name group are alcohol or sugar free. Consult your pharmacist.

Prescribed for

Sneezing, watery eyes, runny nose, itchy or scratchy throat, nasal congestion, and other symptoms of the common cold, allergies, and other upper respiratory conditions.

General Information

The basic formula that appears in each of these antihistamine-decongestant combinations is the same: an antihistamine is used to relieve allergy symptoms and a decongestant to treat the symptoms of either a cold or allergy.

Most of these products are taken several times a day, while others are long-acting and are taken once or twice a day. Since nothing can cure a cold or allergy, the best you can hope to achieve from a cold and allergy remedy is relief from symptoms.

Cautions and Warnings

The antihistamines in these products may cause **drowsiness**. Decongestants may cause **anxiety** and **nervousness** and may interfere with sleep.

People who are **allergic** to antihistamines or decongestants should use these products with caution. Check with your doctor or pharmacist for further information.

People with **narrow-angle glaucoma, prostate disease, certain stomach ulcers,** and **bladder obstruction** should not use these products. People having **asthma attacks** and those taking a **monoamine oxidase inhibitor (MAOI)** for depression or high blood pressure should not take these products. People with serious **liver disease** and **those taking erythromycin, ketoconazole, or itraconazole** should not take terfenadine.

Possible Side Effects

▼ Most common: restlessness, nervousness, sleeplessness, drowsiness, sedation, excitation, dizziness, poor coordination, and upset stomach.

▼ Less common: low blood pressure, heart palpitations, rapid heartbeat and abnormal heart rhythms, chest pain, anemia, fatigue, confusion, tremors, headache, irritability, euphoria (feeling high), tingling or heaviness in the hands, tingling in the feet or legs, blurred or double

---

Possible Side Effects *(continued)*

vision, convulsions, hysterical reaction, ringing or buzzing in the ears, fainting, increase or decrease in appetite, nausea, vomiting, diarrhea or constipation, frequent urination, difficulty urinating, early menstrual periods, loss of sex drive, breathing difficulties, wheezing with chest tightness, stuffed nose, itching, rash, unusual sensitivity to the sun, chills, excessive perspiration, and dry mouth, nose, or throat.

Drug Interactions

• Combining these products with alcoholic beverages, antianxiety drugs, tranquilizers, or narcotic pain relievers may lead to excessive drowsiness or difficulty concentrating.

• These products should be avoided if you are taking an MAOI for depression or high blood pressure because the MAOI may cause a very rapid rise in blood pressure or increase side effects such as dry mouth and nose, blurred vision, and abnormal heart rhythms.

• The decongestant component of these products may interfere with the normal effects of blood-pressure-lowering medications and can aggravate diabetes, heart disease, hyperthyroid disease, high blood pressure, prostate disease, stomach ulcer, and urinary blockage.

• If your doctor has prescribed one of these products, do not self-medicate with an additional over-the-counter drug for the relief of cold symptoms. This combination may aggravate high blood pressure, heart disease, diabetes, or thyroid disease.

Food Interactions

These drugs are best taken on an empty stomach but may be taken with food if they upset your stomach.

Usual Dose

Specific dosages vary depending on the product you are taking. Generally, these antihistamine-decongestant combinations are taken every 4–12 hours.

Overdosage

The main symptoms of overdose are drowsiness, chills, dry

mouth, fever, nausea, nervousness, irritability, rapid or irregular heartbeat, chest pain, and urinary difficulties. Most cases are not severe but should be treated by inducing vomiting as soon as possible with ipecac syrup—available at any pharmacy. Then call your local poison control center for more information and/or take the victim to a hospital emergency room. ALWAYS bring the prescription bottle or container with you.

Special Information

Since the antihistamine component in most of these products may slow your central nervous system, you must use extra caution while doing anything that requires concentration, such as driving a car or operating hazardous machinery.

Call your doctor if your side effects are severe or become intolerable. There are so many different cold and allergy products available that one is sure to be the right combination for you.

If you forget to take a dose of your medication, take it as soon as you remember. If it is almost time for your next dose, skip the dose you forgot and continue with your regular schedule. Do not take a double dose.

Special Populations

Pregnancy/Breast-feeding
Though animal studies have shown that some antihistamines, used mainly against nausea and vomiting, may cause birth defects, the ingredients in these products have not been proven to cause birth defects or other problems in pregnant women. Do not take any of these products without your doctor's knowledge.

Small amounts of antihistamine or decongestant drugs pass into breast milk and may affect a nursing infant. Nursing mothers who must use these products should bottle-feed their infants.

Seniors
Seniors are more sensitive to the side effects of these medications. Confusion; difficult or painful urination; dizziness; drowsiness; feeling faint; dry mouth, nose, or throat; nightmares or excitability; nervousness; restlessness; and irritability are more likely to occur among older adults.

Generic Name

Apraclonidine (ah-prah-KLON-ih-dene)

Brand Name

Iopidine

Type of Drug

Sympathomimetic.

Prescribed for

Post-surgical increases in eye pressure; also prescribed as
additional short-term treatment in people who are using
other glaucoma medicines.

General Information

Apraclonidine hydrochloride reduces both elevated and normal fluid pressure inside the eye and selectively blocks
certain nerve endings without acting as a local anesthetic.
The exact way it works is not known, but apraclonidine, like
other drugs that reduce eye pressure, may work by decreasing the production of eye fluid. This agent can be used after
laser eye surgery to prevent permanent damage to the eye
nerve caused by sharp increases in eye pressure. Apraclonidine has a minimal effect on the heart and blood vessels. The
drug starts to work within 1 hour after it is put into the eye and
reaches its maximum effect in 3 to 5 hours.

Cautions and Warnings

Do not use apraclonidine if you are **allergic** to it or to
clonidine. This drug can cause an allergic-like reaction, including **red eye, swelling of the lid and white of the eye,
itching, burning,** and the **feeling of something in your eye**. If
this happens, stop using the drug and call your doctor. Taking
this drug with a **monoamine oxidase inhibitor (MAOI)** may
result in severe side effects—do not combine them.

Using this medicine with other **eye-pressure-lowering
drugs** may not provide additional benefit: Other drugs work
in the same way and a further effect may not be possible.

The ability of apraclonidine to lower eye pressure decreases over time. Most **people continuously benefit for less than 1 month.**

People with **kidney or liver disease** should be monitored by their doctors while taking this medicine.

Possible Side Effects

▼ Most common: eye redness, itching, tearing, eye discomfort, lid swelling, dry mouth, feeling of something in your eye, headache, and weakness.

▼ Less common: blanching of the eye; upper lid elevation; dilated pupils; blurred vision and other eye disorders; allergic reactions; lid crusting; abnormal vision; eye pain; abdominal pain; diarrhea; stomach discomfort; vomiting; dry mouth or nose; nasal burning; runny nose; sore throat; worsening asthma; constipation and nausea; slow heartbeat; heart palpitations; abnormal heart rhythms; chest pain; fainting; swelling; difficulty sleeping; irritability; reduced sex drive; pain, numbness, or tingling in the hands or feet; clammy or sweaty palms; taste changes; a feeling of having a head cold; and skin rash.

Drug Interactions

• Apraclonidine can reduce pulse and blood pressure. If you are also taking drugs to treat high blood pressure or other cardiovascular drugs, check your pulse and blood pressure.

• MAOI drugs can slow the breakdown of apraclonidine and increase the chance of drug side effects. This combination should be avoided.

Food Interactions

None known.

Usual Dose

Adult: 1–2 drops in the affected eye 3 times a day.

Overdosage

Exaggerated side effects, especially those that affect the nervous system, are symptoms of overdose. Call your local poison control center for more information. ALWAYS take the prescription bottle or container with you if you go to the emergency room.

Special Information

Apraclonidine can cause dizziness and tiredness. Be careful doing anything that requires concentration, coordination, or alertness while taking this medication.

To administer eyedrops, lie down or tilt your head backward and look at the ceiling. Hold the dropper above your eye, hold out your lower lid to make a small pouch, and drop the medicine inside while looking up. Release the lower lid and keep your eye open. Do not blink for about 30 seconds. Press gently on the bridge of your nose at the inside corner of your eye for about a minute to help circulate the medicine around your eye. To prevent infection, do not touch the dropper tip to your finger or eyelid. Wait 5 minutes before using any other eyedrop or ointment.

If you forget a dose of apraclonidine, take it as soon as you remember. If it is almost time for your next dose, take one dose as soon as you remember and then go back to your regular schedule. Do not take a double dose.

Special Populations

Pregnancy/Breast-feeding

In animal studies, apraclonidine was toxic to embryos when given by mouth. There are no studies of this drug in pregnant women; it should be used with caution during pregnancy.

It is not known if this drug passes into breast milk, but nursing mothers should bottle-feed their babies while using it.

Seniors

Seniors may use this medicine without special precautions.

Generic Name

Astemizole (uh-STEM-ih-zole)

Brand Name

Hismanal

Type of Drug

Antihistamine.

Prescribed for

Stuffy and runny nose, itchy eyes, and scratchy throat caused by seasonal allergy, and for other symptoms of allergy such as rash, itching, and hives.

General Information

Astemizole is a non-sedating antihistamine. It is often prescribed for people who find other antihistamines unacceptable because of the drowsiness and tiredness they cause.

Cautions and Warnings

Astemizole should not be taken by people who have had an **allergic** reaction to it in the past.

People with **asthma** or other **deep-breathing problems, glaucoma, stomach ulcer,** or other **stomach problems** should avoid astemizole because it may aggravate these conditions.

In high doses (20 or 30 mg a day) or cases of drug overdose, astemizole may cause **serious abnormal heart rhythms or other possibly fatal cardiac effects**. It should not be taken by people with **serious liver disease** or by **those taking erythromycin, ketoconazole,** or **itraconazole.**

Possible Side Effects

The most important side effects of astemizole are the rare cardiac consequences that most often occur in people with liver disease and those taking erythromycin, ketoconazole, or itraconazole. Dizziness or fainting may be the first sign of a cardiac problem with astemizole.

▼ Most common: headache; nervousness; weakness; upset stomach; nausea; vomiting; dry mouth, nose, or throat; cough; stuffed nose; changes in bowel habits; sore throat; and nosebleeds. In studies, astemizole was found to cause the same degree of drowsiness as placebo (sugar pill). About half of the other antihistamines sold in the U.S. also cause a similar degree of drowsiness. Most commonly used antihistamines cause more sedation than astemizole. Astemizole may also cause increased appetite or weight gain.

▼ Less common: hair loss, allergic reaction (symptoms include rash, itching, hives, and breathing difficulties), depression, sleeplessness, muscle aches, menstrual irregularities, increased sweating, tingling in the hands or feet, frequent urination, and visual disturbances. A few people taking this drug have developed liver damage.

Drug Interactions

- Antihistamines such as astemizole may decrease the effects of anticoagulant (blood-thinning) drugs.
- People combining astemizole and erythromycin, keto-conazole, or itraconazole have developed life-threatening cardiac side effects, though this is rare. Do not take any of these drugs with astemizole.

Food Interactions

Take astemizole 1 hour before or 2 hours after meals.

Usual Dose

Adult and Child (age 12 and over): 10 mg once a day.
Child (under age 12): not recommended.

Overdosage

Astemizole overdose is likely to cause serious cardiac effects or increased side effects. Overdose victims should be given ipecac syrup—available at any pharmacy—to make them vomit; they should then be taken to a hospital emergency room. ALWAYS bring the prescription bottle or container with you.

Special Information

Dizziness or fainting may be the first sign of serious drug side effects; call your doctor at once if you experience these or any other unusual side effects while taking astemizole.

If you forget to take a dose of astemizole, take it as soon as you remember. If it is almost time for your next dose, skip the forgotten dose and continue with your regular schedule. Do not take a double dose.

Special Populations

Pregnancy/Breast-feeding

Though no damage to the fetus was found in animal studies, astemizole should be used by pregnant women only if it is absolutely necessary.

It is not known if astemizole passes into breast milk. Nursing mothers who must use this drug should bottle-feed their infants.

Seniors

Seniors may be more sensitive to the side effects of astemizole and should be treated with the minimum effective dose, 10 mg a day.

Generic Name

Atenolol (ah-TEN-uh-lol) G

Brand Name

Tenormin

Combination Products

Generic Ingredients: Atenolol + Chlorthalidone G
Tenoretic   Tenoretic 100
Tenoretic 50

Type of Drug

Beta-adrenergic blocking agent.

Prescribed for

High blood pressure, abnormal heart rhythms, angina pectoris, prevention of second heart attack and migraine headache, alcohol withdrawal, stage fright and other anxieties, and bleeding from the esophagus.

General Information

Atenolol is one of 15 beta-adrenergic blocking drugs, or beta blockers, that interfere with the action of a specific part of the nervous system. Beta receptors are found all over the body and affect many body functions. This accounts for the usefulness of beta blockers against a wide variety of conditions. The oldest of these drugs, propranolol, affects all types of beta-adrenergic receptors. Newer, more refined beta blockers like atenolol affect only a portion of that system, making them more useful in treating cardiovascular disorders and less useful for other conditions. Other of the newer beta blockers act as mild stimulants to the heart or have particular characteristics that make them better for specific purposes or certain people.

Cautions and Warnings

People with **angina** who take atenolol for high blood pressure risk aggravating their angina if they suddenly stop taking the drug. These people should have their drug dosage reduced gradually over 1 to 2 weeks.

Atenolol should be used with caution if you have **liver or**

kidney disease, because your ability to eliminate this drug from your body may be impaired.

Atenolol reduces the amount of blood the heart pumps. This reduction in blood flow may aggravate the condition of people with **poor circulation** or **circulatory disease**.

If you are undergoing **major surgery**, your doctor may want you to stop taking atenolol at least 2 days before surgery to permit the heart to respond more acutely to stresses that can occur during the procedure. This practice is still controversial and may not be appropriate for all surgeries.

Possible Side Effects

Side effects are relatively uncommon and usually mild; they usually develop early in the course of treatment and are rarely a reason to stop taking atenolol.

▼ Most common: impotence.

▼ Less common: unusual tiredness or weakness, slow heartbeat, heart failure (symptoms include swelling of the legs, ankles, or feet), dizziness, breathing difficulties, bronchospasm, depression, confusion, anxiety, nervousness, sleeplessness, disorientation, short-term memory loss, emotional instability, cold hands and feet, constipation, diarrhea, nausea, vomiting, upset stomach, increased sweating, urinary difficulties, cramps, blurred vision, skin rash, hair loss, stuffy nose, facial swelling, aggravation of lupus erythematosus (chronic condition affecting the body's connective tissue), itching, chest pain, back or joint pain, colitis, drug allergy (symptoms include fever and sore throat), and liver toxicity.

Drug Interactions

• Atenolol may interact with surgical anesthetics to increase the risk of heart problems during surgery. Some anesthesiologists recommend having gradually stopped the drug by 2 days before surgery.

• Atenolol may interfere with the normal signs of low blood sugar and with oral antidiabetic drugs.

• Atenolol increases the blood-pressure-lowering effects of other blood-pressure-reducing agents, including clonidine, guanabenz, and reserpine; and calcium channel blockers, such as nifedipine.

• Aspirin-containing drugs, indomethacin, sulfinpyrazone, and estrogen drugs may interfere with the blood-pressure-lowering effect of atenolol.

• Cocaine may reduce the effectiveness of all beta blockers.

• Atenolol may worsen the problem of cold hands and feet associated with taking ergot alkaloids, used to treat migraine headaches. Gangrene is a possibility in people taking both an ergot and atenolol.

• Atenolol will counteract thyroid hormone replacements.

• Calcium channel blockers, flecainide, hydralazine, oral contraceptives, propafenone, haloperidol, phenothiazine tranquilizers—molindone and others—quinolone antibacterials, and quinidine may increase the amount of atenolol in the bloodstream and lead to increased atenolol effects.

• Atenolol should not be taken within 2 weeks of taking a monoamine oxidase inhibitor (MAOI) antidepressant.

• Cimetidine increases the amount of atenolol absorbed into the bloodstream from oral tablets.

• Atenolol may interfere with the effectiveness of some antiasthma drugs, including theophylline and aminophylline, and especially ephedrine and isoproterenol.

• Combining atenolol with phenytoin or digitalis drugs may result in excessive slowing of the heart, possibly causing heart block (disruption of the electrical impulses that control heart rate).

• If you stop smoking while taking atenolol, your dose may have to be reduced because your liver will break down the drug more slowly.

Food Interactions

None known.

Usual Dose

Adult: starting dose—50 mg a day, taken all at once. The daily dose may be gradually increased up to 200 mg. Maintenance dose—50–200 mg once a day. People with kidney disease may need only 50 mg every other day.

Senior: Older adults should be treated more cautiously and may need lower doses.

Overdosage

Symptoms of overdose include changes in heartbeat—

unusually slow, unusually fast, or irregular—severe dizziness or fainting, breathing difficulties, bluish-colored fingernails or palms, and seizures. The victim should be taken to a hospital emergency room. ALWAYS bring the prescription bottle or container with you.

Special Information

Atenolol is meant to be taken continuously. When ending atenolol treatment, dosage should be reduced gradually over a period of about 2 weeks. Do not stop taking this drug unless directed to do so by your doctor: Abrupt withdrawal may cause chest pain, breathing difficulties, increased sweating, and unusually fast or irregular heartbeat.

Call your doctor at once if you develop back or joint pain, breathing difficulties, cold hands or feet, depression, skin rash, or changes in heartbeat. Atenolol may produce an undesirable lowering of blood pressure, leading to dizziness or fainting; call your doctor if this happens. Call your doctor if you experience persistent or bothersome anxiety, diarrhea, constipation, impotence, headache, itching, nausea or vomiting, nightmares or vivid dreams, upset stomach, insomnia, stuffy nose, frequent urination, unusual tiredness, or weakness.

Atenolol may cause drowsiness, light-headedness, dizziness, or blurred vision. Be careful when driving or performing complex tasks.

It is best to take atenolol at the same time each day. If you forget a dose, take it as soon as you remember. If you take atenolol once a day and it is within 8 hours of your next dose, skip the dose you forgot and continue with your regular schedule. If you take atenolol twice a day and it is within 4 hours of your next dose, skip the one you forgot and continue with your regular schedule. Never take a double dose.

Special Populations

Pregnancy/Breast-feeding

Infants born to women who took a beta blocker while pregnant had lower birth weights, low blood pressure, and reduced heart rates. Atenolol should be avoided by pregnant women and women who might become pregnant while taking it. When the drug is considered crucial by your doctor, its potential benefits must be carefully weighed against its risks.

Atenolol passes into breast milk in concentrations greater than those found in the mother's bloodstream. Nursing mothers should avoid taking atenolol.

Seniors

Seniors may absorb and retain more atenolol, and may require less of the drug to achieve results. Your doctor should adjust your dosage to meet your individual needs. Seniors taking atenolol may be more likely to suffer from cold hands and feet, reduced body temperature, chest pain, general feelings of ill health, sudden breathing difficulties, increased sweating, or changes in heartbeat.

Generic Name

Atorvastatin (ah-tor-vuh-STAT-in)

Brand Name

Lipitor

Type of Drug

Cholesterol-lowering agent (HMG-CoA reductase inhibitor).

Prescribed for

High blood-cholesterol, LDL-cholesterol, and triglyceride levels, in conjunction with a low-cholesterol diet program. It is also prescribed to slow the progression of atherosclerosis (hardening of the arteries), reduce the risk of death in people with heart disease, and treat inherited blood-lipid problems or problems associated with diabetes or kidney disease.

General Information

Atorvastatin calcium is one of several cholesterol-lowering drugs that work by inhibiting an enzyme called HMG-CoA reductase. They interfere with the natural process for manufacturing cholesterol in your body, altering that process in order to produce a harmless by-product. Studies have closely related high blood-fat levels—total cholesterol, LDL cholesterol, and triglycerides—to heart and blood-vessel disease. Drugs that reduce levels of any of these blood fats and increase HDL cholesterol—"good" cholesterol—have been assumed for several years to reduce the risk of death and heart attack. Recently, medication in this class has been proven to slow the formation of blood-vessel plaque—associated with atherosclerosis—and reduce the risk of heart attack and death related to heart disease.

Atorvastatin reduces total triglyceride, cholesterol, and LDL-cholesterol counts while increasing HDL cholesterol. A very small amount of the drug actually reaches the body's circulation. Most is broken down and eliminated by the liver; 10% to 20% of the drug is released from the body through the kidneys. A significant blood-fat-lowering response is seen after 1 to 2 weeks of treatment. Blood-fat levels are lowest within 4 to 6 weeks after taking atorvastatin and remain at or close to that level as long as you continue to take the drug. The effect is known to persist for 4 to 6 weeks after you stop taking it.

Atorvastatin generally does not benefit anyone under age 30, so it is not usually recommended for children. It may, under special circumstances, be prescribed for teenagers in the same dose as adults.

Cautions and Warnings

Do not take atorvastatin if you are **allergic** to it or to any other HMG-CoA reductase inhibitor.

People with a history of **liver disease** and **those who drink large amounts of alcohol** should avoid drugs in this group because they may aggravate or cause liver disease. Your doctor should take a blood sample to test your liver function every month or so during the first year of treatment.

Atorvastatin causes **muscle aches and/or muscle weakness** in a small number of people, which may be a sign of a more serious condition.

At dosages between 50 and 100 or more times the maximum human dose, atorvastatin has caused central nervous system lesions, liver tumors, and male infertility in lab animals. The importance of this information for humans is not known.

Possible Side Effects

Most people who take atorvastatin tolerate it quite well.
- ▼ Most common: headache.
- ▼ Common: muscle ache.

Possible Side Effects *(continued)*

▼ Less common: stomach gas, upset stomach, itching, rash, allergy, and infection.

▼ Rare: Effects can occur in virtually any body part or system. Report anything unusual to your doctor.

Drug Interactions

• The cholesterol-lowering effects of atorvastatin and cholestyramine are additive when the drugs are taken together. Take atorvastatin 1 hour before or 4 hours after cholestyramine. Colestipol reduces the amount of atorvastatin in your blood by about 25%.

• Antacids may reduce the amount of atorvastatin absorbed by the blood. Take these medications at least 1 hour apart.

• Itraconazole can increase atorvastatin levels by 20 times. Avoid this combination by temporarily stopping atorvastatin if you take itraconazole. Erythromycin increases the amount of atorvastatin in your blood by about 40%, possibly increasing the risk of drug side effects.

• Taking atorvastatin with oral contraceptives increases the amount of hormone in the bloodstream. This may lead to unwanted hormone side effects. If you must take both drugs, talk to your doctor about lowering the dose of your contraceptive pill to a lower dose product.

• Atorvastatin may increase the effects of warfarin or digoxin. If you take either of these drugs with atorvastatin you should be periodically checked by your doctor.

• The combination of cyclosporine, erythromycin, gemfibrozil, or niacin with atorvastatin may cause severe muscle ache or degeneration or other muscle problems. These combinations should be avoided.

• Propranolol can interfere with the action of atorvastatin, reducing its effectiveness.

Food Interactions

None known. Continue your low-cholesterol diet while taking this medicine.

Usual Dose

Adult: 10–40 mg at bedtime.

Senior: 10–20 mg at bedtime.

Your daily dosage of atorvastatin should be adjusted monthly, based on how well the drug is working to reduce your blood cholesterol.

Overdosage

There are 2 known cases of atorvastatin overdose, neither of which caused symptoms or problems. A person suspected of having consumed an overdose of atorvastatin should be taken to a hospital emergency room for evaluation and treatment. ALWAYS bring the prescription bottle or container with you.

Special Information

Call your doctor if you develop blurred vision or muscle ache, pain, tenderness, or weakness, especially if you are also feverish or feel sick.

Atorvastatin is always prescribed in combination with a low-fat diet. Be sure to follow you doctor's dietary instructions, since both diet and medication are necessary to treat your condition.

Do not take more cholesterol-lowering medication than your doctor has prescribed or stop taking the medication without your doctor's knowledge.

Atorvastatin may cause unusual sensitivity to the sun. Use sunscreen and wear protective clothing while in the sun until you determine if you are affected.

If you forget to take a dose of atorvastatin, take it as soon as you remember. If it is almost time for your next dose, skip the one you forgot and continue with your regular schedule. Do not take a double dose.

Special Populations

Pregnancy/Breast-feeding

Pregnant women and those who might become pregnant absolutely must not take atorvastatin. Cholesterol is essential to the health and development of a fetus. Anything that interferes with that process will damage the developing brain and nervous system.

Since hardening of the arteries is a long-term process, you should be able to stop this medication during pregnancy without developing atherosclerosis. If you become pregnant while taking atorvastatin, stop the drug immediately and call your doctor.

Atorvastatin may pass into breast milk. Women taking atorvastatin should bottle-feed their infants.

Seniors
Seniors may be more sensitive to the effects of atorvastatin and are likely to require less of the drug than do younger adults. Be sure to report any side effects to your doctor.

Generic Name

Atovaquone (ah-TOE-vuh-quone)

Brand Name
Mepron 🔲

Type of Drug
Anti-infective.

Prescribed for
Pneumocystis carinii pneumonia (PCP) in people who cannot take trimethoprim and sulfamethoxazole.

General Information
Atovaquone is an anti-infective with specific activity against PCP, an infection commonly associated with AIDS. In studies comparing atovaquone with TMP-SMZ, a trimethoprim-sulfamethoxazole combination, approximately 60% of people with PCP improved on each drug. However, more people died of PCP and other infections while being treated with atovaquone. Of those who died, most had less atovaquone in their bloodstream than did those who lived. In studies comparing oral atovaquone with intravenous pentamidine for treating PCP in people with AIDS, both drugs were equally effective, at 14%. Again, there was a direct correlation between the amount of atovaquone in the blood and survival: Of people with less than 5 mcg of drug per ml of blood, 60% died; of those with 5 or more mcg of drug per ml of blood, only 9% died. In clinical trials of atovaquone for PCP using doses of 750 mg 3 times a day, average blood levels were almost 14 mcg per ml of blood, well above the threshold level of 5. The

drug stays in the body for several days and is eliminated through breakdown by the liver.

Cautions and Warnings

Do not take atovaquone if you are or may be **allergic** to it or to any of the product's components.

This drug has not been studied for PCP prevention or for severe PCP, or in those who are failing on TMP-SMZ.

Atovaquone does not work against any infection other than PCP. People with PCP who have bacterial, viral, fungal, or other infections of the lung may continue to worsen despite atovaquone therapy. If this happens, it may be a sign that another kind of infecting organism is the cause. Your doctor will have to prescribe additional medicine.

Since atovaquone absorption is so strongly influenced by food, people who **cannot eat sufficiently** may not be able to absorb enough drug, and may have to take intravenous treatments of other PCP anti-infectives while taking atovaquone.

Possible Side Effects

It may be difficult to detect atovaquone-related side effects because they often resemble the underlying medical condition of people who generally take this medicine. Overall, only 4% to 7% of people stopped taking the drug because of side effects, a much smaller percentage than occurs with other PCP treatments. This drug has not been associated with any life-threatening or fatal side effects.

▼ Most common: rash, nausea, diarrhea, headache, vomiting, fever, sleeplessness, weakness, itching, oral fungal infections, abdominal pain, upset stomach, appetite loss, constipation, cough, dizziness, pain, increased sweating, anxiety, sinus inflammation, and runny nose.

▼ Less common: changes in sense of taste, low blood sugar, and low blood pressure.

Drug Interactions

• Atovaquone may increase levels of warfarin, oral antidiabetes drugs, digoxin, and other drugs that bind strongly to blood proteins.

• Rifampin and rifabutin may reduce blood levels of atovaquone, possibly diminishing its effectiveness.

• Taking atovaquone with TMP-SMZ has resulted in reduced blood levels of TMP-SMZ. This should not reduce TMP-SMZ's effectiveness.

• Taking atovaquone with zidovudine (AZT) causes the body to drastically reduce the rate at which zidovudine is eliminated from the body. For most people, this is not a problem.

Food Interactions

Atovaquone is highly fat-soluble. Its absorption into the blood is intensely affected by food: A high-fat meal can increase the amount absorbed by 300%. Take atovaquone with food or meals to improve drug absorption.

Usual Dose

750 mg 2 times a day for 3 weeks, taken with food.

Overdosage

There is little experience with atovaquone overdose; symptoms are likely to be exaggerated drug side effects. If the overdose is taken without food in the victim's stomach, the amount absorbed may not be enough to be harmful. Call your local poison control center or hospital emergency room for more information. If you go to the hospital, ALWAYS bring the prescription bottle or container with you.

Special Information

Taking atovaquone regularly and with food is essential to the drug's effectiveness. If you cannot eat 2 meals a day, your doctor may have to prescribe another PCP treatment.

Call your doctor if you develop any persistent or bothersome side effects.

If you forget a dose, take it as soon as you remember. If it is almost time for your next dose, space your remaining doses equally throughout the rest of the day so that you can still take a total daily dose of 1500 mg, or 2 tsp.

Special Populations

Pregnancy/Breast-feeding

In animal studies, atovaquone has affected fetal development in doses that are roughly equal to human doses. If you are pregnant this drug should be used only if the potential risks and benefits have been carefully weighed by you and your doctor. If you are not pregnant, use effective contraception while taking atovaquone.

It is not known if atovaquone passes into breast milk or if the drug affects a nursing infant. In animal studies, atovaquone was found in breast milk at levels equal to $\frac{1}{3}$ of those in the blood. Nursing mothers should bottle-feed their babies while taking atovaquone.

Seniors
This drug has not been tested systematically in people over age 65. Seniors, especially those with kidney, heart, or liver disease, may be more sensitive to atovaquone side effects. Report any unusual side effects to your doctor.

Atrovent

see **Ipratropium**, page 525

Augmentin

see **Penicillin Antibiotics**, page 846

Brand Name
Auralgan Otic

Generic Ingredients
Antipyrine + Benzocaine + Glycerin

Other Brand Names
Allergen Ear Drops   Otocalm Ear
Auroto Otic Solution

Type of Drug
Analgesic.

Prescribed for
Earache.

General Information

Auralgan is a combination product containing benzocaine, a local anesthetic that deadens nerves inside the ear that transmit painful impulses; antipyrine, an analgesic that provides additional pain relief; and glycerin, which removes any water present in the ear. This drug is often used to treat painful conditions caused by water in the ear canal, such as "swimmer's ear." Auralgan does not contain antibiotics and should not be used to treat any infection or condition other than the one for which it is prescribed.

Cautions and Warnings

Do not use the product if you are **allergic** to any of the ingredients.

Possible Side Effects

▼ Most common: local irritation.

Drug Interactions

• Do not apply any other medicines at the same time as Auralgan.

Food Interactions

None known.

Usual Dose

Place drops of Auralgan in the ear canal until the canal is filled. Saturate a piece of cotton with Auralgan, and put it in the ear canal to keep the drug from leaking out. Leave the drug in the ear for several minutes. Repeat 3–4 times per day.

Overdosage

Auralgan overdose is not likely to cause serious effects. Call your local poison control center for more information.

Special Information

Before using the product, warm the medicine bottle to body temperature by holding it in your hand for several minutes. Do not warm the bottle to a temperature above normal body temperature. Protect the bottle from light.

Call your doctor if you develop a burning or itching feeling or if the pain does not go away after 2-4 days of treatment.

If you forget a dose of Auralgan, take it as soon as you remember. If it is almost time for your next dose, skip the dose you forgot and continue with your regular schedule.

Special Populations

Pregnancy/Breast-feeding
Pregnant and breast-feeding women may use this product without special restriction.

Seniors
Seniors may use this product without restriction.

Axid

see **Nizatidine**, page 800

Generic Name
Azithromycin (uh-ZIH-throe-MYE-sin)

Brand Name
Zithromax

Type of Drug
Macrolide antibiotic.

Prescribed for
Upper and lower respiratory tract infections, skin infections, and sexually transmitted diseases in adults; middle ear infections in children; also prescribed for tonsillitis and pharyngitis in children when other drugs are not effective.

General Information
Azithromycin dihydrate is an azalide antibiotic, a subgroup of the macrolide antibiotics. Drugs in the macrolide group also include dirithromycin, erythromycin, and clarithromycin and are either bactericidal (bacteria-killing) or bacteriostatic (inhibiting bacterial growth) depending on the organism in question and the amount of antibiotic present.

Azithromycin is rapidly absorbed from the gastrointestinal tract and distributed to all parts of the body. Because the action of this antibiotic depends on its concentration within the invading bacteria, it is crucial that you follow your doctor's directions regarding the spacing of doses as well as the number of days you should continue taking the medication. The effectiveness of this antibiotic may be severely reduced if these instructions are not followed.

Cautions and Warnings

Do not take azithromycin if you are **allergic** to it or any macrolide antibiotic.

Azithromycin is excreted primarily through the liver. People with **liver disease or damage** should consult their doctors. Those on long-term therapy with this drug should have periodic blood tests.

Colitis (bowel inflammation) (see "Possible Side Effects") has been associated with all antibiotics including azithromycin.

Azithromycin is considered appropriate only for the treatment of more mild forms of pneumonia in non-hospitalized patients. People with other underlying conditions, those who are immune-compromised, and those who contract pneumonia in a hospital or other institutional setting probably should be treated with other antibiotics.

Possible Side Effects

▼ Most side effects are mild and will go away once you stop taking azithromycin.

▼ Most common: nausea, vomiting, stomach cramps, stomach gas, and diarrhea. Colitis (symptoms include severe abdominal cramps and severe, persistent, and possibly bloody diarrhea) may develop after taking azithromycin.

▼ Less common: heart palpitations, chest pain, hairy tongue, vaginal irritation, kidney inflammation, dizziness, headache, fainting, tiredness, unusual sensitivity to the sun, rash, and swelling.

▼ Rare: Macrolide antibiotics such as azithromycin have been asociated with serious abnormal heart rhythms.

Drug Interactions

• Azithromycin may increase warfarin's anticoagulant (blood-thinning) effects in people who take it regularly, especially seniors. People taking anticoagulants who must also take azithromycin may need their anticoagulant dose reduced.

• Azithromycin may interfere with the elimination of theophylline from the body. People taking this combination should be carefully monitored by their doctors for changes in blood-theophylline levels.

• Pimozide should not be taken by anyone also taking an amacrolide antibiotic. Two people died while taking this combination.

• Antacid products containing aluminum or magnesium may delay the absorption of azithromycin into the blood. Separate your antacid dose from your azithromycin dose by at least 1 hour.

Food Interactions

Food cuts the amount of azithromycin absorbed into the blood by half. Take it on an empty stomach, 1 hour before or 2 hours after meals.

Usual Dose

Respiratory Tract Infections, Skin Infections, and Sexually Transmitted Diseases
Adult (age 16 and over): 500 mg as a single dose on day 1, then 250 mg once a day on days 2–5 of treatment. Some sexually transmitted diseases are treated with a single dose of 1000 mg.

Middle Ear Infections
Child (age 6 months and over): 100–400 mg on day 1, then 50–200 mg on days 2–5 of treatment. Actual dose depends on body weight.

Tonsillitis and Pharyngitis
Child (age 2 and over): 100–500 mg a day for 5 days. Actual dose depends on body weight.

Overdosage

Azithromycin overdose may cause severe side effects, especially nausea, vomiting, stomach cramps, and diarrhea. Call your local poison control center or hospital emergency room for more information.

Special Information

Call your doctor if you develop nausea, vomiting, diarrhea, stomach cramps, or severe abdominal pain.

Take azithromycin at the same time each day to help you remember. If you forget a dose of azithromycin, take it as soon as you remember. If it is almost time for your next dose, skip the dose you forgot and go back to your regular schedule.

Remember to complete the full course of therapy prescribed by your doctor, even if you feel perfectly well after only 1 or 2 days of treatment.

Special Populations

Pregnancy/Breast-feeding

It is not known if azithromycin passes into the circulation of a fetus. This medication should be taken by pregnant women only if it is clearly needed.

Other macrolide antibiotics pass into breast milk but it is not known if this is true of azithromycin. Nursing mothers who must take this drug should bottle-feed their infants.

Seniors

Seniors, except those with liver disease, may generally use this drug without restriction or dose adjustment. Seniors who have pneumonia or are especially sickly or debilitated probably should be treated with other medications.

Azmacort

see **Corticosteroids, Inhalers,** page 262

Brand Name

Azo Gantrisin

Generic Ingredients

Phenazopyridine + Sulfisoxazole G

Other Brand Names

Azo-Sulfisoxazole

Type of Drug

Urinary anti-infective.

Prescribed for

Urinary tract infections.

General Information

Azo Gantrisin is one of many combination products used to treat urinary tract infections. The primary active ingredient is the sulfa drug sulfisoxazole. The other ingredient, phenazopyridine, is added to relieve urinary tract pain.

Cautions and Warnings

Do not take Azo Gantrisin if you know you are **allergic** to it, to other sulfa drugs, to salicylates, or to similar agents, or if you have a condition called **porphyria**. Azo Gantrisin should not be used by people with advanced **kidney disease**.

Possible Side Effects

▼ Most common: headache; itching; rash; sensitivity to bright light, particularly sunlight; nausea; vomiting; abdominal pains; tiredness; hallucinations; dizziness; ringing in the ears; chills; and not feeling well.

▼ Less common: reduced white-blood-cell and platelet counts, changes in other blood components, itchy eyes, arthritis-type pain, diarrhea, loss of appetite, stomach cramps or pains, hearing loss, drowsiness, fever, hair loss, yellowing of the skin and/or whites of the eyes, and reduction of sperm count.

Drug Interactions

• When Azo Gantrisin is taken with an anticoagulant (blood-thinning) drug, any diabetes drug, methotrexate, phenylbutazone, salicylates, phenytoin, or probenecid, it will cause unusually large amounts of these drugs to be released into the bloodstream, possibly producing symptoms of overdose. If you must take Azo Gantrisin for an extended period, your physician should reduce the dosage of these drugs. Also, avoid large doses of vitamin C.

Food Interactions

Sulfa drugs should be taken with a full glass of water on an empty stomach, but they can be taken with food if they upset your stomach.

Usual Dose

Starting dose—4–6 tablets. Maintenance dose—2 tablets every 4 hours. Take each dose with a full glass of water.

Overdosage

Give the overdose victim ipecac syrup, available in any pharmacy, to induce vomiting as soon as possible. Follow package directions. Take the victim to a hospital emergency room. ALWAYS bring the prescription bottle or container with you.

Special Information

Azo Gantrisin can cause a severe reaction to strong sunlight: Avoid prolonged sun exposure.

Sore throat, fever, unusual bleeding or bruising, rash, and feeling tired are early signs of serious blood disorders and should be reported to your doctor immediately.

The phenazopyridine ingredient in Azo Gantrisin is an orange-red dye and will discolor the urine. This is a normal effect of the drug, but if you are diabetic, the dye may interfere with testing your urine for sugar. This dye may also appear in your sweat and tears. Note that this dye may discolor certain types of contact lenses.

If you miss a dose of Azo Gantrisin, take it as soon as possible. If it is almost time for your next dose, skip the dose you forgot and continue with your regular schedule. Do not take a double dose.

Special Populations

Pregnancy/Breast-feeding

This drug may cause birth defects or interfere with fetal development. Check with your doctor before taking it if you are or might be pregnant.

The sulfa ingredient in this combination may pass into breast milk and can cause problems in infants suffering from G6PD deficiency, a rare genetic disorder. Other infants are usually not affected by this drug.

Seniors

Seniors may take this drug without special restriction.

Generic Name

Baclofen (BAK-loe-fen) [G]

Brand Name

Lioresal

Type of Drug

Skeletal muscle relaxant.

Prescribed for

Muscle spasms of multiple sclerosis (MS) and spinal cord injury or disease; may also be used to treat trigeminal neuralgia (tic douloureux), muscle spasm side effects of psychoactive drugs, and hiccups that do not respond to other treatment.

General Information

Baclofen may work by interfering with nervous system reflexes at the spinal cord, although it may also have some effect outside the spinal cord. Baclofen is chemically similar to a natural nerve transmitter known as GABA; baclofen's effect on muscle spasm may be related to its effect on GABA nerve receptors. Baclofen depresses the central nervous system. It is quickly absorbed into the bloodstream after it is swallowed, but the rate of absorption may decrease as dosage increases. Baclofen passes out of the body through the kidneys.

Cautions and Warnings

Do not take baclofen if you are **allergic** or sensitive to it. It should not be taken for muscle spasm resulting from **rheumatic disease, stroke, cerebral palsy,** or **Parkinson's disease** because its benefit in these situations has not been proven. The condition of people with **epilepsy** or **psychotic disorders** may worsen while taking baclofen.

About 4% of women with MS who take baclofen for less than 1 year develop **ovarian cysts** that usually disappear on their own. This is within the normal range—1% to 5%—for developing ovarian cysts.

Abruptly stopping baclofen may lead to **hallucinations** and **seizure**. Dosage should always be gradually reduced, except in cases of severe side effects.

Possible Side Effects

Baclofen may affect lab tests for liver function and may raise blood sugar levels.

▼ Most common: drowsiness, low blood pressure, weakness, dizziness, light-headedness, nausea and vomiting, headache, and sleeplessness.

▼ Less common: frequent urination, fatigue or lethargy, confusion, euphoria, excitement, depression, hallucinations, tingling in the hands or feet, muscle pain, ringing or buzzing in the ears, coordination difficulties, tremors, rigidity, weakness, loss of muscle tone, unusual eye movement and other muscle-control problems, double vision, pinpoint or wide-open pupils, breathing difficulties, heart palpitations, dry mouth, appetite loss, changes in sense of taste, abdominal pain, diarrhea, bedwetting, difficulty urinating, painful urination, impotence, blood in the urine, rash, itching, swelling of the ankle, excessive sweating, weight gain, and stuffy nose.

▼ Rare: Slurred speech, blurred vision, seizure, fainting, chest pain, and testing positive for blood in the stool.

Drug Interactions

• Avoid alcoholic beverages and other nervous system depressants while taking baclofen.

• Combining a monoamine oxidase inhibitor (MAOI) antidepressant with baclofen may cause drowsiness, nervous system depression, and low blood pressure.

• Combining a tricyclic antidepressant with baclofen may lead to severe muscle weakness.

• Baclofen may increase blood sugar. Diabetics may need to increase the dosage of their antidiabetic drugs to account for this effect.

• Combining blood-pressure-lowering drugs with baclofen may lead to dizziness or fainting due to severe lowering of blood pressure.

Food Interactions

None known.

Usual Dose

Adult and Child: 15 mg a day for 3 days, gradually increased until the desired effect is achieved, usually at 40–80 mg a day. People with kidney disease require lower doses.

Overdosage

Symptoms of baclofen overdose include vomiting, loss of muscle tone, twitching, convulsions, pinpoint or wide-open pupils, drowsiness, blurred or double vision, breathing difficulties, seizure, and coma. Overdose victims should be taken to a hospital emergency room for treatment. ALWAYS bring the prescription bottle or container with you.

Special Information

Baclofen is a nervous system depressant. Take care when driving or doing anything that requires concentration and physical coordination.

Call your doctor if you develop a frequent urge to urinate, painful urination, constipation, nausea, headache, sleeplessness, or persistent confusion.

Do not stop taking baclofen on your own. Abruptly stopping this drug may lead to hallucinations or seizure.

Your pharmacist may prepare a baclofen liquid by grinding the tablets and mixing the powder with sugar syrup. This mixture should be kept in the refrigerator and can be used for 1 month.

If you forget a dose of baclofen, take it immediately—if you remember within 1 hour of your scheduled time. If you do not remember until more than 1 hour later or you forget it completely, skip the dose you forgot and continue with your regular schedule. Do not take a double dose.

Special Populations

Pregnancy/Breast-feeding

Baclofen increases the chances of certain birth defects in lab animals. Pregnant women should only take baclofen after carefully weighing its possible benefits against its risks with their doctor.

Baclofen taken by mouth passes into breast milk. Nursing mothers who must take this drug should bottle-feed their babies or receive the drug by injection directly into the spinal cord, because baclofen administered by injection does not pass into breast milk.

Seniors

Seniors may be more sensitive to nervous system side effects including hallucinations, depression, drowsiness, and confusion. Report anything unusual to your doctor.

Bactroban

*see **Mupirocin**, page 739*

Generic Name

Becaplermin (beh-CAP-ler-min)

Brand Name

Regranex

Type of Drug

Human growth factor.

Prescribed for

Diabetic foot and leg ulcers.

General Information

Becaplermin is a type of human growth factor. Though originally obtained from human blood platelets, it is manufactured by using recombinant DNA technology. When applied to a wound, becaplermin stimulates tissue to heal faster than it would on its own. This is especially important to diabetics, for whom wounds may be a major problem and lead to amputation of a foot or leg. Since becaplermin works best when there is still an adequate supply of blood to the affected area, it may not work for people with diabetes that has already caused extensive tissue damage.

In studies, becaplermin compared favorably to placebo (sugar pill) and to good ulcer care alone. The best results are achieved when good ulcer care is applied to the wound along with the drug.

Cautions and Warnings

Do not use becaplermin if you are **sensitive or allergic** to it or any of its components including its paraben preservative. Do not apply this drug to **cancerous skin**.

This drug is intended only for wound application. **Do not swallow it**. The effect of becaplermin on exposed joints, tendons, and ligaments is not known.

Possible Side Effects

▼ Less common: rash.

Drug Interactions

• It is not known if becaplermin interacts with other drugs applied to the skin. Avoid combining topical drugs, if possible.

Usual Dose

Adult (age 16 and over): Measure the proper amount of becaplermin gel and apply it carefully once a day. Spread the gel evenly over the wound in a thickness of about $\frac{1}{16}$ of an inch. Cover the gel and wound with a moist gauze pad. The exact amount to be applied depends on the size of the ulcer, which should be re-checked every 1 or 2 weeks by your doctor. Each square inch of ulcer surface requires about $\frac{2}{3}$ of an inch of becaplermin gel.

Child (age 15 and under): not recommended.

Overdosage

Applying more becaplermin to a wound than is prescribed is not harmful. In case of accidental ingestion, call your local hospital emergency room or poison control center.

Special Information

Wash your hands before applying becaplermin to a wound. Do not allow the tip of the medication tube to touch any part of the ulcer or anything else. Squeeze the proper amount of becaplermin gel onto a clean surface such as wax paper. Use a cotton swab, tongue depressor, or other aid to apply the gel to your wound.

After the gel has been on the wound for 12 hours, gently rinse it with saline or plain water to remove any remaining gel and cover it with another moist gauze pad.

Store this medication in your refrigerator; do not let it freeze.

Applying more becaplermin to a wound than is prescribed will neither damage it nor help it to heal more quickly.

Special Populations

Pregnancy/Breast-feeding

It is not known if becaplermin affects the fetus. It should be used during pregnancy only when it is absolutely necessary.

It is not known if becaplermin passes into breast milk. Nursing mothers should be careful when using becaplermin or any medication.

Seniors
Seniors may take this drug without special precaution.

Generic Name

Benazepril (ben-AY-zuh-pril)

Brand Name
Lotensin

Type of Drug
Angiotensin-converting enzyme (ACE) inhibitor.

Prescribed for
High blood pressure.

General Information
Benazepril hydrochloride belongs to the class of drugs known as angiotensin-converting enzyme (ACE) inhibitors. ACE inhibitors prevent the conversion of a hormone called angiotensin I to another hormone called angiotensin II, a potent blood-vessel constrictor. Preventing this conversion relaxes blood vessels, thus reducing blood pressure and relieving symptoms of heart failure by making it easier for a failing heart to pump blood through the body. Benazepril also affects the production of other hormones and enzymes that participate in the regulation of blood-vessel dilation; this action probably increases the drug's effectiveness. Benazepril starts working in 1 hour and continues to work for about 24 hours.

Some people who start taking benazepril after they are already on a diuretic (agent that increases urination) experience a rapid drop in blood pressure after their first dose or when their dosage is increased. To prevent this from happening, your doctor may tell you to stop taking your diuretic 2 or 3 days before starting benazepril or to increase your salt intake during that time. The diuretic may then be restarted gradually.

Cautions and Warnings

Do not take benazepril if you have had an **allergic reaction** to it in the past.

Benazepril occasionally causes very **low blood pressure**.

Benazepril may affect **kidney function**. Your doctor should check your urine for protein content during the first few months of treatment. Dosage adjustment is necessary if you have reduced kidney function.

Benazepril can affect white-blood-cell counts, possibly increasing your susceptibility to **infection**. Your doctor should monitor your blood counts periodically.

Possible Side Effects

▼ Most common: dizziness, tiredness, headache, nausea, and chronic cough. The cough usually goes away a few days after you stop taking the medication.

▼ Rare: low blood pressure, chest pain, dizziness when rising from a sitting or lying position, fainting, heart palpitations, difficulty sleeping, tingling in the hands or feet, vomiting, constipation, abdominal pain, blood in the stool, itching, rash, flushing, anxiety, nervousness, reduced sex drive, impotence, muscle and joint aches, arthritis, asthma, bronchitis, breathing difficulties, weakness, increased sweating, urinary tract infection, and swelling of the arms, legs, lips, tongue, face, and throat.

Drug Interactions

• The blood-pressure-lowering effect of benazepril is additive with diuretics and beta blockers. Any other drug that causes a rapid drop in blood pressure should be used with caution if you are taking benazepril.

• Benazepril may increase blood-potassium levels, especially if taken with dyazide or other potassium-sparing diuretics.

• Benazepril may increase the effect of lithium; this combination should be used with caution.

• Antacids may reduce the amount of benazepril absorbed into the blood. Take these medications at least 2 hours apart.

• Capsaicin may trigger or aggravate the cough associated with benazepril therapy.

• Indomethacin may reduce the blood-pressure-lowering effects of benazepril.

• Phenothiazine tranquilizers and antivomiting drugs may increase the effects of benazepril.

• Combining allopurinol and benazepril increases the risk of side effects. Avoid this combination.

• Benazepril increases blood levels of digoxin, which may increase the chance of digoxin-related side effects.

Food Interactions

You may take benazepril with food if it upsets your stomach.

Usual Dose

10–40 mg 1–2 times a day. People with poor kidney function may need less medication to lower blood pressure.

Overdosage

The principal effect of benazepril overdose is a rapid drop in blood pressure, as evidenced by dizziness or fainting. Take the overdose victim to a hospital emergency room immediately. ALWAYS bring the prescription bottle or container with you.

Special Information

Benazepril can cause swelling of the face, lips, hands, and feet. This swelling can also affect the larynx (throat) and tongue and interfere with breathing. If this happens, go to a hospital at once. Call your doctor if you develop a sore throat, mouth sores, abnormal heartbeat, sudden difficulty breathing, chest pain, persistent rash, or loss of taste perception.

You may get dizzy if you rise to your feet too quickly from a sitting or lying position. Avoid strenuous exercise and/or very hot weather because heavy sweating or dehydration can cause a rapid drop in blood pressure.

While taking benazepril, avoid over-the-counter diet pills, decongestants, and other stimulants that can raise blood pressure.

If you take benazepril once a day and forget a dose, take it as soon as you remember. If it is within 8 hours of your next dose, skip the dose you forgot and continue with your regular schedule. If you take it twice a day and miss a dose, take it right away. If it is within 4 hours of your next dose, take one dose immediately and another in 5 or 6 hours, and then go back to your regular schedule. Never take a double dose.

Special Populations

Pregnancy/Breast-feeding

When taken during the last 6 months of pregnancy, ACE inhibitors have caused low blood pressure, kidney failure, slow formation of the skull, and death in fetuses. Women who are or might become pregnant should not take any ACE inhibitor drugs. Sexually active women of childbearing age who must take benazepril must use an effective contraceptive method to prevent pregnancy. If you become pregnant, stop taking the medication and call your doctor immediately.

Relatively small amounts of benazepril pass into breast milk, and the effect on a nursing infant is likely to be small. However, nursing mothers who must take this drug should consider bottle-feeding. Infants, especially newborns, are more susceptible than adults to the drug's effects.

Seniors

Seniors may be more sensitive to the effects of this drug because of age-related losses in kidney or liver function. Dosage must be individualized to your needs.

Generic Name

Benztropine (BENZ-troe-pene) Ⓖ

Brand Name

Cogentin

The information in this profile also applies to the following drugs:

Generic Ingredient: Biperiden
Akineton

Generic Ingredient: Ethopropazine
Parsidol

Generic Ingredient: Procyclidine
Kemadrin

Generic Ingredient: Trihexyphenidyl Ⓖ
Artane   Trihexy-2
Artane Sequels   Trihexy-5

Type of Drug

Anticholinergic.

Prescribed for

Parkinson's disease; also used to prevent and manage uncontrolled muscle spasms caused by phenothiazines and other drugs.

General Information

Benztropine mesylate has an action on the body similar to that of atropine sulfate, but its side effects are less frequent and less severe. Benztropine counteracts the effects of acetylcholine, one of the body's major transmitters of nerve impulses. Benztropine can reduce muscle spasms by about 20%. This property makes the drug useful in treating Parkinson's disease and other diseases associated with spasms of skeletal muscles. Benztropine also reduces other symptoms of Parkinson's disease, such as drooling.

Cautions and Warnings

Benztropine should be used with caution if you have **narrow-angle glaucoma, stomach ulcers, heart disease, obstructions in the gastrointestinal tract, prostatitis,** or **myasthenia gravis**.

Benztropine reduces the ability to perspire and can interfere with the body's heat-control mechanisms. When taken in hot weather—especially by seniors, chronically ill people, alcoholics, and people with nervous system disease—or by people who work in hot environments, this effect may lead to **heat exhaustion** or **heatstroke**. In severe instances, it can be fatal.

Possible Side Effects

▼ Most common: urinary difficulties including painful urination, constipation, blurred vision, and increased sensitivity to bright light.

▼ Less common: rash, disorientation, confusion, memory loss, hallucinations, psychosis, agitation, nervousness, delusions, delirium, paranoia, listlessness, depression, drowsiness, euphoria (feeling high), excitement, light-headedness, dizziness, headache, weakness, giddiness, heaviness or tingling in the hands or feet, rapid heartbeat,

---

Possible Side Effects *(continued)*

palpitations, mild reduction in heart rate, low blood
pressure, dizziness when rising quickly from a sitting or
lying position, dry mouth including extreme dryness,
swollen glands, nausea, vomiting, upset stomach, interference with normal bowel function, duodenal ulcer,
double vision, dilated pupils, glaucoma, muscle weakness or cramping, high temperature, flushing, decreased
sweating, heatstroke, and difficulty in achieving and
keeping an erection.

Drug Interactions

• Side effects may increase if benztropine is taken with
antihistamines, phenothiazines, antidepressants, or other anticholinergic drugs. Benztropine should be used with caution
by people taking barbiturates. Avoid alcoholic beverages.

• Benztropine may reduce the absorption and effect of
some drugs, including levodopa, haloperidol, and phenothiazines.

• Combining amantadine with benztropine may result in
excessive side effects.

Food Interactions

These drugs—except procyclidine—are best taken on an
empty stomach, although they may be taken with food if they
upset your stomach.

Usual Dose

Benztropine: 0.5–6 mg a day.

Biperiden: 2–8 mg a day.

Ethopropazine: 50–600 mg a day.

Procyclidine: 2.5–5 mg 3 times a day after meals.

Trihexiphenidyl: 1–2 mg to start, increased gradually to 6–10
mg daily. This drug may be taken in sustained-release form, a
convenient way to take a high daily dosage once maintenance levels have been reached.

Overdosage

Symptoms of benztropine overdose include clumsiness or

unsteadiness; severe drowsiness; severe dryness of the mouth, nose, or throat; hallucinations; mood changes; breathing difficulties; rapid heartbeat; and unusually warm and dry skin. Victims should be taken to a hospital emergency room at once. ALWAYS bring the prescription bottle or container with you.

Special Information

Dry mouth can be relieved by chewing gum or sucking hard candy. Be aware that dry mouth may lead to cavities and gum disease. It is important that you maintain good oral hygiene to prevent dental problems while taking benztropine.

A stool softener, like docusate, will usually relieve constipation. Sunglasses will reduce the irritation brought on by bright lights.

Benztropine may cause drowsiness and blurred vision. Take care while driving or performing other tasks that require concentration and reliable vision. Avoid alcohol and nervous system depressants.

Call your doctor if you develop confusion, rash, eye pain, or a pounding heartbeat.

Benztropine will make you less tolerant of hot weather because it makes you sweat less. Limit your exposure to heat to reduce the chance of developing heat exhaustion or heatstroke.

If you take benztropine several times a day and you forget a dose, take it as soon as you remember. If it is within 2 hours of your next dose, skip the dose you forgot and continue with your regular schedule. Do not take a double dose. If you take your benztropine twice a day and forget a dose, take it as soon as you remember. If it is within 4 hours of your next dose, take one dose immediately and take the next two doses 8 hours apart. Then continue with your regular schedule.

Special Populations

Pregnancy/Breast-feeding

Drugs of this type have not been proven to be a cause of birth defects or of other problems in pregnant women. However, women who are or may become pregnant while taking benztropine should discuss changing medication with their doctor because of the possibility of birth defects.

Benztropine may reduce the amount of breast milk produced by a nursing mother. Infants are also particularly sensitive to benztropine; nursing mothers who must take this drug should bottle-feed their babies.

Seniors

Seniors who take benztropine on a regular basis may be more sensitive to side effects, including a predisposition to developing glaucoma, confusion, disorientation, agitation, and hallucinations.

Generic Name

Bepridil (bep-RIH-dil)

Brand Name

Vascor

Type of Drug

Calcium channel blocker.

Prescribed for

Angina pectoris.

General Information

Bepridil hydrochloride is one of many calcium channel blockers available in the U.S. These drugs block the passage of calcium, an essential factor in muscle contraction, into the heart and smooth muscles. Such blockage of calcium interferes with the contraction of these muscles, which in turn dilates (widens) the veins and vessels that supply blood to them. This action has several beneficial effects. Because arteries are dilated, they are less likely to spasm. In addition, because blood vessels are dilated, both blood pressure and the amount of oxygen used by the heart muscles are reduced. Bepridil is therefore useful in treating not only high blood pressure but also angina pectoris (brief attacks of chest pain), a condition related to poor oxygen supply to the heart muscles. Other calcium channel blockers are prescribed for abnormal heart rhythm, heart failure, cardiomyopathy (loss of blood-pumping ability due to damaged heart muscle), and diseases that involve blood-vessel spasm, such as migraine headache and Raynaud's syndrome.

Bepridil affects the movement of calcium only into muscle cells; it has no effect on calcium in the blood.

Cautions and Warnings

Do not take this drug if you have had an **allergic reaction** to it.

Bepridil should be used with extreme caution if you have a history of problems related to **heart rhythm**. It has caused serious derangement of heart rhythm and has affected white-blood-cell counts; therefore, it is usually reserved only for people who do not respond to other treatments.

Low blood pressure may occur, especially in people also taking a beta blocker.

Use bepridil with caution if you have **heart failure**, since the drug can worsen the condition. Bepridil may cause **angina** when treatment is first started, when dosage is increased, or if the drug is rapidly withdrawn. This can be avoided by reducing dosage gradually.

Studies have shown that people taking calcium channel blockers—usually those taken several times a day, not those taken only once daily—have a greater chance of having a **heart attack** than do people taking beta blockers or other medications for the same purposes. Discuss this with your doctor to be sure you are receiving the best possible treatment.

Calcium channel blockers can affect **blood platelets**, leading to possible bruising, black-and-blue marks, and bleeding.

People with serious **liver disorders** should use this product with care because it is primarily eliminated from the body by breakdown in the liver. Drug dosage should be reduced.

People with **kidney problems** need to have their bepridil dosage adjusted because elements of the drug pass out of the body through the kidneys.

Possible Side Effects

Side effects produced by calcium channel blockers are generally mild and rarely cause people to stop taking them.

▼ Most common: diarrhea, nausea, and light-headedness.

▼ Less common: abnormal heart rhythms; very slow or very rapid heartbeat; breathing difficulties; coughing or wheezing, which may be signs of lung congestion or

Possible Side Effects *(continued)*

heart failure; constipation; headache; and unusual tiredness or weakness.

▼ Rare: low blood pressure, fainting, and swelling in
the ankles, feet, or legs. Other rare side effects can affect
a wide variety of body systems. Call your doctor if
anything unusual develops.

Drug Interactions

• Bepridil may interact with beta-blocking drugs to cause
heart failure, very low blood pressure, or an increased incidence of angina. However, in many cases these drugs have
been taken together with no problem.

• Bepridil may, in rare instances, increase the effects of
anticoagulant (blood-thinning) drugs.

• Some calcium channel blockers may increase the amount
of digoxin in the blood, but this interaction does not occur
with bepridil.

• Additional drug interactions occur with other members of
this class but have not been seen with bepridil.

Food Interactions

Taking bepridil with food has a minor effect on the absorption
of the drug. You may take it with food if it upsets your
stomach.

Usual Dose

200–400 mg a day in 2 doses. Do not stop taking this drug
abruptly: The dosage should be gradually reduced over a
period of time.

Overdosage

Overdose of bepridil can cause nausea, dizziness, weakness,
drowsiness, confusion, slurred speech, very low blood pressure, reduced heart efficiency, and unusual heart rhythms.
Victims of a bepridil overdose should be taken to a hospital
emergency room. ALWAYS bring the prescription bottle or
container with you.

Special Information

Call your doctor if you develop swelling in the arms or legs, breathing difficulties, abnormal heartbeat, increased heart pain, dizziness, constipation, nausea, light-headedness, or very low blood pressure.

If you forget to take a dose of bepridil, take it as soon as you remember. If it is almost time for your next dose, skip the dose you forgot and continue with your regular schedule. Do not take a double dose.

Special Populations

Pregnancy/Breast-feeding
Very high doses of bepridil have been found to affect the development of animal fetuses in laboratory studies. Bepridil has not caused human birth defects, but women who are or might be pregnant should take it only with their doctor's approval. When the drug is considered crucial by your doctor, its potential benefits must be carefully weighed against its risks.

Bepridil passes into breast milk, but has caused no problems among breast-fed infants. However, if you must take bepridil, you should consider the potential effect on your infant before nursing.

Seniors
No problems have been reported in seniors. However, older adults are likely to have age-related reduction in kidney or liver function. This factor should be taken into account by your doctor when determining the dosage of this medication. Follow your doctor's directions and report any side effects at once. Seniors require more frequent monitoring by their doctors after treatment has started.

Generic Name

Betaine (BEE-tane)

Brand Name

Cystadane

Type of Drug

Homocystine antagonist.

Prescribed for

Homocystinuria.

General Information

Homocystinuria is a group of 3 disorders of the metabolism characterized by too much homocystine in the blood and urine. People with this problem tend to have skeletal problems, problems with the lens of the eye, and blood-clotting problems that can cause heart pain or heart attack. Virtually all people treated with betaine experience a decrease of homocystine in their blood. When used together with other homocystinuria treatments, including folate and vitamins B_{12} and B_6, betaine's effect has been additive to those treatments. Betaine starts working in several days and has been used for several years without any reduction in its effect. Infants and young children have been treated successfully with betaine; in fact, most of the patients treated with betaine have been children. The effects of homocystinuria can be devastating in children and include developmental problems, lethargy, seizures, and eye problems.

Cautions and Warnings

None known.

Possible Side Effects

Side effects from betaine are uncommon but can include nausea, upset stomach, diarrhea, choking if the powder is inhaled, and bad odors. Reported psychological changes from betaine are questionable.

Drug Interactions

None known. Betaine has been used successfully together with folate and vitamins B_{12} and B_6.

Food Interactions

None known.

Usual Dose

Adult and Child: 3 g twice a day. Dosage for children under age 3 may be started at about 50 mg per lb. a day, and then increased in weekly 50-mg steps. Dosage should be increased in all patients until homocystine is either undetectable in the blood or present in small amounts; doses up to 20 g a day have been required. Carefully measure all doses with the scoop provided. Each level scoopful is equal to 1 g of betaine.

Overdosage

In one animal study, betaine was deadly at doses greater than 4.5 g per lb. of body weight, but humans have been safely and successfully treated at doses up to 20 g a day. Call your poison control center or a hospital emergency room for more information.

Special Information

Shake the bottle lightly before removing the cap to loosen the powder. Protect the powder from moisture.

Mix each dose with 4 to 6 oz. of water until it dissolves completely, then drink it at once. Do not use the product if the final solution is either not clear or colored, or if the powder does not completely dissolve.

If you forget a dose of betaine, take it as soon as you remember. If it is almost time for your next dose, skip the dose you forgot and continue with your regular schedule. Tell your doctor about any missed doses. He or she may want to check your homocystine levels if too many doses have been skipped.

Special Populations

Pregnancy/Breast-feeding
The effect of betaine on pregnant women and nursing mothers is not known. This drug should only be used during pregnancy if it is absolutely necessary.

Seniors
Seniors may use this medicine without special precaution.

Generic Name

Betaxolol (bay-TAX-uh-lol)

Brand Names

Betoptic   Kerlone
Betoptic S

Type of Drug

Beta-adrenergic blocking agent.

Prescribed for

High blood pressure and glaucoma.

General Information

Betaxolol hydrochloride is one of 15 beta-adrenergic blocking drugs, or beta blockers, which interfere with the action of a specific part of the nervous system. Beta receptors are found all over the body and affect many body functions. This accounts for the usefulness of beta blockers in a wide variety of conditions. The oldest of these drugs, propranolol, affects all types of beta-adrenergic receptors. Newer, more refined beta blockers affect only a portion of that system, making them more useful in treating cardiovascular disorders and less useful for other purposes. Other of the newer beta blockers act as mild stimulants or have particular characteristics that make them better for specific purposes or certain people.

Applied as eyedrops, betaxolol reduces ocular pressure (pressure inside the eye) by slowing the production of eye fluids and by slightly increasing the rate at which these fluids flow through and leave the eye. Beta blockers produce a greater drop in ocular pressure than either pilocarpine or epinephrine—other glaucoma drugs—and may be combined with these or other drugs to produce a more pronounced drop in pressure.

Unlike other beta-blocker eyedrops, betaxolol eyedrops do not strongly affect lung function or heart rate and are often prescribed for people who cannot use timolol or levobunolol.

Cautions and Warnings

You should be cautious about taking betaxolol if you have **asthma, severe heart failure,** a **very slow heart rate,** or **heart block** (disruption of the electrical impulses that control heart rate) because the drug may aggravate these conditions. Compared with other beta blockers, betaxolol has less of an effect on pulse and bronchial muscles—which affect asthma—and less of a rebound effect when discontinued; it also produces less tiredness, depression, and intolerance to exercise.

People with **angina** who take betaxolol for high blood

pressure risk aggravating their angina if they suddenly stop taking the drug. These people should have their betaxolol dosage reduced gradually over 1 to 2 weeks.

Liver or kidney problems may reduce your ability to eliminate betaxolol from your body.

Betaxolol reduces the amount of blood your heart pumps with each beat. This reduction in blood flow may aggravate the condition of people with **poor circulation** or **circulatory disease**.

If you are undergoing **major surgery**, your doctor may want you to stop taking betaxolol at least 2 days before to permit the heart to respond more acutely to stresses that can occur during the procedure. This practice is still controversial and may not be appropriate for all surgeries.

Betaxolol eyedrops should be avoided by people who cannot take oral beta-blocking drugs such as propranolol.

Possible Side Effects

Side effects are relatively uncommon and usually mild; normally they develop early in the course of treatment and are rarely a reason to stop taking betaxolol.

▼ Most common: impotence.

▼ Less common: unusual tiredness or weakness, slow heartbeat, heart failure (symptoms include swelling of the legs, ankles, or feet), dizziness, breathing difficulties, bronchospasm, depression, confusion, anxiety, nervousness, sleeplessness, disorientation, short-term memory loss, emotional instability, cold hands and feet, constipation, diarrhea, nausea, vomiting, upset stomach, increased sweating, urinary difficulties, cramps, blurred vision, skin rash, hair loss, stuffy nose, facial swelling, aggravation of lupus erythematosus (chronic condition affecting the body's connective tissue), itching, chest pain, back or joint pain, colitis, drug allergy (symptoms include fever and sore throat), and liver toxicity.

Drug Interactions

• Betaxolol may interact with surgical anesthetics to increase the risk of heart problems during surgery. Some anesthesiologists recommend having gradually stopped the drug by 2 days before surgery.

• Betaxolol may interfere with the normal signs of low blood sugar and with the action of oral antidiabetes drugs.

• Betaxolol increases the blood-pressure-lowering effects of other blood-pressure-reducing agents, including clonidine, guanabenz, and reserpine; and calcium channel blockers, such as nifedipine.

• Aspirin-containing drugs, indomethacin, sulfinpyrazone, and estrogen drugs may interfere with the blood-pressure-lowering effect of betaxolol.

• Cocaine may reduce the effectiveness of all beta blockers.

• Betaxolol may worsen the problem of cold hands and feet associated with taking ergot alkaloids, used to treat migraine headache. Gangrene is a possibility in people taking both an ergot and betaxolol.

• Betaxolol will counteract thyroid hormone replacements.

• Calcium channel blockers, flecainide, hydralazine, oral contraceptives, propafenone, haloperidol, phenothiazine tranquilizers—molindone and others—quinolone antibacterials, and quinidine may increase the amount of betaxolol in the bloodstream and lead to increased betaxolol effects.

• Betaxolol should not be taken within 2 weeks of taking a monoamine oxidase inhibitor (MAOI) antidepressant.

• Cimetidine increases the amount of betaxolol absorbed into the bloodstream from oral tablets.

• Betaxolol may lessen the effectiveness of some anti-asthma drugs, including theophylline and aminophylline, and especially ephedrine and isoproterenol.

• Combining betaxolol with phenytoin or digitalis drugs can result in excessive slowing of the heart, possibly causing heart block.

• If you stop smoking while taking betaxolol, your dose may have to be reduced because your liver will break down the drug more slowly afterward.

• If you use other glaucoma eye medications, separate your doses to avoid physically combining them.

• Small amounts of betaxolol eyedrops are absorbed into the bloodstream and may interact with other drugs in the same way as oral beta blockers, although this is unlikely.

Food Interactions

None known.

Usual Dose

Tablets: 5–20 mg once a day. People with kidney failure should take 5 mg to start.

Eyedrops: 1 drop in the affected eye twice a day.

Overdosage

Symptoms of overdose are changes in heartbeat—unusually slow, unusually fast, or irregular—severe dizziness or fainting, breathing difficulties, bluish-colored fingernails or palms, and seizures. The victim should be taken to a hospital emergency room. ALWAYS bring the prescription bottle or container with you.

Special Information

Betaxolol is meant to be taken continuously. When ending betaxolol treatments, dosage should be reduced gradually over a period of about 2 weeks. Do not stop taking this drug unless directed to do so by your doctor: Abrupt withdrawal may cause chest pain, breathing difficulties, increased sweating, and unusually fast or irregular heartbeat.

Call your doctor at once if you develop back or joint pain, breathing difficulties, cold hands or feet, depression, skin rash, or changes in heartbeat. Betaxolol may produce an undesirable lowering of blood pressure, leading to dizziness or fainting; call your doctor if this happens to you. Also call your doctor if you experience persistent or bothersome anxiety, diarrhea, constipation, impotence, headache, itching, nausea or vomiting, nightmares or vivid dreams, upset stomach, trouble sleeping, stuffy nose, frequent urination, unusual tiredness, or weakness.

Betaxolol may cause drowsiness, light-headedness, dizziness, or blurred vision. Be careful when driving or performing complex tasks.

It is best to take betaxolol at the same time each day. If you forget a dose, take it as soon as you remember. If you take betaxolol once a day and it is within 8 hours of your next dose, skip the dose you forgot and continue with your regular schedule. If you take betaxolol twice a day and it is within 4 hours of your next dose, skip the one you forgot and continue with your regular schedule. Never take a double dose.

To administer eyedrops, lie down or tilt your head backward and look at the ceiling. To prevent infection, keep the dropper from touching your fingers, eyelids, or any surface. Hold the dropper above your eye and drop the medication inside your lower lid while looking up and gently pulling your lower lid down. Release the lower lid, keeping your eye open. Do not blink for 30 seconds. Press gently on the bridge of your nose at the inside corner of your eye for 1 minute; this will help circulate the medication around your eye. Wait at least 5 minutes before using any other eyedrops.

If you forget a dose of betaxolol eyedrops, administer it as soon as you remember. If it is almost time for your next dose, skip the dose you forgot and continue with your regular schedule. Do not take a double dose.

Special Populations

Pregnancy/Breast-feeding

Infants born to women who took a beta blocker while pregnant had lower birth weights, low blood pressure, and reduced heart rates. Betaxolol should be avoided by pregnant women and women who might become pregnant while taking it. When the drug is considered crucial by your doctor, its potential benefits must be carefully weighed against its risks.

Beta blockers pass into breast milk in varying concentrations, although problems in nursing infants are rare. Still, nursing mothers taking betaxolol should bottle-feed their babies.

Seniors

Seniors may absorb and retain more betaxolol, and may require less of the drug to achieve results. Your doctor should adjust your dosage to meet your individual needs. Seniors taking betaxolol may be more likely to suffer from cold hands and feet, reduced body temperature, chest pain, general feelings of ill health, sudden breathing difficulties, increased sweating, or changes in heartbeat.

Biaxin

see *Clarithromycin*, page 207

Generic Name

Bicalutamide (BYE-kal-UTE-uh-mide)

Brand Name

Casodex

The information in this profile also applies to the following drugs:

Generic Ingredient: Nilutamide
Nilandron

Type of Drug

Antiandrogen.

Prescribed for

Prostate cancer.

General Information

Bicalutamide is prescribed together with another hormone product for prostate cancer. Bicalutamide competes with testosterone and other natural androgens (male hormones) by binding to the same places in body tissue where androgens normally bind. Prostate cancer is androgen sensitive and responds to treatments that counteract the effects of androgen or remove the sources of androgen.

Cautions and Warnings

Do not take bicalutamide if you are **allergic** to it or any ingredient in the product. Almost 40% of men taking this drug as single therapy for prostate cancer develop **breast pain and enlargement**. Bicalutamide may **reduce sperm count**.

Two of every 100 people taking the related drug nilutamide develop interstitial pneumonitis (symptoms include **cough, chest pain, fever,** and **breathing difficulties**). Report any symptoms to your doctor at once.

People taking nilutamide or flutamide may develop **liver inflammation**. Call your doctor if you experience any signs of liver damage (severe itching, dark-colored urine, flu, tiredness, appetite loss, yellowing of skin or whites of the eyes, abdominal pain, and stomach or intestinal problems).

Isolated cases of **aplastic anemia** (a potentially fatal blood disorder) have been reported in people taking nilutamide, but the relationship between drug and disease is not established.

Possible Side Effects

▼ Most common: bicalutamide—hot flashes. Nilutamide—pain, headache, weakness, back or abdominal pain,

Possible Side Effects *(continued)*

nausea, constipation, flushing, sleeplessness, breathing difficulties, difficulty seeing in the dark, loss of testicle function, and breast swelling and tenderness.

▼ Common: diarrhea, constipation, nausea, pain, back pain, weakness, and pelvic pain.

▼ Less common: vomiting, abdominal pains, chest pain, flu symptoms, high blood pressure, swelling in the ankles or lower legs, high blood sugar, weight loss, dizziness, tingling in the hands or feet, sleeplessness, sweating, rash, nighttime urination, blood in the urine, urinary or other infection, impotence, breast swelling or pain, painful urination, anemia, difficulty breathing, bone pain, and headache.

▼ Rare: fever, neck pain, chills, blood infection, heart pain, heart failure, upset stomach, rectal bleeding, blood in the stool, dry mouth, dehydration, gout, arthritis, muscle pain, leg cramps, anxiety, depression, reduced sex drive, confusion, muscle spasm, nervousness, tiredness, dry skin, itching, hair loss, and feeling the need to urinate.

Drug Interactions

• Bicalutamide increases the effect of oral anticoagulant (blood-thinning) drugs like warfarin. Dosage adjustment may be necessary.

Food Interactions

None known.

Usual Dose

Bicalutamide
　　Adult: 50 mg once a day, morning or night.

Nilutamide
　　Adult: 300 mg a day, reduced to 150 mg a day after 30 days.

Overdosage

All studies of bicalutamide used doses of 200 mg a day or less, and no toxic dose has been established. Symptoms of flutamide overdose include slow breathing, poor muscle coordination, reduced activity, teariness, appetite loss, vomiting, and tiredness.

In one case of massive nilutamide overdose, a 79-year-old man took 13,000 mg of the drug. There were no signs or symptoms of a toxic effect and drug treatment was resumed 30 days later.

Overdose victims should be taken to a hospital emergency room, where vomiting may be induced. ALWAYS bring the prescription bottle or container with you.

Special Information

Treatment with bicalutamide should always be started at the same time as a luteinizing hormone-releasing hormone agent such as leuprolide or goserelin. Do not stop taking either drug without your doctor's knowledge.

For maximum effect, nilutamide treatment should be started on the same day or day after surgical castration. Nilutamide can also be used together with leuprolide.

Up to half of people taking nilutamide can have problems adapting to darkness, ranging from a few seconds to a few minutes. This can be a problem especially when driving at night or through tunnels. Wearing tinted glasses will minimize this effect.

Bicalutamide should be taken at the same time each day for best results. If you forget a dose of bicalutamide, take it as soon as you remember. If it is almost time for your next dose, skip the dose you forgot and continue with your regular schedule. Call your doctor if you forget to take more than one dose.

Special Populations

Pregnancy/Breast-feeding

This drug is not intended for use by women. However, it is important to keep in mind that bicalutamide may harm the fetus if taken during pregnancy.

Seniors

Seniors may take this drug without special precautions.

Generic Name

Bisoprolol (bye-SOPE-roe-lol)

Brand Name

Zebeta

Combination Products

Generic Ingredients: Bisoprolol + Hydrochlorothiazide
Ziac

Type of Drug

Beta-adrenergic blocking agent.

Prescribed for

High blood pressure, angina pectoris, and abnormal heart rhythms. The bisoprolol-hydrochlorothiazide combination is used only for high blood pressure.

General Information

Bisoprolol fumarate is one of 15 beta-adrenergic blocking drugs, or beta blockers, which interfere with the action of a specific part of the nervous system. Beta receptors are found all over the body and affect many body functions. This accounts for the usefulness of beta blockers in a wide variety of conditions. The oldest of these drugs, propranolol, affects all types of beta-adrenergic receptors. Newer, more refined beta blockers affect only a portion of that system, making them more useful in treating cardiovascular disorders and less useful for other purposes. Other of the newer beta blockers act as mild stimulants to the heart or have particular characteristics that make them better for specific purposes or certain people.

Bisoprolol is available in a single-tablet combination with hydrochlorothiazide, a diuretic that also lowers blood pressure.

Cautions and Warnings

People with **angina** who take bisoprolol for high blood pressure risk aggravating their angina if they suddenly stop taking the drug. These people should have their dosage reduced gradually over 1 to 2 weeks.

Bisoprolol should be used with caution if you have **liver or kidney disease**, because your ability to eliminate the drug from your body may be impaired.

Bisoprolol reduces the amount of blood pumped by the heart with each beat. This reduction in blood flow may aggravate the condition of people with **poor circulation** or **circulatory disease**.

If you are undergoing **major surgery**, your doctor may want you to stop taking bisoprolol at least 2 days before surgery to permit the heart to respond more acutely to stresses that can occur during the procedure. This practice is still controversial and may not be appropriate for all surgeries.

Possible Side Effects

Side effects are relatively uncommon and usually mild; normally they develop early in the course of treatment and are rarely a reason to stop taking bisoprolol.

▼ Most common: impotence.

▼ Less common: unusual tiredness or weakness, slow heartbeat, heart failure (symptoms include swelling of the legs, ankles, or feet), dizziness, breathing difficulties, bronchospasm, depression, confusion, anxiety, nervousness, sleeplessness, disorientation, short-term memory loss, emotional instability, cold hands and feet, constipation, diarrhea, nausea, vomiting, upset stomach, increased sweating, urinary difficulties, cramps, blurred vision, skin rash, hair loss, stuffy nose, facial swelling, aggravation of lupus erythematosus (disease of the body's connective tissue), itching, chest pain, back or joint pain, colitis, drug allergy (symptoms include fever and sore throat), and liver toxicity.

Drug Interactions

• Bisoprolol may interact with surgical anesthetics to increase the risk of heart problems during surgery. Some anesthesiologists recommend having gradually stopped the drug by 2 days before surgery.

• Bisoprolol may interfere with the normal signs of low blood sugar and with the action of oral antidiabetes drugs.

• Bisoprolol increases the blood-pressure-lowering effects of other blood-pressure-reducing agents, including clonidine, guanabenz, and reserpine; and calcium channel blockers, such as nifedipine.

• Aspirin-containing drugs, indomethacin, sulfinpyrazone, and estrogen drugs may interfere with the blood-pressure-lowering effect of bisoprolol.

• Cocaine may reduce the effectiveness of all beta blockers.

• Bisoprolol may worsen the problem of cold hands and feet associated with taking ergot alkaloids, used to treat migraine headaches. Gangrene is a possibility in people taking both an ergot and bisoprolol.

• Bisopropol will counteract thyroid hormone replacements.

• Calcium channel blockers, flecainide, hydralazine, oral contraceptives, propafenone, haloperidol, phenothiazine tranquilizers—molindone and others—quinolone antibacterials, and quinidine may increase the amount of bisoprolol in the bloodstream and lead to increased bisoprolol effects.

• Bisoprolol should not be taken within 2 weeks of taking a monoamine oxidase inhibitor (MAOI) antidepressant.

• Cimetidine increases the amount of bisoprolol absorbed into the bloodstream from oral tablets.

• Bisoprolol may lessen the effectiveness of some anti-asthma drugs, including theophylline and aminophylline, and especially ephedrine and isoproterenol.

• Combining bisoprolol with phenytoin or digitalis drugs may result in excessive slowing of the heart, possibly causing heart block.

• If you stop smoking while taking bisoprolol, your dose may have to be reduced because your liver will break down the drug more slowly afterward.

Food Interactions

None known.

Usual Dose

Adult: starting dose—5 mg once daily. The daily dose may be gradually increased up to 20 mg. Maintenance dose—5–10 mg once daily. People with kidney or liver disease may need only 2.5 mg a day to start.

Senior: Seniors should be treated more cautiously; they may respond to lower doses.

Overdosage

Symptoms of overdose include changes in heartbeat—unusually slow, unusually fast, or irregular—severe dizziness or fainting, breathing difficulties, bluish-colored fingernails or palms, and seizures. The victim should be taken to a hospital emergency room. ALWAYS bring the prescription bottle or container with you.

Special Information

Bisoprolol is meant to be taken continuously. When ending bisoprolol treatment, dosage should be lowered gradually over a period of about 2 weeks. Do not stop taking this drug unless directed to do so by your doctor: Abrupt withdrawal may cause chest pain, breathing difficulties, increased sweating, and unusually fast or irregular heartbeat.

Call your doctor at once if you develop back or joint pain, breathing difficulties, cold hands or feet, depression, skin rash, or changes in heartbeat. Bisoprolol may produce an undesirable lowering of blood pressure, leading to dizziness or fainting; call your doctor if this happens to you. Also call your doctor if you experience persistent or bothersome anxiety, diarrhea, constipation, impotence, headache, itching, nausea or vomiting, nightmares or vivid dreams, upset stomach, trouble sleeping, stuffed nose, frequent urination, unusual tiredness, or weakness.

Bisoprolol may cause drowsiness, dizziness, blurred vision, or light-headedness. Be careful when driving or performing complex tasks.

It is best to take bisoprolol at the same time every day. If you forget a dose, take it as soon as you remember. If it is within 8 hours of your next dose, skip the dose you forgot and continue with your regular schedule. Do not take a double dose.

Special Populations

Pregnancy/Breast-feeding

Infants born to women who took a beta blocker while pregnant had lower birth weights, low blood pressure, and reduced heart rates. Bisoprolol should be avoided by pregnant women and women who might become pregnant while taking it. When the drug is considered crucial by your doctor, its potential benefits must be carefully weighed against its risks.

It is not known if bisoprolol passes into breast milk. Nursing mothers taking bisoprolol should bottle-feed their babies.

Seniors

Seniors may absorb and retain more bisoprolol and may require less of the drug to achieve results. Your doctor should adjust your dosage to meet your individual needs. Seniors taking bisoprolol may be more likely to suffer from cold hands and feet, reduced body temperature, chest pain, general feelings of ill health, sudden breathing difficulties, increased sweating, or changes in heartbeat.

Generic Name

Bitolterol (bye-TOL-ter-ol)

Brand Name

Tornalate

Type of Drug

Bronchodilator.

Prescribed for

Asthma and bronchospasm.

General Information

Bitolterol mesylate is currently available only as an inhalant, but may be taken in combination with other medication to control your asthma. The drug starts working 3 to 4 minutes after it is taken and continues to work for 5 to 8 hours. It can be used as necessary to treat asthma attacks or on a regular basis to prevent them. Each dose of bitolterol inhalant delivers 0.37 mg of medication.

Cautions and Warnings

Bitolterol should be used with caution by people with a history of **angina pectoris** (condition characterized by brief attacks of chest pain), **heart disease, high blood pressure, stroke, seizures, diabetes, prostate disease,** or **glaucoma.**

Using excessive amounts of bitolterol can lead to increased breathing difficulties, rather than relief. In the most extreme cases, people have had heart attacks after using excessive amounts of inhalant.

Possible Side Effects

Bitolterol's side effects are similar to those associated with other bronchodilator drugs.

Possible Side Effects *(continued)*

▼ Most common: tremors, cough, and dry or sore throat.

▼ Common: restlessness, weakness, anxiety, shakiness and nervousness, tension, sleeplessness, dizziness and fainting, headache, pallor, sweating, nausea, vomiting, and muscle cramps.

▼ Less common: light-headedness, angina, abnormal heart rhythm, heart palpitations, breathing difficulties, bronchospasm, and flushing.

▼ Rare: abnormalities in liver tests, white-blood-cell counts, and tests for urine protein. The importance of these reactions is not known.

Drug Interactions

• Bitolterol's effects may be enhanced by monoamine oxidase inhibitor (MAOI) antidepressants, thyroid drugs, other bronchodilators, and some antihistamines.

• Bitolterol is antagonized by beta-blocking drugs, such as propranolol.

• Bitolterol may antagonize the effects of blood-pressure-lowering drugs, especially reserpine, methyldopa, and guanethidine.

• The chances of cardiotoxicity may be increased in people taking both bitolterol and theophylline.

Food Interactions

None known.

Usual Dose

Adult and Child (age 12 and over): to treat an attack—2 inhalations at an interval of at least 1–3 minutes, followed by a third inhalation, if needed. To prevent an attack—2 inhalations every 8 hours.

Do not take more than 3 puffs in 6 hours or 2 every 4 hours.

Overdosage

Bitolterol overdose can result in exaggerated side effects, including heart pain and high blood pressure, although the pressure can drop to a low level after a short period of elevation. People who inhale too much bitolterol should see a doctor or go to a hospital emergency room, where they will probably be given a beta-blocking drug such as atenolol or metoprolol to counter the bronchodilator's effects.

Special Information

The drug should be inhaled during the second half of your inward breath. This will allow the medicine to reach more deeply into your lungs.

Be sure to follow your doctor's directions for the use of bitolterol. Using more than you need can lead to drug tolerance and actually worsen your symptoms. If your condition worsens rather than improves after taking bitolterol, stop taking it and call your doctor at once.

Call your doctor at once if you develop chest pains, rapid heartbeat, palpitations, muscle tremors, dizziness, headache, or facial flushing, or if you still have trouble breathing after using the medicine.

If a dose of bitolterol is forgotten, take it as soon as you remember. If it is almost time for your next dose, skip the dose you forgot and continue with your regular schedule. Do not take a double dose.

Special Populations

Pregnancy/Breast-feeding
Bitolterol should be used by a pregnant or breast-feeding woman only when it is absolutely necessary. The potential benefit of using this medication must be carefully weighed against its risks.

It is not known if bitolterol passes into breast milk. Nursing mothers who take this drug must look for side effects in their infants. They may want to consider bottle-feeding their infants.

Seniors
Seniors are more sensitive to the effects of this drug. Follow your doctor's directions and report any side effects at once.

Generic Name

Brimonidine (brim-ON-ih-dene)

Brand Name

Alphagan

Type of Drug

Alpha agonist.

Prescribed for

Glaucoma and ocular hypertension (high pressure inside the eye).

General Information

Brimonidine tartrate stimulates alpha-2 receptors in the eye and lowers pressure inside the eye. The maximum effect occurs 2 hours after the drops are administered in the eye. Brimonidine reduces the amount of aqueous humor (liquid) produced inside the eye and increases the rate at which fluid flows out of the eyeball. That portion of brimonidine that finds its way into the bloodstream is broken down by the liver.

Cautions and Warnings

Do not use this drug if you are **sensitive** or **allergic** to it.

People with **kidney or liver disease** should use this drug with caution. People with **cardiovascular disease** should exercise caution with this medication because it can affect blood pressure. It should be used with caution in people with **depression, cerebral or coronary insufficiency, Raynaud's disease,** and **dizziness or fainting when rising from a sitting or lying position.**

Some loss of effect from brimonidine may occur over time. Your doctor should check your eye pressure periodically to make sure the drug is still working.

Possible Side Effects

▼ Most common: dry mouth; redness, burning, and stinging of the eye; headache; blurred vision; sensation of something in the eye; drowsiness; and eye allergy and itching.

▼ Common: staining or erosion of the cornea, unusual sensitivity to bright light, eyelid redness or swelling, eye pain or ache, dry eye, respiratory symptoms, dizziness, eye irritation, upset stomach, weakness, abnormal vision, and muscle pain.

▼ Less common: crusty deposit on the eyelid, eye bleeding, abnormal taste sensation, sleeplessness, eye

---

Possible Side Effects *(continued)*

discharge, high blood pressure, anxiety, heart palpitations, dry nose, and fainting.

Drug Interactions

• Brimonidine may enhance the effects of alcohol, barbiturates, sedatives, anesthetics, beta-blocking drugs, blood-
pressure-lowering drugs, and cardiac glycosides.
• Tricyclic antidepressants can increase the breakdown of
brimonidine.

Usual Dose

Adult: 1 drop in the affected eye every 8 hours, 3 times a
day.

Overdosage

Overdose victims should be taken to a hospital emergency
room for treatment. ALWAYS bring the prescription bottle or
container with you.

Special Information

If you wear soft contact lenses, wait at least 15 minutes
between the time you put the drops in your eye and when you
put your lenses in.

To self-administer eyedrops, lie down or tilt your head
backward. Hold the dropper above your eye and drop the
medicine inside your lower lid while looking up. To prevent
possible infection, do not allow the dropper to touch your
fingers, eyelids, or any surface. Release the lower lid, keeping
your eye open. Do not blink for 30 seconds. Press gently on
the bridge of your nose at the inside corner of your eye for 1
minute. This will help circulate the medication around your
eye. Wait at least 5 minutes before using any other eyedrops.

Brimonidine may make you drowsy. Be careful while driving or doing anything else that requires concentration while
you are taking this drug.

It is important that brimonidine be used according to your
doctor's directions. If you forget a dose of brimonidine, take it
as soon as you remember. If it is almost time for your next
dose, skip the dose you forgot and continue with your regular
schedule. Do not take a double dose.

Special Populations

Pregnancy/Breast-feeding
A small amount of brimonidine can find its way into the
bloodstream and may pass into the blood of the developing
fetus. It is not known if this drug passes into breast milk.
Pregnant women and nursing mothers should use this medicine with care.

Seniors
Seniors may use brimonidine without special precaution.

Generic Name

Bromfenac (BROM-fen-ak)

Brand Name
Duract

Type of Drug
Nonsteroidal anti-inflammatory drug (NSAID).

Prescribed for
Pain relief.

General Information
Bromfenac sodium is one of 16 NSAIDs, which are used to
relieve pain and inflammation. We do not know exactly how
NSAIDs work, but part of their action may be due to their
ability to inhibit the body's production of a hormone called
prostaglandin as well as the action of other body chemicals,
including cyclooxygenase, lipoxygenase, leukotrienes, and
lysosomal enzymes. NSAIDs are generally absorbed into the
bloodstream quickly. Pain relief comes within 1 hour after
taking the first dose of bromfenac, but its anti-inflammatory
effect takes several days to 2 weeks to become apparent and
may take a month or more to reach maximum effect. Bromfenac is broken down in the liver and eliminated through the
kidneys.

Cautions and Warnings
People **allergic** to bromfenac or any other NSAID and those

with a history of **asthma** attacks brought on by an NSAID, iodides, or aspirin should not take bromfenac.

Bromfenac may cause **gastrointestinal (GI) bleeding, ulcers,** and **stomach perforation**. This may occur at any time, with or without warning, in people who take bromfenac regularly. People with a history of **active GI bleeding** should be cautious about taking any NSAID. People who develop bleeding or ulcers and continue NSAID treatment should be aware of the possibility of developing more serious side effects.

Bromfenac may affect platelets and **blood clotting** at high dosages, and should be avoided by people with clotting problems and by those taking warfarin.

People with **heart problems** who use bromfenac may experience swelling in their arms, legs, or feet.

Bromfenac may be toxic to the **kidney** or **liver**. Report any unusual side effects to your doctor, who might need to periodically test your kidney function.

Bromfenac may make you unusually sensitive to the effects of the sun.

Possible Side Effects

▼ Most common: diarrhea, nausea, vomiting, constipation, stomach gas, stomach upset or irritation, and appetite loss—especially during the first few days of treatment.

▼ Less common: stomach ulcers, GI bleeding, hepatitis, gallbladder attacks, painful urination, poor kidney function, kidney inflammation, blood and protein in the urine, dizziness, fainting, nervousness, depression, hallucinations, confusion, disorientation, tingling in the hands or feet, light-headedness, itching, increased sweating, dry nose and mouth, heart palpitations, chest pain, breathing difficulties, and muscle cramps.

▼ Rare: severe allergic reactions including closing of the throat, fever and chills, changes in liver function, jaundice (yellowing of the skin or whites of the eyes), and kidney failure. People who experience such effects must be promptly treated in a hospital emergency room or doctor's office.

NSAIDs have caused severe skin reactions; if this happens to you, see your doctor immediately.

Drug Interactions

• Bromfenac may increase the effects of oral anticoagulant (blood-thinning) drugs such as warfarin. If you take this combination, your doctor might have to reduce your anticoagulant dosage.

• Taking bromfenac with cyclosporine may increase the kidney-related effects of both drugs. Methotrexate side effects may be increased in people also taking bromfenac.

• Bromfenac may reduce the blood-pressure-lowering effect of beta blockers and loop diuretics.

• Bromfenac may increase phenytoin blood levels, leading to increased side effects. Lithium blood levels may be increased in people taking bromfenac.

• Bromfenac blood levels may be affected by cimetidine.

• Probenecid may interfere with the elimination of bromfenac from the body, increasing the chances for bromfenac side effects.

• Aspirin and other salicylates may decrease the amount of bromfenac in your blood. These drugs should never be combined with bromfenac.

Food Interactions

Take bromfenac with food or a magnesium/aluminum antacid if it upsets your stomach. However, taking bromfenac with high-fat food interferes with the drug's absorption into the blood and may make doses of 50 mg necessary.

Usual Dose

Adult: 25 mg every 6–8 hours, up to 150 mg a day.
Senior: Starting dosage—⅓–½ the adult dose.

Overdosage

People have died from NSAID overdoses. The most common symptoms of overdose are drowsiness, nausea, vomiting, diarrhea, abdominal pain, rapid breathing, rapid heartbeat, increased sweating, ringing or buzzing in the ears, confusion, disorientation, stupor, and coma. Take the victim to a hospital emergency room at once. ALWAYS bring the prescription bottle or container with you.

Special Information

Take each dose with a full glass of water and do not lie down for 15 to 30 minutes afterward.

Bromfenac may make you drowsy and/or tired: Be careful when driving or operating hazardous equipment. Do not take any over-the-counter products containing acetaminophen or aspirin while taking bromfenac. Avoid alcoholic beverages.

Contact your doctor if you develop rash or itching, visual disturbances, weight gain, breathing difficulties, fluid retention, hallucinations, black or tarry stools, persistent headache, or any unusual or intolerable side effect.

If you forget to take a dose, take it as soon as you remember. If you take several doses a day and it is within 4 hours of your next dose, skip the dose you forgot and continue with your regular schedule. Do not take a double dose.

Special Populations

Pregnancy/Breast-feeding

NSAIDs may cross into fetal blood circulation. They have not been found to cause birth defects, but animal studies indicate that they may affect the fetal heart during the second half of pregnancy. A pregnant woman should not take bromfenac without her doctor's approval, particularly during the last 3 months of pregnancy. When the drug is considered crucial by your doctor, its potential benefits must be carefully weighed against its risks.

NSAIDs may pass into breast milk but have caused no problems in breast-fed infants, except for seizures in a baby whose mother was taking the NSAID indomethacin. There is a possibility that a nursing mother taking bromfenac could affect her baby's heart or cardiovascular system. If you must take bromfenac, bottle-feed your baby.

Seniors

Seniors may be more susceptible to bromfenac side effects, especially ulcer disease.

Generic Name

Bupropion (bue-PROE-pee-on)

Brand Names

Wellbutrin	Zyban
Wellbutrin SR	

Type of Drug

Antidepressant and smoking deterrent.

Prescribed for

Depression and nicotine addiction.

General Information

Bupropion hydrochloride is normally used to treat severe or major depression only after other drugs have been tried without success. This is because of the higher-than-normal risk of developing seizures while taking bupropion. Bupropion is chemically different from other antidepressants; it is actually similar to diethylpropion, an appetite suppressant.

It is not known how bupropion works as a smoking deterrent, but it is thought that this feature has to do with the drug's effect on key hormone systems in the brain. Studies of bupropion in smoking cessation found that people taking 150 to 300 mg a day of the drug were able to stop smoking for 4 weeks of the 7-week study. The people in these studies were not depressed.

Bupropion is not likely to work until you have taken it for 3 to 4 weeks. The drug takes about 2 weeks to clear from your system after you have stopped taking it.

Cautions and Warnings

People with **seizure disorders**, people who have had a seizure in the past, and people with **bulimia** or **anorexia nervosa** should be very careful about taking bupropion because they are at a greater than normal risk of having a seizure. About 4 of every 1,000 people taking bupropion in dosages up to 450 mg a day will develop a seizure. This is approximately 4 times the seizure rate associated with other antidepressants. The chance of developing a seizure increases by about 10 times with dosages between 450 and 600 mg a day. About half of all people who developed a seizure on bupropion had a risk factor such as a history of head injury, a previous seizure, or a nervous system tumor, or were taking another drug associated with increased seizure risk.

People with **unstable heart disease** or a recent **heart attack** should take this drug with caution because of possible side effects. Many people taking bupropion experience some **restlessness, agitation, anxiety,** and **sleeplessness**, especially soon after they start taking the drug. Some even require

sleeping pills to counter this effect, and others find the
stimulation so severe that they have to stop taking bupropion.

People taking bupropion may experience **hallucinations,
delusions,** or **psychotic episodes**. Dosage reduction or drug
withdrawal is usually necessary to manage these reactions.
One-quarter of the people who take bupropion **lose their
appetite** and 5 or more lbs. of body weight. Most other
antidepressants cause weight gain, which may simply be
related to the improvement in mood brought on by the
antidepressant. People who have lost weight because of their
depression should be cautious about taking bupropion.

People switching from bupropion to a **monoamine oxidase
inhibitor (MAOI)** antidepressant, or vice versa, should allow
at least 2 weeks to pass between stopping one drug and
starting the other.

In animal studies, bupropion caused **liver damage and
tumors**, but these effects have not been seen in humans.
People with **kidney or liver disease** require less bupropion at
the beginning of treatment. Dosage should be increased
cautiously.

Treatment with an antidepressant other than bupropion
should be seriously considered for people with a history of
drug abuse because of the mild stimulation associated with
bupropion. These people may require larger-than-usual
dosages, but are still susceptible to seizures at these higher
dosages.

Severely depressed people are more likely to attempt
suicide; therefore, they should not be given a large number of
bupropion tablets at one time.

Possible Side Effects

▼ Most common: dry mouth, dizziness, rapid heartbeat, headache including migraine, excessive sweating,
nausea, vomiting, constipation, appetite loss, weight
changes, sedation, agitation, sleeplessness, and tremors.

▼ Less common: upset stomach, diarrhea, increased
appetite, menstrual complaints, impotence, urinary difficulties, slowness of movement, salivation, muscle spasms,
warmth, uncontrolled muscle movement, compulsion
to move around or change positions, abnormal heart
rhythms, blood-pressure changes, heart palpitations,

Possible Side Effects *(continued)*

fainting, itching, redness and rash, confusion, hostility, loss of concentration, reduced sex drive, anxiety, delusions, euphoria (feeling high), fatigue, joint pain, fever or chills, respiratory infection, and visual, taste, and hearing disturbances.

Many other side effects have been reported with bupropion, but their link to the drug is not well established. About 1 in 10 have to stop taking bupropion because of intolerable side effects.

Drug Interactions

• Carbamazepine may reduce blood concentrations of bupropion.

• People taking both bupropion and levodopa experience increased side effects. People taking levodopa should have their bupropion dosage increased more slowly and gradually than others.

• Combining bupropion with ritonavir may lead to significant increases in the amount of bupropion in the blood, increasing the risk of side effects.

• Phenelzine, an MAOI, increases the risk of bupropion side effects. Allow at least 2 weeks to pass between stopping an MAOI and starting bupropion.

• The combination of bupropion and other drugs that increase the risk of seizures—including tricyclic antidepressants, haloperidol, lithium, loxapine, molindone, phenothiazine tranquilizers, and thioxanthene tranquilizers—should be avoided.

Food Interactions

Bupropion may be taken with food if it upsets your stomach.

Usual Dose

Depression
    Adult: 200–450 mg a day divided into 3 or 4 daily doses; normal daily dosage is 300 mg.
    Child (under age 18): not recommended.

Smoking Cessation
    Adult: 150 mg twice a day; treatment should begin while you are still smoking.
    Child (under age 18): not recommended.

Overdosage

Symptoms of bupropion overdose are likely to include severe side effects such as seizures—present in fully ⅓ of all overdoses—hallucinations, loss of consciousness, and abnormal heart rhythms. Most people recover without a serious problem from bupropion overdose, although death has occurred in people taking massive overdoses of bupropion together with other drugs. Overdose victims should be taken to an emergency room at once. ALWAYS bring the prescription bottle or container with you.

Special Information

Do not stop taking bupropion without your doctor's supervision. Suddenly stopping the drug may precipitate withdrawal reactions and side effects.

Call your doctor if you experience agitation or excitement, restlessness, confusion, difficulty sleeping, fast or abnormal heart rhythm, severe headache, seizure, rash, fainting, or any unusually persistent or severe side effect.

To reduce the risk of a seizure, take bupropion in 3 or 4 equal doses each day. The total daily dosage should not exceed 450 mg; single doses should not exceed 150 mg.

Bupropion may make you tired, dizzy, or light-headed. Be careful when driving or performing tasks requiring concentration and coordination.

Alcohol, tranquilizers, and other nervous-system depressants will increase the depressant effects of this drug. Alcohol also increases the risk of a seizure.

If you forget a dose of bupropion, take it as soon as you remember. If it is almost time for your next dose, take 1 dose as soon as you remember and another in 3 or 4 hours, then go back to your regular schedule. Do not take a double dose.

Special Populations

Pregnancy/Breast-feeding

There is no information on the use of bupropion during pregnancy. Pregnant women should take bupropion only if it is absolutely necessary. Pregnant women trying to stop smoking should use non-drug methods until their pregnancy is completed.

Bupropion passes into breast milk. Nursing mothers who must use bupropion should bottle-feed their babies because of the severe side effects caused by this drug.

Seniors

No special problems have been reported in seniors. However, older adults are likely to have age-related reduction in kidney and/or liver function, which should be taken into account when determining dosage.

BuSpar

see **Buspirone**, page 139

Generic Name

Buspirone (bue-SPYE-rone)

Brand Name

BuSpar

Type of Drug

Minor tranquilizer and antianxiety drug.

Prescribed for

Anxiety; also prescribed for the aches, pains, fatigue, and cramps of premenstrual syndrome (PMS).

General Information

Although it is chemically distinct from the benzodiazepines, the most widely prescribed antianxiety drugs in the U.S., buspirone hydrochloride has a potent antianxiety effect. It is approved by the Food and Drug Administration (FDA) for short-term relief of anxiety, but it may apparently be used safely for longer periods of time—more than 4 weeks. The exact way in which buspirone works is not known, but it seems to lack the addiction dangers associated with other antianxiety drugs, including the benzodiazepines. It neither severely depresses the nervous system nor acts as an anti-convulsant or muscle relaxant, as other antianxiety drugs do. Minor improvement will be apparent after only 7 to 10 days of drug treatment, but the maximum effect does not occur until 3 to 4 weeks after starting treatment.

Cautions and Warnings

Do not take buspirone if you are **allergic** to it.

Buspirone should be used cautiously by people with **liver or kidney disease**.

Buspirone does not have any antipsychotic effect and should not be taken for symptoms of **psychosis**.

Although buspirone has not shown a potential for drug abuse, you should be aware of this possibility.

Possible Side Effects

▼ Most common: dizziness, nausea, headache, fatigue, nervousness, light-headedness, and excitement.

▼ Common: heart palpitations, muscle aches and pains, tremors, rash, sweating, and clamminess.

▼ Less common: sleeplessness, chest pain, rapid heartbeat, low blood pressure, fainting, stroke, heart attack, heart failure, dream disturbances, difficulty concentrating, euphoria (feeling high), anger or hostility, depression, depersonalization or disassociation, fearfulness, loss of interest, hallucinations, suicidal tendencies, claustrophobia, stupor, slurred speech, intolerance to noise, and intolerance to cold temperatures.

▼ Rare: ringing or buzzing in the ears, a "roaring" sensation in the head, sore throat, red and itchy eyes, changes in sense of taste, changes in sense of smell, inner ear problems, eye pain, sensitivity to bright light, dry mouth, stomach or intestinal upset or cramps, diarrhea, constipation, stomach gas, changes in appetite, excess salivation, urinary difficulties, menstrual irregularity, pelvic inflammatory disease, muscle cramps and spasms, numbness, tingling in the hands or feet, bedwetting, poor coordination, involuntary movements, slowed reaction time, rapid breathing, shortness of breath, chest congestion, changes in sex drive, itching, facial swelling or flushing, easy bruising, hair loss, dry skin, blisters, fever, feeling unwell, unusual bleeding or bruising, voice loss, very slow heartbeat, hypertention (high blood pressure), seizures and psychotic reactions, blurred vision, stuffy nose, pressure on the eyes, thyroid abnormalities, irritable colon, bleeding from the rectum, burning of the tongue, periodic menstrual spotting, pain-

---

Possible Side Effects *(continued)*

ful urination, muscle weakness, nosebleeds, delayed ejaculation and impotence in men, thinning of the nails, and
hiccups.

Drug Interactions

• Combining buspirone with a monoamine oxidase inhibitor (MAOI) antidepressant may produce severe hypertension
and may be dangerous.

• The effects of combining buspirone with other drugs that
work in the central nervous system (CNS) are not known. Do
not take other tranquilizers or antianxiety or psychoactive
drugs with buspirone unless prescribed by a doctor familiar
with your complete medical history.

• Combining buspirone and haloperidol results in high
blood levels of haloperidol, increasing the risk of side effects.

• Studies show that buspirone is not affected by alcohol,
but this combination should still be used with caution because buspirone causes drowsiness and dizziness.

• The combination of buspirone and trazodone may cause
liver inflammation.

Food Interactions

Food tends to double the amount of drug absorbed into the
bloodstream, although it decreases the rate at which the drug
is absorbed. This drug may be taken either with or without
food, but for the most consistent results, always take your
dose at the same time of day in the same way—that is, with
or without food.

Usual Dose

Starting dosage—15 mg a day in 3 divided doses. Dosage
may be increased gradually to 60 mg a day.

Overdosage

Symptoms of overdose are nausea, vomiting, dizziness,
drowsiness, pinpointed pupils, and upset stomach. To date,
no deaths have been caused by buspirone overdose. There is
no specific antidote—go to a hospital emergency room.
ALWAYS bring the prescription bottle or container with you.

Special Information

Buspirone may cause nervous-system depression, drowsiness, and dizziness. Be careful while driving or operating hazardous equipment. Avoid other CNS drugs and alcoholic beverages because they will enhance buspirone's effects.

Contact your doctor if you become restless, develop uncontrolled or repeated movements of the head, face, or neck, or have any intolerable side effects. About 1 out of 10 people who were included in drug studies had to stop taking buspirone because of side effects.

If you forget to take a dose of buspirone, take it as soon as you remember. If it is almost time for your next dose, skip the dose you forgot and go back to your regular schedule. Do not take a double dose.

Special Populations

Pregnancy/Breast-feeding

Make sure your doctor knows if you are or might be pregnant or if you will be breast-feeding while taking this drug.

Buspirone has not been found to cause birth defects. When the drug is considered crucial by your doctor, its potential benefits must be carefully weighed against its risks.

It is not known how much buspirone passes into breast milk. Consider the risk of side effects on a nursing infant.

Seniors

Several hundred seniors participated in drug evaluation studies without any unusual problems. However, the effect of this drug in seniors is not well known, and special problems may surface, particularly in those with kidney or liver disease.

Generic Name

Butenafine (bue-TEN-uh-fene)

Brand Name

Mentax

Type of Drug

Antifungal.

Prescribed for

Athlete's foot.

General Information

Butenafine hydrochloride works by blocking the natural synthesis of a chemical—ergosterol—essential to the fungal cell membrane (outer skin). Butenafine may actually kill the fungus if enough of it is present. Some butenafine is absorbed through the skin into the bloodstream, but the exact extent of absorption is not known.

Cautions and Warnings

Do not use butenafine if you are **sensitive or allergic** to it.

Possible Side Effects

▼ Common: rash, burning, stinging, worsening of the infection, swelling, irritation, and itching.

Drug Interactions

• When you apply butenafine to the skin, do not combine it with any other medication.

Usual Dose

Adult and Child (age 12 and over): Apply enough to cover the affected area and surrounding skin once a day for 4 weeks. Wash your hands after each application.

Child (under age 12): not recommended.

Overdosage

Call your local poison control center or hospital emergency room in case of accidental ingestion.

Special Information

This drug may irritate sensitive skin. Call your doctor if this happens, since another medication may be more appropriate for you. Also call your doctor if you experience any of these symptoms: redness, itching, burning, blistering, swelling, or oozing.

Athlete's foot is relatively common and may be caused by a number of different kinds of fungi. Do not use this drug without your doctor's knowledge.

Butenafine is to be applied only to your skin. It should not be applied to other areas, including the eyes, nose, mouth, or vagina.

If you apply the cream after bathing, be sure that your feet are completely dry, especially the areas between your toes.

As is often the case when using an anti-infective, your symptoms may begin to improve before you have completed the full course of treatment. Be sure to use all of the medication as directed. Also, follow your doctor's instructions about the kind of bandage or dressing to use.

Call your doctor if the condition does not improve after 4 weeks of using the cream.

Special Promotions

Pregnancy/Breast-feeding
There are no studies of butenafine use by pregnant women. It should only be used if absolutely necessary.

It is not known if this drug passes into breast milk after being applied to the skin.

Seniors
Seniors may use this medication without special precaution.

Generic Name

Butoconazole (BUE-toe-KON-uh-zole)

Brand Name

Femstat

Type of Drug

Antifungal.

Prescribed for

Fungal infection in the vagina.

General Information

Butoconazole nitrate is used as a vaginal cream. About 5% of each dose is absorbed into the bloodstream. Butoconazole may also be applied to the skin to treat common fungal infection; it is effective against this type of infection, but the exact mechanism of action is not known.

Cautions and Warnings

Do not use butoconazole if you know you are **allergic** to it.

Proper diagnosis is essential for effective treatment. Do not use this product without first consulting your doctor.

Possible Side Effects

▼ Most common: vaginal burning, itching, and irritation.

▼ Rare: vaginal discharge, swelling of the vulva, soreness, and itchy fingers.

Drug Interactions

None known.

Usual Dose

One applicator's worth of cream into the vagina at bedtime for 3–6 days. Pregnant women should use it for 6 days and only during the last 6 months of pregnancy.

Special Information

When using the vaginal cream, insert the contents of the applicator high into the vagina. Be sure to complete the full course of treatment as prescribed. Call your doctor if you develop burning or itching.

Refrain from sexual intercourse or use a condom while using this product to avoid reinfection. Using sanitary napkins during treatment may prevent butoconazole from staining your clothing.

If you forget to take a dose of butoconazole, take it as soon as you remember. If it is almost time for your next dose, skip the dose you forgot and continue with your regular schedule. Do not take a double dose.

Special Populations

Pregnancy/Breast-feeding

Pregnant women should avoid using this product because the use of a vaginal applicator may cause problems. If use is necessary, it must begin during the first 3 months of pregnancy. The effect of butoconazole on the fetus is not known.

It is not known if butoconazole passes into breast milk. Nursing mothers using this product should watch their infants for side effects.

Seniors

Seniors may take this medication without special restriction. Follow your doctor's directions and report any side effects at once.

Calan SR

see **Verapamil**, page 1153

Generic Name

Calcitonin (KAL-sih-TONE-in)

Brand Names

Calcimar   Miacalcin

Type of Drug

Peptide hormone.

Prescribed for

Osteoporosis (condition characterized by loss of bone mass due to depletion of minerals, especially calcium) in women who have gone through menopause; also prescribed for Paget's disease of bone.

General Information

Produced within the thyroid gland, calcitonin is a naturally occurring hormone that has a role in regulating calcium and bone production and maintenance. It also directly affects calcium in the body through its action on the kidneys and gastrointestinal tract. The calcitonin used in this drug comes from salmon, which is essentially identical to human calcitonin, except that it is much more potent. Calcitonin helps to strengthen bone by driving calcium into it and also slows the natural process of resorption by which bone is broken down. People with osteoporosis have low bone mass and a deteriorated bone structure, causing bone to be brittle and easily broken. People with osteoporosis also experience fractures of the vertebrae (bones that compose the spinal column) associated with back pain and a loss of height. Calcitonin helps reverse these situations. Calcitonin has been available for some years as an injection, but the development of a calcitonin nasal spray makes the drug easier to use and more accessible to the average person.

Cautions and Warnings

This drug should not be used if you are sensitive or **allergic** to salmon-calcitonin. Allergic reactions to calcitonin are possible because it is a naturally derived hormone. Although serious allergic reactions were reported with the injectable form of salmon-calcitonin, none have been experienced to date with the nasal spray.

Changes in the lining of your nose are possible with extended use of this product. Periodic nasal examinations are recommended.

Possible Side Effects

▼ Most common: stuffy nose, runny nose, and other nasal symptoms; and back pain.

▼ Less common: flu-like symptoms, red rash, muscle ache, joint problems, sinus irritation, upper respiratory infection, bronchial spasm, high blood pressure, angina pain, upset stomach, constipation, abdominal pain, nausea, diarrhea, cystitis, dizziness, tingling in the hands or feet, eye tearing, swollen lymph glands, and infections.

▼ Rare: depression; fatigue; swelling around the eyes; red eyes; fever; skin ulcers; eczema; baldness; itching; sweating; arthritis; stiffness; sore throat; bronchitis; pneumonia; coughing; breathing difficullties; changes in senses of taste and smell, including phantom smells; rapid heartbeat; heart palpitation; heart attack; vomiting; stomach gas; increased appetite; stomach irritation; dry mouth; hepatitis; thirst; gallstones; weight gain; goiter; overactive thyroid; blood in the urine; urinary infection; fainting; migraines; nerve pain; agitation; hearing loss; ringing or buzzing in the ears; earache; blurred vision; floaters (floating particles) in eye fluid; flushing; stroke; vein irritation; anemia; sleeplessness; anxiety; and appetite loss.

Food and Drug Interactions

None known.

Usual Dose

Adult: 1 spray (200 IU) a day.

Child: Information is lacking on the use of this drug in children.

Overdosage

No cases of overdose from calcitonin nasal spray have been reported and no adverse effects have been reported after high doses. Call your local poison control center for more information. Overdose victims should be taken to a hospital emergency room for treatment. ALWAYS bring the prescription bottle or container with you.

Special Information

Alternate nostrils daily when using calcitonin nasal spray.

Before you take your first dose, you must activate the pump. Hold the bottle upright and press the two white arms toward the bottle 6 times until a faint spray is emitted. Once you have seen the spray, the pump is activated and ready to be used. It is not necessary to reactivate the pump every day.

If you forget a dose of calcitonin nasal spray, take it as soon as you remember. If it is almost time for the next dose, skip the dose you forgot and continue with your regular schedule. Call your doctor if you forget to take your calcitonin for two or more days, or if you develop a severe nose irritation or any other unusual or intolerable symptom.

Special Populations

Pregnancy/Breast-feeding

Animal studies have associated injectable salmon-calcitonin with low birth weight, but calcitonin does not cross into the blood of the fetus. This drug is recommended for use during pregnancy only if its possible benefits outweigh its risks.

Animal studies have shown that calcitonin reduces the amount of milk produced, but it is not known if calcitonin passes into breast milk. Nursing mothers who must use calcitonin should discuss bottle-feeding their babies with their doctors.

Seniors

Studies of salmon-calcitonin have included people up to age 77. Seniors may use this product without special precaution.

Generic Name

Captopril (KAP-toe-pril) Ⓖ

Brand Name

Capoten

Combination Products

Generic Ingredients: Captopril + Hydrochlorothiazide
Capozide

Type of Drug

Angiotensin-converting enzyme (ACE) inhibitor; antihypertensive.

Prescribed for

High blood pressure and congestive heart failure; also used to treat diabetic kidney disease and high blood pressure associated with other medical conditions, such as scleroderma and Takayasu's disease. Captopril combined with the diuretic hydrochlorothiazide is used to treat high blood pressure.

General Information

Captopril belongs to the class of drugs known as angiotensin-converting enzyme inhibitors. ACE inhibitors work by preventing the conversion of a hormone called angiotensin I to another hormone called angiotensin II, a potent blood-vessel constrictor. Preventing this conversion relaxes blood vessels, helps to reduce blood pressure, and relieves the symptoms of heart failure by making it easier for a failing heart to pump blood through the body. Captopril also affects the production of other hormones and enzymes that participate in the regulation of blood-vessel dilation, which probably contributes to the drug's effectiveness. Captopril usually begins working about 1 hour after it is taken.

 People who are already taking a diuretic (agent that increases urination) may experience a rapid blood-pressure drop after their first dose of captopril or when their captropril dose is increased. To prevent this, your doctor may tell you to stop taking your diuretic or to increase your salt intake 2 or 3 days before starting captopril. The diuretic may then be restarted gradually. Heart-failure patients beginning captopril treatment generally have already been taking digoxin and a diuretic.

In addition to its labeled uses, captopril has been studied in the diagnosis of certain kidney diseases and of primary aldosteronism, and in the treatment of rheumatoid arthritis, swelling and fluid accumulation, Bartter's syndrome, Raynaud's disease, and post-heart-attack treatment when the function of the left ventricle is affected.

Cautions and Warnings

Do not take captopril if you are **allergic** to it. Although not common, captopril may cause very **low blood pressure**. It may also affect your kidneys, especially if you have **congestive heart failure**. Your doctor should check your urine for protein content during the first few months of captopril treatment. Captopril may cause a decline in kidney function. Dosage adjustment of captopril is necessary if you have **reduced kidney function** because the drug is generally eliminated from the body via the kidneys.

Captopril may affect **white-blood-cell counts**, possibly increasing your susceptibility to infection. Your doctor should monitor your blood counts periodically.

Possible Side Effects

▼ Most common: rash, itching, and cough that usually goes away a few days after you stop taking the drug.

▼ Less common: dizziness, tiredness, sleep disturbances, headache, tingling in hands or feet, chest pain, heart palpitations, feeling unwell, abdominal pain, nausea, vomiting, diarrhea, constipation, appetite loss, dry mouth, breathing difficulties, and hair loss.

▼ Rare: fever, angina (symptoms include chest tightness and pain), heart attack, stroke, low blood pressure, dizziness when rising from a sitting or lying position, abnormal heart rhythms, sleeping difficulties, hepatitis and jaundice, blood in the stool, unusual skin sensitivity to the sun, flushing, nervousness, reduced sex drive, muscle cramps or weakness, muscle ache, arthritis, bronchitis or other respiratory infections, sinus irritation, weakness, confusion, depression, increased sweating, kidney

---

Possible Side Effects *(continued)*

problems, urinary infection, blurred vision, and swelling of the arms, legs, lips, tongue, face, and throat.

Drug Interactions

• The blood-pressure-lowering effect of captopril is additive with diuretic drugs and beta blockers. Any other drug that causes a rapid blood-pressure drop should be used with caution if you are taking captopril.

• Captopril may increase blood-potassium levels, especially when taken with dyazide or other potassium-sparing diuretics.

• Captopril may increase the effects of lithium; this combination should be used with caution.

• Antacids may reduce the amount of captopril absorbed into the blood. Separate doses of these 2 medications by at least 2 hours.

• Capsaicin may trigger or aggravate the cough associated with captopril.

• Indomethacin may reduce the blood-pressure-lowering effect of captopril.

• Phenothiazine tranquilizers and antivomiting agents may increase the effects of captopril.

• Probenecid increases blood levels of captopril, thus increasing the drug's effect as well as the chance of side effects.

• The combination of allopurinol and captopril increases the chance of an adverse drug reaction.

• Captopril may increase blood levels of digoxin, which may increase the chance of digoxin-related side effects.

Food Interactions

Captopril is affected by food in the stomach and should be taken on an empty stomach, or at least 1 hour before or 2 hours after a meal.

Usual Dose

Adult: 75 mg a day to start. Dosage may be increased to 450 mg a day in divided doses, if needed. Dosage must be tailored to your needs. People with poor kidney function must take lower doses.

Child: approximately 0.15 mg per lb. of body weight, 3 times a day.

Overdosage

The principal effect of captopril overdose is a rapid drop in blood pressure, which may lead to dizziness or fainting. Take the overdose victim to a hospital emergency room immediately. ALWAYS bring the prescription bottle or container with you.

Special Information

Captopril may cause swelling of the face, lips, hands, and feet. This swelling may also affect the larynx (throat) and tongue, and interfere with breathing. If this happens, go to a hospital emergency room at once. Call your doctor if you develop a sore throat, mouth sores, abnormal heartbeat, chest pain, a persistent rash, or losses in the sense of taste.

You may get dizzy if you rise to your feet too quickly from a sitting or lying position. Avoid strenuous exercise and/or very hot weather because heavy sweating or dehydration may lead to a rapid drop in blood pressure.

Avoid over-the-counter stimulants that can raise blood pressure while taking captopril, including diet pills and decongestants.

If you forget to take a dose of captopril, take it as soon as you remember. If it is within 4 hours of your next dose, take 1 dose immediately and another in 5 or 6 hours, then go back to your regular schedule. Do not take a double dose.

Special Populations

Pregnancy/Breast-feeding
When taken during the last 6 months of pregnancy, ACE inhibitors have caused injury to the fetus and the newborn, including low blood pressure, kidney failure, slow skull formation, and death. Women who are or might be pregnant should not take any ACE inhibitors. Sexually active women taking captopril must use an effective contraceptive method to prevent pregnancy, or use an alternative drug. If you become pregnant, stop taking captopril and call your doctor immediately.

Relatively small amounts of captopril pass into breast milk, and the effect on a nursing infant has not been determined. Mothers who must take this drug should consider bottle-feeding with formula because infants, especially newborns, are more susceptible to this drug's side effects than adults.

Seniors

Seniors may be more sensitive to the effects of captopril because of normal age-related declines in kidney or liver function. Dosage must be tailored to individual needs.

Generic Name

Carbamazepine (car-bam-AH-zuh-pene)

Brand Names

Atretol	Tegretol
Depitol	Tegretol-XR
Epitrol	

Type of Drug

Anticonvulsant.

Prescribed for

Seizure disorders, trigeminal neuralgia, and other neuralgias; also used to treat some forms of severe pain; certain psychiatric disorders including depression, bipolar disorder in people who cannot tolerate lithium or antipsychotic drugs alone, intermittent explosive disorder, post-traumatic stress disorder, psychotic disorders, and schizophrenia; withdrawal from alcohol, cocaine, or benzodiazepine-type drugs including diazepam; restless leg syndrome; and non-hereditary chorea in children. Carbamazepine has been used with only limited success to treat diabetes insipidus.

General Information

Carbamazepine was first approved for the relief of the severe pain of trigeminal neuralgia. Over the years, though, it has gained greater acceptance for seizure control, especially in people whose seizures are not controlled by phenytoin, phenobarbital, or primidone, or who have suffered severe side effects from these drugs. Carbamazepine is not a simple pain reliever and should not be taken for everyday aches and pains. It carries potentially fatal side effects.

Carbamazepine is well absorbed into the bloodstream, but different dosages of tablet and liquid forms are needed to maintain carbamazepine blood levels. Liquid carbamazepine must be taken 3 times a day, regular carbamazepine tablets only twice a day, and long-acting tablets once daily. Do not change your dosage schedule without first checking with your doctor.

Cautions and Warnings

Carbamazepine should not be used if you have a history of **bone marrow depression** or if you are sensitive or **allergic** to this drug or to any tricyclic antidepressant. Monoamine oxidase inhibitor **(MAOI) antidepressants** should be discontinued 2 weeks before carbamazepine treatment is begun.

Carbamazepine may cause severe, possibly **life-threatening blood reactions**. Your doctor should have a complete blood count done before you start taking this drug and repeat these tests weekly during the first 3 months of treatment, and then every month for the next 2 to 3 years. Unexplained fever or infection may be a sign that a blood reaction is developing.

Carbamazepine may aggravate **glaucoma** and should be used with caution by people with this condition. This drug may activate underlying **psychosis, confusion**, or **agitation**, especially in older adults.

Possible Side Effects

▼ Most common: dizziness, drowsiness, unsteadiness, nausea, and vomiting. Other common side effects are blurred or double vision, confusion, hostility, headache, and severe water retention.

▼ Less common: mood and behavior changes, especially in children. Hives, itching, rash, and other allergic reactions may also occur.

▼ Rare: chest pain, fainting, breathing difficulties, continuous back-and-forth eye movements, slurred speech, depression, restlessness, nervousness, muscle rigidity, ringing or buzzing in the ears, trembling, uncontrolled body movement, hallucinations, darkening of the stool or urine, yellowing of the skin or whites of the eyes, mouth sores, unusual bleeding or bruising, unusual tiredness or weakness, changes in urination patterns—more frequent or suddenly decreased urine production, swelling of the feet or lower legs, numbness, tingling, pain or weakness in the hands or feet, pain, tenderness, a bluish discoloration of the legs or feet, and swollen glands.

Drug Interactions

• The level of carbamazepine in the blood may be increased by cimetidine, danazol, diltiazem, isoniazid, propoxyphene, erythromycin-type antibiotics except azithromycin, fluoxetine, fluvoxamine, mexiletine, nicotinamide, terfenadine, troleandomycin, or verapamil, leading to possible carbamazepine toxicity. Consult your doctor.

• Carbamazepine may decrease the effectiveness of oral contraceptives and cause breakthrough bleeding.

• Charcoal tablets or powder, phenobarbital and other barbiturates, phenytoin, and primidone may decrease the amount of carbamazepine absorbed into the bloodstream. In addition, studies show that phenobarbital, which is a breakdown product of primidone, may be increased by combining primidone with carbamazepine.

• Carbamazepine decreases the effect of acetaminophen, the anticoagulant (blood thinner) warfarin, and theophylline, prescribed for asthma. Dosages of these drugs may need to be increased to achieve the desired effects. Other drugs counteracted by carbamazepine are cyclosporine, dacarbazine, digitalis drugs, disopyramide, doxycycline, haloperidol, levothyroxine, and quinidine.

• When combining carbamazepine with other drugs to control seizure, including felbamate, hydantoins, succinimides, and valproic acid, outcome is difficult to predict because the action of these drugs can be affected in different ways. Combination treatments to control seizures must be customized to each patient.

• If carbamazepine is taken together with lithium, increased nervous system toxicity may occur.

Food Interactions

Take carbamazepine with food if it causes stomach upset.

Usual Dose

Adult and Child (age 13 and over): 400–1200 mg a day, depending on the condition being treated. Usual maintenance dose is 400–800 mg a day in 2 divided doses.

Child (age 6–12): 200–1000 mg a day, or 10–15 mg per lb. of body weight a day, divided into 3–4 equal doses.

Overdosage

Carbamazepine is a potentially lethal drug. The lowest single lethal dose known is 60 g. Adults have survived single doses of 30 g and children have survived single doses of 5 to 10 g. Overdose symptoms appear 1 to 3 hours after the drug is taken. The most prominent symptoms are irregularity or difficulty in breathing, rapid heartbeat, changes in blood pressure, shock, loss of consciousness or coma, convulsions, muscle twitching, restlessness, uncontrolled body movements, drooping eyelids, psychotic mood changes, nausea, vomiting, and reduced urination.

Successful treatment depends on prompt elimination of the drug from the body: Give the victim ipecac syrup—available at any pharmacy—to make him or her vomit. The victim must then be taken immediately to a hospital emergency room for treatment. ALWAYS bring the prescription bottle or container with you.

Special Information

Carbamazepine may cause dizziness and drowsiness. Take care while driving or operating hazardous equipment.

Call your doctor at once if you develop a yellow discoloration of the skin or whites of the eyes, unusual bleeding or bruising, abdominal pain, pale stools, dark urine, impotence, mood changes, nervous system symptoms, swelling, fever, chills, sore throat, or mouth sores. These may be signs of a potentially fatal reaction to the drug.

Do not stop taking carbamazepine abruptly without your doctor's advice. If you forget to take a dose, however, skip the dose you forgot and go back to your regular schedule. If you miss more than 1 dose in a day, call your doctor.

Special Populations

Pregnancy/Breast-feeding

Carbamazepine causes birth defects in animal studies. However, women taking this drug for a seizure problem should continue taking it because of the possibility that stopping the drug will cause a seizure, which could be just as dangerous to the fetus. If possible, anticonvulsant drugs should be stopped before pregnancy begins.

Carbamazepine passes into breast milk in concentrations of about 60% of the concentration in the mother's bloodstream and may affect a nursing infant. Nursing mothers who must take carbamazepine should bottle-feed their babies.

Seniors

Seniors are more likely to develop carbamazepine-induced heart problems, psychosis, confusion, or agitation.

Cardizem CD

see **Diltiazem**, page 324

Cardura

see **Doxazosin**, page 350

Generic Name

Carisoprodol (kar-ih-SOP-roe-dol) Ⓖ

Brand Name

Soma

Type of Drug

Skeletal muscle relaxant.

Prescribed for

Pain and discomfort associated with sprain, strain, and back problems.

General Information

Carisoprodol is one of several drugs prescribed as part of a coordinated program of rest, physical therapy, and other treatments. Carisoprodol does not have a direct effect on muscle spasm, the source of pain in these conditions. In animals, carisoprodol interferes with central nerves that cause the muscles to go into spasm, but this effect has not been confirmed in humans. This drug begins working within 30 minutes after it is taken and lasts for 4 to 6 hours.

Cautions and Warnings

Do not take carisoprodol if you are sensitive or **allergic** to it or to meprobamate, or if you have **acute intermittent porphyria** (hereditary condition characterized by metabolic imbalance of the liver). A few people experience unusual side effects within a few minutes or hours of taking their first dose of carisoprodol. They may include extreme weakness, temporary loss of use of the arms and legs, dizziness, muscle weakness, temporary loss of vision, double vision, dilated pupils, agitation, joint pain, euphoria (feeling high), confusion, and disorientation.

People can become **dependent** on this drug and may experience withdrawal (symptoms include abdominal cramps, sleeplessness, chills, headache, and nausea) after taking it for an extended period of time, especially if they are addicted to other substances or addiction-prone.

People with **kidney or liver disease** should use carisoprodol with care.

Possible Side Effects

▼ Common: drowsiness.

▼ Less common: rapid heartbeat; dizziness or lightheadedness; fainting; depression; large hive-like swellings on the face, eyelids, mouth, lips, or tongue; breathing difficulties; chest tightness and/or wheezing; allergic fever; stinging or burning eyes; headache; unusual stimulation; trembling; upset stomach or abdominal cramps; hiccups; and nausea or vomiting.

▼ Rare: visual changes including blurred or double vision, clumsiness or unsteadiness, aplastic anemia (symptoms include breathing difficulties, chest tightness and/or wheezing, sores or white spots on the lips or mouth, swollen or painful glands, unusual bleeding or bruising, and unusual tiredness or weakness), low counts of white blood cells and other blood components, severe rash with or without fever, chills, and muscle cramps or pain.

Drug Interactions

• Avoid alcoholic beverages, sleeping pills, tranquilizers, and other nervous system depressants while taking carisoprodol.

Food Interactions

You may take carisoprodol with food if it upsets your stomach.

Usual Dose

Adult: 350 mg 3–4 times a day and at bedtime.
Child (under age 12): not recommended.

Overdosage

Symptoms of carisoprodol overdose include slurred speech, stupor, coma, shock, and breathing difficulties. In rare cases, carisoprodol overdose is fatal. The effects of a carisoprodol overdose are amplified by alcohol and other nervous system depressants. Victims should be taken to a hospital emergency room for treatment at once. ALWAYS bring the prescription bottle or container with you.

Special Information

Carisoprodol may adversely affect your ability to concentrate and slow your physical reactions. Be careful when driving a car or doing anything else that requires concentration and alertness.

Avoid alcohol and other nervous system depressants while taking carisoprodol.

Call your doctor if you become dizzy or faint while taking carisoprodol, or if you develop a rapid or pounding heartbeat.

If you forget a dose of carisoprodol, take it immediately—if you remember within 1 hour of your scheduled time. If you do not remember until more than 1 hour later or you forget it completely, skip the dose you forgot and continue with your regular schedule. Do not take a double dose.

Special Populations

Pregnancy/Breast-feeding

There is no information on the safety of carisoprodol during pregnancy. Pregnant women should not use this drug unless they have thoroughly discussed its risks and benefits with their doctor.

Carisoprodol concentrations in breast milk are 2 to 4 times higher than blood concentrations. Nursing mothers should avoid this drug because it may affect their babies.

Seniors

Seniors with kidney or liver disease should be careful about taking carisoprodol; it may cause sleepiness or affect the ability to concentrate.

Generic Name

Carteolol (car-TEE-uh-lol)

Brand Names

Cartrol   Ocupress

Type of Drug

Beta-adrenergic blocking agent.

Prescribed for

High blood pressure, angina pectoris, and glaucoma.

General Information

Carteolol hydrochloride is one of 15 beta-adrenergic blocking drugs, or beta blockers, that interfere with the action of a specific part of the nervous system. Beta receptors are found all over the body and affect many body functions. This accounts for the usefulness of beta blockers against a wide variety of conditions. The oldest of these drugs, propranolol, affects all types of beta-adrenergic receptors. Newer, more refined beta blockers affect only a portion of that system, making them more useful in treating cardiovascular disorders and less useful for other purposes. Other of the newer beta blockers act as mild stimulants to the heart or have particular characteristics that make them better for specific purposes or certain people.

When applied as eyedrops, carteolol reduces ocular pressure (pressure inside the eye) by slowing the production of eye fluids and by slightly increasing the rate at which these fluids flow through and leave the eye. Carteolol produces a greater drop in ocular pressure than either pilocarpine or epinephrine—other glaucoma drugs—and may be combined with these or other drugs to produce a more pronounced drop in pressure.

Cautions and Warnings

You should be cautious about taking carteolol if you have **asthma, severe heart failure, a very slow heart rate,** or **heart block** (disruption of the electrical impulses that control heart rate) because the drug may aggravate these conditions. Compared with many other beta blockers, carteolol has less of an effect on your pulse and bronchial muscles—which affect asthma—and less of a rebound effect when discontinued; it also produces less tiredness, depression, and intolerance to exercise.

People with **angina** who take carteolol for high blood pressure risk aggravating their angina if they suddenly stop taking the drug. These people should have their drug dosage reduced gradually over 1 to 2 weeks.

Carteolol should be used with caution if you have **liver or kidney disease** because the ability to eliminate the drug from your body may be impaired.

Carteolol reduces the amount of blood pumped by the heart with each beat. This reduction in blood flow may aggravate the condition of people with **poor circulation** or **circulatory disease**.

If you are undergoing **major surgery**, your doctor may want you to stop taking carteolol at least 2 days before surgery to permit the heart to respond more acutely to stresses that can occur during the procedure. This practice is still controversial and may not hold true for all surgeries.

Carteolol eyedrops should be avoided by people who cannot take oral beta-blocking drugs such as propranolol.

Possible Side Effects

Side effects are relatively uncommon and usually mild; normally they develop early in the course of treatment and are rarely a reason to stop taking carteolol.

▼ Most common: impotence.

▼ Less common: unusual tiredness or weakness, slow heartbeat, heart failure (symptoms include swelling of the legs, ankles, or feet), dizziness, breathing difficulties, bronchospasm, depression, anxiety, nervousness, sleeplessness, disorientation, short-term memory loss, emotional instability, cold hands and feet, constipation, diarrhea, nausea, vomiting, upset stomach, increased sweating, urinary difficulties, cramps, blurred vision, skin rash, hair loss, stuffy nose, facial swelling, aggravation of lupus erythematosus (chronic condition affecting the body's connective tissue), itching, chest pain, back or joint pain, colitis, and drug allergy (symptoms include fever and sore throat).

Drug Interactions

• Carteolol may interact with surgical anesthetics to increase the risk of heart problems during surgery. Some anesthesiologists recommend having gradually stopped the drug by 2 days before surgery.

• Carteolol may interfere with the normal signs of low blood sugar and with the action of oral antidiabetes drugs.

• Carteolol increases the blood-pressure-lowering effects of other blood-pressure-reducing agents, including clonidine, guanabenz, and reserpine; and calcium channel blockers, such as nifedipine.

• Aspirin-containing drugs, indomethacin, sulfinpyrazone, and estrogen drugs may interfere with the blood-pressure-lowering effect of carteolol.

• Cocaine may reduce the effectiveness of all beta blockers.

• Carteolol may worsen the problem of cold hands and feet associated with ergot alkaloids, used to treat migraine headache. Gangrene is a possibility in people taking both an ergot and carteolol.

• Carteolol will counteract thyroid hormone replacements.

• Calcium channel blockers, flecainide, hydralazine, oral contraceptives, propafenone, haloperidol, phenothiazine tranquilizers—molindone and others—quinolone antibacterials, and quinidine may increase the amount of carteolol in the bloodstream and lead to increased carteolol effects.

• Carteolol should not be taken within 2 weeks of taking a monoamine oxidase inhibitor (MAOI) antidepressant.

• Cimetidine increases the amount of carteolol absorbed into the bloodstream from oral tablets.

• Carteolol may reduce the effect of some antiasthma drugs, including theophylline and aminophylline, and especially ephedrine and isoproterenol.

• Combining carteolol with phenytoin or digitalis drugs may result in excessive slowing of the heart, possibly causing heart block.

• If you stop smoking while taking carteolol, your dose may have to be reduced because your liver will break down the drug more slowly afterward.

• If you use other glaucoma eye medications, separate your dose to avoid physically combining them.

• Small amounts of carteolol eyedrops are absorbed into the bloodstream and may interact with other drugs in the same way as oral beta blockers, although it is unlikely.

Food Interactions

None known.

Usual Dose

Tablets: 2.5–10 mg once a day. Taking more than 10 mg a day is not likely to improve the drug's effect. People with poor kidney function may need to take their dose as infrequently as once every 72 hours.

Eyedrops: 1 drop in the affected eye 1–2 times a day.

Overdosage

Symptoms of overdose include: changes in heartbeat—unusually slow, unusually fast, or irregular—severe dizziness or fainting, breathing difficulties, bluish-colored fingernails or palms, and seizures. The victim should be taken to a hospital emergency room. ALWAYS bring the prescription bottle or container with you.

Special Information

Carteolol should be taken continuously. When ending carteolol treatment, dosage should be lowered gradually over a period of about 2 weeks. Do not stop taking this drug unless directed to do so by your doctor. Abrupt withdrawal may cause chest pain, breathing difficulties, increased sweating, and unusually fast or irregular heartbeat.

Call your doctor at once if you develop back or joint pain, breathing difficulties, cold hands or feet, depression, skin rash, or changes in heartbeat. This drug may produce an undesirable lowering of blood pressure, leading to dizziness or fainting; call your doctor if this happens to you. Call your doctor if you experience persistent or bothersome anxiety, diarrhea, constipation, impotence, headache, itching, nausea or vomiting, nightmares or vivid dreams, upset stomach, trouble sleeping, stuffy nose, frequent urination, unusual tiredness, or weakness.

Carteolol can cause drowsiness, light-headedness, dizziness, or blurred vision. Be careful when driving or performing complex tasks.

It is best to take carteolol at the same time each day. If you forget a dose of carteolol tablets, take it as soon as you remember. If you take you take carteolol once a day and it is within 8 hours of your next dose, skip the dose you forgot and continue with your regular schedule. If you take carteolol twice a day and it is within 4 hours of your next dose, skip the one you forgot and continue with your regular schedule. Never take a double dose.

To administer the eyedrops, lie down or tilt your head backward and look at the ceiling. To prevent possible infection, do not allow the dropper to touch your fingers, eyelids, or any surface. Hold the dropper above your eye and drop the medicine inside your lower lid while looking up and gently pulling your lower lid down. Release the lower lid, keeping your eye open. Do not blink for 30 seconds. Press gently on the bridge of your nose at the inside corner of your eye for 1 minute; this will help circulate the medication around your eye. Wait at least 5 minutes before using any other eyedrops.

If you forget a dose of carteolol eyedrops, administer it as soon as you remember. If it is almost time for your next dose, skip the one you forgot and continue with your regular schedule. Do not take a double dose.

Special Populations

Pregnancy/Breast-feeding
Infants born to women who took a beta blocker while pregnant had lower birth weights, low blood pressure, and reduced heart rates. Carteolol should be avoided by pregnant women and women who might become pregnant while taking it. When the drug is considered crucial by your doctor, its potential benefits must be carefully weighed against its risks.

It is not known if carteolol passes into breast milk. Nursing mothers taking carteolol should bottle-feed their babies.

Seniors
Seniors may absorb and retain more carteolol, and may require less of the drug to achieve results. Your doctor should adjust your dosage to meet your individual needs. Seniors taking carteolol may be more likely to suffer from cold hands and feet, reduced body temperature, chest pain, general feelings of ill health, sudden breathing difficulties, increased sweating, or changes in heartbeat.

Generic Name

Carvedilol (car-VAY-dil-al)

Brand Name

Coreg

Type of Drug

Alpha-beta-adrenergic blocker.

Prescribed for

Heart failure; also used to treat high blood pressure, congestive heart failure, angina pain, and cardiomyopathy.

General Information

Carvedilol is the first beta blocker to be approved by the FDA for the treatment of heart failure. Carvedilol blocks both the alpha- and beta-adrenergic portions of the central nervous system. This unique combination of actions produces the following effects on the body: It reduces the amount of blood pumped with each heartbeat and also decreases the responsiveness of the heart to various kinds of stimulation that normally cause tachycardia (very rapid heartbeat). Carvedilol's beta-blocking effects begin within an hour of taking the first dose; maximum blood pressure lowering occurs after 1 or 2 weeks. The drug also causes blood vessels to widen and makes it easier for the heart to pump blood more efficiently. People with heart failure have traditionally been warned against taking beta-blocking drugs, but a study reported in late 1995 suggests that carvedilol provides an important benefit for people with heart failure. Carvedilol was approved in 1997 to treat the disease, for which there is no cure other than a heart transplant. Other beta blockers may also be helpful in treating heart failure.

Because carvedilol blocks alpha-nervous-system receptors, it causes a greater drop in blood pressure when you are standing than when you are lying down. Consequently, carvedilol increases the risk of dizziness when rising quickly from a sitting or lying position more than do other drugs.

Cautions and Warnings

Carvedilol causes **liver injury** in about 1 of every 100 people who take it. Those who already have **severe liver disease** should not take this medication. Call your doctor at once if you develop signs of liver damage (symptoms include severe itching, dark-colored urine, flu, appetite loss, and yellowing of the skin or whites of the eyes). Check with your doctor about continuing carvedilol if you are having **general anesthesia**; heart function that is depressed by anesthetics can worsen if carvedilol is used at the same time.

Carvedilol can mask signs of **low blood sugar** and may increase the effects of insulin or oral antidiabetes drugs, making it more difficult to recover from the effects of low blood sugar.

Carvedilol can mask symptoms of an **overactive thyroid gland**. Abruptly stopping carvedilol can bring on an attack of hyperthyroidism.

Possible Side Effects

Most carvedilol side effects are considered mild or moderate.

▼ Most common: dizziness, sleepiness or sleeplessness, diarrhea, abdominal pain, slow heartbeat, dizziness when rising from a sitting or lying position, swelling of the hands or feet, sore throat, breathing difficulties, tiredness, back pain, urinary infection, viral infection, high blood-triglyceride levels, and low blood-platelet counts.

▼ Less common: extra heartbeats; palpitation; blood-pressure changes; fainting; reduced blood supply to the arms and legs (symptoms include aches, cramps, pain, or tiredness on walking, or in the foot, thigh, hip, or buttocks); tingling in the hands or feet; reduced feeling; depression; nervousness; constipation; stomach gas; liver irritation; cough; male impotence and reduced sex drive; itching; rash; visual difficulties; ringing or buzzing in the ears; high blood cholesterol, sugar, or uric acid; anemia; weakness; hot flushes; leg cramps; dry mouth; not feeling well; sweating; and muscle ache.

▼ Rare: angina pain, abnormal heart rhythms, heart failure, migraine, neuralgia, confusion, forgetfulness, slight paralysis, asthma, allergy, bronchial spasm, blood in the urine, frequent urination, hair loss, hearing loss, weight gain, sugar in the urine, loss of kidney function, and changes in potassium levels.

Drug Interactions

• Carvedilol increases the effects of insulin and oral antidiabetes drugs. People taking this combination must monitor their blood sugar levels regularly. Call your doctor if there is any change from your normal pattern.

• Carvedilol increases the effects of verapamil, diltiazem, and similar calcium-channel blocking drugs.

• Carvedilol increases the blood-pressure-lowering effect of clonidine. People taking this combination may need less clonidine to control their pressure.

• Carvedilol increases the amount of digoxin in the blood by about 15% when the drugs are taken together. Digoxin dosages may have to be adjusted when you are starting, taking, or stopping carvedilol.

• Cimetidine increases the amount of carvedilol absorbed into the blood by about 30%, but it may not affect you.

• Rifampin increases the breakdown of carvedilol and reduces the amount of carvedilol in the blood by about 70%. Dosage adjustment is necessary if you combine these medicines.

Food Interactions

Food slows the rate at which carvedilol is absorbed into the blood. Take carvedilol with food to reduce the risk of dizziness or fainting.

Usual Dose

Heart Failure
Adult: 3.125 mg 2 times a day for 2 weeks. Dose may be doubled every 2 weeks to the highest level tolerated. Maximum daily dose is 25 mg 2 times a day in people weighing less than 187 lbs., and 50 mg twice a day in people who weigh more.

High Blood Pressure and Cardiomyopathy
Adult: 6.25 mg twice a day to start, increased to 25 mg twice a day if needed.
Child: not recommended.

Overdosage

Carvedilol overdose may cause very low blood pressure

(symptoms include dizziness and fainting), slow heartbeat, and other heart problems including shock and heart attack. Breathing difficulties, bronchial spasm, vomiting, periods of unconsciousness, and seizures may also develop. Three cases of overdose are known—including a child age 2; all victims fully recovered. Overdose victims must be taken to a hospital emergency room for treatment. ALWAYS bring the prescription bottle or container with you.

Special Information

Carvedilol is meant to be taken continuously. Do not stop taking it unless directed to do so by your doctor; abrupt withdrawal may cause chest pain, breathing difficulties, increased sweating, and unusually fast or irregular heartbeat. The dose should be gradually reduced over a period of about 2 weeks.

People taking carvedilol may become dizzy and even faint on standing. If this happens to you, sit or lie down until you feel better. Carvedilol can also cause drowsiness, lightheadedness, or blurred vision. Be careful when driving or performing complex tasks.

Contact lens wearers are more likely to experience dry eyes if taking carvedilol.

It is best to take carvedilol at the same time each day. If you forget a dose, take it as soon as you remember. If it is within 4 hours of your next dose, skip the dose you forgot and continue with your regular schedule. Do not take a double dose.

Special Populations

Pregnancy/Breast-feeding

While animal studies indicate that carvedilol passes into the fetal bloodstream and may interfere with pregnancy, there is no information on humans available. This drug should be taken during pregnancy only if its possible benefits outweigh its risks.

It is not known if carvedilol passes into human breast milk, though it passes into rat breast milk. Beta-blocking drugs like carvedilol may affect babies' hearts. Nursing mothers who must take this drug should bottle-feed their babies.

Seniors

Seniors break down carvedilol less efficiently than do younger adults and may have 50% more in their blood than do younger people. Older adults may be more likely to develop drug side effects, especially dizziness.

Ceftin

see *Cephalosporin Antibiotics, page 169*

Cefzil

see *Cephalosporin Antibiotics, page 169*

Type of Drug

Cephalosporin Antibiotics

(CEF-uh-loe-SPOR-in)

Brand Names

Generic Ingredient: Cefaclor
Ceclor   Ceclor Pulvules
Ceclor CD

Generic Ingredient: Cefadroxil Ⓖ
Duricef

Generic Ingredient: Cefixime
Suprax

Generic Ingredient: Cefpodoxime Proxetil
Vantin

Generic Ingredient: Cefprozil
Cefzil

Generic Ingredient: Ceftibuten
Cedax

Generic Ingredient: Cefuroxime Axetil
Ceftin

Generic Ingredient: Cephalexin G
Keflex

Generic Ingredient: Cephalexin Hydrochloride
Keftab

Generic Ingredient: Cephradine G
Velosef

Generic Ingredient: Loracarbef
Lorabid

Prescribed for

Bacterial infections.

General Information

These antibiotics are all related to cephalosporin C, which was isolated from the *Cephalosporium acremonium* fungus discovered in the sea near Sardinia in 1948. Over the years, researchers have manipulated the cephalosporin C molecule, which is similar to penicillin, to produce more than 20 different antibiotic drugs. The cephalosporin antibiotics included in *The Pill Book* may be taken orally as a liquid, tablet, or capsule. Injectable cephalosporins are not included.

The most common infections can be treated with almost all of these antibiotics, but they are not interchangeable. Your doctor will take their differences into account when selecting the most appropriate antibiotic for a particular infection.

Cautions and Warnings

Approximately 5% of people with an **allergy to penicillin** may also be allergic to cephalosporin. Be sure your doctor knows about any penicillin allergy. The most common allergic reaction to a cephalosporin is a hivelike condition with redness over large areas of the body. Other sensitivity reactions to the cephalosporins may include skin rash, fever, and joint aches or pain. Such reactions generally begin after a few days of taking the antibiotic and resolve within a few days after the antibiotic is stopped.

Prolonged or repeated use of a cephalosporin antibiotic may lead to the overgrowth of a fungus or bacteria that is not susceptible to the antibiotic, causing a **secondary infection**.

Occasionally, people taking a cephalosporin may develop drug-related **colitis**. Call your doctor if you develop diarrhea while taking one of these medicines.

People with **kidney disease** who receive high doses of a cephalosporin antibiotic may have a seizure, though this is rare. Call your doctor at once if this happens.

The dosage of some cephalosporins must be adjusted for people with **poor kidney function**.

Possible Side Effects

Most cephalosporin side effects are quite mild.

▼ Most common: abdominal pain and gas, upset stomach, nausea, vomiting, diarrhea, itching, and rash.

▼ Less common: headache, dizziness, tiredness, tingling in the hands or feet, seizure, confusion, drug allergy, fever, joint pain, chest tightness, redness, muscle aches and swelling, appetite loss, and changes in taste perception. Colitis may develop because of changes in the bacteria normally found in the gastrointestinal tract.

Cefaclor may cause serum sickness (symptoms include fever, joint pain, and rash).

Cephalosporins may cause changes in some blood cells, but this problem is not generally seen with the oral forms. Some cephalosporins have caused kidney problems, liver inflammation, and jaundice, but these are also rarely a problem with oral cephalosporins.

Drug Interactions

- The cephalosporins should not be taken with erythromycin or tetracycline because of possible conflicting antibacterial action.
- Some cephalosporin antibiotics may increase the blood-thinning effects of anticoagulant drugs.
- Probenecid may increase blood levels of the cephalosporins.
- Cephalosporins may cause a false-positive test result for sugar in the urine with Clinitest tablets or similar products. Enzyme-based tests like Tes-Tape and Clinistix are not affected.
- Cefuroxime may cause a false-positive test result for blood sugar.

Food Interactions

Generally, the cephalosporins may be taken with food or milk if they upset your stomach.

Food interferes with the absorption of cephalexin, ceftibuten, and cefaclor into the blood. These drugs should be taken on an empty stomach, 1 hour before or 2 hours after meals.

Cefpodoxime and cefuroxime should be taken with food to increase the amount of drug absorbed into the blood.

Cefadroxil, cefixime, cefprozil, cephradine, and loracarbef may be taken without regard to food or meals.

Usual Dose

Cefaclor
    Adult: 250 mg every 8 hours, or 375–500 mg every 12 hours.
    Child: 9 mg per lb. of body weight a day, to 2–3 equal doses.

Cefadroxil
    Adult: 1–2 g a day, in 1–2 doses.
    Child: 13 mg per lb. of body weight a day, in 1–2 doses.

Cefixime
    Adult: 400 mg a day, in 1–2 doses.
    Child: 3½ mg per lb. of body weight a day, in 1–2 doses.

Cefpodoxime Proxetil
    Adult and Child (age 13 and over): 200–400 mg a day, in 1–2 doses.
    Child (age 5 months–12 years): 2½–5 mg per lb. of body weight a day. Maximum daily dose for middle ear infections is 400 mg; 200 mg for sore throat or tonsillitis.

Cefprozil
    Adult: 250–1000 mg a day.
    Child (age 6 months–12 years): 13 mg per lb. of body weight every 12 hours.

Ceftibuten
    Adult and Child (age 12 and over): 400 mg once a day for 10 days.
    Child: 4 mg per lb. of body weight, up to 400 mg, once a day for 10 days.

Cefuroxime
    Adult and Child (age 12 and over): 125–500 mg every 12 hours.
    Child (under age 12): 125–250 mg every 12 hours.

Cephalexin
    Adult: 250–1000 mg every 6 hours. Some urinary infections may be treated with 500 mg every 12 hours.
    Child: 11–23 mg per lb. of body weight a day. The dose may be increased to 46 mg per lb. of body weight for middle-ear infections.

Cephradine
    Adult: 250–500 mg every 6–12 hours.
    Child (9 months and over): 11–45 mg per lb. of body weight a day, in 2–4 doses.

Loracarbef
    Adult and Child (age 13 and over): 200–400 mg every 12 hours.
    Child (age 6 months–12 years): 6.5–13 mg per lb. of body weight a day.

Overdosage

The most common symptoms of cephalosporin overdose are nausea, vomiting, and upset stomach. These can often be treated with milk or antacid. Cephalosporin overdoses are generally not serious; contact a hospital emergency room or local poison control center for more information.

Special Information

Like all antibiotics, cephalosporins will make you feel better in 2 or 3 days. However, to obtain the maximum benefit from any antibiotic, you must take the full course of treatment prescribed by your doctor.

    Proper diagnosis is key to the effectiveness of any antibiotic medicine: Do not take any antibiotic without first consulting your doctor.

    If you miss a dose of a cephalosporin that you take once a day and it is almost time for your next dose, take the dose you forgot right away and your next one 10 to 12 hours later. Then go back to your regular schedule.

    If you take the medication 2 times a day, take the dose you forgot right away and the next dose 5 to 6 hours later. Then go back to your regular schedule.

    If you take the medication 3 or more times a day, take the dose you missed right away and your next dose 2 to 4 hours later. Then go back to your regular schedule.

    Most cephalosporin liquids must be kept in the refrigerator

to maintain their strength. Only cefixime liquid does not require refrigeration. All of the liquid cephalosporins have a very limited shelf life. Do not keep any of these liquids beyond the 10 days to 2 weeks specified on the label. Follow your pharmacist's product storage instructions, and consult your pharmacist if you are unsure about the drug's shelf life.

Special Populations

Pregnancy/Breast-feeding

These drugs are considered to be relatively safe during pregnancy, though there is little information available about the newer members of the group. Cephalosporin antibiotics should be taken only if the potential benefit outweighs any harm they could cause.

Small amounts of most cephalosporin antibiotics pass into breast milk. Nursing mothers who must take a cephalosporin antibiotic should bottle-feed their babies to avoid possible problems; these drugs may cause infant diarrhea and may interfere with the identification of an offending bacteria if the baby gets sick.

Seniors

Seniors with reduced kidney function should be regularly monitored for possible antibiotic side effects. Otherwise, seniors may take oral cephalosporin antibiotics without special restriction. Be sure to report any unusual side effects to your doctor.

Generic Name

Cerivastatin (suh-RIH-vuh-stat-in)

Brand Name

Baycol

Type of Drug

Cholesterol-lowering agent (HMG-CoA reductase inhibitor).

Prescribed for

High blood-cholesterol and LDL-cholesterol levels, in conjunction with a low-cholesterol diet program. It is also prescribed to slow the progression of atherosclerosis (hardening of the arteries), reduce the risk of death in people with heart disease, and treat inherited blood-lipid problems or lipid problems associated with diabetes or kidney disease.

General Information

Cerivastatin sodium is one of several cholesterol-lowering drugs that work by inhibiting an enzyme called HMG-CoA reductase. They interfere with the natural process for manufacturing cholesterol in your body, altering that process in order to produce a harmless by-product. Studies have closely related high blood-fat levels—total cholesterol, LDL cholesterol, and triglycerides—to heart and blood-vessel disease. Drugs that reduce levels of these blood fats and increase HDL cholesterol—"good" cholesterol—have been assumed for several years to reduce the risk of death and heart attack. Recently, medication in this class has been proven to slow the formation of blood-vessel plaque—associated with atherosclerosis—and reduce the risk of heart attack and death related to heart disease.

Cerivastatin reduces cholesterol and LDL-cholesterol counts while increasing HDL cholesterol. A very small amount of the drug actually reaches the body's circulation. Most is broken down and eliminated by the liver; 10% to 20% of the drug is released from the body through the kidneys. A significant blood-fat-lowering response is seen after 1 to 2 weeks of treatment. Blood-fat levels are lowest within 4 to 6 weeks after taking cerivastatin and remain at or close to that level as long as you continue to take the drug. The effect is known to persist for 4 to 6 weeks after you stop taking it.

Cerivastatin generally does not benefit anyone under age 30, so it is not usually recommended for children. It may, under special circumstances, be prescribed for teenagers in the same dose as adults.

Cautions and Warnings

Do not take cerivastatin if you are **allergic** to it or to any other HMG-CoA reductase inhibitor.

People with a history of **liver disease** and **those who drink large amounts of alcohol** should avoid drugs in this group because they may aggravate or cause liver disease. Your doctor should take a blood sample to test your liver function every month or so during the first year of treatment.

Cerivastatin causes **muscle aches and/or muscle weakness**

in a small number of people, which may be a sign of a more serious condition.

People with moderate or severe **kidney failure** should receive a lower daily dose of cerivastatin.

Possible Side Effects

Most people who take cerivastatin tolerate it quite well.

▼ Most common: headache.

▼ Common: nausea, vomiting, diarrhea, stomach cramps or pain, stomach gas, itching, and rash.

▼ Less common: constipation; heartburn; upset stomach; muscle aches, cramps, or pain; dizziness; eye irritation; and blurred vision.

▼ Rare: taste changes; dry mouth; acid regurgitation; leg, shoulder, or local pain; joint pain; sleeplessness; tingling in the hands or feet; chest pain; and hair loss. Other effects can occur in virtually any part of the body. Report anything unusual to your doctor.

Drug Interactions

• The cholesterol-lowering effects of cerivastatin and colestipol or cholestyramine are additive. Take cerivastatin 1 hour before or 4 hours after either of these drugs.

• Cerivastatin may increase the effects of warfarin or digoxin. If you take either of these drugs with cerivastatin you should be periodically checked by your doctor.

• The combination of cyclosporine, erythromycin, gemfibrozil, or niacin with cerivastatin can cause severe muscle aches or degeneration or other muscle problems. These combinations should be avoided.

• Propranolol can interfere with the action of cerivastatin, reducing its effectiveness.

• The effect of cerivastatin can be reduced by combining it with isradipine or propranolol.

• Itraconazole can increase HMG-CoA reductase inhibitor levels by 20 times. Avoid this combination by temporarily stopping cerivastatin if you take itraconazole.

Food Interactions

Take cerivastatin with food to maximize the amount of drug absorbed. Continue your low-cholesterol diet while taking it.

Usual Dose

Adult: 0.3 mg a day, usually at bedtime. People with kidney failure—0.2 mg at bedtime.

Overdosage

Anyone suspected of having taken an overdose of cerivastatin should be taken to a hospital emergency room for evaluation and treatment. The effects of cerivastatin overdose are not well understood since only a few cases have actually occurred and all victims recovered.

Special Information

Call your doctor if you develop blurred vision or muscle aches, pain, tenderness, or weakness, especially if you are also feverish or feel sick.

Cerivastatin is always prescribed in combination with a low-fat diet. Be sure to follow your doctor's dietary instructions, because both diet and medication are necessary to treat your condition.

Cerivastatin may cause unusual sensitivity to the sun. Use sunscreen and wear protective clothing while in the sun until you determine if you are affected.

Do not take more cholesterol-lowering medication than your doctor has prescribed or stop taking the medication without your doctor's knowledge.

If you forget to take a dose of cerivastatin, take it as soon as you remember. If it is almost time for your next dose, skip the one you forgot and continue with your regular schedule. Do not take a double dose.

Special Populations

Pregnancy/Breast-feeding

Pregnant women and those who might become pregnant must not take cerivastatin. Cholesterol is essential to the health and development of a fetus—anything that interferes with that process will damage the developing brain and nervous system.

Hardening of the arteries is a long-term process, so you should be able to temporarily stop taking cerivastatin during pregnancy without developing atherosclerosis. If you become pregnant while taking cerivastatin, stop taking the drug and call your doctor.

Cerivastatin may pass into breast milk. Women taking

cerivastatin should bottle-feed their infants to avoid interfering with the baby's development.

Seniors

Seniors may take cerivastatin without special precaution. Be sure to report any side effects to your doctor.

Generic Name

Cetirizine (seh-TERE-ih-zene)

Brand Name

Zyrtec

Type of Drug

Antihistamine.

The information in this profile also applies to the following drug:

Generic Ingredient: Fexofenadine
Allegra

Prescribed for

Stuffy and runny nose, itchy eyes, and scratchy throat caused by seasonal and year-round allergy, and for other symptoms of allergy such as rash, itching, and hives; also prescribed for chronic itching and for asthma when attacks are allergy-triggered. Fexofenadine is used only for sneezing, stuffy and runny nose, scratchy throat and mouth, and itchy, watery, and red eyes caused by seasonal allergies.

General Information

Antihistamines generally work by blocking the release of histamine (chemical released by body tissue during an allergic reaction) from the cell at the H_1 histamine receptor site, drying up secretions of the nose, throat, and eyes. Cetirizine causes less sedation than older antihistamines and appears to be just as effective. It is widely used by people who wish to avoid the drowsiness and tiredness caused by older antihistamines.

Cautions and Warnings

Do not take cetirizine if you are **allergic** or **sensitive** to it.

People with **kidney disease** should receive reduced dosage of cetirizine because they cannot clear the drug rapidly from their bodies.

Possible Side Effects

▼ Occasional side effects include headache, nervousness, weakness, upset stomach, nausea, vomiting, sore throat, nosebleeds, cough, stuffy nose, changes in bowel habits, and dry mouth, nose, or throat.

Drug Interactions

• Cetirizine is less likely than other antihistimines to interact with other drugs because it causes less sedation.

Food Interactions

Take cetirizine on an empty stomach, 1 hour before or 2 hours after food or meals; it may be taken with food or milk if it upsets your stomach.

Usual Dose

Cetirizine
  Adult (age 12 and over): 5–10 mg once a day. Reduced dosage is necessary in people with kidney disease.
    Child (age 6–11): 10 mg a day.
    Child (age 2–5): 5 mg a day.

Fexofenadine
  Adult (age 12 and over): 60 mg twice a day. People with kidney disease should take 60 mg a day.
    Child: not recommended.

Overdosage

Drug overdose is likely to cause severe side effects. Overdose victims should be given ipecac syrup—available at any pharmacy—to make them vomit and be taken to a hospital emergency room. ALWAYS bring the prescription bottle or container with you.

Special Information

Report sore throat, unusual bleeding, bruising, tiredness, weakness, or any other unusual side effect to your doctor. Cetirizine is less sedating than most antihistamines yet may still cause drowsiness and should not be combined with alcohol or other nervous system depressants.

If you forget to take a dose of cetirizine, take it as soon as you remember. If it is almost time for your next dose, skip the one you forgot and continue with your regular schedule. Do not take a double dose.

Special Populations

Pregnancy/Breast-feeding

Antihistamines have not been proven to cause birth defects in humans. In animal studies, cetirizine in doses several times larger than the human dose resulted in reduced birth weight and increased death rates. Do not take any antihistamine without your doctor's knowledge if you are or might become pregnant—especially during the last 3 months of pregnancy, because newborns may have severe reactions to antihistamines.

Small amounts of antihistamine pass into breast milk and may affect a nursing infant. Nursing mothers who must take cetirizine should bottle-feed their infants.

Seniors

Seniors may take cetirizine without special precaution.

Generic Name

Chlordiazepoxide

(klor-dye-az-uh-POX-ide) G

Brand Names

Libritabs   Librium

Type of Drug

Benzodiazepine tranquilizer.

Prescribed for

Anxiety, tension, fatigue, and agitation; also prescribed for irritable bowel syndrome and panic attacks.

General Information

Chlordiazepoxide is a member of the group of drugs known

as benzodiazepines. These drugs have some activity as anti-anxiety agents, anticonvulsants, or sedatives. Some are more suited to a specific role because of differences in their chemical makeup that give them greater activity in a certain area; others have particular characteristics that make them more desirable for certain functions. Often, individual drugs are limited by the applications for which their research has been sponsored.

Benzodiazepines work by a direct effect on the brain. They can relax you and make you more tranquil or sleepier, or they can slow nervous system transmissions in such a way as to act as an anticonvulsant: The exact effect differs according to drug and dosage. Many doctors prefer benzodiazepines to other drugs that can be used to similar effect because they tend to be safer, have fewer side effects, and are usually as effective, if not more so.

Cautions and Warnings

Do not take chlordiazepoxide if you know you are **sensitive** or **allergic** to it or another member of the group, including clonazepam.

Chlordiazepoxide can aggravate narrow-angle **glaucoma**, but you may take it if you have open-angle glaucoma. Check with your doctor.

Other conditions in which chlordiazepoxide should be avoided are severe **depression**, severe **lung disease**, **sleep apnea** (intermittent cessation of breathing during sleep), **liver disease, drunkenness,** and **kidney disease**. In each of these conditions, the depressive effects of chlordiazepoxide may be enhanced and/or could be detrimental to your overall situation.

Chlordiazepoxide should not be taken by **psychotic patients**, because it is not effective for them and can trigger unusual excitement, stimulation, and rage.

Chlordiazepoxide is not intended for more than 3 to 4 months of continuous use. Your condition should be reassessed before continuing chlordiazepoxide beyond that time.

Chlordiazepoxide may be **addictive**: You can experience drug withdrawal symptoms if you suddenly stop taking it after as little as 4 to 6 weeks of treatment. Withdrawal generally begins with increased feelings of anxiety; it continues with tingling in the extremities, sensitivity to bright lights or to the sun, long periods of sleep or sleeplessness, a metallic taste, flu-like illness, fatigue, difficulty concentrating, restlessness, appetite loss, nausea, irritability, headache, dizziness, sweating, muscle tension or cramps, tremors, and feeling uncomfortable or ill at ease. Other major withdrawal symptoms include confusion, abnormal perception of movement, depersonalization, paranoid delusions, hallucinations, psychotic reactions, muscle twitching, seizures, and memory loss.

Possible Side Effects

Weakness and confusion may occur, especially in seniors and in those who are sickly.

▼ Most common: mild drowsiness during the first few days of therapy.

▼ Less common: depression, lethargy, disorientation, headache, inactivity, slurred speech, stupor, dizziness, tremor, constipation, dry mouth, nausea, inability to control urination, sexual difficulties, irregular menstrual cycle, changes in heart rhythm, low blood pressure, fluid retention, blurred or double vision, itching, rash, hiccups, nervousness, inability to fall asleep, and occasional liver dysfunction. If you experience any of these symptoms, stop taking the medicine and contact your doctor immediately.

▼ Rare: diarrhea, coated tongue, sore gums, vomiting, changes in appetite, difficulty swallowing, increased salivation, upset stomach, incontinence, changes in heart rate, blood pressure changes, palpitations, swelling, stuffy nose, difficulty hearing, hair loss, hairiness, increased sweating, fever, tingling in the hands or feet, breast pain, muscle disturbances, breathing difficulties, changes in blood components, and joint pain.

Drug Interactions

• Chlordiazepoxide is a central-nervous-system depressant. Avoid alcohol, other tranquilizers, narcotics, barbiturates, monoamine oxidase inhibitors (MAOIs), antihistamines, and antidepressants. Taking chlordiazepoxide with these drugs may result in excessive depression, tiredness, sleepiness, breathing difficulties, or related symptoms.

• Smoking may reduce the effectiveness of chlordiazepoxide by increasing the rate at which it is broken down by the body.

• The effects of chlordiazepoxide may be prolonged when it is taken with cimetidine, oral contraceptives, disulfiram, fluoxetine, isoniazid, ketoconazole, metoprolol, probenecid, propoxyphene, propranolol, rifampin, or valproic acid.

• Theophylline may reduce chlordiazepoxide's sedative effects.

• If you take antacids, separate them by at least 1 hour from your chlordiazepoxide dose to prevent them from interfering with the passage of chlordiazepoxide into the bloodstream.

• Chlordiazepoxide may increase blood levels of digoxin and the chances for digoxin toxicity.

• Levodopa's effectiveness may be reduced by chlordiazepoxide.

• Phenytoin blood concentrations may be increased when taken with chlordiazepoxide, resulting in possible phenytoin toxicity.

Food Interactions

Chlordiazepoxide is best taken on an empty stomach but may be taken with food if it upsets your stomach.

Usual Dose

Adult: 5–100 mg a day. This range is due to individual response related to age, weight, disease severity, and other characteristics.

Child (age 6 and over): may be given if deemed appropriate by a doctor. Starting dose—5 mg 2–4 times a day. Maintenance dose—up to 30–40 mg a day for some children, but must be individualized to obtain maximum benefit.

Child (under age 6): not recommended.

Overdosage

Symptoms of overdose are confusion, sleepiness, poor coordination, lack of response to pain such as a pin prick, loss of reflexes, shallow breathing, low blood pressure, and coma. The victim should be taken to a hospital emergency room. ALWAYS bring the prescription bottle or container with you.

Special Information

Chlordiazepoxide can cause tiredness, drowsiness, inability to concentrate, or similar symptoms. Be careful if you are driving, operating machinery, or performing other activities that require concentration.

If you forget a dose of chlordiazepoxide, take it as soon as you remember. If it is almost time for your next dose, skip the dose you forgot and continue with your regular schedule. Do not take a double dose.

Special Populations

Pregnancy/Breast-feeding

Chlordiazepoxide may cross into the fetal circulation and may cause birth defects if taken during the first 3 months of pregnancy. Avoid chlordiazepoxide while pregnant.

Chlordiazepoxide may pass into breast milk. Because infants break down the drug more slowly than do adults, they may accumulate enough chlordiazepoxide in their systems to produce undesirable effects. Nursing mothers who must take chlordiazepoxide should bottle-feed their babies.

Seniors

Seniors, especially those with liver or kidney disease, are more sensitive to the effects of chlordiazepoxide and generally require smaller doses to achieve the same effect. Follow your doctor's directions and report any side effects at once.

Generic Name

Chlorpheniramine Maleate

(KLOR-fen-ERE-uh-mene MAL-ee-ate) G

Brand Names

Chlorpheniramine E.R.	Pro-Hist-8
Chlor-Phen	

The information in this profile also applies to the following drugs:

Generic Ingredient: Azatadine Maleate
Optimine

Generic Ingredient: Brompheniramine Maleate G

Bromatane	Nasahist-B
Colhist	ND-Stat
Cophene-B	Rohist

Generic Ingredient: Cyproheptadine Hydrochloride G
Periactin

Generic Ingredient: Dexchlorpheniramine Maleate G
Polaramine   Polarmine Repetabs

Generic Ingredient: Tripelennamine Hydrochloride G
PBZ   PBZ-SR

Type of Drug

Antihistamine.

Prescribed for

Stuffy and runny nose, itchy eyes, and scratchy throat caused by seasonal allergy, and other symptoms of allergy such as rash, itching, and hives.

General Information

Antihistamines generally work by blocking the release of histamine (chemical released by body tissue during an allergic reaction) from the body cells at the H_1 histamine receptor site, drying up secretions of the nose, throat, and eyes.

Cautions and Warnings

Do not use chlorpheniramine maleate if you are **allergic** to it.

Use chlorpheniramine maleate with care if you have a history of **thyroid disease, heart disease, high blood pressure,** or **diabetes.** Chlorpheniramine maleate should be avoided or used with extreme care if you have **narrow-angle glaucoma, stomach ulcer or other stomach problems, enlarged prostate,** or **problems passing urine.** It should not be used by people who have **deep-breathing problems** such as **asthma.**

Possible Side Effects

▼ Less common: rash or itching, sensitivity to bright light, increased sweating, chills, lowered blood pressure, headache, rapid heartbeat, sleeplessness, dizziness, disturbed coordination, confusion, restlessness, nervousness, irritability, euphoria (feeling high), tingling in the hands or feet, blurred or double vision, ringing in the ears, upset stomach, appetite loss, nausea, vomiting, constipation, diarrhea, urinary difficulties, chest tight-

> **Possible Side Effects** *(continued)*
>
> ness, wheezing, stuffy nose, and dryness of the mouth, nose, or throat. Young children may also develop nervousness, irritability, tension, and anxiety.

Drug Interactions

• Chlorpheniramine maleate should not be taken with a monoamine oxidase inhibitor (MAOI) antidepressant, because the combination may cause severe side effects.

• The effects of tranquilizers, benzodiazepines, sedatives, and sleeping medications will be increased when any of these drugs is combined with chlorpheniramine maleate. It is extremely important for your doctor to know if you are taking any other medication with chlorpheniramine maleate so that the dosage of that medication can be properly adjusted.

• Be extremely cautious when drinking alcoholic beverages while taking chlorpheniramine maleate, which enhances the intoxicating and sedating effects of alcohol.

Food Interactions

You may take chlorpheniramine maleate with food if it upsets your stomach.

Usual Dose

Azatadine
1–2 mg twice a day.

Brompheniramine
   Adult and Child (age 13 and over): 4 mg 3–4 times a day.
   Child (age 6–12): 2–4 mg 3–4 times a day; do not take more than 12 mg a day.
   Child (under age 6): ¼ mg per lb. of body weight a day, in divided doses.

Chlorpheniramine
   Adult and Child (age 13 and over): 4-mg tablet every 4–6 hours; do not take more than 24 mg a day.
   Child (age 6–12): 2-mg tablet every 4–6 hours; do not take more than 8 mg a day.
   Child (age 2–5): 1 mg every 4–6 hours; do not take more than 4 mg a day.

Chlorpheniramine, Sustained-release
 Adult and Child (age 13 and over): 8–12 mg at bedtime, or every 8–12 hours during the day.
 Child (age 6–12): 8 mg during the day or at bedtime.
 Child (under age 6): not recommended.

Cyproheptadine
 Adult and Child (age 15 and over): do not exceed 32 mg a day.
 Child (age 7–14): 4 mg 2–3 times a day; do not exceed 16 mg a day.
 Child (age 2–6): 2 mg 2–3 times a day; do not exceed 12 mg a day.

Dexchlorpheniramine
 Adult and Child (age 12 and over): 2 mg every 4–6 hours.
 Child (age 6–11): 1 mg every 4–6 hours.
 Child (age 2–5): 0.5 mg every 4–6 hours.

Dexchlorpheniramine, Sustained-release
 Adult and Child (age 12 and over): 4–6 mg every 8–10 hours and at bedtime.
 Child (age 6–11): 4 mg once a day and at bedtime.
 Child (under age 6): not recommended.

Tripelennamine
 Adult and Child (age 12 and over): 25–50 mg every 4–6 hours; do not take more than 600 mg a day. Adults may take up to 3 100-mg, sustained-release tablets a day, although this much is not usually needed.
 Child (under age 12): 2 mg per lb. of body weight a day in divided doses; no more than 300 mg should be given a day.

Overdosage

Symptoms of overdose include depression or stimulation, especially in children; dry mouth; fixed or dilated pupils; flushing of the skin; and upset stomach. Overdose victims should be made to vomit as soon as possible with ipecac syrup—available at any pharmacy—to remove excess drug from the stomach. Follow directions on the package label and be sure to prevent victims from inhaling their own vomit. Take the victim to a hospital emergency room immediately if the victim is unconscious or if you cannot induce vomiting. ALWAYS bring the prescription bottle or container with you.

Special Information

Chlorpheniramine maleate may cause tiredness or loss of concentration: Be extremely cautious when driving or doing anything that requires close attention.

If you forget a dose of chlorpheniramine maleate, take it as soon as you remember. If it is almost time for your next dose, skip the one you forgot and continue with your regular schedule. Do not take a double dose.

Special Populations

Pregnancy/Breast-feeding

While antihistamines have not been proven to cause birth defects in humans, animal studies have shown that some antihistamines may cause birth defects. Do not take any antihistamine without your doctor's knowledge if you are or might be pregnant. This is especially important during the last 3 months of pregnancy, because newborns may have severe reactions to antihistamines.

Small amounts of some antihistimines pass into breast milk and may cause side effects in infants. Nursing mothers who must take chlorpheniramine maleate should bottle-feed their infants.

Seniors

Seniors are more sensitive to antihistamine side effects, particularly confusion, difficult or painful urination, dizziness, drowsiness, feeling faint, nightmares, excitability, nervousness, restlessness, irritability, and dry mouth, nose, or throat.

Generic Name

Chlorpromazine (klor-PROE-muh-zene) Ⓖ

Brand Name

Thorazine*

The information in this profile also applies to the following drugs:

Generic Ingredient: Fluphenazine Hydrochloride
Permitil   Prolixin

Generic Ingredient: Mesoridazine Besylate
Serentil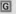

Generic Ingredient: Thioridazine Hydrochloride Ⓖ
Mellaril   Mellaril-S

Generic Ingredient: Trifluoperazine Hydrochloride Ⓖ
Stelazine

Some products in this brand-name group are alcohol or sugar free. Consult you pharmacist.

Type of Drug

Phenothiazine antipsychotic.

Prescribed for

Psychotic disorders, moderate to severe depression with anxiety, agitation or aggressiveness in disturbed children, alcohol withdrawal, intractable pain, and senility; may also be used to relieve nausea, vomiting, hiccups, restlessness, and apprehension before surgery or other procedures.

General Information

Chlorpromazine—and the other drugs listed above—is one of the phenothiazines, a group of drugs that act upon a portion of the brain called the hypothalamus. Phenothiazines affect parts of the hypothalamus that control metabolism, body temperature, alertness, muscle tone, hormone balance, and vomiting, and may be used to treat problems related to any of these functions. Chlorpromazine is available in suppositories and as liquid for those who have trouble swallowing tablets.

Cautions and Warnings

Chlorpromazine may depress the **cough reflex**. People have accidentally choked to death because the cough reflex failed to protect them. Because of its effect in reducing vomiting, chlorpromazine may obscure symptoms of disease or toxicity due to overdose of another drug.

Do not take chlorpromazine if you are **allergic** to it or any phenothiazine drug. Do not take it if you have very **low blood pressure, Parkinson's disease,** or any **blood, liver, kidney, or heart disease**.

Use chlorpromazine with caution and under your doctor's strict supervision if you have **glaucoma, epilepsy, ulcers,** or **urinary difficulties.**

Avoid exposure to **extreme heat,** because this drug may upset your body's normal temperature-control mechanism.

Do not allow the liquid forms of this drug to come in contact with your skin, because they are highly irritating.

Possible Side Effects

▼ Most common: drowsiness, especially during the first or second week of therapy. If drowsiness becomes troublesome, contact your doctor.

▼ Less common: changes in blood components including anemias, raised or lowered blood pressure, abnormal heart rate, heart attack, and faintness or dizziness.

▼ Rare: itching; swelling; unusual sensitivity to bright light; red skin or rash; stuffy nose; headache; nausea; vomiting; appetite loss; changes in body temperature; loss of facial color; excessive salivation or perspiration; constipation; diarrhea; urinary and bowel changes; worsening of glaucoma; blurred vision; weakening of eyelid muscles; spasms in bronchial or other muscles; increased appetite; excessive thirst; changes in the coloration of skin, particularly in areas exposed to the sun; breast enlargement in women; false-positive pregnancy tests; changes in menstrual flow; impotence; and changes in sex drive in males.

Jaundice (symptoms include yellowing of the whites of the eyes or skin) may appear; when it does it is usually within the first 2 to 4 weeks of treatment. Normally it goes away when the drug is discontinued, but there have been cases when it has not. If you develop jaundice or symptoms such as fever and general feelings of ill health, contact your doctor immediately.

Phenothiazines may produce extrapyramidal side effects, including spasm of the neck muscles, rolling back of the eyes, convulsions, difficulty swallowing, and symptoms associated with Parkinson's disease. These side effects seem very serious but usually disappear after the drug has been withdrawn; however, symptoms affecting the face, tongue, or jaw may persist for as long as several years, especially in older adults with a history of brain damage. If you experience extrapyramidal effects, contact your doctor immediately.

Chlorpromazine may cause an unusual increase in psychotic symptoms or may cause paranoid reactions, tiredness, lethargy, restlessness, hyperactivity, confusion

Possible Side Effects *(continued)*

at night, bizarre dreams, sleeplessness, depression, and euphoria (feeling high).

Drug Interactions

• Be cautious about taking chlorpromazine with barbiturates, sleeping pills, narcotics or other tranquilizers, or any other drug that may produce a depressive effect. Avoid alcoholic beverages for the same reason.

• Aluminum antacids may interfere with the absorption of phenothiazine drugs into the bloodstream, reducing their effectiveness.

• Chlorpromazine may reduce the effects of bromocriptine and appetite suppressants.

• Anticholinergic drugs may reduce the effectiveness of chlorpromazine and increase the chance of side effects.

• The blood-pressure-lowering effect of guanethidine may be counteracted by phenothiazine drugs.

• Taking lithium together with a phenothiazine drug may lead to disorientation, loss of consciousness, or uncontrolled muscle movements.

• Combining propranolol and a phenothiazine drug may lead to unusually low blood pressure.

• Blood concentrations of tricyclic antidepressants may increase if they are taken together with a phenothiazine drug. This can lead to antidepressant side effects.

Food Interactions

Take liquid chlorpromazine with fruit juice or other liquids. You may also take it with food if it upsets your stomach.

Usual Dose

Adult: 30–1000 mg or more a day, individualized according to your disease and response.

Child (age 6 months and over): 0.25 mg per lb. of body weight every 4–6 hours, up to 200 mg or more a day, depending on disease, age, and response.

Overdosage

Overdose symptoms include depression, extreme weakness, tiredness, lowered blood pressure, agitation, restlessness, uncontrolled muscle spasms, convulsions, fever, dry mouth, abnormal heart rhythms, and coma. The victim should be taken to a hospital emergency room immediately. ALWAYS bring the prescription bottle or container with you.

Special Information

Call your doctor at once if you develop sore throat, fever, rash, weakness, visual problems, tremors, muscle movements or twitching, yellowing of the skin or whites of the eyes, or darkening of the urine.

This drug may cause drowsiness. Use caution when driving or operating hazardous equipment. Avoid alcoholic beverages.

Chlorpromazine may cause unusual sensitivity to the sun and may turn your urine reddish-brown to pink.

If dizziness occurs, avoid rising quickly from a sitting or lying position and avoid climbing stairs. Use caution in hot weather, because this drug may make you more prone to heat stroke.

If you are using sustained-release capsules, do not chew them or break them: Swallow them whole. Liquid forms of phenothiazines must be protected from light. Do not take them out of the opaque bottles in which they are dispensed.

If you take chlorpromazine more than once a day and forget to take a dose, take it right away if you remember within an hour. If you do not remember within an hour, skip the dose you forgot and continue with your regular schedule. If you take just 1 dose a day and forget a dose, skip the dose you forgot and continue your regular schedule the next day. Never take a double dose.

Special Populations

Pregnancy/Breast-feeding

Infants born to women taking this drug have experienced side effects—including jaundice and nervous system effects—immediately after birth. Check with your doctor about taking chlorpromazine if you are or might be pregnant.

This drug may pass into breast milk and affect a nursing infant. Consider bottle-feeding your baby if you must take chlorpromazine.

Seniors

Seniors are more sensitive to the effects of this drug and usually achieve desired results with lower dosages. Seniors are also more likely to develop side effects. Some experts feel that seniors should receive ½ to ¼ the usual adult dose.

Generic Name

Chlorzoxazone (klor-ZOX-uh-zone) Ⓖ

Brand Names

Paraflex   Remular-S
Parafon Forte DSC

Type of Drug

Skeletal muscle relaxant.

Prescribed for

Pain and spasm of muscular conditions, including strain, sprain, bruising, and lower back problems.

General Information

Chlorzoxazone is one of several drugs used to treat pain associated with muscle ache, strain, or a bad back. It provides only temporary relief and is not a substitute for other types of therapy, such as rest, surgery, and physical therapy.

Chlorzoxazone acts primarily on the spinal cord level and on areas of the brain, acting as a mild sedative. This results in fewer spasms, less pain, and greater mobility. It does not directly relax tense muscles.

Cautions and Warnings

Do not take chlorzoxazone if you are **allergic** to it or if you have a condition known as **porphyria** (hereditary condition characterized by abdominal pain, psychoses, and nervous system disorders).

People with **poor liver or kidney function** should take this drug with caution because it is broken down by the liver and passes out of the body in the urine.

Chlorzoxazone may worsen **depression** or interact with other drugs that cause nervous system depression (see "Drug Interactions").

Because it is possible to become **dependent** on this drug, people with a history of substance abuse should take chlorzoxazone with caution.

Possible Side Effects

▼ Most common: dizziness, drowsiness, and light-headedness.

▼ Less common: headache, stimulation, stomach cramps or pain, diarrhea, constipation, heartburn, nausea, and vomiting.

▼ Rare: stomach or intestinal bleeding (symptoms include black or tarry stools and vomiting blood or material that resembles coffee grounds); rapid drop in white-blood-cell count (symptoms include fever with or without chills, sore throat, and sores or white spots on the lips or mouth); unusual tiredness or weakness; liver inflammation (symptoms include yellowing of the skin or whites of the eyes); allergic reaction (symptoms include changes in facial color, rash, hives, itching, rapid or irregular breathing, breathing difficulties, chest tightness, and wheezing); large hive-like swellings on the face, eyelids, mouth, or tongue; and skin rash.

Drug Interactions

• The depressive effects of chlorzoxazone may be enhanced by taking it with alcohol, tranquilizers, sleeping pills, or other nervous system depressants. Avoid these combinations.

Food Interactions

Take this drug with food if it upsets your stomach. Chlorzoxazone tablets may be crushed and mixed with food.

Usual Dose

Adult: 250–750 mg 3–4 times a day.
Child: 125–500 mg 3–4 times a day.

Do not take more medication than is prescribed.

Overdosage

Early signs of chlorzoxazone overdose may include nausea, vomiting, diarrhea, drowsiness, dizziness, light-headedness, and headache. Victims may also feel sluggish or sickly and lose the ability to move their muscles. Breathing may become slow or irregular, and blood pressure may drop. Contact a doctor immediately or go to a hospital emergency room for treatment. ALWAYS bring the prescription bottle or container with you.

Special Information

Chlorzoxazone may make you drowsy or reduce your ability to concentrate. Be extremely careful while driving or operating hazardous equipment. Avoid alcoholic beverages.

A breakdown product of chlorzoxazone may turn your urine orange to purple-red; this is not dangerous.

Call your doctor if you develop drowsiness, weakness, an allergic reaction, breathing difficulties, black or tarry stools, vomiting of material that resembles coffee grounds, liver problems, or any other severe or bothersome side effect.

If you miss a dose of chlorzoxazone by more than an hour, skip the dose you forgot and continue with your regular schedule. Do not take a double dose.

Special Populations

Pregnancy/Breast-feeding

This drug has not been found to cause birth defects. Nevertheless, pregnant women and women who might become pregnant should not take chlorzoxazone without their doctor's approval.

It is not known if chlorzoxazone passes into breast milk, and this drug has not caused problems among breast-fed infants. However, you should consider the potential effect on your infant if you breast-feed while taking this drug.

Seniors

Seniors, especially those with severe liver disease, are more sensitive to the effects of chlorzoxazone because they retain it in their bodies longer than younger people. Follow your doctor's directions and report any side effects at once.

Generic Name

Cholestyramine (kol-es-TYE-rah-mene)

Brand Names

Prevalite   Questran Lite
Questran

The information in this profile also applies to the following drugs:

Generic Ingredient: Colestipol
Colestid

Type of Drug

Anti-hyperlipidemic (blood-fat reducer).

Prescribed for

High blood-cholesterol levels, generalized itching associated with bile duct obstruction—cholestyramine only—colitis, digitalis or thyroid overdose, and pesticide poisoning.

General Information

Cholestyramine resin lowers blood-cholesterol levels by removing bile acids from the biliary system. Since the body uses cholesterol to make bile acids—needed to digest fat— the only way fat digestion can continue is to make more bile acid from blood cholesterol. This results in lower blood-cholesterol levels beginning 4 to 7 days after cholestyramine is begun.

Cholestyramine works entirely within the bowel and is never absorbed into the bloodstream. Though usually given 3 to 4 times a day, there appears to be no advantage to taking it more often than 2 times a day. The cholesterol-lowering effect of cholestyramine may be increased when taken with an HMG-CoA inhibitor or nicotinic acid.

In some kinds of hyperlipidemia, colestipol may be more effective in lowering total blood cholesterol than clofibrate. There are 6 different types of hyperlipidemia. Check with your doctor as to the kind you have and the proper drug treatment for your condition.

Cautions and Warnings

Do not use cholestyramine if you are **sensitive** to it or if your bile duct is blocked. The powder form should not be taken dry; doing so may result in the inhalation of powder into your lungs or a clogged esophagus.

Cholestyramine may cause or worsen **constipation** and **hemorrhoids**. Most constipation is mild but some people may need to stop the medication or take less of it.

Possible Side Effects

▼ Most common: constipation, which may be severe
and result in bowel impaction. Hemorrhoids may be
worsened.

▼ Less common: abdominal pain and bloating, and
bleeding disorders or black-and-blue marks due to interference with the absorption of vitamin K, a necessary
factor in the clotting process. One person developed
night-blindness because the medication interfered with
vitamin A absorption into the blood. Other side effects
include belching, gas, nausea, vomiting, diarrhea, heartburn, and appetite loss. Your stool may have an unusual
appearance because of a high fat-level.

▼ Rare: rash, irritation of the tongue and anus, osteoporosis, black stools, stomach ulcer, dental bleeding,
hiccups, a sour taste in your mouth, pancreas inflammation, ulcer attack, gallbladder attack, itching, backache,
muscle and joint pain, arthritis, headache, anxiety, dizziness, fatigue, ringing or buzzing in the ears, fainting,
tingling in the hands or feet, blood in the urine, frequent
or painful urination, an unusual urine odor, swollen
glands, swelling of the arms or legs, and shortness of
breath.

Drug Interactions

• Cholestyramine interferes with the absorption of virtually
all other oral drugs including acetaminophen, amiodarone,
aspirin, cephalexin, chenodiol, clindamycin, clofibrate, corticosteroids, diclofenac, iron, digitalis drugs, furosemide,
gemfibrozil, glipizide, hydrocortisone, imipramine (an antidepressant), methyldopa, mycophenolate, nicotinic acid, penicillin, phenobarbital, phenytoin, piroxicam, propranolol,
tetracycline, thiazide diuretics, thyroid drugs, tolbutamide,
trimethoprim, warfarin and other anticoagulant (blood-
thinning) drugs, and vitamins A, D, E, and K.

• Take all other medications at least 1 hour before or 4 to 6
hours after taking cholestyramine.

Food Interactions

Take this medication before meals. It may be mixed with
soda, water, juice, cereal, or pulpy fruits—such as applesauce

or crushed pineapple. Cholestyramine bars should be thoroughly chewed and taken with plenty of fluids.

Usual Dose

Cholestyramine: 4 g (1 packet) taken 1–6 times a day.

Colestipol: 5–30 g (1–6 packets) a day in 2–4 divided doses.

Overdosage

The most severe effect of overdose is bowel impaction. Take the overdose victim to a hospital emergency room for evaluation and treatment. ALWAYS bring the prescription bottle or container with you.

Special Information

Do not swallow the granules or powder in their dry form. Prepare each packet of powder by mixing it with soup, cereal, or pulpy fruit or by adding the powder to a 6-oz. glass of liquid such as a carbonated beverage. Some of the drug may stick to the sides of the glass; this should be rinsed with liquid and drunk.

Constipation, stomach gas, nausea, and heartburn may occur and then disappear with continued use of this medication. Call your doctor if these side effects continue or if you develop unusual problems such as bleeding from the gums or rectum.

If you miss a dose of cholestyramine, skip it and continue on your regular schedule. Do not take a double dose.

Special Populations

Pregnancy/Breast-feeding

Cholestyramine is not absorbed into the blood and will not directly affect the fetus. However, it may prevent the absorption of vitamins A, D, and E and other nutrients essential to the fetus' proper development, even when you take a prenatal vitamin supplement.

Cholestyramine will not affect a nursing infant. However, reductions in the absorption of vitamins A, D, and E and other nutrients may make your milk less nutritious. Nursing mothers who must take cholestyramine should bottle-feed their infants.

Seniors

Seniors are more likely to experience side effects with cholestyramine, especially those relating to the bowel.

Generic Name

Ciclopirox (sye-kloe-PERE-ox)

Brand Name

Loprox

Type of Drug

Antifungal.

Prescribed for

Fungal and yeast infections of the skin, including athlete's foot and candidiasis.

General Information

Ciclopirox olamine slows the growth of a wide variety of fungus organisms and yeasts, and kills many others. The drug penetrates the skin very well and is present in levels sufficient to kill or inhibit most fungus organisms. In addition, it penetrates the hair, hair follicles, and skin sweat glands.

Cautions and Warnings

Do not use this product if you are **allergic** to it.

Possible Side Effects

▼ Common: burning, itching, and stinging at the application site.

Drug Interactions

None known.

Usual Dose

Apply enough of the cream or lotion to cover affected areas and massage it into the skin twice a day.

Overdosage

If this drug is accidentally swallowed, the victim may become nauseated and have an upset stomach. Call your local poison control center or hospital for more information.

Special Information

Clean the affected areas before applying ciclopirox, unless otherwise directed by your doctor.

This product is quite effective and can be expected to relieve symptoms within the first week of use. Follow your doctor's directions for the complete 2- to 4-week course of treatment to gain maximum benefit from this product. If stopped too soon, the medication may not have eliminated the fungus completely; this can lead to a relapse.

Call your doctor if the affected area burns, stings, or becomes red after you use this product. Also, notify your doctor if your symptoms do not clear up after 4 weeks of treatment; by then it is unlikely that the cream will be effective at all.

If you forget a dose of ciclopirox, apply it as soon as you remember. Do not apply more than prescribed to make up for the missed dose.

Special Populations

Pregnancy/Breast-feeding

Ciclopirox may pass to the fetus in very small amounts. However, there is no proof that it causes damage to the fetus. When the drug was given by mouth to animals in doses 10 times the amount normally applied to the skin, it was found to be nontoxic to fetuses.

Ciclopirox is not known to pass into breast milk. As with all drugs, caution should be exercised when using ciclopirox during pregnancy and while breast-feeding.

Seniors

Seniors may use this drug without special restriction.

Generic Name

Cimetidine (sih-MET-ih-dene) G

Brand Name

Tagamet   Tagamet HB

Type of Drug

Histamine H_2 antagonist.

Prescribed for

Ulcers of the stomach and duodenum (upper intestine); also used to treat upset stomach, gastroesophageal reflux disease (GERD), benign stomach ulcer, bleeding in the stomach and duodenum, colorectal cancer, prevention of stress ulcer, hyperparathyroidism, fungal infections of the hair and scalp, herpesvirus infection, excessive hairiness in women, chronic itching of unknown cause, skin reactions, warts, acetaminophen overdose, and other conditions characterized by the production of large amounts of gastric fluids. Cimetidine may be prescribed when it is desirable to stop the production of stomach acid during surgery.

General Information

Cimetidine, approved in 1977, was the first histamine H_2 antagonist used in the U.S. Cimetidine works against ulcers and other gastrointestinal (GI) conditions by actually turning off the system that produces stomach acid and other secretions.

Cimetidine is effective in treating the symptoms of ulcer and preventing complications of the disease, although an ulcer that does not respond to another histamine H_2 antagonist will probably not respond to cimetidine because all these drugs work in exactly the same way. Histamine H_2 antagonists differ only in their potency. Cimetidine is the least potent; 1000 mg are roughly equal to 300 mg of either nizatidine or ranitidine, or 40 mg of famotidine. All these drugs have roughly equivalent success rates in treating ulcer disease and all carry comparable chances of side effects.

Cautions and Warnings

Do not take cimetidine if you have ever had an **allergic** reaction to it or to any histamine H_2 antagonist. Cimetidine has a mild antiandrogen effect, which probably causes the **painful, swollen breasts** that some people experience after taking this drug for a month or more.

People with **kidney or liver disease** should take cimetidine with caution because it is broken down in the liver and passes out of the body through the kidneys.

The fact that symptoms are alleviated by cimetidine does not preclude the possibility of **stomach cancer**, which can have symptoms similar to other GI disorders. Make sure your doctor screens for possible malignancy.

Some people—mostly very ill people—may experience confusion, agitation, psychosis, hallucinations, depression, anxiety, or disorientation. When these symptoms do occur, it is usually within 2 or 3 days of starting cimetidine treatment. Normally they stop 3 to 4 days after discontinuing the drug. Call your doctor if this happens to you.

Possible Side Effects

Most people taking cimetidine do not experience serious side effects.

▼ Most common: mild diarrhea, dizziness, rash, painful breast swelling, nausea and vomiting, headache, confusion, drowsiness, hallucinations, and impotence.

▼ Less common: liver inflammation, peeling or red and swollen rash, breathing difficulties, tingling in the hands or feet, delirious feelings, and oozing fluid from the nipples.

▼ Rare: Cimetidine may affect white blood cells or blood platelets. Some symptoms of these effects are unusual bleeding or bruising, unusual tiredness, and weakness. Other rare side effects are inflammation of the pancreas, reversible hair loss, abnormal heart rhythms, heart attack, reversible muscle or joint pains, and reversible drug reactions.

Drug Interactions

• The effects of cimetidine may be reduced if it is taken with an antacid. This minor interaction may be avoided by separating cimetidine from antacid doses by about 3 hours. Other drugs that may reduce the absorption of cimetidine are metoclopramide and anticholinergic drugs, including trihexyphenidyl hydrochloride, oxybutynin, and benztropine mesylate.

• Cigarette smoking has been shown to reverse the healing effect cimetidine has on ulcers.

• Cimetidine may increase the side effects of a variety of drugs by preventing their breakdown or elimination from the body, possibly leading to drug toxicity. These drugs include alcohol; aminophylline; oral antidiabetes drugs; benzodiazepine tranquilizers and sleeping pills, except lorazepam, oxazepam, and temazepam; caffeine; calcium channel blockers; carbamazepine; carmustine; chloroquine; flecainide; fluorouracil; labetalol; lidocaine; metoprolol; metronidazole; moricizine; mexiletine; narcotic pain relievers; ondansetron; pentoxifylline; phenytoin; procainamide; propafenone; propranolol; quinine; quinidine; tacrine; theophylline drugs, except dyphylline; triamterene; tricyclic antidepressants; valproic acid; and warfarin, a blood-thinning drug.

• Drugs whose absorption may be decreased by cimetidine are iron, indomethacin, fluconazole, ketoconazole, and tetracycline antibiotics.

• Enteric-coated tablets should not be taken with cimetidine. The change in stomach acidity will cause the tablets to disintegrate prematurely in the stomach.

• The effects of digoxin and tocainide may decrease while you are taking cimetidine.

Food Interactions

None known.

Usual Dose

Adult: 400–800 mg at bedtime; 300 mg 4 times a day with meals and at bedtime; or 400 mg 2 times a day. To treat GERD—400 mg 4 times a day. Do not exceed 2400 mg a day.

Seniors: Smaller doses may be as effective for seniors or patients with impaired kidney function.

Overdosage

Symptoms of cimetidine overdose are usually exaggerated side effects, but little else is known. Two deaths occurred in people who reportedly took 40,000 mg (40 g) of cimetidine at once. Your local poison control center may advise giving the victim ipecac syrup—available at any pharmacy—to induce vomiting and remove any drug remaining in the stomach. Victims who have definite symptoms should be taken to a hospital emergency room. ALWAYS bring the prescription bottle or container with you.

Special Information

You must take cimetidine exactly as directed and follow your doctor's instructions regarding diet and other treatment in order to get the maximum benefit from the drug.

Cigarettes are known to be associated with stomach ulcers and will reverse the effect of cimetidine on stomach acid.

Call your doctor at once if any unusual side effects develop, especially unusual bleeding or bruising, unusual tiredness, diarrhea, dizziness, rash, or hallucinations. Black, tarry stools or vomiting material that resembles coffee grounds may indicate your ulcer is bleeding.

If you miss a dose of cimetidine, take it as soon as possible. If it is almost time for your next dose, skip the dose you forgot and continue with your regular schedule. Do not take a double dose.

Special Populations

Pregnancy/Breast-feeding
Studies with laboratory animals reveal no damage to the fetus, although cimetidine does pass into the fetal blood. When cimetidine is considered crucial, its potential benefits must be carefully weighed against its risks.

Large amounts of cimetidine pass into breast milk. Nursing mothers who must take this drug should bottle-feed their babies.

Seniors
Seniors respond well to cimetidine. They may need less medication to achieve results, because the drug is eliminated through the kidneys and kidney function tends to decline with age. Older adults may be more susceptible to cimetidine side effects, especially confusion and other nervous system effects (see "Cautions and Warnings").

Cipro

see *Fluoroquinolone Anti-infectives*, page 433

Generic Name

Cisapride (CIS-uh-pride)

Brand Name
Propulsid

Type of Drug
Gastrointestinal (GI) stimulant.

Prescribed for

Nighttime heartburn caused by gastroesophageal reflux disease (GERD).

General Information

Cisapride restores the normal ability of the stomach and intestines to move food through the GI tract. It does this by stimulating the release of the hormone acetylcholine at key nerve endings throughout the GI tract. Stimulating movement of the GI tract increases pressure in the lower esophagus and helps to pull through any stomach contents that might have refluxed (come back up into the lower esophagus). People with GERD have about half of the normal lower-esophageal pressure; cisapride restores that pressure to normal levels. Cisapride increases the rate at which food moves through the stomach. This is helpful in treating nighttime heartburn caused by GERD. Cisapride has no consistent effect on daytime heartburn, regurgitation (casting up of undigested food from the stomach), or changes in the esophagus, and it does not work as an antacid. Cisapride is related to metoclopramide but is more specific and targeted in its effects.

Cautions and Warnings

Cisapride should be avoided by people with **stomach or intestinal bleeding**, **bowel obstruction or perforation**, or other **conditions in which increasing GI tract activity could be harmful**. Rare cases of serious **abnormal heart rhythms** have occurred in people taking cisapride. Animal studies indicate that high doses of cisapride may lead to infertility in women.

Possible Side Effects

▼ Most common: headache, diarrhea, abdominal pain, nausea, constipation, and runny nose.

▼ Less common: upset stomach, stomach gas, sinus inflammation, upper respiratory infection, coughing, pain, fever, urinary infection, frequent urination, sleeplessness, anxiety, nervousness, rash, itching, viral infection, joint pain, changes in vision, and vaginal irritation.

▼ Rare: dizziness, vomiting, sore throat, chest pain, back pain, depression, dehydration, muscle aches, dry

---

Possible Side Effects *(continued)*

mouth, tiredness, heart palpitations, migraine, tremors,
swelling in the feet or legs, seizure, uncontrollable muscle
movements, rapid heartbeat, liver inflammation, hepatitis, and reduced counts of white blood cells and blood
platelets.

Drug Interactions

• Combining cisapride with ketoconazole (an antifungal)
results in serious heart abnormalities because unusually
high blood levels of cisapride develop. Itraconazole, miconazole
administered intravenously, fluconazole, clarithromycin, erythromycin, and troleandomycin also do this and should not be
combined with cisapride.

• Cisapride's stimulating effect on the GI tract interferes
with the absorption of most oral drugs into the bloodstream
by speeding them through the system before they can be
adequately absorbed. Your doctor should check to be sure
that other drugs you are taking are not affected.

• When cimetidine and cisapride are taken together, the
amount of both drugs absorbed into the blood is increased.
Cisapride also increases the amount of ranitidine absorbed.

• Cisapride may increase the effects of anticoagulant (blood-
thinning) drugs. Your anticoagulant dosage may need to be
adjusted or you may have to stop taking cisapride. Cimetidine
may increase the amount of cisapride absorbed into the bloodstream; cisapride, in turn, increases the amount of cimetidine
absorbed into the blood. Your doctor will have to adjust these
drug combinations to fit your needs.

• Anticholinergic drugs including atropine, benztropine,
donnatal, oxybutynin, and trihexyphenidyl interfere with the
effects of cisapride.

Food Interactions

Take cisapride 15 minutes before meals and at bedtime.

Usual Dose

4–80 mg a day.

Overdosage

Symptoms of overdose include stomach rumbling, stomach

gas, and frequent stools and urination. Other possible symptoms are droopy eyelids, tremors, convulsions, breathing difficulties, catatonic reaction, loss of muscle tone, and diarrhea. Doses as low as 80 mg per lb. of body weight have been lethal in animal studies. Overdose victims should be taken to a hospital emergency room. ALWAYS bring the prescription bottle or container with you.

Special Information

Take cisapride with care if you take a benzodiazepine tranquilizer or sleeping medication; avoid alcoholic beverages while taking cisapride.

Call your doctor if any side effects become intolerable, bothersome, or interfere with regular activities.

If you forget a dose of cisapride, take it as soon as you remember, as long as it is before a meal. If it is almost time for your next dose, skip the one you forgot and continue with your regular schedule. Do not take a double dose.

Special Populations

Pregnancy/Breast-feeding

Animal studies indicate that cisapride may be harmful to the fetus. There are no conclusive studies of this drug in people. When this drug is considered crucial by your doctor, its potential benefits must be carefully weighed against its risks.

Cisapride passes into breast milk in 5% of the concentration found in the blood. Nursing mothers taking cisapride should observe their infants for possible side effects.

Seniors

Seniors generally have more cisapride in the blood since it takes longer to remove the medication from their bodies. Nevertheless, the usual dose is the same and side effects are about as common in seniors as in other adults.

Generic Name

Clarithromycin (klah-rith-roe-MYE-sin)

Brand Name

Biaxin

Type of Drug

Macrolide antibiotic.

Prescribed for

Mild to moderate infections of the upper and lower respiratory tract; also prescribed for duodenal ulcers—with omeprazole—and skin and other infections including membrane attack complex (MAC).

General Information

Clarithromycin is a member of the macrolide group of antibiotics. Drugs in this group also include erythromycin, dirithromycin, and azithromycin and are either bactericidal (bacteria-killing) or bacteriostatic (inhibiting bacterial growth) depending on the organism in question and the amount of antibiotic present.

In ulcer disease, clarithromycin is used to fight *Helicobacter pylori* infection, which is present in almost all ulcers and most gastritis.

Clarithromycin is rapidly absorbed into the blood and distributed through the bloodstream to all parts of the body. Because the action of this antibiotic depends on its concentration within the invading bacteria, it is important for you to follow your doctor's directions regarding spacing of doses and the number of days you must take the medication. Clarithromycin's effectiveness may be severely reduced if these instructions are not followed. Clarithromycin may be prescribed to prevent MAC.

Cautions and Warnings

Do not take clarithromycin if you are **allergic** to it or any macrolide antibiotic.

Clarithromycin is primarily eliminated from the body through the liver and kidneys. People with **severe kidney disease** may require dose adjustments. Liver disease generally does not call for an adjustment.

Colitis (bowel inflammation)—see "Possible Side Effects" for symptoms—has been associated with all antibiotics including clarithromycin.

Possible Side Effects

Most side effects are mild and will go away once you stop taking clarithromycin.

▼ Most common: nausea, vomiting, upset stomach,

Possible Side Effects *(continued)*

changes in sense of taste, stomach cramps, stomach gas, and headache. Colitis (symptoms include severe abdominal cramps and severe, persistent, and possibly bloody diarrhea) may develop after taking clarithromycin.

Drug Interactions

• Clarithromycin may increase the anticoagulant (blood-thinning) effects of warfarin in people who take it regularly, especially older adults. People taking this combination must be carefully monitored by their doctors.

• Clarithromycin may raise blood levels of carbamazepine. People taking this combination should be carefully monitored by their doctors for changes in blood-carbamazepine levels.

• Two deaths have been reported in people combining clarithromycin and pimozide. Pimozide should not be used by people taking a macrolide antibiotic.

• Clarithromycin may raise blood levels of theophylline, possibly leading to a theophylline overdose. It can increase the effects of caffeine, which is chemically related to theophylline.

• Clarithromycin may also increase blood levels of digoxin, cyclosporine, ergot alkaloids, tacrolimus, and triazolam when clarithromycin is taken with one of these drugs, possibly leading to drug side effects.

• Clarithromycin may increase blood levels of terfenadine and astemizole (non-sedating antihistamines). This drug interaction may lead to serious cardiac side effects and should be avoided.

• Combining clarithromycin and cisapride may produce serious abnormal heart rhythms, some fatal.

• Combining fluconazole and clarithromycin increases the amount of clarithromycin in the blood.

• Combining zidovudine (an AIDS drug—also known as AZT) with clarithromycin may reduce the amount of zidovudine in the bloodstream.

Food Interactions

Clarithromycin can be taken without regard to food or meals. It may be taken with milk.

Usual Dose

Adult: 250–500 mg every 12 hours. Dosage must be reduced in people with severe kidney disease.

Child: 3.4 mg per lb. of body weight every 12 hours, up to 250–500 mg a dose, depending on the offending organism.

Overdosage

Clarithromycin overdose may cause severe side effects, especially nausea, vomiting, stomach cramps, and diarrhea. Call your local poison control center or hospital emergency room for more information.

Special Information

Call your doctor if you develop nausea, vomiting, diarrhea, stomach cramps, or severe abdominal pain.

Clarithromycin suspension must be shaken well before each dose. Do not store it in the refrigerator.

Clarithromycin may be gentler on the digestive tract than erythromycin.

Remember to complete the full course of treatment as prescribed by your doctor, even if you feel well after only a few days of clarithromycin use.

Take clarithromycin at the same time each day to help you remember. If you forget a dose, take it as soon as you remember. If it is within 4 hours of your next dose, skip the dose you forgot and go back to your regular schedule.

Special Populations

Pregnancy/Breast-feeding

In animal studies, clarithromycin has affected the fetus. Pregnant women should take clarithromycin only if no alternative is available.

Other macrolide antibiotics pass into breast milk, but it is not known if this is true of clarithromycin. Nursing mothers should use this drug with caution.

Seniors

Seniors may take the usual dosage of clarithromycin. Those with severe kidney disease require a dosage adjustment.

Claritin

see **Loratadine**, page 608

Claritin-D

see *Antihistamine-Decongestant Combination Products,*
page 66

Generic Name

Clemastine (KLEH-mas-tene)

Brand Name

Tavist

Type of Drug

Antihistamine.

Prescribed for

Stuffy and runny nose, itchy eyes, and scratchy throat caused
by seasonal allergy and for other symptoms of allergy such
as rash, itching, and hives.

General Information

Antihistamines generally work by blocking the release of
histamine (chemical released by body tissue during an allergic reaction) from cells at the H_1 histamine receptor site,
drying up secretions of the nose, throat, and eyes. Clemastine
fumarate is distinguished from many other antihistamines in
that it is somewhat less sedating. It is not less sedating than
astemizole or loratadine—the newest and least sedating of
this group.

Cautions and Warnings

Clemastine should not be taken if you are **allergic** to it. People
with asthma or other deep-breathing problems, glaucoma,
or **stomach ulcers or other stomach problems** should avoid
clemastine because its side effects can aggravate these problems.

Possible Side Effects

▼ Most common: headache, weakness, nervousness,
stomach upset, nausea, vomiting, cough, stuffy nose,

Possible Side Effects *(continued)*

changes in bowel habits, sore throat, nosebleeds, and dry mouth, nose, or throat.

▼ Less common: drowsiness, hair loss, allergic reaction (symptoms include rash, itching, hives, and breathing difficulties), depression, sleeplessness, menstrual irregularities, muscle aches, sweating, tingling in the hands or feet, frequent urination, and visual disturbances.

Drug Interactions

• Combining clemastine with alcohol, tranquilizers, sleeping pills, or other nervous system depressants may increase the depressant effects of clemastine. Do not combine these drugs.

• The effects of oral anticoagulant (blood-thinning) drugs may be decreased by clemastine. Do not take this combination without your doctor's knowledge.

• Monoamine oxidase inhibitor (MAOI) antidepressants may increase the drying and other effects of clemastine. This combination can also worsen urinary difficulties.

Food Interactions

Clemastine is best taken on an empty stomach at least 1 hour before or 2 hours after eating; it may be taken with food if it upsets your stomach.

Usual Dose

Adult and Child (age 12 and over): 1.34 mg 2 times a day or 2.68 mg up to 3 times a day. Do not take more than 8.04 mg— 7 tablets of Tavist-1 or 3½ tablets of Tavist—daily.

Child (under age 12): not recommended.

Overdosage

Clemastine overdose is likely to cause severe side effects. Overdose victims should be given ipecac syrup—available at any pharmacy—to induce vomiting and then be taken to a hospital emergency room for treatment. ALWAYS bring the prescription bottle or container with you.

Special Information

Clemastine may make it difficult for you to concentrate or

perform complex tasks such as driving a car. Be sure to report any unusual side effects to your doctor.

If you forget to take a dose of clemastine, take it as soon as you remember. If it is almost time for your next dose, skip the one you forgot and continue with your regular schedule. Do not take a double dose.

Special Populations

Pregnancy/Breast-feeding

Antihistamines have not been proven to cause birth defects in humans. Do not take any antihistamines without your doctor's knowledge if you are or might be pregnant. Antihistamines should be avoided especially during the last 3 months of pregnancy, because newborns may have severe reactions to antihistamines.

Small amounts of clemastine pass into breast milk and may affect a nursing infant. Nursing mothers who must take clemastine should bottle-feed their infants.

Seniors

Seniors are more sensitive to side effects such as confusion; difficult or painful urination; dizziness; drowsiness; feeling faint; dry mouth, nose, or throat; nightmares; excitability; nervousness; restlessness; and irritability.

Generic Name

Clindamycin (klin-duh-MYE-sin) Ⓖ

Brand Name

Cleocin

Type of Drug

Antibiotic.

Prescribed for

Bacterial infections. Clindamycin vaginal cream is used to treat bacterial vaginosis. Topical clindamycin is used to treat acne and rosacea.

General Information

Clindamycin is one of the few oral drugs that is effective

against anaerobic organisms (bacteria that grow only in the absence of oxygen and are frequently found in infected wounds, lung abscesses, abdominal infections, and infections of the female genital tract). It is also effective against the organisms usually treated by penicillin or erythromycin.

Clindamycin may be useful for treating certain skin or soft tissue infections where susceptible organisms are present. It kills the bacteria that frequently cause acne. Another topical antimicrobial, azelaic acid, works on these bacteria and also normalizes skin processes that can worsen acne.

Cautions and Warnings

Do not take clindamycin if you are **allergic** to it or to lincomycin, another antibiotic.

Clindamycin can cause a severe intestinal irritation called **colitis**, which can be fatal. Signs of colitis are diarrhea, blood in the stool, and abdominal cramps. Colitis can be provoked by any form of this drug, including products applied to the skin and the vaginal cream. Because of this, clindamycin should be reserved for serious infections involving organisms known to be affected by the drug. It should not be used for treatment of the common cold and other moderate infections, or for infections that can be treated successfully with other drugs.

Clindamycin should be used with caution if you have **kidney or liver disease**.

Possible Side Effects

▼ Most common: oral—stomach pain; nausea; vomiting; diarrhea, in up to 30 percent of people who take this drug; and pain when swallowing. Topical—skin dryness, redness, burning, and peeling; oily skin; and itching. Vaginal—cervicitis, vaginitis, and irritation.

▼ Less common: oral—itching; rash; signs of serious drug sensitivity, such as difficulty in breathing and yellowing of the skin or the whites of the eyes; colitis, indicated by severe and persistent—possibly bloody—diarrhea and severe abdominal cramps; occasional effects on components of the blood; and joint pain. Topical—diarrhea, abdominal pain, colitis, and gastrointestinal upset. Vaginal—nausea, vomiting, diarrhea, constipation, abdominal pain, dizziness, headache, and fainting.

Drug Interactions

• Clindamycin and erythromycin may antagonize each other; these drugs should not be taken together.

• The absorption of clindamycin capsules into the blood-stream is delayed by Kaolin-Pectin Suspension, prescribed for diarrhea.

Food Interactions

Take the oral medication with a full glass of water or with food to prevent irritation of the stomach and intestine.

Usual Dose

Capsules
   Adult: 150–450 mg every 6 hours.
   Child: 4–11 mg per lb. of body weight a day, in divided doses. No child should be given less than 37.5 mg 3 times a day, regardless of weight.

Topical Lotion
Apply enough to cover the affected area(s) lightly twice a day.

Vaginal Cream
Insert one applicator's worth at bedtime for 7 consecutive days.

Special Information

Unsupervised use of clindamycin can lead to secondary infections from susceptible organisms, such as fungi. As with any antibiotic treatment, take this drug for the full course of therapy as indicated by your physician.

If you develop severe diarrhea or abdominal pain, call your doctor at once.

Women using the vaginal cream should refrain from vaginal intercourse until the course of treatment is complete.

If you miss a dose of oral clindamycin, take it as soon as possible. If it is almost time for your next dose, double that dose and go back to your regular dosage schedule.

Special Populations

Pregnancy/Breast-feeding
This drug crosses into fetal blood circulation but has not been found to cause birth defects. When the drug is considered crucial by your doctor, its potential benefits must be carefully weighed against its risks.

Clindamycin passes into breast milk but has caused no problems among breast-fed infants. You should consider bottle-feeding your baby if taking clindamycin by mouth.

Seniors
Seniors with other illnesses may be unable to tolerate diarrhea and other clindamycin side effects. Be sure to report any clindamycin complications at once.

Generic Name

Clofibrate (cloe-FIH-brate) [G]

Brand Name
Atromid-S

Type of Drug
Anti-hyperlipidemic (blood-fat reducer).

Prescribed for
High blood levels of triglycerides; also prescribed for high cholesterol and LDL cholesterol levels and for diabetes insipidus.

General Information
Although we do not know exactly how clofibrate works, we do know that it works on both blood cholesterol and triglycerides by interfering with the natural systems that make these blood fats and by increasing the rate at which they are removed from the body.

While clofibrate is used to lower cholesterol and LDL cholesterol levels, it is less predictable and effective than other cholesterol-lowering medications. It is usually prescribed for people whose blood fats remain high despite changes in diet, weight control, and exercise. Clofibrate is generally much more effective in reducing blood triglycerides than cholesterol. Clofibrate has also been used to treat diabetes insipidus; however, this condition is usually treated with other drugs.

Lower blood-fat levels are considered beneficial in reducing the risk of heart disease. But people with high cholesterol and low triglycerides should not take clofibrate because it is most effective in lowering triglycerides.

Clofibrate is only part of the therapy for high blood-fat levels. Diet and weight control are also very important. This drug is not a substitute for exercise or dietary restrictions that have been prescribed by your doctor.

Cautions and Warnings

Clofibrate causes **liver cancer** in rats.

It should be used with caution if you are **allergic** to the drug or if you have **cirrhosis of the liver, heart disease, gallstones**—clofibrate users have twice the risk of developing gallstones as people who do not take this drug—**liver disease,** an **underactive thyroid,** or **stomach ulcer.**

People with **kidney disease** may take clofibrate as long as the daily dosage is calibrated for the degree of kidney function loss.

Clofibrate does not reduce the number of fatal heart attacks. A 1978 study suggests that taking clofibrate regularly for many years increases the risk of dying from noncardiac causes, but this has not been confirmed by more recent research. Another clofibrate study shows an increase in side effects, including abnormal heart rhythms and intermittent leg pains due to blood-vessel spasm. Clofibrate should be used only by people whose other efforts to solve their triglyceride or cholesterol problems have not worked.

Possible Side Effects

▼ Most common: nausea.

▼ Less common: vomiting; loose stools; upset stomach; gas; abdominal pain; liver enlargement; gastric irritation; mouth sores; headache; dizziness; tiredness; cramped muscles; aching and weakness; rash; itching; brittle hair or hair loss; abnormal heart rhythms; blood clots in the lungs or veins; gallstones, especially in people who have taken clofibrate for a long time; decreased sex drive; and impotence.

If you suffer from angina pectoris (condition characterized by brief attacks of chest pain), clofibrate may increase or decrease this pain. It may cause you to produce smaller quantities of urine than usual and has

---

Possible Side Effects *(continued)*

been associated with blood in the urine, tiredness, weakness, drowsiness, and mildly increased appetite and weight gain. Some experts claim that clofibrate causes stomach ulcer, stomach bleeding, arthritis-like symptoms, uncontrollable muscle spasm, increased perspiration, blurred vision, breast enlargement, and effects on the blood.

Drug Interactions

• If you are taking an anticoagulant (blood thinner) and get a new prescription for clofibrate, your anticoagulant dosage may have to be reduced by up to one-half. It is essential that your doctor know that you are taking both drugs so that the proper dosage adjustments can be made.

• Taking clofibrate with an anticholesterol drug such as lovastatin or pravastatin may result in a reaction that leads to skeletal muscle destruction.

• The effect of chenodiol may be reduced when it is taken together with clofibrate.

• Clofibrate may increase the effects of oral antidiabetics and any drug used to treat diabetes insipidus including carbamazepine, chlorpropamide, desmopressin, diuretics, and hormone replacement products.

• Contraceptive drugs may interfere with the effectiveness of clofibrate.

• Probenecid may increase the effectiveness and side effects of clofibrate.

• Rifampin may increase the rate at which clofibrate is broken down in the liver, reducing its effectiveness.

• Clofibrate may interfere with a number of blood tests. Make sure your doctor knows that you are taking the drug before any blood tests are done.

Food Interactions

Take this drug with food or milk to prevent upset stomach.

Usual Dose

2000 mg a day.

Overdosage

Overdose symptoms are most likely to be severe side effects.

Take the overdose victim to a hospital emergency room.
ALWAYS bring the prescription bottle or container with you.

Special Information

Call your doctor if you develop chest pain, breathing difficulties, abnormal heart rates, severe stomach pain with nausea
and vomiting, fever and chills, sore throat, swelling of the
legs, weight gain, blood in the urine, changes in urinary
habits, or if other side effects become intolerable.

Follow your diet; limit your intake of alcoholic beverages.

Clofibrate should be stored at room temperature in a dry
place—not in a bathroom medicine cabinet—to protect this
drug's soft gelatin covering.

Regular visits to your doctor are necessary while taking
clofibrate to be sure that the drug is still working and to be
screened with blood counts and liver function tests, which
may uncover possible side effects.

If you forget a dose of clofibrate, take it as soon as possible.
If it is almost time for your next dose, skip the one you forgot
and continue with your regular schedule. Do not take a
double dose.

Special Populations

Pregnancy/Breast-feeding

Pregnant women should not take clofibrate because large
amounts of this drug pass into the bloodstream of the fetus,
which cannot break it down. If you are planning to become
pregnant, stop taking clofibrate several months before trying
to conceive.

Clofibrate passes into breast milk. Nursing mothers who
must take clofibrate should bottle-feed their infants.

Seniors

Seniors generally may take clofibrate without special restriction. Age-related loss of kidney function may require your
doctor to adjust your daily dosage.

Generic Name

Clonazepam (klon-AH-zeh-pam)

Brand Name

Klonopin

Type of Drug

Anticonvulsant.

Prescribed for

Petit mal and other seizure; also prescribed for panic attacks, periodic leg movements during sleep, speaking difficulty associated with Parkinson's disease, acute manic episodes, nerve pain, and schizophrenia.

General Information

Clonazepam is a member of the family of drugs known as benzodiazepines; this group also includes diazepam, chlordiazepoxide, flurazepam, and triazolam. Unlike the other benzodiazepines, clonazepam is not used as a sedative or hypnotic. It is used only to control petit mal seizures in people who have not responded to other drug treatments, such as ethosuximide. Clonazepam is generally considered safe and effective for such seizures and shares many of the same side effects, precautions, and interactions as its benzodiazepine cousins.

Unfortunately, people commonly become tolerant to the effects of clonazepam within about 3 months of starting it. This happens because of the body's natural tendency to become more efficient in breaking the drug down and eliminating it from circulation. Your doctor may have to raise your clonazepam dosage periodically to maintain the drug's effect.

Cautions and Warnings

Do not take clonazepam if you are **sensitive** or **allergic** to it or another benzodiazepine.

When stopping clonazepam treatments, it is essential that the drug be discontinued gradually to allow for safe withdrawal. Abrupt discontinuance of any benzodiazepine, including clonazepam, may lead to **drug withdrawal symptoms**. In the case of clonazepam, the withdrawal symptoms can include severe seizures. Other symptoms include tremors, abdominal cramps, muscle cramps, vomiting, and increased sweating.

Clonazepam should be used with caution if you have a chronic **respiratory illness**, since the drug tends to increase salivation and other respiratory secretions and can make breathing more labored. Other conditions in which benzodiazepines should be avoided are severe **depression**, severe

lung disease, **sleep apnea** (intermittent cessation of breathing during sleep), **liver disease**, **alcoholism**, and **kidney disease**. These conditions may exacerbate the depressive effects of benzodiazepines, and such effects may be detrimental to your overall condition.

Clonazepam can aggravate **narrow-angle glaucoma**, but if you have open-angle glaucoma, you may take it. Check with your doctor.

Possible Side Effects

▼ Most common: drowsiness, poor muscle control, and behavioral changes.

▼ Rare: abnormal eye movement, loss of voice and/or the ability to express a thought, double vision, coma, a glassy-eyed appearance, headache, temporary paralysis, labored breathing, shortness of breath, slurred speech, tremors, dizziness, fainting, confusion, depression, forgetfulness, hallucination, increased sex drive, hysteria, sleeplessness, psychosis, suicidal acts, chest congestion, stuffy nose, heart palpitations, hair loss or gain, rash, swelling of the face or ankles, increase or decrease in appetite or body weight, coated tongue, constipation, diarrhea, involuntary passing of feces, dry mouth, stomach irritation, nausea, sore gums, difficulty urinating, pain upon urination, bed-wetting, nighttime urination, muscle weakness or pain, reduced red- and white-blood-cell and platelet levels, enlarged liver, liver inflammation, dehydration, a deterioration in general health, fever, and swollen lymph glands.

Drug Interactions

• The depressant effects of clonazepam are increased by tranquilizers, sleeping pills, narcotic pain relievers, antihistamines, alcohol, monoamine oxidase inhibitors (MAOIs), tricyclic antidepressants, and other anticonvulsants.

• The combination of valproic acid and clonazepam may produce severe petit mal seizures.

• Phenobarbital or phenytoin may reduce clonazepam's effectiveness by increasing the rate at which it is eliminated from the body.

• Smoking may reduce clonazepam's effectiveness.

• Clonazepam treatment may increase the requirement for

other anticonvulsant drugs in people who suffer from multiple types of seizures.

• The effects of clonazepam may be prolonged when it is taken with cimetidine, oral contraceptives, disulfiram, fluoxetine, isoniazid, ketoconazole, metoprolol, probenecid, propoxyphene, propranolol, rifampin, or valproic acid.

• Theophylline may reduce clonazapam's sedative effects.

• If you take antacids, separate them from your clonazepam dose by at least 1 hour to prevent them from interfering with the passage of clonazepam into the bloodstream.

• Clonazepam may increase blood levels of digoxin and the chances for digoxin toxicity.

• The effect of levodopa may be decreased if it is taken with clonazepam.

Food Interactions

Clonazepam is best taken on an empty stomach but may be taken with food if it upsets your stomach.

Usual Dose

Adult and Child (age 10 and over): starting dose—0.5 mg 3 times a day. The dose is increased by 0.5–1 mg every 3 days until seizures are controlled or side effects develop. The maximum daily dose is 20 mg. Other uses for clonazepam involve doses from 0.5–16 mg a day, depending on the condition being treated and its severity.

Child (under age 10, or below 66 lbs.): starting dose—0.004–0.013 mg per lb. of body weight a day. The dosage can be increased gradually to a maximum of 0.045–0.09 mg per lb. of body weight.

The dosage of clonazepam must be reduced in people with impaired kidney function because this drug is released from the body primarily via the kidneys.

Overdosage

Clonazepam overdose may cause confusion, coma, poor reflexes, sleepiness, low blood pressure, labored breathing, and other depressive effects. If the overdose is discovered within a few minutes and the victim is still conscious, it may be helpful to make him or her vomit with ipecac syrup—available at any pharmacy—to remove any remaining medication from the stomach. All victims of clonazepam overdose must be taken to a hospital emergency room. ALWAYS bring the prescription bottle or container with you.

Special Information

Clonazepam may interfere with your ability to drive a car or perform other complex tasks because it can cause drowsiness and difficulty in concentrating.

Your doctor should perform periodic blood counts and liver function tests while you are taking this drug to check for possible side effects.

Do not suddenly stop taking clonazepam, because doing so could result in severe seizures. The dosage must be discontinued gradually by your doctor.

If you miss a dose and it is within an hour of that dose time, take it right away. Otherwise, skip the dose you forgot and go back to your regular schedule. Do not take a double dose.

Carry identification or wear a bracelet indicating that you have a seizure disorder for which you take clonazepam.

Special Populations

Pregnancy/Breast-feeding

Clonazepam crosses into the fetal circulation and can affect the fetus. Clonazepam should be avoided by women who are or might be pregnant. When the drug is considered crucial by your doctor, its potential benefits must be carefully weighed against its risks.

Some reports suggest a strong link between anticonvulsant drugs and birth defects, though most of the information pertains to phenytoin and phenobarbital, not clonazepam. It is also possible that the epileptic condition itself or genetic factors common to people with seizure disorders may figure in the higher incidence of birth defects.

Mothers taking clonazepam should bottle-feed their infants because of the chance that the drug will pass into their breast milk and affect the baby.

Seniors

Seniors, especially those with liver or kidney disease, are more sensitive to the effects of this drug—especially dizziness and drowsiness—and may require smaller doses. Follow your doctor's directions and report any side effects at once.

Generic Name

Clonidine (KLAH-nih-dene) Ⓖ

Brand Name

Catapres

Type of Drug

Antihypertensive.

Prescribed for

High blood pressure, including hypertensive emergency (diastolic blood pressure over 120); also used for excess sweating, childhood growth delay, attention-deficit hyperactivity disorder (ADHD), Tourette's syndrome, migraine headache, ulcerative colitis, painful or difficult menstruation, flushing related to menopause, diagnosis of pheochromocytoma (adrenal gland tumor), diabetic diarrhea, smoking cessation, methadone and opiate detoxification, withdrawal from alcohol and benzodiazepines such as Valium, nerve pain following herpes attack, and allergic reactions in the presence of asthma triggered by external sources. Clonidine by epidural injection has been used to treat cancer pain in people who cannot tolerate epidural narcotic analgesics.

General Information

Clonidine acts in the brain to stimulate a set of nerve endings called alpha-adrenergic receptors. Initially, this stimulation causes a minor increase in blood pressure. But once clonidine produces its major effect on alpha receptors in the brain, it causes dilation (widening) of certain blood vessels, thus decreasing blood pressure. Clonidine works very quickly, causing a decline in blood pressure within 1 hour. Beyond its blood-pressure-lowering effects, the other effects of clonidine may be traced to its stimulation of alpha receptors throughout the body.

Cautions and Warnings

Do not take clonidine or any product that contains clonidine if you are **allergic** to the drug. People who have had a **recent heart attack** or have **chronic kidney failure, cardiac insufficiency,** or **disease of blood vessels in the brain** should avoid clonidine.

Some people develop a **tolerance** of their clonidine dosage. If this happens, your blood pressure may increase and your doctor may have to prescribe a higher dose.

If you abruptly stop taking clonidine, you may experience an **unusual increase in blood pressure** accompanied by **agitation, headache,** and **nervousness**. These effects can be reversed by resuming clonidine therapy or by taking another drug to lower your blood pressure. Never stop taking clonidine without your doctor's knowledge. Abruptly stopping this drug may cause severe reactions, possibly even death. Be sure you always have an adequate supply of clonidine on hand.

Animal studies of clonidine show a tendency toward degeneration of the retina. People taking this drug on a regular basis should have their **eyes examined regularly**.

If you are going to have **surgery**, your doctor will continue your clonidine therapy until about 4 hours before surgery and resume it as soon as possible afterward.

People who develop **skin sensitivity** (symptoms include rash, itching, and swelling) to Catapres-TTS, the transdermal patch form of clonidine, may find that they experience the same reactions with oral clonidine.

Possible Side Effects

Tablets

▼ Most common: dry mouth, drowsiness, constipation, and sedation.

▼ Common: dizziness, headache, and fatigue. These effects tend to diminish within 4 to 6 weeks.

▼ Less common: appetite loss, swelling or pain in the glands of the throat, nausea, vomiting, weight gain, blood-sugar elevation, breast pain or enlargement, worsening of congestive heart failure, heart palpitations, rapid heartbeat, dizziness when rising quickly from a sitting or lying position, painful blood-vessel spasm, abnormal heart rhythms, electrocardiogram changes, feeling unwell, changes in dream patterns, nightmares, difficulty sleeping, hallucinations, delirium, anxiety, depression, nervousness, restlessness, headache, rash, hives, thinning or loss of scalp hair, difficult or painful urination, nighttime urination, retaining urine, decrease or loss of sex drive, weakness, muscle or joint pain, leg cramps,

Possible Side Effects *(continued)*

increased alcohol sensitivity, dryness and burning of the
eyes, dry nose, loss of color, and fever.

Transdermal Patch
   ▼ Most common: dry mouth and drowsiness.
   ▼ Less common: constipation, nausea, changes in
sense of taste, dry throat, fatigue, headache, lethargy,
changes in sleep patterns, nervousness, dizziness, impotence, sexual difficulties, and mild skin reactions including itching, swelling, contact dermatitis, discoloration,
burning, peeling, throbbing, white patches, and generalized rash. Rashes of the face and tongue have also
occurred but cannot be specifically tied to transdermal
clonidine.

Drug Interactions

• Avoid alcohol, barbiturates, sedatives, and tranquilizers
because clonidine's depressive effect will increase the depressive effects of these drugs.

• Antidepressants including tricyclic antidepressants, some
appetite suppressants, estrogens, stimulants, indomethacin
and other nonsteroidal anti-inflammatory drugs (NSAIDs),
and prazosin may counteract the effects of clonidine.

• Taking clonidine together with a beta blocker may increase the severity of a drug-withdrawal reaction and rebound high blood pressure. In addition, this combination
may actually cause blood pressure to rise.

• Combining verapamil and clonidine may lead to very low
blood pressure and atrioventricular (AV) block (abnormality in
the heartbeat patterns).

Food Interactions

Clonidine tablets are best taken on an empty stomach, but
may be taken with food if they upset your stomach.

Usual Dose

Tablets
   Adult: high blood pressure—100 mcg twice a day to start;
may be raised by 100–200 mcg a day until maximum control
is achieved. Dosage must be tailored to individual needs. It is

recommended that no one take more than 2400 mcg a day. Other uses—100–900 mcg a day, or up to 0.8 mcg per lb. of body weight in divided doses.

Senior: Start with a lower dose and increase more slowly.

Child: 5–25 mcg a day for every 2.2 lbs. of body weight, divided into 4 doses given every 6 hours.

Transdermal Patch

Adult: 100 mcg delivered daily from a patch applied once every 7 days. Up to 2 300-mcg patches may be needed to control blood pressure. Transdermal dosage exceeding 600 mcg a day has not been shown to increase effectiveness.

Child: not recommended.

Overdosage

Symptoms of clonidine overdose are slow heartbeat, nervous system depression, very slow breathing or no breathing at all, low body temperature, pinpoint pupils, seizures, lethargy, agitation, irritability, nausea, vomiting, abnormal heart rhythms, mild increases in blood pressure followed by a rapid drop in blood pressure, dizziness, weakness, loss of reflexes, and vomiting. Victims should be taken to a hospital emergency room immediately. ALWAYS bring the prescription bottle or container with you.

Special Information

Clonidine causes drowsiness in about a third of people who take it. Be extremely careful while driving or operating any hazardous appliance or machine. This effect is prominent during the first few weeks of clonidine therapy, then tends to decrease.

Do not take over-the-counter cough and cold medications unless directed by your doctor.

Call your doctor if you become depressed or have vivid dreams or nightmares while taking clonidine, or if you develop swelling in your feet or legs, paleness or coldness in your fingertips or toes, or any other persistent or bothersome side effect.

Apply the transdermal patch to a hairless area of skin such as the upper arm or torso. Use a different skin site each time. If the patch becomes loose, apply the supplied adhesive directly over it. If the patch falls off before 7 days are up, apply a new one. Do not remove the patch while bathing.

If you miss a dose of oral clonidine, take it as soon as

possible and then go back to your regular schedule. If you miss 2 or more consecutive doses, consult your doctor; missed doses may cause your blood pressure to go up and cause severe adverse effects. Do not take a double dose.

Special Populations

Pregnancy/Breast-feeding

Animal studies show that clonidine may damage the fetus in doses as low as ⅓ the maximum human dose. Clonidine passes into the fetal bloodstream. Women who are or might be pregnant should only take clonidine after talking with their doctor about the risks and possible benefits of taking it.

Clonidine passes into breast milk, but no effects on nursing infants have been noted. Nursing mothers should avoid this drug or bottle-feed their babies.

Seniors

Seniors are more susceptible to the effects of this drug and should begin with lower-than-normal doses.

Generic Name

Clorazepate (klor-AZ-uh-pate) G

Brand Names

Tranxene-SD   Tranxene-T-Tab

Type of Drug

Benzodiazepine tranquilizer.

Prescribed for

Anxiety, tension, fatigue, and agitation; also prescribed for irritable bowel syndrome and panic attacks.

General Information

Clorazepate dipotassium is a member of a group of drugs known as benzodiazepines, used as antianxiety agents, as anticonvulsants, or as sedatives. Some are more suited to a specific role because of differences in their chemical makeup that give them greater activity in a certain area; others have particular characteristics that make them more desirable for certain functions. Often, individual drugs are limited by the applications for which their research has been sponsored.

Benzodiazepines all directly affect the brain. They can relax you and make you more tranquil or sleepier, or they can slow nervous system transmissions in such a way as to act as an anticonvulsant: The exact effect varies according to drug and dosage. Many doctors prefer benzodiazepines to other drugs that can be used to similar effect because they tend to be safer, have fewer side effects, and usually work as well, if not better.

Cautions and Warnings

Do not take clorazepate if you know you are **sensitive** or **allergic** to it or to another benzodiazepine drug, including clonazepam.

Clorazepate can aggravate **narrow-angle glaucoma**, but you may take it if you have open-angle glaucoma. Check with your doctor.

Other conditions in which clorazepate should be avoided are: severe **depression**, severe **lung disease, sleep apnea** (intermittent cessation of breathing during sleep), **liver disease, drunkenness,** and **kidney disease**. In each of these conditions, the depressive effects of clorazepate may be enhanced and/or could be detrimental to your overall condition.

Clorazepate should not be taken by **psychotic patients** because it is not effective for them and can trigger unusual excitement, stimulation, and rage.

Clorazepate is not intended to be used for more than 3 to 4 months at a time. Your doctor should reassess your condition before continuing your prescription beyond that time.

Clorazepate may be **addictive**. You can experience drug withdrawal symptoms if you suddenly stop taking it after as little as 4 to 6 weeks of treatment. Withdrawal generally begins with increased feelings of anxiety; it continues with tingling in the extremities, sensitivity to bright lights or to the sun, long periods of sleep or sleeplessness, a metallic taste, flulike illness, fatigue, difficulty concentrating, restlessness, appetite loss, nausea, irritability, headache, dizziness, sweating, muscle tension or cramps, tremors, and feeling uncomfortable or ill at ease. Other major withdrawal symptoms include confusion, abnormal perception of movement, depersonalization, paranoid delusions, hallucinations, psychotic reactions, muscle twitching, seizures, and memory loss.

Possible Side Effects

Weakness and confusion may occur, especially in seniors and in those who are more sickly.

▼ Most common: mild drowsiness during the first few days of therapy.

▼ Less common: confusion, depression, lethargy, disorientation, headache, inactivity, slurred speech, stupor, dizziness, tremors, constipation, dry mouth, nausea, inability to control urination, sexual difficulties, irregular menstrual cycle, changes in heart rhythm, low blood pressure, fluid retention, blurred or double vision, itching, rash, hiccups, nervousness, inability to fall asleep, and occasional liver dysfunction. If you have any of these symptoms, stop taking the medicine and contact your doctor immediately.

▼ Rare: diarrhea, coated tongue, sore gums, vomiting, appetite changes, difficulty swallowing, increased salivation, upset stomach, changes in sex drive, urinary difficulties, changes in heart rate, palpitations, swelling, stuffy nose, difficulty hearing, hair loss or gain, sweating, fever, tingling in the hands or feet, breast pain, muscle disturbances, breathing difficulties, changes in blood components, and joint pain.

Drug Interactions

• Clorazepate is a central-nervous-system depressant. Avoid alcohol, other tranquilizers, narcotics, barbiturates, monoamine oxidase inhibitors (MAOIs), antihistamines, and antidepressants. Taking clorazepate with these drugs may result in excessive depression, tiredness, sleepiness, breathing difficulties, or related symptoms.

• Smoking may reduce the effectiveness of clorazepate by increasing the rate at which it is broken down by the body.

• The effects of clorazepate may be prolonged when it is taken together with cimetidine, oral contraceptives, disulfiram, fluoxetine, isoniazid, ketoconazole, metoprolol, probenecid, propoxyphene, propranolol, rifampin, or valproic acid. Theophylline may reduce clorazepate's sedative effects.

• If you take antacids, separate them from your clorazepate dose by at least 1 hour to prevent them from interfering with the absorption of clorazepate into the bloodstream.

- Clorazepate may increase blood levels of digoxin and the chances of digoxin toxicity.
- The effect of levodopa may be decreased if it is taken together with clorazepate.
- Combining clorazepate with phenytoin may increase phenytoin blood concentrations and the chances of phenytoin toxicity.

Food Interactions

Clorazepate is best taken on an empty stomach, but it may be taken with food if it upsets your stomach.

Usual Dose

Immediate-release
   Adult and Child (age 9 and over): 15–60 mg daily. The average dose is 30 mg in divided quantities, but dosage must be adjusted to individual response for maximum effect.
   Child (under age 9): not recommended.

Sustained-release
   Adult: The sustained-release form of clorazepate may be given as a single dose, either 11.25 or 22.5 mg, once every 24 hours.
   Child: not recommended.

Overdosage

Symptoms of overdose are confusion, sleepiness, poor coordination, lack of response to pain such as a pin prick, loss of reflexes, shallow breathing, low blood pressure, and coma. The victim should be taken to a hospital emergency room. ALWAYS bring the prescription bottle or container with you.

Special Information

Clorazepate can cause tiredness, drowsiness, inability to concentrate, or similar symptoms. Be careful if you are driving, operating machinery, or performing other activities that require concentration.

People taking clorazepate for more than 3 or 4 months at a time may develop drug withdrawal reactions if the medication is stopped suddenly (see "Cautions and Warnings").

If you forget a dose of clorazepate, take it as soon as you remember. If it is almost time for your next dose, skip the dose you forgot and continue with your regular schedule. Do not take a double dose.

Special Populations

Pregnancy/Breast-feeding

Clorazepate may cross into fetal circulation and may cause birth defects if taken during the first 3 months of pregnancy. Avoid this drug if you are or might be pregnant.

Clorazepate may pass into breast milk. Since infants break down the drug more slowly than adults, they may accumulate enough clorazepate in their systems to produce undesirable effects. Nursing mothers who must take clorazepate should bottle-feed their babies.

Seniors

Seniors, especially those with liver or kidney disease, are more sensitive to the effects of clorazepate and generally require smaller doses to achieve the same effect. Follow your doctor's directions and report any side effects at once.

Generic Name

Clotrimazole (kloe-TRIM-uh-zole) Ⓖ

Brand Names

Lotrimin   Mycelex

Type of Drug

Antifungal.

Prescribed for

Fungal infections of the mouth, skin, and vaginal tract.

General Information

Clotrimazole is useful against a wide variety of fungus organisms that other drugs do not affect. The exact way in which clotrimazole produces its effect is not known.

Cautions and Warnings

If clotrimazole causes local **itching** and/or **irritation**, stop using it. Do not use clotrimazole in your eyes. **Proper diagnosis** is essential for effective treatment. Do not use this product without first consulting your doctor.

Possible Side Effects

Side effects do not occur very often and are usually mild.
▼ Most common: cream or solution—redness, stinging, blistering, peeling, itching, and swelling of local areas. Vaginal tablets—mild burning, skin rash, mild cramps, frequent urination, and burning or itching in a sexual partner. Lozenges—stomach cramps or pain, diarrhea, nausea, and vomiting.

Drug Interactions

None known.

Food Interactions

The oral form of clotrimazole is best taken on an empty stomach, at least 1 hour before or 2 hours after meals. However, you may take it with food as long as you allow the tablet to dissolve in your mouth like a lozenge.

Usual Dose

Topical Cream and Solution: Apply to affected areas morning and night.

Vaginal Cream: 1 applicator's worth at bedtime for 7–14 days.

Vaginal Tablet: 1 tablet inserted into the vagina at bedtime for 7 days, or 2 tablets a day for 3 days.

Lozenge: 1 lozenge 5 times a day for 2 weeks or more.

Overdosage

This drug is not well absorbed into the blood. Call your local poison control center for more information.

Special Information

If treating a vaginal infection, you should refrain from sexual activity or be sure that your partner wears a condom until the treatment is finished. Call your doctor if burning or itching develops or if the condition does not show improvement within 7 days.

If you are using the vaginal cream, you may want to wear a sanitary napkin to avoid staining your clothing.

Dissolve the lozenge slowly in the mouth.

This medicine must be taken on consecutive days. If you forget to take a dose of oral clotrimazole, take it as soon as you remember. Do not double your dose.

Special Populations

Pregnancy/Breast-feeding

No problems have been found in infants born to women who used clotrimazole during their pregnancies. Women who are or might be pregnant should talk to their doctors about the medication's risks and benefits. Women who are in the first 3 months of pregnancy should use this drug only if directed to do so by their doctors. If you are pregnant, your doctor may want you to insert vaginal tablets by hand rather than use a vaginal applicator.

This drug is poorly absorbed into the bloodstream and is not likely to pass into breast milk. Nursing mothers need not worry about adverse effects on their infants while taking clotrimazole.

Seniors

Seniors may use this medication without special restriction.

Generic Name

Clozapine (KLOE-zuh-pene)

Brand Name

Clozaril

Type of Drug

Antipsychotic.

Prescribed for

Severe schizophrenia that does not respond to other medication.

General Information

Clozapine is a unique antipsychotic that has the capacity to treat people who do not respond to other drugs or who suffer from severe side effects of those drugs. Chemically, it is a distant cousin of the benzodiazepine tranquilizers and anticonvulsants, but it works by a mechanism that differs from those of other antipsychotic drugs.

A very small number of people who take clozapine develop a rapid drop in their white-blood-cell count, a condition called agranulocytosis. This effect usually reverses itself when the drug is stopped, but the drug must be stopped AS SOON AS IT IS DISCOVERED. An unusually large number of people who have developed clozapine agranulocytosis in the U.S. are of Eastern European Jewish descent, but the association is not very strong. Most cases of agranulocytosis occur between week 4 and week 10 of treatment. It is essential that blood samples be taken approximately every week and for 4 weeks after the drug is stopped to watch for this effect. Also, because of the possibility of agranulocytosis, no one should start taking clozapine until he or she has tried at least 2 other antipsychotic medicines to make sure that nothing else will work.

Some people taking antipsychotic drugs develop tardive dyskinesia, a potentially irreversible condition marked by uncontrollable movements. Tardive dyskinesia has not been seen in patients taking clozapine, a major advantage of this drug over other antipsychotic medicines. However, there is still a possibility that this set of symptoms could occur with clozapine.

Cautions and Warnings

Women, seniors, people with **serious illnesses,** those who are **emaciated,** those with a history of **diseases affecting the white blood cells,** or those who are taking **other medication** that could affect white blood cells may be more susceptible to clozapine agranulocytosis. There is no easy way to know who is likely to develop clozapine agranulocytosis.

About 5% of people taking the drug experience a **seizure** in the first year of treatment. Seizure is most likely to occur at higher drug doses.

People with **heart disease** should be carefully monitored while on clozapine because of possible cardiac risks.

A more serious set of side effects, known as **neuroleptic malignant syndrome (NMS),** includes a high fever and has been associated with clozapine when it is used together with lithium or other drugs. The symptoms that constitute NMS include muscle rigidity, mental changes, irregular pulse or blood pressure, increased sweating, and abnormal heart rhythm. NMS is potentially fatal and requires immediate medical attention.

Use this drug with caution if you have **glaucoma, prostate problems**, or **liver, kidney, or heart disease**.

Clozapine may interfere with mental or physical abilities because of the **sedation** it usually causes during the first few weeks of treatment.

Possible Side Effects

▼ Most common: rapid heartbeat, low blood pressure, dizziness, fainting, drowsiness or sedation, salivation, and constipation.

▼ Less common: headache, tremor, sleep disturbance, restlessness, slow muscle motions, absence of movement, agitation, convulsions, rigidity, restlessness, confusion, sweating, dry mouth, visual disturbances, high blood pressure, nausea, vomiting, heartburn or abdominal discomfort, fever, and weight gain.

▼ Rare: agranulocytosis (symptoms include fever with or without chills, sore throat, and sores or white spots on the lips or mouth) and other changes in blood components, electrocardiogram changes, fatigue, sleeplessness, rapid movements, general weakness, muscle weakness, lethargy, slurred speech, tremors, depression, seizure, tardive dyskinesia (symptoms include lip smacking or puckering, puffing of the cheeks, rapid or wormlike tongue movement, uncontrolled chewing motions, and uncontrolled arm and leg movements), NMS (symptoms include convulsions, breathing difficulties, and back, neck, or leg pain), muscle spasm, angina, diarrhea, abnormal liver function, appetite loss, loss of bladder control, abnormal ejaculation, frequent or infrequent urination, the feeling of having to urinate, breathing difficulties, sore throat, stuffy nose, and numbness or soreness of the tongue.

Drug Interactions

• Clozapine's anticholinergic effects—blurred vision, dry mouth, and confusion—may be enhanced by interaction with other anticholinergics, such as tricyclic antidepressants like amitriptyline.

• Drugs that reduce blood pressure may enhance the blood-pressure-lowering effects of clozapine.

• Alcohol and other nervous system depressants, including benzodiazepines and other antianxiety drugs, may enhance clozapine's sedative actions. There is at least one known case of a patient dying while taking a combination of diazepam and clozapine.

• Clozapine may increase blood levels of digoxin, warfarin, heparin, and phenytoin.

• The combination of lithium and clozapine may cause seizures, confusion, and NMS (see "Cautions and Warnings").

• Cigarette smoking may increase the rate at which the liver breaks down clozapine, altering dosage requirements. This is usually a problem only if a person changes his or her smoking habits while taking the drug.

Food Interactions

None known.

Usual Dose

Starting dose—25 mg 2 times a day. Maintenance dose—generally, 300–450 mg a day. Dosage may be increased gradually to a daily maximum of 900 mg if required.

Overdosage

Usual symptoms of overdose are delirium, drowsiness, changes in heart rhythm, unusual excitement, nervousness, restlessness, hallucinations, excessive salivation, dizziness or fainting, slow or irregular breathing, and coma. Overdose victims must be taken to a hospital emergency room immediately. ALWAYS bring the prescription bottle or container with you.

Special Information

Clozapine may cause a fever during the first few weeks of treatment. Generally, the fever is not important, but it may occasionally be necessary to stop treatment due to persistent fever, a decision that would be made by your doctor.

Regular blood tests are necessary to monitor blood composition for any changes that might be caused by clozapine.

Call your doctor at once if you develop lethargy or weakness, a flu-like infection, sore throat, feelings of ill health, sweating, muscle rigidity, mental changes, irregular pulse or blood pressure, mouth ulcers, or dry mouth that lasts for more than 2 weeks. Dry mouth, a common side effect of clozapine, may be countered by using gum, candy, ice, or a saliva substitute such as Orex or Moi-Stir.

Do not stop taking clozapine without your doctor's knowledge and approval, because a gradual dosage reduction may be necessary to prevent side effects.

Avoid alcohol or any other nervous system depressant while taking clozapine.

Some of the side effects of clozapine—drowsiness, blurred vision, or seizures—may interfere with the performance of complex tasks like driving or operating hazardous equipment.

While taking clozapine, rapidly rising from a sitting or lying position may cause you to become dizzy or faint.

If you take clozapine twice a day and forget a dose, take it as soon as you remember. If it is almost time for your next dose, take one dose as soon as you remember and another in 5 or 6 hours, then go back to your regular schedule. If you take clozapine 3 times a day and forget a dose, take it as soon as you remember. If it is almost time for your next dose, take one dose as soon as you remember and another in 3 or 4 hours, then go back to your regular schedule. Never take a double dose.

Special Populations

Pregnancy/Breast-feeding
This drug should be used during pregnancy only if your doctor determines that it is absolutely necessary.

Clozapine may pass into breast milk. Nursing mothers who must take this drug should bottle-feed their babies.

Seniors
Seniors may be more sensitive than younger adults to the side effects of clozapine, such as dizziness on rapidly rising from a sitting or lying position, confusion, and excitability. Older men are also more likely to have prostate problems, a reason to be cautious with clozapine.

Generic Name

Codeine (KOE-dene) Ⓖ

Brand Name
Only available in generic form.

The information in this profile also applies to the following drug:

Generic Ingredient: Fentanyl
Duragesic

Type of Drug

Narcotic.

Prescribed for

Relief of moderate pain and cough suppression.

General Information

Codeine is a narcotic drug with pain-relieving and cough-suppressing activity. As an analgesic it is useful for mild to moderate pain. The pain-relieving effect of 30 mg to 60 mg of codeine is equal to approximately 650 mg, or 2 tablets, of aspirin. Codeine may be less active than aspirin for types of pain associated with inflammation because aspirin reduces inflammation and codeine does not. Codeine suppresses the cough reflex but does not cure the underlying cause of the cough. In fact, sometimes it may not be desirable to overly suppress a cough because cough suppression reduces your ability to naturally eliminate excess mucus produced during a cold or allergy attack. Other narcotic cough suppressants are stronger than codeine, but codeine remains the best cough medication available today.

Fentanyl is a potent pain reliever that can be substituted for other narcotic drugs, though drug dosage must be individualized to your specific needs. The patch form of fentanyl was developed because it has a shorter length of action than any other narcotic pain reliever. The patch delivers fentanyl to the bloodstream at a steady rate so that a new patch need only be applied about once every 3 days. The liquid and lozenge forms of fentanyl are given to children being prepared for surgery. These forms should only be used under controlled circumstances because of the chance of side effects and overdose if too much medication is taken. Low doses of fentanyl relieve pain and larger doses cause a loss of consciousness and breathing difficulties.

Cautions and Warnings

Do not take narcotics if you know you are **allergic** or **sensitive** to them. Use narcotics with extreme caution if you suffer from **asthma** or other **breathing problems.** Long-term use of narcotics may cause drug **dependence or addiction.** Narcotics may make it difficult to monitor the progress of people who have suffered head injuries. Narcotic pain relievers should be used with caution in these patients.

Possible Side Effects

▼ Most common: light-headedness, dizziness, sleepiness, nausea, vomiting, appetite loss, and sweating. If these occur, ask your doctor about lowering your codeine dose. Most of these side effects disappear if you simply lie down.

▼ Less common: euphoria (feeling high), headache, agitation, uncoordinated muscle movement, minor hallucinations, disorientation and visual disturbances, dry mouth, constipation, flushing of the face, rapid heartbeat, palpitations, faintness, urinary difficulties or hesitancy, reduced sex drive or impotence, itching, rash, anemia, lowered blood sugar, and yellowing of the skin or whites of the eyes. Narcotic analgesics may aggravate convulsions in those who have had convulsions in the past.

More serious side effects of codeine are shallow breathing or breathing difficulties.

Drug Interactions

• Avoid combining narcotics with alcohol, sleeping medications, tranquilizers, or other depressant drugs.

• Combining a narcotic pain reliever with any other medication that lowers blood pressure can lead to excessive blood-pressure lowering. Avoid this combination.

• Combining cimetidine with a narcotic pain reliever may cause confusion, disorientation, breathing difficulties, and seizure.

Food Interactions

Codeine may be taken with food to reduce upset stomach. The fentanyl patch may be used without regard to food.

Usual Dose

Codeine
  Adult: 15–60 mg 4 times a day for relief of pain; 10–20 mg every few hours as needed to suppress cough.

Child: 1–2 mg per lb. of body weight in divided doses for relief of pain; 0.5–0.75 mg per lb. of body weight in divided doses to suppress cough.

Fentanyl Patch
Apply to a clean and non-irritated patch of skin as directed, usually once every 3 days.

Overdosage

Symptoms of narcotic overdose are breathing difficulties or slowing of respiration, extreme tiredness progressing to stupor and then coma, pinpoint pupils, no response to pain stimulation, cold and clammy skin, slowing of heartbeat, lowering of blood pressure, convulsions, and cardiac arrest. The victim should be taken to a hospital emergency room immediately. ALWAYS bring the prescription bottle or container with you.

Special Information

Codeine is a respiratory depressant and affects the central nervous system (CNS), producing sleepiness, tiredness, or inability to concentrate. Be careful if you are driving, operating hazardous machinery, or performing other functions requiring concentration. Avoid alcohol while taking codeine because it enhances these effects.

Call your doctor if you develop breathing difficulties, constipation, dry mouth, or any other side effect that is prominent or persistent.

Apply the fentanyl patch only to non-irritated skin on a flat surface of the upper body. Hair at the application site should be clipped or cut, not shaved, before applying the patch. Do not use oils, soaps, lotions, alcohol, or anything else that might irritate the skin before applying the patch.

If you forget a dose of codeine, take it as soon as you remember. If it is almost time for your next dose, skip the one you forgot and continue with your regular schedule. Never take a double dose.

Special Populations

Pregnancy/Breast-feeding
No studies of this medication have been done in pregnant women and no reports of human birth defects exist, but animal studies show that quantities of codeine may cause

problems in a fetus. Women who are or might be pregnant should talk to their doctors about the risks of taking codeine versus its possible benefits.

Like all narcotics, fentanyl is not recommended during pregnancy because the drug passes into the circulation of the fetus. If given to a pregnant woman before cesarean section, fentanyl may cause drowsiness in newborns.

Narcotics pass into breast milk at different rates. Nursing mothers who must take codeine should bottle-feed their infants.

Excessive use of any narcotic, including codeine, during pregnancy or breast-feeding may cause drug dependence in infants. Narcotics may also cause breathing difficulties in infants during delivery.

Seniors

Seniors are more likely to be sensitive to side effects of codeine and should be treated with the smallest effective dose.

Generic Name

Colchicine (KOLE-chih-sene) G

Type of Drug

Antigout.

Prescribed for

Gouty arthritis; may also be prescribed for Mediterranean fever; cirrhosis of the liver; biliary cirrhosis; Behçet's disease; pseudogout (condition caused by calcium deposits); amyloidosis; very low blood-platelet count (also known as ITP); skin reactions, including scleroderma, psoriasis, and other conditions; and nerve disability associated with chronic progressive multiple sclerosis.

General Information

While no one knows exactly how colchicine works, it appears to help people with gout by reducing their inflammatory response to uric acid crystals that form inside joints and by interfering with the body's mechanism for making uric acid.

Unlike drugs that affect uric acid levels, colchicine does not block the progression of gout to chronic gouty arthritis; it will, however, relieve the pain of acute attacks and lessen the frequency and severity of attacks. It has no effect on other kinds of pain.

Cautions and Warnings

Do not use colchicine if you suffer from any serious **blood, kidney, liver, stomach, or cardiac conditions**.

Vomiting, abdominal pain, diarrhea, nausea, kidney damage, and **blood in the urine** may occur with colchicine, especially at maximum doses. This can worsen existing gastrointestinal (GI) or other conditions. Stop taking the medication and call your doctor if you develop one of these symptoms.

The **weakness** that people develop while taking colchicine is frequently related to high levels of colchicine in the blood caused by poor kidney function and improves without treatment 3 to 4 weeks after the drug is stopped. This reaction is often mistaken for other conditions.

Periodic **blood counts** should be done if you are taking colchicine for long periods of time.

Colchicine interferes with the absorption of vitamin B_{12} by affecting the lining of the GI tract.

Colchicine may affect the process of **sperm** generation in men.

The safety and effectiveness for **use by children** have not been established.

Possible Side Effects

▼ Common: vomiting, diarrhea, and abdominal pain may occur if you take maximum doses of colchicine for an acute gout attack. You may also experience severe diarrhea, kidney and blood-vessel damage, blood in the urine, and reduced urination.

▼ Less common: hair loss, skin rash, appetite loss, and muscle and nerve weakness.

▼ Rare: with long-term colchicine therapy—reduced white-blood-cell and platelet counts, nerve inflammation, blood-clotting problems, skin rash, and other reactions. Colchicine may interfere with sperm formation.

Drug Interactions

- Colchicine interferes with the absorption of vitamin B_{12}.
- Colchicine may increase sensitivity to central-nervous-system depressants, such as tranquilizers and alcohol.
- The following drugs may reduce colchicine's effectiveness: anticancer drugs, bumetanide, diazoxide, thiazide diuretics, ethacrynic acid, furosemide, mecamylamine, pyrazinamide, and triamterene.
- Taking phenylbutazone with colchicine increases the chance of side effects.

Food Interactions

None known.

Usual Dose

Acute Gout Attack: 1–1.2 mg. This dose may be followed by 0.5–1.2 mg every 1–2 hours until pain is relieved or nausea, vomiting, or diarrhea occurs. The total dose needed to control pain and inflammation during an attack varies from 4–8 mg.

Prevention of Gout Attack: 0.5–1.8 mg daily. In mild cases, 0.5 mg or 0.6 mg may be taken 3–4 days a week.

Familial Mediterranean Fever: 1–3 mg a day.

Cirrhosis of the Liver: 1 mg a day for 5 days each week.

Biliary Cirrhosis: 0.6 mg 2 times a day.

Amyloidosis: 0.5 mg 1–2 times a day.

Behçet's Disease: 0.5–1.5 mg a day.

Pseudogout: 0.6 mg 2 times a day.

ITP: 1.2–1.8 mg a day for 2 weeks or more.

Scleroderma: 1 mg a day.

Other Skin Disorders: up to 1.8 mg a day, depending on the specific condition.

Overdosage

The lethal dose is estimated at 65 mg, although people have died after taking as little as 7 mg at once. Usually 1 to 3 days pass between the time that an overdose is taken and symptoms begin. Overdose symptoms start with nausea, vomiting, stomach pain, diarrhea—which may be severe and bloody—and burning sensations in the throat or stomach or on the skin. If you think you are experiencing overdose symptoms, contact your doctor immediately, or go to a hospital emergency room. ALWAYS bring the prescription bottle or container with you.

Special Information

Call your doctor if you develop skin rash, sore throat, fever, unusual bleeding or bruising, tiredness, or numbness or tingling. Seniors are more likely to develop drug side effects and should use this drug with caution.

Stop taking maximum doses of colchicine as soon as gout pain is relieved and reduce your dose to a maintenance level if your doctor has prescribed it for gout prevention. Stop taking the drug entirely and contact your doctor at the first sign of nausea, vomiting, stomach pain, or diarrhea.

If you forget a dose of colchicine, take it as soon as possible. If it is almost time for your next dose, skip the dose you forgot and continue with your regular schedule. Do not take a double dose.

Special Populations

Pregnancy/Breast-feeding

Colchicine can harm the fetus. Pregnant women should not take it unless the benefits clearly outweigh the potential risks.

It is not known if colchicine passes into breast milk. No problems with nursing infants are known, but you should consider bottle-feeding your baby if you must take colchicine.

Seniors

Seniors and sick people are more likely to develop side effects and should use colchicine with caution.

Type of Drug

Contraceptives

Brand Names

Generic Ingredients: Low-Dose Estrogen + Low-Dose Progestin, Single-Phase Combination

Brevicon	Nelova 0.5/35 E
Genora 0.5/35	Nelova 1/35 E
Genora 1/35	Nelova 1/50 M
Genora 1/50	Norethin 1/50 M
Loestrin 21 1.5/30	Norinyl 1+35
Loestrin 21 1/20	Norinyl 1+50
Loestrin Fe 1.5/30	Ortho-Novum 1/35
Loestrin Fe 1/20	Ortho-Novum 1/50
Modicon	Ovcon-35
N.E.E. 1/35	

Generic Ingredients: Low-Dose Estrogen + Intermediate-Dose Progestin, Single-Phase Combination

Demulen 1/35	Nordette
Desogen	Ortho-Cept
Levlen	Ortho-Cyclen
Lo/Ovral	

Generic Ingredients: Intermediate-Dose Estrogen + Low-Dose Progestin, Single-Phase Combination
Ovcon-50

Generic Ingredients: Intermediate-Dose Estrogen + Intermediate-Dose Progestin, Single-Phase Combination
Demulen 1/50

Generic Ingredients: Intermediate-Dose Estrogen + High-Dose Progestin, Single-Phase Combination
Ovral

Generic Ingredients: Low-Dose Estrogen + Low-Dose Progestin, 2-Phase Combination

Nelova 10/11	Ortho-Novum 10/11

Generic Ingredients: Low-Dose Estrogen + Low-Dose Progestin, 3-Phase Combination

Ortho-Novum 7/7/7	Tri-Norinyl
Tri-Levlen	Triphasil

Generic Ingredient: Low-Dose Progestin, Mini-Pill
Ovrette

Generic Ingredient: High-Dose Progestin, Mini-Pill
Micronor   Nor-Q.D.

Generic Ingredient: Progestin Implant System
Norplant System

Generic Ingredient: Progesterone, Intrauterine Insert
Progestasert

Prescribed for

Prevention of pregnancy, endometriosis, excessive menstruation, and cyclic withdrawal bleeding.

General Information

Oral contraceptives—"the Pill"—are synthetic hormones containing either a progestin hormone alone or a progestin hormone combined with an estrogen hormone. These hormones are similar to naturally occurring female hormones that control the menstrual cycle and prepare a woman's body to accept a fertilized egg. Natural hormones cannot be used as contraceptives because very large doses would be needed. Synthetic hormones are much more potent and are effective at much smaller doses.

Once an egg has been fertilized and is implanted (accepted) in the womb, no more eggs are released from the ovaries until the pregnancy is over. Oral contraceptives interfere with the natural processes of human reproduction: They may prevent sperm from reaching the unfertilized egg, prevent the acceptance of a fertilized egg in the womb, and/or prevent ovulation (the release of an unfertilized egg from the ovaries).

Oral contraceptives provide a very high rate of protection from pregnancy. They are from 97% to 99% effective, depending upon which product is used and how closely instructions for taking the medication are followed. With no contraceptive at all, the normal pregnancy rate is 60% to 80%.

The many different kinds of combination products available contain different amounts of estrogen and progestin, and different hormone products. Contraceptives with the smallest amounts of estrogen may be less effective in some women than others. In general, to keep side effects to a minimum, the contraceptive that contains the least amount of hormone but is effective is preferred.

The mini-pill, a progestin-only product, may cause irregular menstrual cycles and may be less effective than estrogen-progestin combinations. Mini-pills may be recommended to older women or women who should avoid estrogens (see "Cautions and Warnings").

Single-phase products provide constant amounts of estrogen and progestin throughout the entire month-long pill cycle. In 2-phase combinations, the amount of estrogen remains at a steady low level throughout the cycle, and the progestin first increases and then decreases. This variation in progestin is to allow normal changes to take place in the uterus. The newest combination products are 3-phase combinations. Throughout the cycle, the estrogen portion remains the same but progestin amounts change to create a 3-part wave pattern. This 3-part pattern is meant to simulate the normal hormone cycle and reduce breakthrough bleeding. Breakthrough bleeding may occur with the older combination products from day 8 through 16 of the cycle. The amount of estrogen in these new products is considered to be in the low category.

Levonorgestrel, a progestin, is used in implants that provide effective contraception for up to 5 years after surgical implantation under the skin of the upper arm. Levonorgestrel implants should be replaced at least once every 5 years. They can be removed at any time, reversing the contraceptive effect. The intrauterine insert provides a continuous flow of progestin, and effective contraception, for about 1 year. The hormones contained in both the implant and the intrauterine systems are the same type as progestin-only mini-pills, and are associated with many of the same side effects and precautions as oral contraceptives.

Every woman using or considering a contraceptive, whether it is a pill, an implant, or insert, should be fully aware of the problems associated with contraceptive drugs. The highest risk occurs in women over age 35 who smoke and have high blood pressure.

Cautions and Warnings

You should not use contraceptive drugs if you are or might be **pregnant** or if you have or have had **blood clots** of the veins or arteries, **stroke**, any **blood-coagulation disorder**, known or suspected **cancer of the breast or sex organs, liver cancer,** or **irregular or scanty menstrual periods**. Contraceptive drugs may cause some **eye problems.** Call your doctor at once if you develop visual difficulties of any kind.

Your doctor should carefully consider the risks of contraceptive drugs if you are **physically immobile** or if you have **asthma, cardiac insufficiency, epilepsy, migraine headaches, kidney problems,** a strong **family history of breast cancer, benign breast disease, diabetes, endometriosis, gallbladder disease** or **gallstones, liver problems** including jaundice, **high blood cholesterol, high blood pressure, estrogen or progestin intolerance, depression, tuberculosis,** or **varicose veins.**

There is an increased risk of **heart attack** in women who have taken oral contraceptives for more than 10 years, or who are between age 40 and 49 and have other coronary risk factors, including smoking, obesity, high blood pressure, diabetes, and high blood cholesterol. This risk remains even after the medication is stopped. Women who use oral contraceptives and **smoke** are 5 times more likely to have a heart attack as nonsmokers taking contraceptives, and 10 to 12 times more likely to have a heart attack than nonsmoking women who are not on the Pill.

Women with a history of **headaches, high blood pressure,** and **varicose veins** should avoid estrogen-containing products. Older women and women who have experienced side effects from estrogen also should not take estrogen products.

Oral contraceptives may mask the onset of **menopause.**

Progestin-only products carry an increased risk of **blood-clotting** problems, but the exact risk is not well understood.

Possible Side Effects

▼ Common: Ideally, oral contraceptives will have virtually no side effects. Your doctor will choose a product suited to you, but may have to change products from time to time depending on the side effects you develop. If you are taking too much estrogen, for example, you may experience nausea, bloating, high blood pressure, migraine, or breast tenderness. If you have too little estrogen, you may develop early or mid-cycle breakthrough bleeding, spotting, or reduced periodic flow. Too much progestin is associated with weight gain and increased appetite, tiredness or weakness, low periodic flow, acne, depression, breast regression, and oily scalp. Too little

Possible Side Effects *(continued)*

progestin is associated with late breakthrough bleeding, excessive periodic bleeding, and no period at all.

▼ Less common: abdominal cramps, infertility after discontinuance of the drug, breast tenderness, weight change, headache, rash, vaginal itching and burning, general vaginal infection, nervousness, dizziness, depression, cataract, changes in sex drive, hair loss, and unusual sensitivity to the sun.

▼ Rare: Women who take oral contraceptives are more likely to develop several serious conditions, including blood clots in the deep veins, stroke, heart attack, liver cancer, gallbladder disease, and high blood pressure. Women who smoke cigarettes are at much higher risk for some of these adverse effects.

Drug Interactions

• Rifampin decreases the effectiveness of oral contraceptives, as may barbiturates, phenylbutazone, phenytoin, ampicillin, neomycin, penicillin, tetracycline, chloramphenicol, sulfa drugs, griseofulvin, nitrofurantoin, tranquilizers, and antimigraine drugs.

• Oral contraceptives may reduce the breakdown of certain benzodiazepine tranquilizers and sleeping pills, caffeine, metoprolol, corticosteroids, theophylline drugs, and tricyclic antidepressants, increasing the amount of these drugs in the blood and the chances for side effects and toxicities.

• Oral contraceptives may increase the toxic effect of acetaminophen on your liver. In addition, acetaminophen effectiveness may be reduced by oral contraceptives. Oral contraceptives may reduce the effect of anticoagulant (blood-thinning) drugs, although an increased effect of anticoagulants has also been reported. Discuss this combination with your doctor.

• Oral contraceptives may decrease the effects of salicylate pain relievers including aspirin, clofibrate, lorazepam, oxazepam, and temazepam by increasing the rate at which they are broken down by the liver.

• Oral contraceptives may increase blood-cholesterol (blood-fat) levels and may interfere with blood tests for thyroid function and blood sugar.

Food Interactions

None known.

Usual Dose

The first day of bleeding is the first day of the menstrual cycle. Beginning on the 5th day of the menstrual cycle, 1 pill a day for 20–21 days according to the number of pills supplied by the manufacturer. If menstrual flow has not begun 7 days after taking the last pill, begin the next month's cycle of pills.

Some manufacturers recommend starting the pills on a Sunday, to make it easy to remember to take them. In this case, start taking your pills on the first Sunday after your period begins. If menstruation begins on a Sunday, take the first pill that day.

Progestin-only mini-pills are taken once a day, 365 days a year.

Overdosage

Overdosage may cause nausea and withdrawal bleeding in adult females. Accidental overdosage in children who take their mothers' pills has not caused serious adverse effects; however, overdose victims should be taken to a hospital emergency room for evaluation and treatment. ALWAYS bring the prescription package with you.

Special Information

Use a backup method of birth control to be sure to prevent pregnancy in the first 3 weeks after you begin taking oral contraceptives.

Take your pill at the same time each day to establish a routine and ensure maximum contraceptive protection.

Call your doctor immediately if you develop sudden, severe abdominal pains; severe or sudden headache; pain in the chest, groin, or leg, especially the calf; sudden slurring of speech; changes in vision; or weakness, numbness, or unexplained pain in the arms or legs; or if you start coughing up blood, lose coordination, or become suddenly short of breath.

Other problems that may develop and require medical attention are bulging eyes; changes in vaginal bleeding; fainting; frequent or painful urination; a gradual increase in blood pressure; breast lumps or secretions; depression; yellowing of the whites of the eyes or skin; rash; redness or irritation; upper abdominal swelling, pain, or tenderness; an unusual or dark-colored mole; thick, white vaginal discharge; or vaginal itching or tenderness. Other symptoms associated with contraceptive drugs require medical attention only if they are unusually bothersome or persistent.

See your doctor for a check-up every 6 to 12 months.

Some manufacturers include 7 inert or iron pills in their packaging, to be taken on days when the drug is not taken. These products, which have the number 28 as part of their brand name, should be taken every day.

For single or 2-phase combinations: If you forget to take a pill for 1 day, take 2 pills the following day. If you miss 2 consecutive days, take 2 pills for the next 2 days. Then return to your schedule of 1 pill a day. If you miss 3 consecutive days, do not take any pills for the next 7 days and use another form of contraception; then start a new cycle.

For 3-phase combinations: If you forget to take a pill for 1 day, take 2 pills the following day. If you miss 2 consecutive days, take 2 pills for the next 2 days. Then return to your schedule of 1 pill a day. If you forget to take a pill for 3 days in a row, stop taking the drug and use an alternate means of contraception until your period comes. ALWAYS use a backup contraceptive method for the remainder of your cycle if you forget even 1 pill of a 3-phase combination.

Forgetting to take a pill reduces your protection. If you keep forgetting to take your pills, you should use another means of birth control.

If you must take any drugs listed in "Drug Interactions," use a backup contraceptive method during that cycle to prevent accidental pregnancy.

It is important to maintain good dental hygiene while taking contraceptive drugs and to brush and floss carefully because of the chance that the drug will make you more susceptible to some infections. See your dentist regularly while taking a contraceptive. Check with your dentist if you notice swelling or bleeding of your gums.

You may be more sensitive to the sun while taking oral contraceptives.

You may become intolerant to contact lenses because of minor changes in the shape of your eyes.

All oral contraceptive prescriptions must come with a "patient package insert" for you to read. It gives detailed information about the drug and is required by federal law.

Special Populations

Pregnancy/Breast-feeding

Oral contraceptives cause birth defects and may interfere with fetal development. They are not safe for use during pregnancy.

Oral contraceptives reduce the amount of breast milk produced and may also affect its quality. Some of the hormone passes into breast milk, but the effect on a nursing infant is not known. Do not breast-feed while you are taking oral contraceptives.

Type of Drug

Corticosteroids (kor-tih-koe-STER-oids)

Brand Names

Generic Ingredient: Betamethasone
Celestone

Generic Ingredient: Cortisone Acetate [G]
Cortone Acetate

Generic Ingredient: Dexamethasone [G]
Decadron   Dexone
Dexameth   Hexadrol

Generic Ingredient: Hydrocortisone [G]
Cortef   Hydrocortone
Cortenema

Generic Ingredient: Methylprednisolone [G]
Medrol

Generic Ingredient: Prednisolone [G]
Delta-Cortef   Prelone

Generic Ingredient: Prednisone [G]
Deltasone   Prednicen-M
Liquid Pred   Prednisone Intensol
Meticorten   Sterapred
Orasone   Sterapred DS
Panasol-S

Generic Ingredient: Triamcinolone Ⓖ

Aristocort   Kenacort

Atolone

Prescribed for

A wide variety of disorders from rash to cancer, including adrenal disease, adrenal hormone replacement, bursitis, arthritis, severe skin reactions including psoriasis and other rashes, severe or disabling allergies, asthma, drug or serum sickness, severe respiratory diseases including pneumonitis, blood disorders, gastrointestinal (GI) disease including ulcerative colitis, and inflammation of the nerves, heart, or other organs. Dexamethasone is also used to treat mountain sickness, vomiting, bronchial disease in premature babies, excessive hairiness, and hearing loss associated with bacterial meningitis. Dexamethasone has been used to detect and manage depression, although this use is controversial.

General Information

Natural corticosteroids are hormones produced by the adrenal gland which affect almost all body systems. The major differences among the corticosteroids are potency of medication and variation in some secondary effects. Choosing one corticosteroid for a specific disease is usually a matter of doctor preference and past experience. Using 5 mg of prednisone as the basis for comparison, equivalent doses of other corticosteroids are: 0.6 mg to 0.75 mg of betamethasone, 25 mg of cortisone, 0.75 mg of dexamethasone, 20 mg of hydrocortisone, 4 mg of methylprednisolone, 5 mg of prednisolone, and 4 mg of triamcinolone.

Cautions and Warnings

If you are **allergic** to one corticosteroid, you are probably allergic to all corticosteroids and should avoid using them.

Corticosteroids may mask symptoms of an **infection**. Because these drugs compromise the immune system, new infections may occur during corticosteroid treatment; when this happens, a relatively minor infection that would respond to ordinary treatment can turn into a major problem. Corticosteroids may impair immune response to **hepatitis B**, prolonging recovery. They may reactivate dormant **amebiasis** (amebic infection usually acquired in the tropics). Corticosteroids should not be taken if you have a **fungal blood infection**, because they could actually make it easier for the infection to spread. They should be used with caution by people with **tuberculosis**.

Long-term use of any corticosteroid may increase the chances of developing **cataracts, glaucoma**, or **eye infections**, especially viral or fungal.

Because of the effect of corticosteroids on adrenal glands, it is essential that when the drug is stopped dosage is gradually reduced over a period of time and under a doctor's supervision. If you stop taking a corticosteroid suddenly or without the advice of your doctor, you could experience **adrenal gland failure**, which may have extremely serious consequences.

If you are taking large corticosteroid doses, you should not receive any live virus **vaccine**, because corticosteroids will interfere with the body's normal reaction to the vaccine. Speak with your doctor before receiving any vaccine.

Hydrocortisone and cortisone may lead to **high blood pressure** because of their effect on blood sodium and other electrolytes. The possibility of increased blood pressure is less of a problem with other corticosteroids.

Corticosteroids should be used with caution if you have severe kidney disease.

High-dose or long-term corticosteroid therapy may aggravate or worsen **stomach ulcers**. With prednisone, this is not likely to happen until the total dose reaches 1000 mg. Doses at which this effect occurs vary with the other corticosteroids—150 mg of betamethasone and dexamethasone, 5000 mg of cortisone, 4000 mg of hydrocortisone, 1000 mg of prednisolone, and 800 mg of either triamcinolone and methylprednisolone.

People who have recently stopped taking a corticosteroid and who are going through a period of **stress** may need small doses of a rapid-acting corticosteroid, such as hydrocortisone, to get them through. Call your doctor if you think you might be experiencing this kind of stress-related need.

Use corticosteroids with care if you have had a **recent heart attack**, or if you have **ulcerative colitis, heart failure, high blood pressure, blood-clotting tendencies, thrombophlebitis, osteoporosis, antibiotic-resistant infections, Cushing's disease, myasthenia gravis, metastatic cancer, diabetes, underactive thyroid disease, cirrhosis of the liver,** or **seizure disorders**.

Corticosteroid psychosis (symptoms include euphoria or

feeling high, delirium, sleeplessness, mood swings, personality changes, and severe depression) may develop in people taking doses greater than 40 mg a day of prednisone. These symptoms may also develop with other corticosteroids taken in equivalent doses (see "General Information" for relative equivalencies). Symptoms of corticosteroid psychosis usually develop within 15 to 30 days of beginning corticosteroid treatment. These symptoms may also be linked to other factors, including a family history of psychosis and female gender.

Corticosteroids may also cause a **loss of calcium**, which may result in bone fractures and aseptic necrosis of the femoral and humoral heads (condition in which the large bones in the hip degenerate from loss of calcium).

Prednisone may aggravate existing **emotional instability**.

Corticosteroids may be used for speeding the recovery from attacks of **multiple sclerosis** (MS), but they do not fight the underlying disease or slow its progression.

Corticosteroid products often contain tartrazine dyes to add color and sulfite preservatives, two chemicals to which many people are allergic. Check with your pharmacist to determine if the product you are using contains **tartrazine** or **sulfites**.

Possible Side Effects

▼ Most common: upset stomach, possibly leading to stomach or duodenal ulcer.

▼ Common: water retention, heart failure, potassium loss, muscle weakness, loss of muscle mass, slowed healing of wounds, black-and-blue marks, increased sweating, allergic rash, itching, convulsions, dizziness, and headache.

▼ Less common: irregular menstruation, slowed growth in children particularly after lengthy periods of corticosteroid treatment, adrenal and/or pituitary gland suppression, diabetes, drug sensitivity or allergic reactions, blood clots, insomnia, weight gain, increased appetite, nausea, feeling unwell, euphoria (feeling high), mood swings, personality changes, and severe depression.

Drug Interactions

• Tell your doctor if you are taking any oral anticoagulant (blood-thinning drug). If you begin taking a corticosteroid, your anticoagulant dose may have to be changed.

• Interaction with diuretics—such as hydrochlorothia-zide—may cause loss of blood potassium. Signs of low blood-potassium levels include weakness, muscle cramps, and tiredness; report any of these symptoms to your doctor. Eat high-potassium foods such as bananas, citrus fruits, melons, and tomatoes. Side effects of digitalis drugs may be increased because of low blood potassium.

• Oral contraceptives, estrogens, erythromycin, azithromy-cin, clarithromycin, and ketoconazole may increase the effects of corticosteroids, increasing the chance of corticosteroid side effects.

• Barbiturates, aminoglutethimide, phenytoin and other hydantoin anticonvulsants, rifampin, ephedrine, colestipol, and cholestyramine may reduce corticosteroid effectiveness.

• Corticosteroids may decrease the effects of aspirin and other salicylates, growth hormones, and isoniazid.

• Corticosteroids and theophylline drugs may interact to alter the requirements of either or both drugs. Your doctor will have to determine proper dosage levels for each.

• Corticosteroids may interfere with laboratory tests. Tell your doctor if you are taking any of these drugs so that tests are properly analyzed.

Food Interactions

Take corticosteroids with food or a small amount of antacid to avoid stomach upset. If stomach upset continues, notify your doctor.

Usual Dose

Betamethasone: starting dosage—0.6–7.2 mg a day. Mainte-nance dosage—0.6–7.2 mg a day, depending on response.

Cortisone: starting dosage—25–300 mg a day. Maintenance dosage—25–300 mg a day, depending on response.

Dexamethasone: 0.75–9 mg a day, depending on response and disease being treated. Daily dosage sometimes exceeds 9 mg, although the lowest effective dose is desirable. Stress-ful situations may cause a need for a temporary dosage increase. Dexamethasone may also be given in alternate-day therapy in which twice the usual daily dose is given every other day.

Hydrocortisone: 20–240 mg a day, depending on individual response.

Methylprednisolone: starting dosage—4–48 mg a day, or more. Maintenance dosage—varies according to response and the disease being treated. The lowest effective dose is desirable. Stressful situations may cause a need for a temporary dosage increase. Methylprednisolone may be given in alternate-day therapy in which twice the usual daily dose is given every other day.

Prednisone and Prednisolone: 5–60 mg a day, depending on response and disease being treated. Daily dosage sometimes exceeds 60 mg, although the lowest effective dose is desirable. Stressful situations may cause a need for a temporary dosage increase. Prednisone and prednisolone may be given in alternate-day therapy in which twice the usual daily dose is given every other day.

Overdosage

Symptoms of corticosteroid overdose are anxiety, depression and/or stimulation, stomach bleeding, increased blood sugar, high blood pressure, and water retention. The victim should be taken to a hospital emergency room immediately because stomach pumping, oxygen, intravenous fluid, and other supportive treatments may be necessary. ALWAYS bring the prescription bottle or container with you.

Special Information

Do not stop taking this medication on your own. Suddenly stopping any corticosteroid drug may have severe consequences; the dosage must be gradually reduced by your doctor.

Call your doctor if you develop unusual weight gain, black or tarry stools, swelling of the feet or legs, muscle weakness, vomiting of blood, menstrual irregularity, prolonged sore throat, fever, cold or infection, appetite loss, nausea and vomiting, diarrhea, weight loss, weakness, dizziness, or low blood sugar.

If you forget a corticosteroid dose and you take several doses a day, take the dose you forgot as soon as you can. If it is almost time for your next dose, skip the one you forgot and double the next dose.

If you take only one dose a day and you forget a dose until the next day, skip the dose you forgot and continue with your regular schedule. Do not take a double dose.

If you take a corticosteroid every other day and forget a

dose, take it immediately if you remember it in the morning of your regularly scheduled day. If it is much later in the day, skip the dose you forgot and take it the following morning, then go back to your regular schedule. Do not take a double dose.

Special Populations

Pregnancy/Breast-feeding
Studies have shown that large doses of corticosteroids over long periods may cause birth defects, as may chronic corticosteroid use during the first 3 months of pregnancy. Pregnant women should not take a corticosteroid unless the risks have been carefully considered.

Corticosteroids taken by mouth may pass into breast milk. As long as the daily dose is relatively low—less than 20 mg of prednisone or prednisolone, or less than 8 mg of methylprednisolone—and the drug is being taken for a short time, the amount of drug that appears in breast milk is usually negligible. Nursing mothers taking doses in this low range should either bottle-feed their babies or wait 3 to 4 hours after each corticosteroid dose to nurse or collect breast milk. Mothers taking larger corticosteroid doses should bottle-feed their babies.

Seniors
Seniors are more likely to develop high blood pressure while taking an oral corticosteroid. Older women are more susceptible to osteoporosis (condition characterized by loss of bone mass due to depletion of minerals, especially calcium) associated with large doses of corticosteroids. In seniors, lower corticosteroid doses are desirable because they are as effective and cause fewer problems.

Type of Drug

Corticosteroids, Eye Products
(kor-tih-koe-STER-oids)

Brand Names

Generic Ingredient: Fluorometholone

Flarex

Fluor-Op

FML

FML Forte

FML S.O.P.

Generic Ingredient: Medrysone
HMS

Generic Ingredient: Dexamethasone [G]
AK-Dex   Maxidex
Decadron Phosphate

Generic Ingredient: Prednisolone [G]
AK-Pred   Inflamase Mild
Econopred   Pred Mild
Econopred Plus   Pred Forte
Inflamase Forte

Generic Ingredient: Rimexolone
Vexol

Prescribed for

Allergic and inflammatory conditions of the eye.

General Information

Corticosteroids produce a generalized reduction in inflammation throughout the body. When applied directly to the eye, corticosteroids provide general relief of allergies and irritation by inhibiting the inflammatory response in the eye. Very severe eye conditions that do not respond to eyedrops or ointments may require treatment with oral corticosteroids. Fluorometholone, medrysone, and prednisolone in concentrations up to 0.125% are preferred for long-term treatment because they are least likely to increase intraocular pressure (IOP—pressure inside the eye).

Cautions and Warnings

Do not use corticosteroid eyedrops or eye ointment if you are **allergic** or sensitive to them. They should be used with care if you have **a fungal infection, herpes, tuberculosis, viral infection of the eye, cataracts, glaucoma,** or **diabetes**.

Possible Side Effects

▼ Rare: watery eyes; glaucoma; optic nerve damage; gradual blurring, reduction, or loss of vision; eye pain; nausea; vomiting; eye infection; and eye burning, stinging, or redness.

Drug Interactions

• Corticosteroids applied to the eye may interfere with the effect of antiglaucoma drugs.

• The risk of raising IOP is increased when corticosteroid eyedrops are taken with anticholinergic drugs, especially atropine, over a long period of time.

Usual Dose

Eyedrops: 1–2 drops several times a day.

Ointment: 1 thin strip of ointment in the affected eye(s) several times a day.

Overdosage

Swallowing a container of corticosteroid eyedrops or ointment does not generally produce serious effects; however, call your doctor or local poison control center for information in the event of accidental ingestion.

Special Information

If you forget a dose of corticosteroid eyedrops or ointment, administer it as soon as you remember. If it is almost time for your next dose, skip the one you forgot and continue with your regular schedule.

To administer eyedrops, lie down or tilt your head back. Hold the dropper above your eye, gently squeeze your lower lid to form a small pouch, and release the drop or drops of medication inside your lower lid while looking up. Release the lower lid, keeping your eye open. Do not blink for 40 seconds. Press gently on the bridge of your nose at the inside corner of your eye for 1 minute to help circulate the drug in your eye. To avoid infection, do not touch the dropper tip to your finger, eyelid, or any other surface. Wait at least 5 minutes before using another eyedrop or eye ointment.

To use an eye ointment, tilt your head back and with your index finger gently pull your lower eyelid down to make a small space. Squeeze a thin strip of ointment into the space; ⅓ in. is usually enough. Let go of the lower lid and close your eye for 1 to 2 minutes to allow the medication to circulate in the eye.

Special Populations

Pregnancy/Breast-feeding

Problems have not been found in women using corticosteroid

eyedrops during pregnancy. However, babies born to mothers who used large amounts of corticosteroid eyedrops during pregnancy should be watched for possible effects on the adrenal gland. Women who are or might be pregnant should not use these drugs without first discussing possible benefits and risks with their doctor.

Nursing mothers have used corticosteroid eyedrops without problems.

Seniors
Seniors may use corticosteroid eyedrops without special precaution.

Type of Drug

Corticosteroids, Inhalers

(kor-tih-koe-STER-oids)

Brand Names

Generic Ingredient: Beclomethasone Dipropionate

Beclovent	Vanceril
Vancenase Pockethaler	Vanceril Double Strength

Generic Ingredient: Budesonide
Pulmicort Turbohaler

Generic Ingredient: Flunisolide

AeroBid	AeroBid-M

Generic Ingredient: Triamcinolone Acetonide

Azmacort	Nasacort

Prescribed for

Chronic asthma and bronchial disease.

General Information

Corticosteroid inhalers relieve the symptoms associated with asthma and bronchial disease by reducing inflammation of bronchial mucous membranes, making it easier to breathe. Asthma experts have come to recognize these drugs as essential to asthma treatment because all asthma is, in part, an inflammatory disease. Many believe that virtually all people with asthma should be using an inhaled corticosteroid as part of their regular treatment. Corticosteroid inhalers produce the same effect as oral corticosteroids, with some important differences. Because inhalers bring the drug specifically to the area where it is needed, the same effect is achieved with a much smaller dose and without affecting other parts of the body. In addition, because only a small portion of the drug is absorbed into the bloodstream, corticosteroid inhalers have fewer side effects than oral corticosteroids. Corticosteroid inhalers are meant to be taken regularly to prevent an asthma attack; they will not relieve an acute asthma attack. Generally, corticosteroid inhalers are not recommended for children under age 6.

Cautions and Warnings

Do not use these drugs if you are **allergic** to any corticosteroid.

Corticosteroid inhalers are not meant to be used as the primary treatment of **severe asthma**. They are intended only for people who take prednisone or another oral corticosteroid, or for people who do not respond to other asthma drugs.

Combining an oral corticosteroid with a corticosteroid inhaler may cause **pituitary gland suppression**. The combination of oral and nasal corticosteroids must be used with caution.

Even though these drugs are inhaled, they are potent adrenal corticosteroids. During a period of severe **stress**, you may have to go back to taking oral corticosteroids if the inhaler does not control your asthma. During periods of stress or a **severe asthmatic attack,** people who have stopped using an inhaler should contact their doctor to find out about taking an oral corticosteroid.

Death from **adrenal gland failure** has occurred in asthma patients during and after switching from an oral corticosteroid to a corticosteroid inhaler. Restoration of the body's natural adrenal function takes several months after switching from oral to inhaled corticosteroid therapy.

Corticosteroid inhalers may be associated with immediate or delayed drug reactions, including breathing difficulties, rash, and bronchospasm.

Possible Side Effects

▼ Most common: dry mouth, hoarseness, rash, and bronchospasm.

Possible Side Effects *(continued)*

▼ Rare: cough, wheezing, and facial swelling. Cough and wheezing are probably caused by an ingredient in the inhaler other than the corticosteroid itself; a chemical ingredient that helps disperse the drug around the lungs has been implicated as the cause of these side effects. Newer administration systems that omit this ingredient may minimize the problem.

Deaths caused by adrenal gland failure have occurred in people who took adrenal corticosteroid tablets or syrup and were switched to beclomethasone by inhalation. This is a rare complication and usually results from stopping the liquid or tablets too quickly. They must be stopped gradually, over a long period of time. Adrenal gland suppression has occurred in people taking 38 puffs of beclomethasone, or 40 puffs of triamcinolone, once a day for 1 month, or recommended doses of these drugs for 6 to 12 weeks.

Food and Drug Interactions

None known.

Usual Dose

Beclomethasone
  Adult and Child (age 13 and over): 2 inhalations (84 mcg) 3–4 times a day, or 4 inhalations twice a day. People with severe asthma may take up to 16 inhalations a day.
  Child (age 6–12): 1–2 inhalations 3–4 times a day.

Budesonide
  Adult: starting dose—200–400 mcg twice a day. Do not exceed 800 mcg twice a day.
  Child (age 6 and over): 200 mcg twice a day. Do not exceed 400 mcg twice a day.

Flunisolide
  Adult and Child (age 16 and over): 2 inhalations (500 mcg) morning and evening. Do not exceed 8 inhalations a day.
  Child (age 6–15): 2 inhalations (500 mcg) morning and evening. Do not exceed 4 inhalations a day.

Triamcinolone
   Adult and Child (age 13 and over): 2 inhalations (200 mcg) 3–4 times a day. Do not exceed 16 inhalations a day unless specifically directed by your doctor.
   Child (age 6–12): 1–2 inhalations (100–200 mcg) 3–4 times a day. Do not exceed 12 inhalations a day.

Overdosage

Serious adverse effects are unlikely after accidental ingestion of a corticosteroid inhaler. In extreme situations, excessive use or large amounts of inhaled corticosteroid may cause overdose symptoms that parallel oral corticosteroids; such cases may require gradual discontinuance of the drug. Call your local poison control center or hospital emergency room for more information.

Special Information

People using both a corticosteroid inhaler and a bronchodilator, such as albuterol, should use the bronchodilator first, wait a few minutes, and then use the corticosteroid inhaler. This will allow more corticosteroid to be absorbed.

   These drugs are for preventive therapy only and will not affect an asthma attack. Inhaled corticosteroids must be taken regularly, as directed. Wait at least 1 minute between inhalations.

   To properly take this medication, follow these instructions: Thoroughly shake the inhaler if it is one that must be shaken. Take a drink of water to moisten your throat. Place the inhaler 2 finger-widths away from your mouth and tilt your head back slightly. While activating the inhaler, take a slow, deep breath for 3 to 5 seconds, then hold your breath for about 10 seconds, and finally breathe out slowly. Allow at least 1 minute between puffs. Rinse your mouth after each use to reduce dry mouth and hoarseness.

   If you forget a dose of your inhaler, take it as soon as you remember. If it is almost time for your next dose, skip the dose you forgot and continue with your regular schedule. Do not take a double dose.

Special Populations

Pregnancy/Breast-feeding
Using large amounts of corticosteroids during pregnancy may slow fetal growth. Corticosteroids may cause birth

defects or interfere with fetal development. Check with your doctor before taking any of these drugs if you are or might be pregnant.

Oral corticosteroids may pass into breast milk and cause side effects in nursing infants. It is not known if inhaled corticosteroids find their way into breast milk; nursing mothers should be cautious about using these drugs.

Seniors

Seniors may use corticosteroid inhalers without special restriction. Be sure your doctor knows if you suffer from bone disease, bowel disease, colitis, diabetes, glaucoma, fungal or herpes infections, high blood pressure, high blood cholesterol, an underactive thyroid, or heart, kidney, or liver disease.

Type of Drug

Corticosteroids, Nasal

(kor-tih-koe-STER-oids)

Brand Names

Generic Ingredient: Beclomethasone Dipropionate
Beconase   Vancenase
Beconase AQ   Vancenase AQ

Generic Ingredient: Budesonide
Rhinocort

Generic Ingredient: Dexamethasone Sodium Phosphate
Decadron Phosphate Turbinaire

Generic Ingredient: Flunisolide
Nasalide   Nasarel

Generic Ingredient: Fluticasone Propionate
Flonase

Generic Ingredient: Triamcinolone Acetonide
Nasacort

Prescribed for

Rhinitis (nasal inflammation) associated with seasonal or chronic allergy and other causes; also used to prevent postsurgical recurrence of nasal polyps.

General Information

Nasal corticosteroids are specially formulated for use as a nasal spray. They are used to treat severe symptoms of seasonal allergy that have not responded to other types of drugs, such as decongestants. Nasal corticosteroids work by reducing inflammation of the mucous membranes that line the nasal passages, making it easier to breathe. These drugs may take several days to produce an effect. Do not use these drugs continuously for more than 3 weeks unless you have experienced a definite benefit. Fluticasone and triamcinolone are approved only for allergic rhinitis; other nasal corticosteroids are approved for both allergic and non-allergic rhinitis.

Cautions and Warnings

Do not use a nasal corticosteroid if you are **allergic** to any of its ingredients. On rare occasions, serious and life-threatening drug-sensitivity reactions have occurred.

If your nose is severely congested, you may need to use a nasal decongestant before using a nasal corticosteroid to get the best effect.

Combining prednisone or another oral corticosteroid with a nasal corticosteroid may cause **pituitary gland suppression**, although nasal corticosteroids alone rarely cause this problem. The combination of oral and nasal corticosteroids should be taken with caution and only under your doctor's supervision.

On rare occasions, *Candida* (yeast) infections of the nose and throat develop. If this happens, your corticosteroid may be discontinued and other therapy may be prescribed.

Even though these drugs are taken by inhalation, they should be considered potent adrenal corticosteroid drugs. During a period of severe **stress**, you may have to go back to taking an oral corticosteroid drug if the nasal form does not control your symptoms.

Possible Side Effects

▼ Most common: mild irritation of the nose, nasal passages, and throat; burning; stinging; dryness; and headache.

▼ Less common: light-headedness, nausea, nosebleed or bloody mucus, unusual nasal congestion, bronchial

Possible Side Effects *(continued)*

asthma, sneezing attacks, runny nose, throat discomfort, and loss of the sense of taste.

▼ Rare: ulcers of the nasal passages, watery eyes, sore throat, vomiting, hypersensitivity reactions (symptoms include itching, rash, swelling, bronchospasms, and breathing difficulties), nasal infection, wheezing, perforation of the septal wall between the nostrils, and increased eye pressure.

Very rarely, deaths caused by failure of the adrenal gland have occurred in people taking adrenal corticosteroid tablets or syrup who were switched to a nasal corticosteroid. This is a rare complication and usually results from stopping the liquid or tablets too quickly; they must be stopped gradually, over a long period of time.

Food and Drug Interactions

None known.

Usual Dose

Beclomethasone
   Adult and Child (age 13 and over): 1 spray (42 mcg) in each nostril 2–4 times a day.
   Child (age 6–12): 1 spray (42 mcg) in each nostril 3 times a day.

Budesonide
   Adult and Child (age 6 and over): 2 sprays (64 mcg) in each nostril morning and evening, or 4 sprays in the morning.

Dexamethasone
   Adult and Child (age 13 and over): 2 sprays (168 mcg) in each nostril 3 times a day. Do not exceed 12 sprays a day.
   Child (age 6–12): 1–2 sprays (84–168 mcg) in each nostril 2 times a day. Do not exceed 8 sprays a day.

Flunisolide
   Adult and Child (age 15 and over): 2 sprays (50 mcg) in each nostril 2 times a day to start; may be increased up to 8 sprays a day in each nostril.
   Child (age 6–14): 1 spray (25 mcg) in each nostril 3 times a day, or 2 sprays in each nostril 2 times a day.

Fluticasone

Adult: 2 sprays (100 mcg) in each nostril once a day or divided in 2 doses, to start. Dosage may be reduced in half in a few days, if tolerated.

Child (over age 12): 1 spray (50 mcg) in each nostril once a day; may be increased to 2 sprays a day in each nostril, if needed.

Child (under age 12): not recommended.

Triamcinolone

Adult and Child (age 13 and over): 2 sprays (220 mcg) in each nostril once a day; may be increased to 4 sprays a day in each nostril.

Child (under age 13): not recommended.

Overdosage

Serious adverse effects are unlikely after accidental ingestion of a nasal corticosteroid. Excessive use of large amounts of nasal corticosteroids may cause overdose symptoms and require gradual discontinuation of the drug. Call your local poison control center or hospital emergency room for more information.

Special Information

It may be necessary to clear your nasal passages with a nasal decongestant before using a nasal corticosteroid to allow it to reach the mucous membranes.

Some of these drugs take 10 to 14 days to start working. Beclomethasone, budesonide, and triamcinolone work faster, in 3 to 7 days; in some cases, triamcinolone provides relief in 12 hours. Flunisolide may take up to 3 weeks.

If you are taking more than one spray at a time, wait at least 1 minute between sprays.

Nasal corticosteroids may cause irritation and drying of mucous membranes in the nose. Call your doctor if this effect persists or if symptoms get worse.

Rarely, nasal *Candida* infections have developed in people taking a nasal corticosteroid. These infections may require treatment with an antifungal drug, as well as the discontinuance of the nasal corticosteroid.

People using nasal corticosteroids to prevent the return of nasal polyps after surgery may experience nosebleeds because the drugs can slow healing of the wound.

If you forget a dose of nasal corticosteroid, take it as soon as you remember. If it is almost time for your next dose, skip the dose you forgot and continue with your regular schedule. Do not take a double dose.

Special Populations

Pregnancy/Breast-feeding

Taking large amounts of corticosteroids during pregnancy may slow fetal growth. The small amount of drug absorbed into the blood after nasal application is unlikely to have any effect. Nevertheless, talk with your doctor before taking any drug if you are or might be pregnant.

Dexamethasone passes into breast milk. Nursing mothers who use this drug should bottle-feed their babies. It is not known if other nasal corticosteroids pass into breast milk; nursing mothers should be cautious about using any of these drugs.

Seniors

Seniors may use nasal corticosteroids without special restriction. Be sure your doctor knows if you suffer from bone disease, bowel disease, colitis, diabetes, glaucoma, fungal or herpes infections, high blood pressure, high blood cholesterol, an underactive thyroid, or heart, kidney, or liver disease.

Type of Drug

Corticosteroids, Topical

(kor-tih-koe-STER-oids)

Brand Names

Generic Ingredient: Alclometasone Dipropionate
Aclovate

Generic Ingredient: Amcinonide
Cyclocort

Generic Ingredient: Augmented Betamethasone Dipropionate
Diprolene   Diprolene AF

Generic Ingredient: Betamethasone [G]
Alphatrex   Beta-Val
Betatrex   Diprosone

Maxivate   Valisone
Teladar   Valisone Reduced Strength
Uticort

Generic Ingredient: Clobetasol Propionate
Temovate

Generic Ingredient: Clocortolone Pivalate
Cloderm

Generic Ingredient: Desonide
Desonide   Tridesilon
DesOwen

Generic Ingredient: Desoximetasone 🄶
Topicort   Topicort LP

Generic Ingredient: Dexamethasone
Aeroseb-Dex   Decaspray
Decadron

Generic Ingredient: Diflorasone Diacetate
Florone   Maxiflor
Florone E   Psorcon

Generic Ingredient: Fluocinolone Acetonide
Derma-Smoothe/FS   Synalar
Fluonid   Synalar-HP
Flurosyn   Synemol
FS Shampoo

Generic Ingredient: Fluocinonide 🄶
Fluonex   Lidex-E
Lidex

Generic Ingredient: Flurandrenolide 🄶
Cordran   Cordran SP

Generic Ingredient: Fluticasone Propionate
Cutivate

Generic Ingredient: Halcinonide
Halog   Halog-E

Generic Ingredient: Halobetasol Propionate
Ultravate

Generic Ingredient: Hydrocortisone Ⓖ

1% HC	Dermtex HC with Aloe
Acticort 100	Gynecort
Ala-Cort	Hemril HC
Ala-Scalp	Hi-Cor
Analpram-HC	Hycort
Anucort-HC	Hydrocort
Anumed HC	Hydro-Tex
Anusol-HC	Hytone
Bactine Hydrocortisone	Lacticare-HC
Cetacort	Locoid
CortaGel	Nutracort
Cortaid	Pandel
Cort-Dome	Penecort
Cortenema	Proctocort
Cortifoam	ProctoCream-HC
Cortizone-5	ProctoFoam-HC
Cortizone-10	S-T Cort
Dermacort	Synacort
Dermol HC	Texacort
Dermolate	Westcort

Generic Ingredient: Methylprednisolone Acetate
Medrol Acetate Topical

Generic Ingredient: Mometasone Furoate
Elocon

Generic Ingredient: Prednicarbate
Dermatop

Generic Ingredient: Triamcinolone Acetonide

Aristocort	Kenalog-H
Aristocort A	Kenonel
Delta-Tritex	Triacet
Flutex	Triderm
Kenalog	

Prescribed for

Inflammation, itching, or other local dermatologic (skin) problems; may also be used to treat psoriasis, severe diaper rash, and other conditions.

General Information

Topical (applied to and affecting the skin) corticosteroids are used to relieve the symptoms of rash, itching, or inflammation; they do not treat the underlying cause of skin problems. Topical corticosteroids work by interfering with body mechanisms that produce rash, itching, or inflammation. If you use one of these drugs without discovering the cause of the problem, the condition may return after you stop using the drug. Do not use a topical corticosteroid without your doctor's knowledge because it could cover an important symptom that may be valuable in diagnosing your condition.

Some generic versions of topical corticosteroids vary in their potency from related brand-name forms. Check with your doctor or pharmacist for more information on the interchangeability of these products.

Cautions and Warnings

Do not use a topical corticosteroid as the sole treatment for a **viral disease** of the skin—such as herpes; **fungal infections** of the skin—such as athlete's foot; or **tuberculosis of the skin**. These drugs should not be used in the ear if the **eardrum has been perforated**. Do not use these drugs if you are **allergic** to any component of the aerosol, cream, gel, lotion, ointment, or solution.

Rectal corticosteroid products should not be used if you have any serious **bowel condition**, including bowel perforation, obstruction, abscess, and systemic fungal infection.

The **rectal foam** is not expelled after it has been applied and may result in higher drug blood levels than those associated with rectal enema products. The possibility of systemic (whole-body) side effects is greater when more of the drug finds its way into the blood. If there is no improvement after 2 or 3 weeks of treatment with a rectal corticosteroid, see your doctor.

Using a topical corticosteroid around the eyes for prolonged periods may cause **cataracts** or **glaucoma**.

Children may be more susceptible to serious side effects from topical corticosteroids, especially if they are applied to large areas over long periods. Augmented betamethasone propionate, clobetasol, desoximetasone, fluticasone, and halobetasol are not recommended for use on children's skin.

Possible Side Effects

▼ Most common: burning, itching, irritation, acne, dry and cracking skin, skin tightening, secondary infection,

---

Possible Side Effects *(continued)*

and skin discoloration. These effects are more likely when the treated area is covered with an occlusive bandage (one that prevents contact with water and air).

Significant quantities of corticosteroids may be absorbed through the skin into the bloodstream if large amounts are used over a period of time. This can result in systemic effects and may cause serious problems, particularly in people with liver disease.

Drug Interactions

None known.

Usual Dose

Cream, Ointment, Solution, and Aerosol: Apply a thin film to the skin 2–4 times a day.

Rectal Enema: 100 mg nightly for 21 days.

Rectal Foam: 1 applicator's worth, 1–2 times a day for 2–3 weeks.

Overdosage

Serious adverse effects are unlikely after accidental ingestion of a topical corticosteroid. Wash excess topical corticosteroid off skin. In extreme situations, excessive use of large amounts of topical corticosteroids may cause overdose symptoms and require gradual discontinuation of the drug. Call your local poison control center or hospital emergency room for more information.

Special Information

To prevent secondary infection, clean the skin before applying a topical corticosteroid. Apply a very thin film and rub in gently—effectiveness depends on contact area, not the thickness of the layer applied.

To use a lotion, solution, or gel on your scalp, part your hair and apply a small amount of the medication to the affected area. Rub in gently.

Do not wash, rub, or put clothing on the area until the medication has dried.

Flurandrenolide tape comes with specific directions for use; follow them carefully.

If your doctor instructs you to apply plastic wrap or any other occlusive dressing on top of a topical corticosteroid product, follow directions carefully. These dressings can increase the penetration of the drug into your skin by as much as 10 times, which may be a crucial element in the medication's effectiveness. Occlusive dressings should not be used with augmented betamethasone, betamethasone propionate, clobetasol, halobetasol, or mometasone.

If you are using one of these products for diaper rash, do not use tight-fitting diapers or plastic pants, which can cause too much drug to be absorbed through the skin into the blood.

Your doctor may prescribe a specific form of the product for a specific reason. Do not change forms without your doctor's knowledge; a different form may not be as effective.

If you forget to apply a dose of a topical corticosteroid, do so as soon as you remember. If it is almost time for your next dose, skip the one you forgot and continue with your regular schedule. Do not apply a double dose.

Special Populations

Pregnancy/Breast-feeding

Corticosteroids applied to the skin in large amounts or over long periods of time have been linked to birth defects. Pregnant women should only use these drugs under a doctor's supervision. Over-the-counter hydrocortisone products should not be used for more than a few days without your doctor's knowledge.

Oral corticosteroid drugs pass into breast milk and may interfere with the growth of a nursing infant. Topical corticosteroids are not likely to cause problems, but nursing mothers should not use these drugs except under their doctor's care. If you must apply a corticosteroid to the nipple area, be sure to completely clean the area prior to nursing. Nursing mothers should never use clobetasol.

Seniors

Seniors are more susceptible to high blood pressure and osteoporosis (condition characterized by loss of bone mass due to depletion of minerals, especially calcium) associated with large doses of oral corticosteroids. However, these effects are unlikely with corticosteroids applied to the skin unless a high-potency medication is used over a large area for an extended period.

Brand Name

Cortisporin Otic

Generic Ingredients

Hydrocortisone + Neomycin Sulfate + Polymyxin B Sulfate Ⓖ

Other Brand Names
AK-Spore H.C. Otic
AntibiOtic
Cortatrigen Ear Drops
Drotic
Ear-Eze
LazerSporin-C
Octicair

Otic-Care
OtiTricin
Otocort
Otomycin-HPN Otic
Pediotic
UAD Otic

Type of Drug

Antibiotic-corticosteroid combination.

Prescribed for

Superficial ear infection, ear inflammation or itching, and other problems of the outer ear.

General Information

Cortisporin Otic contains a corticosteroid drug to reduce inflammation and 2 antibiotics to treat local ear infections. This combination can be quite useful for local ear problems because of its dual method of action and its relatively broad, nonspecific applicability.

"Otic" refers to the ear; "ophthalmic" refers to the eye. Cortisporin also makes an ophthalmic suspension and an ophthalmic ointment, both made for use in the eye. Do not confuse these products with Cortisporin Otic—a drug intended for use in the eye must not be used in the ear, and vice versa.

Cautions and Warnings

Do not use this product if you are **sensitive** or **allergic** to any of its ingredients.

Cortisporin Otic is specifically **designed to be used in the ear**. It can be very damaging if accidentally placed into the eye.

Possible Side Effects

Local irritation, such as itching or burning, may occur if you are sensitive or allergic to one of the ingredients in this medication.

Drug Interactions

None known.

Usual Dose

2–4 drops in the affected ear 3–4 times a day.

Overdosage

The amount of drug contained in each bottle of Cortisporin Otic is too small to cause serious problems. Call your doctor, hospital emergency room, or local poison control center for more information.

Special Information

Use only when specifically prescribed by a physician. Overuse of this or similar products can result in the growth of new organisms, such as fungi.

If new infections or new problems appear during the time you are using this medication, stop using the drug and contact your doctor.

When using eardrops, wash your hands, then hold the closed bottle in your hand for a few minutes to warm it to body temperature. Shake well for 10 seconds to mix the suspended antibiotic in the solution. For best results, drops should not be self-administered; they should be given by another person. The person receiving the drops should lie on his or her side with the affected ear facing upward. Fill the dropper and instill the required number of drops directly in the ear canal.

If the drops are being given to an infant, hold the earlobe *down* and back to allow the drops to run in. If the drops are being given to an older child or adult, hold the earlobe *up* and back to allow them to run in. Do not put the dropper into the ear or allow it to touch any part of the ear or bottle. Keep the ear tilted for about 2 minutes after the drops have been put in or insert a soft cotton plug, whichever is recommended by your doctor.

If you forget a dose of Cortisporin Otic, take it as soon as you remember. If it is almost time for your next dose, skip the dose you forgot and continue with your regular schedule. Do not apply a double dose.

Special Populations

Pregnancy/Breast-feeding
Pregnant and breast-feeding women may use this product without special restriction.

Seniors
Seniors may use this product without special restriction.

Coumadin

see **Warfarin**, page 1157

Cozaar

see **Losartan**, page 615

Generic Name

Cromolyn (KROE-muh-lin) G

Brand Names

Crolom	Intal
Gastrocrom	Nasalcrom

Type of Drug

Allergy preventive and antiasthmatic.

Prescribed for

Prevention of severe allergic reactions, including asthma, runny nose, and mastocytosis; also prescribed for food allergies, eczema, dermatitis, chronic itching, and hay fever. It may be used to treat and prevent chronic inflammatory bowel disease; however, other drug products are more effective for this use. Cromolyn eyedrops are used to treat conjunctivitis (pinkeye) and other eye irritations.

General Information

Cromolyn sodium prevents allergy, asthma, and other conditions by stabilizing mast cells, which are a key component in any allergic reaction because they release histamine. Cromolyn prevents the release of histamine and other potent chemicals from mast cells in your body. The drug works only in the areas to which it is applied; only 7% to 8% of an inhaled dose and 1% of a swallowed capsule is absorbed into the blood. Even the oral capsules, which one would normally expect to be absorbed into the blood, treat only gastrointestinal-tract allergies. Cromolyn products must be used on a regular basis to be effective in reducing the frequency and intensity of allergic reactions.

Cautions and Warnings

Cromolyn should never be used to treat an **acute allergy attack**. It is intended only to prevent or reduce the number of allergic attacks and their intensity. Once the proper dosage level has been established for you, reducing that level may result in a recurrence of attacks.

On rare occasions, people have experienced severe **allergic attacks** after taking cromolyn. People allergic to cromolyn should not take any product containing it.

People with **kidney or liver disease** should take reduced dosages of this drug.

Cough or **bronchial spasm** may occasionally occur after the inhalation of a cromolyn dose. Severe bronchospasm is rare.

Cromolyn aerosol should be used with caution in people with **abnormal heart rhythm** or **diseased coronary blood vessels** because of a possible reaction to the propellants used in the product.

Possible Side Effects

▼ Most common: skin rash and itching. Capsules—headache and diarrhea. Most capsule side effects are minor and may be attributable to the underlying condition; a variety have been reported but cannot be tied conclusively to the drug.

Possible Side Effects *(continued)*

▼ Less common: local irritation, including nasal stinging, sneezing, tearing, cough, and stuffy nose; urinary
difficulty; dizziness; headache; joint swelling; a bad taste
in the mouth; nosebleeds; abdominal pain; and nausea.

▼ Rare: severe drug reactions, consisting of coughing,
difficulty in swallowing, hives, itching, breathing difficulties, or swelling of the eyelids, lips, or face.

Drug Interactions

None known.

Food Interactions

Inhaled or swallowed cromolyn products should not be
mixed with any food, juice, or milk. The nasal and eye
products may be taken without regard to food or meals.

Usual Dose

Inhaled Capsules or Solution

   Adult and Child (age 2 and over): starting dose—20 mg 4
times a day. Children under age 5 may inhale cromolyn
powder if their allergies are severe. The solution must be
given with a power-operated nebulizer and face mask. Hand-
held nebulizers are not adequate. To prevent exercise asthma,
20 mg may be inhaled up to 1 hour before exercise.

Aerosol

   Adult and Child (age 5 and over): up to 2 sprays 4 times a
day, spaced equally throughout the day. To prevent exercise
asthma, 2 puffs may be inhaled up to 1 hour before exercise.

Nasal Solution

   Adult and Child (age 6 and over): 1 spray in each nostril 3–6
times a day at regular intervals. First blow your nose, and
then inhale the spray.

Oral Capsules

   Adult: 2 capsules ½ hour before meals and at bedtime.

   Child (age 2–12): 1 capsule (100 mg) 4 times a day ½ hour
before meals and at bedtime. Dosage may be increased to
about 13–18 mg per lb. of body weight in 4 equal doses.

   Child (under age 2): about 10 mg per lb. of body weight a

day, divided into 4 equal doses. This product is recommended in infants and young children only if absolutely necessary.

Eyedrops
   Adult and Child (age 4 and over): 1–2 drops in each eye 4–6 times a day, at regular intervals.

Overdosage

No action is necessary other than medical observation. Call your local poison control center or hospital emergency room for more information.

Special Information

Cromolyn is taken to prevent or minimize severe allergic reactions. It is imperative that you take cromolyn products on a regular basis to provide equal protection throughout the day.

If you are taking cromolyn to prevent seasonal allergies, it is essential that you start taking the medication before you come into contact with the cause of the allergy and that you continue treatment throughout the period during which you will be exposed to the allergy source.

Cromolyn oral capsules should be opened and their contents mixed with about 4 ounces of hot water. Stir until the powder completely dissolves and the solution is completely clear; then fill the rest of the glass with cold water. Drink the entire contents of the glass. Do not mix the solution with food, juice, or milk.

Do not wear soft contact lenses while using cromolyn eyedrops. The lenses may be replaced a few hours after you stop taking the drug.

Call your doctor if you develop wheezing, coughing, severe drug reaction (see "Possible Side Effects"), or skin rash. Other side effects should be reported if they are severe or particularly bothersome.

Call your doctor if your symptoms do not improve or if they worsen while you are taking this drug.

Cromolyn's effectiveness depends on taking it regularly. If you forget a dose of cromolyn, take it as soon as you remember and space the remaining doses equally throughout the rest of the day. Do not take a double dose of this drug. Call your doctor if symptoms of your condition return because you have skipped too many doses.

Special Populations

Pregnancy/Breast-feeding

Animal studies have shown no birth defects related to cromolyn, nor have any individual cases of cromolyn-associated birth defects been reported. Animal studies with very large doses of cromolyn administered directly into a vein have shown some potential for damage to the fetus, however. Women who are or might be pregnant should not use cromolyn unless its advantages have been carefully weighed against its risks.

It is not known if cromolyn passes into breast milk. No drug-related problems have been known to occur, but nursing mothers who use cromolyn should exercise caution.

Seniors

No problems have been reported in seniors. However, older adults are likely to have age-related reduction in kidney and/or liver function. Your doctor should take this factor into account when determining your cromolyn dosage.

Generic Name

Cyclobenzaprine (sye-cloe-BEN-zuh-prene) Ⓖ

Brand Name

Flexeril

Type of Drug

Skeletal muscle relaxant.

Prescribed for

Serious muscle spasm and acute muscle pain; also used to treat fibrositis (muscular rheumatism) characterized by pain, stiffness, and tenderness.

General Information

Cyclobenzoprine hydrochloride is used in the treatment of severe muscle spasms; it is prescribed as part of a coordinated program of rest, physical therapy, and other measures. It is not effective for spastic movement associated with spinal cord or brain disease. Cyclobenzaprine begins working an hour after it is taken and reaches its maximum effect after 1 to 2 weeks of continuous use.

Cautions and Warnings

Do not take cyclobenzaprine if you are **allergic** to it. This drug should not be taken for several weeks following a **heart attack** or by people with **abnormal heart rhythms, heart failure, heart block** (disruption of the electrical impulses that control heart rate), or **hyperthyroidism** (overactive thyroid gland).

Cyclobenzaprine should be avoided by people with **urinary retention, glaucoma**, or **increased eye pressure**. This drug inhibits the flow of saliva and may increase the chances of **cavities** or **gum disease**.

Cyclobenzaprine is intended only for **short-term use** of 2 to 3 weeks. Painful muscle spasm is usually a short-term condition; treatment beyond 2 to 3 weeks is usually not needed.

Cyclobenzaprine is chemically similar to tricyclic antidepressants and may produce some of the more serious side effects associated with those drugs. Abruptly stopping cyclobenzaprine may cause **nausea, headache,** and **feelings of ill health;** this is not a sign of addiction.

Possible Side Effects

▼ Most common: dry mouth, drowsiness, and dizziness.

▼ Less common: muscle weakness, fatigue, nausea, constipation, upset stomach, unpleasant taste, blurred vision, headache, nervousness, and confusion.

▼ Rare: rapid heartbeat, fainting, low blood pressure, abnormal heart rhythms, heart palpitations, disorientation, sleeplessness, depression, unusual sensation, anxiety, agitation, abnormal thoughts and dreams, hallucinations, excitement, vomiting, appetite loss, stomach irritation and pain, diarrhea, stomach gas, thirst, temporary loss of sense of taste, urinary changes, hepatitis, yellowing of the skin or whites of the eyes, sweating, rash, itching, muscle twitching, local weakness, and swelling of the face or tongue.

Many other side effects have been reported by people taking cyclobenzaprine, but their relationship to the drug

---
Possible Side Effects *(continued)*
---
has not been established. Report anything unusual to
your doctor.

Drug Interactions

• The effects of alcohol, sedatives, or other nervous system
depressants may be increased by cyclobenzaprine.

• Cyclobenzaprine may increase some side effects of atropine, ipratropium, and other anticholinergic drugs. These
include blurred vision, constipation, urinary difficulties, dry
mouth, confusion, and drowsiness.

• The combination of cyclobenzaprine and a monoamine
oxidase inhibitor (MAOI) antidepressant may produce very
high fever, convulsions, and possibly death. Do not take these
drugs within 14 days of each other.

• Cyclobenzaprine may increase the effects of haloperidol,
loxapine, molindone, pimozide, anticoagulant (blood-thinning)
drugs, anticonvulsants, thyroid hormones, antithyroid drugs,
phenothiazines, and thioxanthenes. The effects of nasal decongestants such as naphazoline, oxymetazoline, phenylephrine,
and xylometazoline may be increased by cyclobenzaprine.

• Barbiturates and carbamazepine may counteract the effects of cyclobenzaprine.

• Fluoxetine, ranitidine, cimetidine, methylphenidate, es-
tramustine, estrogens, and oral contraceptives may increase
the effects and side effects of cyclobenzaprine.

• Cyclobenzaprine may counteract the effects of clonidine,
guanadrel, and guanethidine.

Food Interactions

None known.

Usual Dose

Adult and Child (age 15 and over): 10 mg 3 times a day; may
be increased up to 60 mg a day.
Child (under age 15): not recommended.

Overdosage

Cyclobenzaprine overdose may cause confusion, loss of concentration, hallucinations, agitation, overactive reflexes, fever
or vomiting, rigid muscles, and other side effects of the drug.

It may also cause drowsiness, low body temperature, rapid or irregular heartbeat and other kinds of abnormal heart rhythms, heart failure, dilated pupils, convulsions, very low blood pressure, stupor, coma, and sweating. Overdose victims must be taken to a hospital emergency room. ALWAYS bring the prescription bottle or container with you.

Special Information

Cyclobenzaprine causes drowsiness, dizziness, or blurred vision in more than 40% of people who take it, which may interfere with the ability to perform complex tasks like driving or operating equipment. Avoid alcohol, sedatives, and other nervous system depressants because they can enhance sedative effects of cyclobenzaprine.

Call your doctor if you develop rash; hives; itching; urinary difficulties; clumsiness; confusion; depression; convulsions; yellowing of the skin or whites of the eyes; swelling of the face, lips, or tongue; or any other persistent or bothersome side effect.

If you forget a dose of cyclobenzaprine, take it as soon as you remember. If you take cyclobenzaprine once a day and it is almost time for your next dose, skip the one you forgot and continue with your regular schedule. If you take cyclobenzaprine twice a day and it is almost time for your next dose, take 1 dose as soon as you remember, another in 5 or 6 hours, and then go back to your regular schedule. If you take cyclobenzaprine 3 times a day and it is almost time for your next dose, take 1 dose as soon as you remember, another in 3 or 4 hours, and then go back to your regular schedule. Never take a double dose.

Special Populations

Pregnancy/Breast-feeding

Animal studies have shown no evidence that cyclobenzaprine harms the fetus. Nevertheless, it should be avoided by pregnant women unless the potential benefits clearly outweigh the risks.

It is not known if cyclobenzaprine passes into breast milk, but antidepressants with a similar chemical structure do pass into breast milk. Nursing mothers who must take this drug should consider bottle-feeding.

Seniors

Seniors are more likely to be sensitive to the effects of cyclobenzaprine. Be sure to report any unusual or bothersome side effects to your doctor.

Generic Name

Cyclosporine (sye-kloe-SPOR-in)

Brand Names

Sandimmune   Neoral

Type of Drug

Immunosuppressant.

Prescribed for

Kidney, heart, or liver transplantation; used without Food and Drug Administration (FDA) approval for bone-marrow, heart-lung, and pancreas transplants; also prescribed for patchy hair loss, rheumatoid arthritis, aplastic anemia, atopic dermatitis, Behçet's disease, cirrhosis of the liver related to bile-duct blockade, ulcerative colitis, dermatomyositis, eye symptoms of Graves' disease, insulin-dependent diabetes, kidney inflammation associated with lupus and other kidney diseases, multiple sclerosis (MS), severe psoriasis and psoriasis-related arthritis, myasthenia gravis, pemphigus, sarcoidosis of the lung, and pyoderma gangrenosum.

General Information

Cyclosporine was the first drug approved in the U.S. to prevent rejection of transplanted organs. A product of fungus metabolism, cyclosporine was proven to be a potent immunosuppressant in 1972 and was first given to human kidney and bone marrow transplant patients in 1978. It selectively inhibits cells known as T-lymphocytes that, as an integral part of the body's defense mechanism, destroy invading cells. Cyclosporine also prevents the production of a substance known as interleukin-II that activates T-lymphocyte cells. In 1995, a new form of cyclosporine called Neoral, a microemulsion, was introduced by its manufacturer. This form is as safe and effective as the original product but is better absorbed into the bloodstream and requires less medication to achieve the same effect. Thus, if you are already taking cyclosporine, your Neoral dosage will be less than that of Sandimmune and must be adjusted by your doctor.

Cautions and Warnings

Cyclosporine should be prescribed only by **doctors experi-**

enced in immunosuppressive therapy and the care of organ-transplant patients. Sandimmune is always used with corticosteroid drugs like prednisone. Neoral has been used with a corticosteroid and azathioprine, an immune suppressant. When combined with other immune suppressants, cyclosporine must be used with great care because oversuppression of the immune system may lead to lymphoma or extreme susceptibility to infection.

Sandimmune, the original oral form of cyclosporine, is poorly absorbed into the bloodstream; it must be taken in a dosage that is 3 times greater than the injectable dosage. People taking this drug by mouth for a long period of time should have their blood checked for **cyclosporine levels** so that the dosage may be adjusted if necessary. Since more Neoral is absorbed into the blood you will probably need less of it. When you first start taking Neoral, your dosage will be about the same as that of the older oral liquid but then will be reduced according to the amount of cyclosporine in your blood. Follow your doctor's directions about drug dosage. **Do not substitute Neoral for Sandimmune**; they are not equivalent to each other.

Cyclosporine causes **kidney toxicosis** (condition due to poisoning)—different from transplant rejection—in 25% to 35% of people taking it to prevent organ rejection. Mild symptoms usually start after about 2 or 3 months of treatment. This effect may be controlled by reducing drug dosage. In one study, clonidine skin patches used before and after surgery decreased toxic risks to the kidney.

Liver toxicosis is seen in about 5% of transplant patients taking cyclosporine. It usually appears in the first month and may be controlled by reducing the dosage.

Convulsions may develop, especially in people also taking high dosages of corticosteroids. Other nervous system side effects are listed below (see "Possible Side Effects").

Cyclosporine may cause **high blood-potassium or uric-acid levels.**

In one study, cyclosporine increased **cholesterol** and other blood-fat levels. It is not known how this affects people who take the drug on a long-term basis.

There is conflicting information on how cyclosporine affects sugar in the body. Kidney-transplant patients taking the drug have developed **insulin-dependent diabetes**, which is related to the dosage of cyclosporine and reverses itself when you stop taking the drug. On the other hand, cyclosporine preserves the function of insulin-producing cells in the pancreas and has allowed many insulin-dependent diabetics to live without taking insulin.

Possible Side Effects

▼ Most common: Cyclosporine is known to be toxic to the kidneys. Your doctor will carefully monitor your kidney function while you are taking cyclosporine. Other side effects are high blood pressure, increased hair growth, and enlargement of the gums. Lymphoma may develop in people whose immune systems are excessively suppressed. Almost 85% of people treated with cyclosporine develop an infection, compared with 94% of people on other immune-system suppressants.

▼ Less common: tremors, cramps, acne, brittle hair or fingernails, convulsions, headache, confusion, diarrhea, nausea or vomiting, tingling in the hands or feet, facial flushing, reduction in blood counts of white cells and platelets, sinus inflammation, swollen and painful male breasts, drug allergy (symptoms include rash, itching, hives, and breathing difficulties), conjunctivitis (pinkeye), fluid retention and swelling, ringing or buzzing in the ears, hearing loss, high blood sugar, and muscle pain.

▼ Rare: blood in the urine, heart attack, itching, anxiety, depression, lethargy, weakness, mouth sores, difficulty swallowing, intestinal bleeding, constipation, pancreas inflammation, night sweats, chest pain, joint pain, visual disturbances, and weight loss.

Drug Interactions

• Cyclosporine should be used carefully with other kidney-toxic drugs including nonsteroidal anti-inflammatory drugs (NSAIDs) such as ibuprofen, naproxen, and others; gentamicin; tobramycin; vancomycin; trimethoprim-sulfamethoxazole; melphalan; amphotericin B; ketoconazole; azapropazon; diclofenac; cimetidine; ranitidine; and tacrolimus.

• Drugs that may increase blood levels of cyclosporine include amiodarone, diltiazem, nicardipine, verapamil, fluconazole, itraconazole, clarithromycin, danazol, erythromycin, methyltestosterone, methylprednisolone—this combination also causes convulsions—allopurinol, bromocriptine, danazol, and metoclopramide. With ketoconazole, this drug interaction may be used by your doctor to reduce your cyclosporine dosage.

• Drugs that decrease cyclosporine levels and may lead to organ rejection include nafcillin, rifabutin, rifampin, carbamazepine, probucol, phenobarbital, and phenytoin.

• Cyclosporine interferes with the body's ability to clear digoxin, prednisolone, and lovastatin. People taking any of these drugs who start on cyclosporine must have their drug dosage reduced.

• Combining colchicine with cyclosporine may lead to liver, kidney, stomach, and other side effects. Avoid this combination.

• Combining cyclosporine with nifedipine may lead to gum overgrowth.

• Cyclosporine increases blood potassium. Excessive blood-potassium levels may be reached if cyclosporine is taken with enalapril, lisinopril, a potassium-sparing diuretic such as spironolactone, salt substitutes, potassium supplements, or high potassium—low sodium—food.

• Cyclosporine prevents the normal body response to live vaccines. People taking cyclosporine should be vaccinated only after specific discussions with their doctors. You must wait for a period of several months to several years after stopping the medication before vaccination may be considered again.

Food Interactions

Sandimmune comes in a castor oil base. Neoral is made as a microemulsion to make it taste a little better; still, you may mix it in a glass—not a paper or plastic cup—with room-temperature orange or apple juice to make it taste better. Chocolate milk may also be used. DO NOT USE GRAPEFRUIT JUICE BECAUSE IT SPEEDS THE BREAKDOWN OF CYCLO-SPORINE. Drink immediately after mixing, then put more juice in the glass and drink it to be sure that the entire dose has been taken. Cyclosporine microemulsion should not be taken with unflavored milk because it may be unpalatable. Cyclosporine capsules—either brand—may be taken with no special procedures.

Eating a fatty—15 g to 45 g of fat—meal within half an hour of taking Neoral may reduce the amount absorbed by 13%.

Cyclosporine may be taken with food if it upsets your stomach.

Usual Dose

In general, the usual dosage of Neoral is lower than Sandimmune but dosage must be individualized for you by your doctor. Do not substitute one brand for the other.

Sandimmune
Adult: The usual oral dosage of cyclosporine is 6–8 mg per lb. of body weight a day. The first dose is given 4–12 hours before the transplant operation or immediately after surgery. This dosage is continued after the operation for 1 or 2 weeks and then slowly reduced to 2.25–4.5 mg per lb. of body weight.
Child: Similar dosages are usually prescribed but, because children tend to release the drug from their bodies faster than adults, larger and more frequent doses may be needed.

Neoral
Adult: The usual oral dosage of Neoral is 3–4 mg per lb. of body weight a day divided into 2 doses. The first dose is given 4–12 hours before the transplant operation or immediately after surgery. This dosage is continued after the operation for 1 or 2 weeks and then slowly reduced to maintain a target amount of cyclosporine in the body.
Child: Similar dosages are usually prescribed but, because children tend to release the drug from their bodies faster than adults, larger and more frequent doses may be needed.

Overdosage

Overdose victims may be expected to develop side effects and symptoms of extreme immunosuppression. Suspected victims must be made to vomit with ipecac syrup—available at any pharmacy—to remove any remaining drug from the stomach, which is recommended up to 2 hours after the overdose was taken. Call your doctor or a poison control center before inducing vomiting. If you must go to a hospital emergency room, ALWAYS bring the prescription bottle or container with you.

Special Information

Call your doctor at the first sign of fever; sore throat; tiredness; weakness; nervousness; unusual bleeding or bruising; tender or swollen gums; convulsions; irregular heartbeat; confusion; numbness or tingling of your hands, feet, or lips; breathing difficulties; severe stomach pain with nausea; or blood in the urine. Other side effects such as shaking or trembling of the hands, increased hair growth, acne, headache, leg cramps, nausea, or vomiting are less serious but should be brought to your doctor's attention, particularly if they are unusually bothersome or persistent.

It is important to maintain good dental hygiene while taking cyclosporine and to use extra care when using your toothbrush or dental floss because of the risk that the drug will make you more susceptible to dental infections. Cyclosporine may cause swollen gums and suppresses the normal body systems that fight infection. See your dentist regularly while taking this drug.

Continue taking your medication as long as your doctor continues to prescribe it. Do not stop taking it without telling your doctor. If you cannot take one of the oral forms, cyclosporine can be given by injection.

Do not keep either brand of the oral liquid in the refrigerator. After the bottle is opened, use the medication within 2 months. At temperatures below 68°F, Neoral can form a gel and a light sediment can form in Sandimmune. These do not affect the potency of either product. They can still be used and are effective.

If you forget to take a dose of cyclosporine, take it as soon as you remember if it is within 12 hours of your regular dose. If not, skip the dose you forgot and continue with your regular schedule. Do not take a double dose.

Special Populations

Pregnancy/Breast-feeding

In animal studies cyclosporine damages the fetus. Though a small number of pregnant women have taken cyclosporine without major problems, it is recommended that pregnant women avoid cyclosporine. When this drug is considered crucial by your doctor, its potential benefits must be carefully weighed against its risks.

Cyclosporine passes into breast milk. Nursing mothers who must take cyclosporine should bottle-feed their infants.

Seniors

Seniors are likely to have age-related decreases in kidney function and may therefore be more susceptible to kidney toxicosis associated with this drug. Otherwise, seniors may take cyclosporine without special restriction.

Cycrin

see **Medroxyprogesterone Acetate**, page 645

Daypro

see **Oxaprozin**, page 821

Generic Name

Delavirdine (deh-LAV-er-dene)

Brand Name

Rescriptor

Type of Drug

Antiviral.

Prescribed for

Human immunodeficiency virus (HIV) infection, in combination with other antiviral drugs.

General Information

Delavirdine mesylate is a non-nucleoside reverse transcriptase inhibitor (NNRTI). Delavirdine inhibits the reverse transcriptase (RT) enzyme, necessary for reproduction of HIV in body cells, by binding directly to RT. If delavirdine is not taken with other antivirals, resistance to the drug may develop as soon as 8 weeks after treatment begins. For this reason, delavirdine is recommended only in combination with other anti-HIV drugs.

HIV that is resistant to one NNRTI is likely to be resistant to other drugs of this type. The possibility of cross-resistance between delavirdine and a protease inhibitor is unlikely because these two drug types act on different kinds of enzymes.

Delavirdine is rapidly absorbed into the blood, with blood levels reaching their peak 1 hour after it is taken. It is broken down in the liver by two different enzyme systems, 3A and 2D6. Delavirdine inhibits the enzymes that break it down, so the period that it stays in the body increases as you continue treatment. Women reach 30% higher delavirdine blood levels than men.

Cautions and Warnings

Delavirdine **drug interactions may be serious or life threatening** (see "Drug Interactions"). Delavirdine is primarily broken down in the liver; people with **liver disease** should use it with caution. People taking delavirdine should have their liver enzymes measured periodically. The chances of developing a **rash** while taking delavirdine are almost 1 in 5. Anyone who develops a severe rash, rash with fever, blisters, mouth sores, eye irritation, swelling, or muscle or joint ache should stop taking delavirdine and call the doctor.

Possible Side Effects

▼ Most common: nausea and rash.
▼ Common: headache and tiredness.
▼ Less common: diarrhea, vomiting, liver irritation, itching. Other reactions may affect almost any part of the body including the heart, nervous system, stomach and intestines, genitals and urinary system, blood and lymph system, muscles and bones, lungs, eyes, ears, and nose.

Drug Interactions

• Some delavirdine drug interactions are potentially serious or life threatening. These interactions occur because of delavirdine's effect on liver enzymes.

• Anticonvulsants, rifabutin, and rifampin may reduce the amount of delavirdine in the blood.

• Antacids and didanosine may reduce the amount of delavirdine in the blood by interfering with its absorption in the blood; take these drugs and delavirdine at least 1 hour apart.

• When delavirdine and clarithromycin are combined, the amount of either drug in the blood may be doubled.

• Delavirdine interferes with the breakdown of the protease inhibitors indinavir and saquinavir. A reduction in the protease inhibitor dosage may be needed.

• Fluoxetine and ketoconazole increase the amount of delavirdine in the blood by about 50%.

• Cimetidine, ranitidine, and similar drugs may reduce the

amount of delavirdine absorbed. Do not combine these drugs
with delavirdine for any length of time.

• Do not take delavirdine with certain antimicrobials, including clarithromycin, dapsone, and rifabutin; benzodiazepine tranquilizers and sleeping medication; cisapride; ergot
drugs; quinidine; and warfarin.

Food Interactions

None known.

Usual Dose

Adult: 400 mg 3 times a day.

Overdosage

No cases of delavirdine overdose are known. Overdose victims should be taken to a hospital emergency room for
treatment. ALWAYS bring the prescription bottle or container
with you.

Special Information

Delavirdine solution is somewhat better absorbed than the
tablets. The amount of drug absorbed from delavirdine tablets can be increased by allowing them to disintegrate in
water and then swallowing the mixture.

People with achlorhydria (absence of stomach acid) should
take delavirdine with an acidic drink, such as orange or
cranberry juice.

Delavirdine does not cure HIV. It will not prevent you from
transmitting the HIV virus to another person; you must still
practice safe sex. People taking delavirdine for HIV can still
develop HIV-related conditions. The long-term effects of delavirdine are not known. People taking this drug should be under
a doctor's care at all times.

If you develop a severe rash, or rash with fever, blisters,
mouth sores, eye irritation, swelling, or muscle or joint ache,
stop taking delavirdine and see your doctor.

Take the medication every day exactly as prescribed. It is
important to follow your doctor's directions and not miss
doses. If you forget to take a dose of delavirdine, take it as
soon as you remember. If it is almost time for your next dose,
skip the dose you forgot and continue with your regular
schedule. Do not take a double dose.

Special Populations

Pregnancy/Breast-feeding
Delavirdine causes birth defects in laboratory animals. Of 7 unplanned pregnancies reported in delavirdine studies, 3 women had ectopic pregnancies, 3 had normal, healthy babies, and one baby was born prematurely with a heart valve defect. However, there are no specific studies of delavirdine in pregnant women. This drug should not be taken unless you have discussed the possible benefits and risks with your doctor.

Delavirdine passes into breast milk in concentrations that are 3 to 5 times the concentrations found in the mother's blood and should not be taken by nursing mothers. In any case, mothers who are HIV positive should bottle-feed their babies to avoid transmitting the virus through their milk.

Seniors
Seniors may take delavirdine without special precaution.

Deltasone

see **Corticosteroids**, *page 253*

Depakote

see **Valproic Acid**, *page 1143*

Generic Name

Desmopressin (dez-moe-PRES-in)

Brand Names

DDAVP   Stimate

Type of Drug

Pituitary hormone replacement.

Prescribed for

Nighttime bed-wetting and diabetes insipidus (central or

cranial diabetes). Desmopressin injection is used for hemophilia A and von Willebrand's disease. Desmopressin has no effect on diabetes mellitus, a condition brought on by the inability to make or use insulin.

General Information

Desmopressin is a synthetic version of the natural antidiuretic hormone (ADH). When ADH is lacking, the body has difficulty retaining fluid. People lacking ADH become very thirsty, make a lot of urine, and still become dehydrated; desmopressin controls these symptoms. When used for nighttime bedwetting, desmopressin should be used in conjunction with behavioral or other nondrug therapies. Desmopressin's effect is stronger than ADH and it lasts longer than the natural hormone; a single dose lasts up to 20 hours.

Cautions and Warnings

People **allergic** to desmopressin should not take this drug.

People using desmopressin should only drink enough fluid to satisfy their thirst. Rarely, people taking it develop **water intoxication**, which can result in seizures.

Heart attacks and strokes after treatment with desmopressin have been reported in people at risk for them, but there is no definite link to desmopressin use.

People using desmopressin should have their **urine checked regularly** by their doctor. Other things your doctor will watch for are how the drug affects your heart, nasal swelling, congestion, and scarring.

Possible Side Effects

▼ Rare: slight increases in blood pressure, loss of sodium, water intoxication (symptoms include coma, confusion, drowsiness, continuing headache, decreased urination, rapid weight gain, and seizures), stomach or abdominal cramps, redness or flushing of the skin, and vulvar pain. A stuffy or runny nose may occur with use of the nasal solution.

Drug Interactions

• Desmopressin may increase the effects of other drugs that raise blood pressure. This only happens with large doses.

• Chlorpropamide and carbamazepine may increase the effects of desmopressin.

Food Interactions

None known.

Usual Dose

Nasal Solution—Nighttime Bed-wetting
   Adult and Child (age 6 and over): 20 mcg—0.2 ml—at bedtime.

Nasal Solution—Diabetes Insipidus
   Adult: 0.1–0.4 ml daily
   Child (age 3 months–12 years): 0.05–0.3 ml a day in 1 or 2 doses.

Tablets
   Adult: Begin with 0.05 mg 2 times a day. Daily dosage should be increased according to individual need, up to 1.2 mg a day divided into 2 or 3 doses.
   Child: Begin with 0.05 mg and adjust according to individual need.

Overdosage

Overdose symptoms are headache, abdominal cramps, nausea, and facial flushing. Call your doctor or a hospital emergency room if you suspect an overdose. Because there is no known antidote to desmopressin, your dosage may be temporarily reduced until overdose symptoms subside.

Special Information

Call your doctor if you develop headache, breathing difficulties, heartburn, nausea, abdominal or stomach cramps, or vulvar pain.
   The Stimate Nasal Solution spray pump must be primed before its first use. To prime the pump, press down 4 times. Stimate delivers 25 doses per bottle. Throw away the bottle after 25 doses have been used, because anything remaining after the 25th dose is likely to deliver less drug than is needed.

Special Populations

Pregnancy/Breast-feeding

Several articles have discussed successful desmopressin treatment of diabetes insipidus in pregnant women without harm to the fetus, but there are no conclusive studies. Synthetic desmopressin does not stimulate contractions. Like all other drugs, desmopressin should only be used by pregnant women when absolutely necessary. One study of nursing mothers using desmopressin nasal spray showed little, if any, change in their breast milk. Although other articles have been published on nursing mothers using desmopressin, there is still little information about desmopressin effects on nursing. Nursing mothers should use this drug with caution and discuss bottle-feeding their baby with their doctor.

Seniors

Seniors may use desmopressin without special precaution. Avoid drinking excessive fluid.

Desogen

see **Contraceptives**, *page 246*

Generic Name

Diazepam (dye-AZ-uh-pam) [G]

Brand Names

Diastat   Valrelease
Diazepam Intensol   Zetran
Valium [S]

The information contained in this profile also applies to the following drugs:

Generic Ingredient: Halazepam
Paxipam

Generic Ingredient: Oxazepam [G]
Serax

Generic Ingredient: Prazepam [G]
Centrax

Type of Drug

Benzodiazepine tranquilizer.

Prescribed for

Anxiety, tension, fatigue, agitation, muscle spasm, and seizures; also prescribed for irritable bowel syndrome and panic
attacks.

General Information

Diazepam and the other drugs named above are *benzodiazepines*, used as antianxiety agents, as anticonvulsants, or as
sedatives. Some are more suited to a specific role because of
differences in chemical makeup that give them greater activity in a certain area; others have particular characteristics that
make them more desirable for certain functions. Often, individual drugs are limited by the applications for which their
research has been sponsored.

Benzodiazepines directly affect the brain. They can relax
you and make you more tranquil or sleepier, or they can slow
nervous system transmissions in such a way as to act as an
anticonvulsant: The exact effect varies according to drug and
dosage. Many doctors prefer benzodiazepines to other drugs
that can be used to similar effect because they tend to be
safer, have fewer side effects, and are usually as effective, if
not more so.

Cautions and Warnings

Do not take diazepam if you know you are **sensitive** or **allergic**
to it or to another benzodiazepine drug, including clonazepam.

Diazepam can aggravate narrow-angle glaucoma, but you
may take it if you have open-angle glaucoma. Check with
your doctor.

Other conditions in which diazepam should be avoided are
severe **depression**, severe **lung disease, sleep apnea** (intermittent cessation of breathing during sleep), **liver disease,
drunkenness,** and **kidney disease**. In all of these conditions,
the depressive effects of diazepam may be enhanced and/or
could be detrimental to your overall condition.

Diazepam should not be taken by **psychotic patients,** because it is not effective for them and can trigger unusual
excitement, stimulation, and rage.

Diazepam is not intended for more than 3 to 4 months of
continuous use. Your condition should be reassessed before
continuing your medication beyond that time.

Diazepam may be **addictive**, and you can experience drug
withdrawal symptoms if you suddenly stop taking it after as

little as 4 to 6 weeks of treatment. Withdrawal symptoms include increased anxiety, tingling in the extremities, sensitivity to bright light or to the sun, long periods of sleep or sleeplessness, a metallic taste, flu-like illness, fatigue, difficulty concentrating, restlessness, loss of appetite, nausea, irritability, headache, dizziness, sweating, muscle tension or cramps, tremors, and feeling uncomfortable. Other major symptoms are confusion, abnormal perception of movement, depersonalization, paranoid delusions, hallucinations, psychotic reactions, muscle twitching, seizures, and memory loss.

Possible Side Effects

▼ Most common: mild drowsiness during the first few days of therapy. Weakness and confusion may occur, especially in seniors and in those who are sickly. If these effects persist, contact your doctor.

▼ Less common: depression, lethargy, disorientation, headache, inactivity, slurred speech, stupor, dizziness, tremors, constipation, dry mouth, nausea, inability to control urination, sexual difficulties, irregular menstrual cycle, changes in heart rhythm, low blood pressure, fluid retention, blurred or double vision, itching, rash, hiccups, nervousness, inability to fall asleep, and occasional liver dysfunction. If you have any of these symptoms, stop taking the drug and contact your doctor at once.

▼ Rare: diarrhea, coated tongue, sore gums, vomiting, changes in appetite, difficulty swallowing, increased salivation, upset stomach, changes in sex drive, urinary difficulties, changes in heart rate, palpitations, swelling, stuffy nose, difficulty hearing, hair loss or gain, sweating, fever, tingling in the hands or feet, breast pain, muscle disturbances, breathing difficulty, changes in blood components, and joint pain.

Drug Interactions

• Diazepam is a central-nervous-system depressant. Avoid alcohol, other tranquilizers, narcotics, barbiturates, monoamine oxidase inhibitors (MAOIs), antihistamines, and antidepressants. Taking diazepam with these drugs may result in excessive depression, drowsiness, or difficulty breathing.

• Smoking may reduce the effectiveness of diazepam by increasing the rate at which it is broken down by the body.

• The effects of diazepam may be prolonged when taken with cimetidine, oral contraceptives, disulfiram, fluoxetine, isoniazid, ketoconazole, rifampin, metoprolol, probenecid, propoxyphene, propranolol, and valproic acid.

• Theophylline may reduce the sedative effects of diazepam.

• If you take antacids, separate them from your diazepam dose by at least 1 hour to prevent them from interfering with the passage of diazepam into the bloodstream.

• Diazepam may increase blood levels of digoxin and the chances for digoxin toxicity.

• Levodopa's effect may be decreased if it is taken with diazepam.

• Combining diazepam and phenytoin may increase phenytoin blood concentrations and the risk of phenytoin toxicity.

Food Interactions

Diazepam is best taken on an empty stomach, but it may be taken with food if it upsets your stomach.

Usual Dose

Solution or Tablets

Adult: 2–40 mg a day. Dosage must be adjusted to individual response for maximum effect.

Senior: Less of the drug is usually required to control tension and anxiety.

Child (6 months and over): 1–2.5 mg 3 or 4 times a day; more may be needed to control anxiety and tension.

Child (under 6 months): not recommended.

Rectal Gel

Adult and Child (age 12 and over): 0.09 mg per lb. of body weight. Approximate dosage: 5 mg if 31–60 lbs., 10 mg if 61–110 lbs., 15 mg if 111–165 lbs., or 20 mg if 166–244 lbs.

Child (age 6–11): 0.14 mg per lb. of body weight. Approximate dosage: 5 mg if 22–40 lbs., 10 mg if 41–82 lbs., 15 mg if 83–121 lbs., or 20 mg if 122–163 lbs.

Child (age 2–5): 0.23 mg per lb. of body weight. Approximate dosage: 5 mg if 13–24 lbs., 10 mg if 25–49 lbs., 15 mg if 50–73 lbs., or 20 mg if 74–97 lbs.

An extra 2.5 mg of the rectal gel may be given if a more precise dosage is needed or as a partial replacement for people who do not retain the full dosage after it is first inserted rectally.

Overdosage

Symptoms of overdose include confusion, sleepiness, poor coordination, lack of response to pain, loss of reflexes, shallow breathing, low blood pressure, and coma. The victim should be taken to a hospital emergency room. ALWAYS bring the prescription bottle or container with you.

Special Information

Diazepam can cause tiredness, drowsiness, inability to concentrate, or similar symptoms. Be careful if you are driving, operating machinery, or performing other activities that require concentration.

People taking diazepam for more than 3 or 4 months at a time may develop drug withdrawal reactions if the medication is stopped suddenly (see "Cautions and Warnings").

If you forget a dose of diazepam, take it as soon as you remember. If it is almost time for your next dose, skip the one you forgot and continue with your regular schedule. Do not take a double dose.

Special Populations

Pregnancy/Breast-feeding

Diazepam may cross into the fetal circulation and may cause birth defects if taken during the first 3 months of pregnancy. Avoid taking any benzodiazepine if you are or might be pregnant.

Diazepam may pass into breast milk. Since infants break down the drug more slowly than do adults, they may accumulate enough diazepam in their systems to produce undesirable effects. Nursing mothers who must take this drug should bottle-feed their babies.

Seniors

Seniors, especially those with liver or kidney disease, are more sensitive to the effects of diazepam and generally require smaller doses to achieve the same effect. Follow your doctor's directions and report any side effects at once.

Generic Name

Diclofenac (dye-CLOE-fen-ak)

Brand Names

Cataflam   Voltaren

Combination Products

Generic Ingredients: Diclofenac + Misoprostol
Arthrotec

Type of Drug

Nonsteroidal anti-inflammatory drug (NSAID).

Prescribed for

Rheumatoid arthritis; osteoarthritis; ankylosing spondylitis; mild to moderate pain; juvenile rheumatoid arthritis; shoulder pain; menstrual pain and cramps; sunburn; eye inflammation after cataract surgery—eyedrops only; and stomach and intestinal irritation and ulcer—in combination with misoprostol.

General Information

Diclofenac sodium is one of 16 NSAIDs, which are used to relieve pain and inflammation. We do not know exactly how NSAIDs work, but part of their action may be due to their ability to inhibit the body's production of a hormone called prostaglandin as well as the action of other body chemicals, including cyclooxygenase, lipoxygenase, leukotrienes, and lysosomal enzymes. NSAIDs are generally absorbed into the bloodstream quickly. Pain relief comes within 1 hour after taking the first dose of diclofenac, but its anti-inflammatory effect takes several days to 2 weeks to become apparent and may take a month or more to reach maximum effect. Diclofenac is broken down in the liver and eliminated through the kidneys.

Cataflam, a newer version of diclofenac, does not contain sodium and is the preferred form for menstrual pain and cramps. Voltaren, the older version of diclofenac, does contain sodium; women taking Cataflam for menstrual problems should not switch to Voltaren. In addition to preventing inflammation after cataract surgery, NSAID eyedrops are used during eye surgery to prevent movement of the eye muscles, and for itching and redness due to seasonal allergies. The combination of diclofenac and misoprostol is used to protect against stomach and intestinal irritation and ulcer.

Cautions and Warnings

People **allergic** to diclofenac or any other NSAID and those with a history of **asthma** attacks brought on by an NSAID, iodides, or aspirin should not take diclofenac.

Diclofenac may cause **gastrointestinal (GI) bleeding, ulcers, and stomach perforation**. This can occur at any time, with or without warning, in people who take diclofenac regularly. People with a history of active **GI bleeding** should be cautious about taking any NSAID. People who develop bleeding or ulcers and continue NSAID treatment should be aware of the possibility of developing more serious side effects.

Diclofenac may affect platelets and **blood clotting** at high doses, and should be avoided by people with clotting problems and by those taking warfarin.

People with **heart problems** who use diclofenac may experience swelling in their arms, legs, or feet.

Diclofenac may cause severe toxic effects to the **kidney**. Report any unusual side effects to your doctor, who might need to periodically test your kidney function.

People taking diclofenac should have their liver function checked periodically.

Diclofenac may make you unusually sensitive to the effects of the sun.

Possible Side Effects

Tablets

▼ Most common: diarrhea, nausea, vomiting, constipation, stomach gas, stomach upset or irritation, and appetite loss, especially during the first few days of treatment.

▼ Less common: stomach ulcers, GI bleeding, hepatitis, gallbladder attacks, painful urination, poor kidney function, kidney inflammation, blood and protein in the urine, dizziness, fainting, nervousness, depression, hallucinations, confusion, disorientation, tingling in the hands or feet, light-headedness, itching, increased sweating, dry nose and mouth, heart palpitations, chest pain, breathing difficulties, and muscle cramps.

▼ Rare: severe allergic reactions including closing of the throat, fever and chills, changes in liver function, jaundice (yellowing of the skin or whites of the eyes), and kidney failure. People who experience such effects must be promptly treated in a hospital emergency room or doctor's office. NSAIDs have caused severe skin reac-

Possible Side Effects *(continued)*

tions; if this happens to you, see your doctor immediately.

Eyedrops
▼ Most common: temporary burning, stinging, or other minor eye irritation.
▼ Less common: nausea, vomiting, viral infections, and eye allergies including persistent redness, burning, itching, or tearing.
▼ Rare: The risk of developing bleeding problems or other systemic (whole-body) side effects is low because only a small amount of the drug is absorbed into the bloodstream.

Drug Interactions

Tablets
• Diclofenac may increase the effects of oral anticoagulant (blood-thinning) drugs such as warfarin. If you take this combination, your doctor might have to reduce your anticoagulant dose.
• Taking diclofenac with cyclosporine may increase the kidney-related side effects of both drugs. Methotrexate side effects may be increased in people also taking diclofenac.
• Diclofenac may reduce the blood-pressure-lowering effect of beta blockers and loop diuretics.
• Diclofenac may increase phenytoin blood levels, leading to increased side effects. Lithium blood levels may be increased in people taking diclofenac.
• Diclofenac blood levels may be affected by cimetidine.
• Probenecid may interfere with the elimination of diclofenac from the body, increasing the chances for diclofenac side effects.
• Aspirin and other salicylates may decrease the amount of diclofenac in your blood. These drugs should never be combined with diclofenac.

Eyedrops
None known.

Food Interactions

Take diclofenac with food or a magnesium/aluminum antacid if it upsets your stomach.

Usual Dose

Tablets
   Adult: 100–200 mg a day.
   Senior: starting dose—⅓–½ the usual dosage.

Eyedrops
1 drop 4 times a day for 2 weeks, beginning 24 hours after cataract surgery.

Overdosage

People have died from NSAID overdoses. The most common signs of overdose are drowsiness, nausea, vomiting, diarrhea, abdominal pain, rapid breathing, rapid heartbeat, increased sweating, ringing or buzzing in the ears, confusion, disorientation, stupor, and coma. Take the victim to a hospital emergency room at once. ALWAYS bring the prescription bottle or container with you.

Special Information

Tablets: Take each dose with a full glass of water and do not lie down for 15 to 30 minutes afterward.

   Diclofenac can make you drowsy and/or tired: Be careful when driving or operating hazardous equipment. Do not take any over-the-counter products containing acetaminophen or aspirin while taking diclofenac. Avoid alcoholic beverages.

   If you are taking Cataflam for menstrual problems, be sure not to substitute Voltaren, which contains sodium.

   Contact your doctor if you develop skin rash or itching, visual disturbances, weight gain, breathing difficulties, fluid retention, hallucinations, black or tarry stools, persistent headache, or any unusual or intolerable side effect.

   If you forget to take a dose, take it as soon as you remember. If you take several doses a day and it is within 4 hours of your next dose, skip the one you forgot and continue with your regular schedule. Do not take a double dose.

Eyedrops: To self-administer the eyedrops, lie down or tilt your head backward. Hold the dropper above your eye and drop the medication inside your lower lid while looking up. To prevent possible infection, do not allow the dropper to touch your fingers, eyelids, or any surface. Release the lower lid, keeping your eye open. Do not blink for 30 seconds. Press gently on the bridge of your nose at the inside corner of your eye for 1 minute. This will help circulate the medication in your eye. Wait at least 5 minutes before using any other eyedrops.

If you forget a dose of your eyedrops, take it as soon as you remember. If it is almost time for your next dose, skip the one you missed and continue with your regular schedule. Do not take a double dose.

Special Populations

Pregnancy/Breast-feeding

NSAIDs may cross into fetal blood circulation. They have not been found to cause birth defects, but animal studies indicate that they may affect a fetal heart during the second half of pregnancy. Pregnant women should not take diclofenac without their doctor's approval, particularly during the last 3 months of pregnancy. When the drug is considered crucial by your doctor, its potential benefits must be carefully weighed against its risks.

NSAIDs may pass into breast milk but have caused no problems in breast-fed infants, except for seizures in a baby whose mother was taking the NSAID indomethacin. There is a possibility that a nursing mother taking diclofenac could affect her baby's heart or cardiovascular system. If you must take diclofenac, bottle-feed your baby.

Seniors

Seniors may be more susceptible to diclofenac side effects, especially ulcer disease.

Generic Name

Dicyclomine (dih-SYE-kloe-mene) Ⓖ

Brand Names

Bemote	Byclomine
Bentyl	Di-Spaz

Type of Drug

Antispasmodic and anticholinergic.

Prescribed for

Irritable bowel, spastic colon, and similar digestive problems.

General Information

Dicyclomine hydrochloride is a member of a very large class of drugs that have been used for many years to calm "nervous stomach." It was once widely prescribed for morning sickness during pregnancy. Dicyclomine and other anticholinergics work by inhibiting the effects of the neurohormone acetylcholine in the gastrointestinal (GI) tract. This effect directly reduces the mobility of the GI tract and slows the production of enzymes and other secretions. Dicyclomine and other members of this drug class may cause dry mouth, reduce sweating, and cause dilation of the pupil—increasing the time it takes for the eyes to adjust to bright light.

Cautions and Warnings

Do not take dicyclomine if you are **allergic** to it or another belladonna-related drug. This drug should be used with caution if you have **heart disease, Down syndrome, reduced mobility of the stomach and lower esophagus, fever, stomach obstruction, glaucoma, acute bleeding, hiatal hernia, intestinal paralysis, myasthenia gravis, kidney or liver dysfunction, rapid heartbeat, high blood pressure, or ulcerative colitis**. Because this drug reduces your ability to sweat, its use in hot weather may cause heat exhaustion.

Possible Side Effects

▼ Common: constipation, decreased sweating, and dry mouth, throat, or skin.

▼ Less common: reduced breast-milk flow, difficulty swallowing, blurred vision, and sensitivity to bright light.

▼ Rare: drug allergy (symptoms include rash, itching, hives, and breathing difficulties), confusion, eye pain, dizziness when rising quickly from a sitting or lying position, a bloated feeling, difficult or painful urination, drowsiness, unusual tiredness or weakness, headache, memory loss, and nausea or vomiting.

Drug Interactions

• Antacids containing calcium or magnesium, citrates, sodium bicarbonate, and carbonic anhydrase inhibitor drugs may slow the rate at which dicyclomine is released from the blood, increasing its therapeutic effect and side effects.

• Do not combine dicyclomine with other anticholinergic

drugs including atropine, belladonna, clidinium, glycopyrrol-ate, hyoscyamine, isopropamide, propantheline, and scopol-amine because of the possibility of intensifying side effects.

• Dicyclomine may reduce stomach acidity and the amount of ketoconazole (an antifungal) absorbed by the blood after it is taken by mouth.

• Dicyclomine may counteract the effect of metoclopra-mide in reducing nausea and vomiting.

• Taking dicyclomine with a narcotic pain reliever may increase the risk of severe constipation.

• Taking this or any drug that slows the movement of stomach and intestinal muscles with a potassium chloride supplement—especially one in wax-matrix tablet form—may lead to excessive irritation of the stomach.

Food Interactions

Take dicyclomine on an empty stomach, a half hour before or 2 hours after a meal.

Usual Dose

Adult: 30–160 mg a day.
Senior: Begin with the lowest possible dosage and increase only as needed.
Child (age 2 and over): 10 mg 3 or 4 times a day.
Child (age 6 months–2 years): 5–10 mg 3 or 4 times a day.
Child (under 6 months): not recommended.

Overdosage

The principal signs of overdose are blurred vision; clumsi-ness; confusion; breathing difficulties; dizziness; drowsiness; dry mouth, nose, or throat; rapid heartbeat; fever; hallucina-tions; weakness; slurred speech; excitement, restlessness, or irritability; warmth; and dry or flushed skin. Overdose victims should be taken to a hospital emergency room at once. ALWAYS bring the prescription bottle or container with you.

Special Information

Children taking dicyclomine may be more likely to develop high body temperature in hot weather and other side effects and should be carefully watched for side effects.

Call your doctor if you develop rash, flushing, eye pain, dry mouth, urinary difficulties, constipation, unusual sensitivity to light, or other side effects that are persistent or bothersome.

Brush and floss your teeth regularly while taking this drug. Because dicyclomine may cause dry mouth, you may be more likely to develop cavities or other dental problems while you are taking it. Ice or hard candy may be used to relieve this side effect.

Constipation may be treated by using a laxative.

Dicyclomine may make you drowsy or tired and cause blurred vision. Be careful when driving or doing other tasks that require concentration or coordination.

If you forget to take a dose of dicyclomine, take it as soon as you remember. If it is almost time for your next dose, skip the dose you forgot and continue with your regular schedule. Do not take a double dose.

Special Populations

Pregnancy/Breast-feeding
A few cases of human malformation were linked to dicyclomine, but studies have shown that the drug has no effect on the fetus. As with all other drugs, dicyclomine should be used during pregnancy only when absolutely necessary.

Dicyclomine should not be used by nursing mothers because, like other drugs in its group, it may reduce the amount of milk produced. Also, a few infants less than age 3 months who were given dicyclomine drops developed breathing difficulties that went away after 20 to 30 minutes.

Seniors
Seniors may be more susceptible to the side effects of this drug, especially memory loss, mental changes, and glaucoma, and may need less medication to get a beneficial effect than do younger adults. Report any problems to your doctor at once.

Generic Name

Didanosine (dye-DAN-oe-zene)

Brand Name
Videx

Type of Drug
Antiviral.

Prescribed for

Acquired immunodeficiency syndrome (AIDS).

General Information

Didanosine, also known as ddI or dideoxyinosine, is approved for people with AIDS who have had long-term zidovudine (AZT) treatment and whose disease is continuing to worsen. Didanosine is also approved for children 6 months and older with AIDS who cannot tolerate or respond to AZT.

Didanosine interferes with the life of the human immunodeficiency virus (HIV) that causes AIDS by interrupting the internal DNA manufacturing process essential to the reproduction of HIV. Didanosine was tested in patients with advanced AIDS. It was approved because of its ability to prolong life and to delay the next AIDS-related opportunistic infection or other AIDS-defining event. Didanosine also was effective in increasing blood levels of CD4 cells, which represent the level of immune function and are considered important indicators of the severity of an AIDS infection.

Cautions and Warnings

The most serious—and potentially fatal—side effects of didanosine are nervous system inflammation and inflammation of the pancreas.

Up to 50% of patients who take didanosine experience symptoms of **nervous system inflammation** and about 33% need to reduce their dosage to control these symptoms. Symptoms generally manifest as numbness, tingling, and pain in the hands and feet. People who already have these signs of nerve damage should not take didanosine.

Potentially fatal **inflammation of the pancreas** has occurred in up to 3% of people taking didanosine. Of people with a history of pancreatic inflammation who take didanosine, 33% are likely to develop this problem again. Symptoms of inflammation of the pancreas include major changes in blood-sugar levels, increased triglyceride blood levels, a drop in blood calcium, nausea, vomiting, and abdominal pain. People who develop pancreatic inflammation must stop taking didanosine.

Liver failure may develop in people taking this drug, 15% to 20% of whom will begin to test abnormally for liver function. A small number of these patients may develop fatal liver disease.

Four children taking didanosine developed **severe eye**

disease, resulting in some loss of sight. The progress of the eye disease slowed or stopped when dosage was reduced. Children taking this drug should have an eye examination every 6 months or if vision starts to worsen.

Didanosine has caused **muscle toxicities** in animals. This has not been seen in humans, but it can occur with other AIDS antiviral drugs.

Kidney and liver disease may interfere with the elimination of didanosine from the body. Reduced doses may be required to accommodate these conditions.

Do not take didanosine if you are **allergic** to it or any ingredient in the didanosine tablet.

Possible Side Effects

▼ Most common: diarrhea, nervous system inflammation, fever, chills, itching, rash, abdominal pain, weakness, pains, headache, nausea, vomiting, infection, pneumonia, and pancreatic inflammation.

▼ Less common: tumors, muscle pain, appetite loss, dry mouth, convulsions, abnormal thought patterns, breathing difficulties, drug allergy, anxiety, nervousness, twitching, confusion, depression, and blood component abnormalities.

▼ Rare: abscesses, skin infections, cysts, dehydration, flu-like symptoms, hernia, neck rigidity, numbness of the hands or feet, chest pain, blood pressure changes, heart palpitations, migraine, dizziness, coldness of the hands or feet, leg pain, colitis, stomach gas, stomach inflammation, ulcers or bleeding, oral fungus infections, personality changes, memory loss, convulsions, dizziness, muscle stiffness, loss of muscle control, poor coordination, loss of bowel control, stroke, feeling unwell, paranoia, paralysis, psychosis, sleep disturbances, speech difficulties, tremors, joint inflammation or pain, swelling in the legs or arms, asthma, bronchitis, cough, nosebleeds, laryngitis, pneumonia, respiratory difficulties, blurred vision, double vision, conjunctivitis, dry eyes, hearing abnormalities, glaucoma, herpes infections of the skin, and sweating,

Almost all children who take didanosine experience side effects. They are likely to experience many of the same reactions as adults, most commonly chills, fever,

---

Possible Side Effects *(continued)*

weakness, appetite loss, nausea and vomiting, diarrhea, liver dysfunction, pains, headache, nervousness, sleeplessness, cough, runny nose, asthma or breathing difficulties, rash, and skin problems.

Drug Interactions

• Other drugs that may cause inflammation of the nervous system such as chloramphenicol, cisplatin, dapsone, disulfiram, ethionamide, glutethimide, gold, hydralazine, isoniazid, metronidazole, nitrofurantoin, ribavirin, and vincristine should be avoided while you are taking didanosine.

• Didanosine should not be taken with zalcitabine.

• Drugs that may cause inflammation of the pancreas, including intravenous pentamidine, should not be taken with didanosine.

• Quinolone anti-infectives, tetracycline antibiotics, and other drugs whose absorption into the bloodstream may be affected by antacids should not be taken within 2 hours of taking didanosine because of its high magnesium and aluminum content.

Food Interactions

Food may prevent the absorption of a dose of didanosine by up to 50%. Take didanosine on an empty stomach.

Usual Dose

Adult: 167–250 mg every 12 hours.
Child: 50–250 mg a day.

Dosage should be adjusted to the patient's level of kidney and liver function.

Overdosage

Didanosine overdose will cause many of the drug's side effects, especially inflammation of the nervous system or pancreas, diarrhea, and liver failure. There is little experience with didanosine overdose and victims should be taken to a hospital emergency room for testing and monitoring. ALWAYS remember to bring the prescription bottle or container with you.

Special Information

Didanosine does not cure AIDS. It will not prevent you from

transmitting the HIV virus to another person; you must still practice safe sex. People may still develop AIDS-related opportunistic infections while taking this drug.

Didanosine may affect components of the blood system. Your doctor should perform blood tests to check for any changes.

People taking didanosine should take good care of their teeth and gums to minimize the possibility of oral infections.

Call your doctor if you develop any of the following symptoms of didanosine toxicity: numbness and pain in the hands and feet, nausea, vomiting, or abdominal pain.

If you are taking didanosine in chewable tablets, be sure to thoroughly chew each tablet. You may also completely dissolve the tablets in about ¼ cup of water and drink the entire mixture immediately. Do not mix didanosine tablets with juice or any other acidic drink.

If you are using the powdered form of didanosine, make a solution by pouring the entire contents of a packet into ½ cup of water. Stir until dissolved and drink immediately. Do not mix didanosine powder with juice or any other acidic drink. For children, your pharmacist will prepare a mixture of 10 mg per ml of didanosine and an equal amount of Mylanta Double Strength Antacid or Maalox TC Antacid. This mixture must be stored in a refrigerator and can be kept for 30 days. Shake well before using. Spilled didanosine should be cleaned immediately to prevent accidental poisoning.

If you forget to take a dose of didanosine, take it as soon as you remember. If it is almost time for your next dose, allow 4 to 8 hours to pass between the dose you took late and your next dose, and then continue with your regular schedule. Call your doctor for more specific advice if you forget to take several doses.

Special Populations

Pregnancy/Breast-feeding

Didanosine was slightly toxic to pregnant animals receiving doses 12 times human levels. There are no studies of pregnant women taking this drug; however, women who are or might become pregnant should only take didanosine if absolutely necessary and should use effective contraception to avoid passing on the virus.

It is not known if didanosine passes into breast milk. In any case, mothers who are HIV positive should bottle-feed their babies to avoid transmitting the virus through their milk.

Seniors

People with reduced kidney or liver function—common in seniors—should receive smaller dosages of didanosine than those with normal function.

Diflucan

*see **Fluconazole**, page 428*

Generic Name

Diflunisal (dye-FLOO-nih-sal)

Brand Name

Dolobid

Type of Drug

Nonsteroidal anti-inflammatory drug (NSAID).

Prescribed for

Rheumatoid arthritis, osteoarthritis, and mild to moderate pain.

General Information

Diflunisal is chemically similar to aspirin and is considered to be a nonsteroidal anti-inflammatory drug (NSAID); it is used to relieve pain and inflammation. We do not know exactly how NSAIDs work, but part of their action may be caused by an ability to inhibit both the body's production of a hormone called prostaglandin and the action of other body chemicals, including cyclooxygenase, lipoxygenase, leukotrienes, and lysosomal enzymes. Diflunisal is absorbed into the bloodstream fairly rapidly. Pain relief comes within 1 hour after taking the first dose, but the drug's anti-inflammatory effect takes several days to 2 weeks to become apparent and may take several months to reach its maximum.

Cautions and Warnings

People who are **allergic** to diflunisal or any other NSAID and those with a **history of asthma** attacks brought on by NSAIDs, by iodides, or by aspirin should not take diflunisal.

This drug can cause **gastrointestinal (GI) bleeding, ulcers, and perforation**. This can occur at any time with or without warning in people who regularly use diflunisal. People with a history of active GI bleeding should be cautious about taking any NSAID. **Minor stomach upset, gas, or distress** is common during the first few days of treatment with diflunisal. People who develop bleeding or ulcers and continue their NSAID treatment should be aware of the possibility of developing more serious drug toxicity.

High doses of diflunisal can affect blood platelets and blood clotting. This drug should be avoided by people with clotting problems and those taking warfarin.

People with heart problems who use diflunisal may find that their **arms, legs, or feet become swollen**.

Diflunisal can cause severe side effects to the **kidney**. Report any unusual side effects to your doctor, who may need to periodically test your kidney function.

Diflunisal can make you **unusually sensitive to the effects of the sun**.

Diflunisal should be used with **caution in children and adolescents**; because it is related to aspirin, it may cause Reye's syndrome.

Possible Side Effects

▼ Most common: diarrhea, nausea, vomiting, constipation, stomach gas, stomach upset or irritation, and appetite loss.

▼ Less common: stomach ulcers, GI bleeding, hepatitis, gallbladder attacks, painful urination, poor kidney function, kidney inflammation, blood and protein in the urine, dizziness, fainting, nervousness, depression, hallucinations, confusion, disorientation, tingling in the hands or feet, light-headedness, itching, increased sweating, dry nose and mouth, heart palpitations, chest pain, breathing difficulties, and muscle cramps.

▼ Rare: severe allergic reactions, including closing of the throat, fever, and chills; changes in liver function; jaundice (symptoms include yellowing of the skin or whites of the eyes), and kidney failure. People who

---

Possible Side Effects *(continued)*

experience such effects must promptly be treated in a hospital emergency room or doctor's office at once. NSAIDs have caused severe skin reactions; if this happens to you, see your doctor immediately.

Drug Interactions

• Diflunisal can increase the effects of oral anticoagulant (blood-thinning) drugs such as warfarin. You may take this combination, but your doctor may have to reduce your anticoagulant dose to take this effect into account.

• Diflunisal may increase acetaminophen blood levels by as much as 50%. This can be a problem for people with liver disease.

• Diflunisal increases the blood levels and effects of thiazide diuretics.

• Combining diflunisal with indomethacin can cause GI bleeding, which can be fatal. Do not take this combination.

Food Interactions

Take diflunisal with food or a magnesium/aluminum antacid if it upsets your stomach.

Usual Dose

Starting dosage—500–1000 mg. Maintenance dosage—250–500 mg every 8–12 hours. Do not take more than 1500 mg a day. Do not crush or chew diflunisal tablets.

Overdosage

People have died from diflunisal overdose. The most common overdose signs are drowsiness, nausea, vomiting, diarrhea, abdominal pain, rapid breathing, rapid heartbeat, increased sweating, ringing or buzzing in the ears, confusion, disorientation, stupor, and coma.

Take the victim to a hospital emergency room at once. ALWAYS bring the prescription bottle or container with you.

Special Information

Take each dose with a full glass of water and do not lie down for 15 to 30 minutes afterward. Diflunisal can make you drowsy and/or tired: Be careful when driving or operating hazardous equipment.

Do not take any over-the-counter products with acetaminophen or aspirin while taking diflunisal; also, avoid alcoholic beverages.

Contact your doctor if you develop rash, itching, visual disturbances, weight gain, breathing difficulties, fluid retention, hallucinations, black stools, or persistent headache. Call your doctor if you develop any unusual or intolerable side effects.

If you forget to take a dose of diflunisal, take it as soon as you remember. If you take several diflunisal doses a day and it is within 4 hours of your next dose, skip the one you forgot and continue with your regular schedule. If you take diflunisal once a day and it is within 8 hours of your next dose, skip the dose you forgot and continue with your regular schedule. Never take a double dose.

Special Populations

Pregnancy/Breast-feeding
Diflunisal may cross into the fetal blood circulation. It has not been found to cause birth defects, but may affect the fetal heart during the last 3 months of pregnancy. If you are or might be pregnant, do not take diflunisal without your doctor's approval; pregnant women should be particularly cautious about using this drug during the last 3 months of pregnancy. When the drug is considered crucial by your doctor, its potential benefits must be carefully weighed against its risks.

Diflunisal passes into breast milk. There is a possibility that a nursing mother taking diflunisal could affect her baby's heart or cardiovascular system. Nursing mothers who must take this drug should bottle-feed their babies.

Seniors
Seniors may be more susceptible to diflunisal side effects, especially ulcer disease.

Type of Drug

Digitalis Glycosides

(dih-jih-TAL-is GLYE-coe-sides) Ⓖ

Brand Names

Generic Ingredient: Digitoxin
Crystodigin

Generic Ingredient: Digoxin
Lanoxicaps   Lanoxin

Prescribed for

Congestive heart failure (CHF) and other heart conditions involving a very rapid heartbeat.

General Information

Digitalis glycosides work directly on heart muscle. They improve the heart's pumping ability or help to control its beating rhythm. People with heart failure very often develop swelling of the lower legs, feet, and ankles; digitalis drugs improve these symptoms by improving blood circulation. Digitoxin is more useful than digoxin for people who have kidney problems because digoxin is removed mostly by the liver, not the kidneys.

Digitalis glycosides are generally used as part of the life-long treatment of CHF.

Cautions and Warnings

Do not use digitalis glycosides if you know you are **allergic or sensitive** to them. Digitalis allergies are rare and are often limited to only one member of the group; another digitalis drug may work in its place.

Digitalis glycosides have been used as part of a treatment for obesity. The possibility of developing fatal heart rhythms while undergoing such treatment makes digitalis glycosides extremely **dangerous as weight-loss medication**. Many **heart disease symptoms** may also be associated with digitalis glycosides. **Report any unusual side effects to your doctor at once**. **Kidney disease** may increase blood levels of all digitalis glycosides except digitoxin. **Liver disease** may increase blood levels of digitoxin. Your dosage may need adjusting.

Long-term use of a digitalis glycoside may cause the body to lose potassium, especially since these drugs are generally used in combination with diuretics (agents that increase urination). For this reason, be sure to eat a balanced diet and high-potassium foods—bananas, citrus fruits, melons, and tomatoes.

Digitalis requirements vary with thyroid status. If you are taking a digitalis glycoside and your thyroid status changes, your doctor will have to change your digitalis dosage.

Possible Side Effects

Adult and Senior

▼ Most common: appetite loss, nausea, vomiting, diarrhea, and blurred or disturbed vision. If you experience any of these problems, call your doctor immediately.

▼ Less common: headache, weakness, apathy, drowsiness, blurred or yellow-tinted vision, seeing halos around bright lights, depression, psychoses, confusion or disorientation, restlessness, hallucinations, delirium, seizure, nerve pain, abnormal heart rhythms, and slow pulse.

▼ Rare: Enlargement of the breasts has been reported after long-term use of a digitalis glycoside. Allergy or sensitivity to digitalis drugs is uncommon.

Child

Children respond differently to digitalis glycosides than do adults. Children are more likely to develop abnormal heart rhythms before they see yellow or green halos or spots and before they develop nausea, vomiting, diarrhea, or stomach pain. Any abnormal heart rhythms that develop while a child is taking a digitalis glycoside should be assumed to be a side effect.

Drug Interactions

• Drugs that may increase the effect of a digitalis glycoside are alprazolam, amiloride aminoglycoside antibiotics, amiodarone, anticholinergic drugs, benzodiazepines, bepredil, captopril, diltiazem, erythromycin, esmolol, felodipine, flecainide, hydroxychloroquine, ibuprofen, indomethacin, itraconazole, nifedipine, omeprazole, propafenone, propantheline, quinidine, quinine, tetracycline, tolbutamide, triamterene, and verapamil.

• Drugs that may decrease the amount of a digitalis glycoside in the blood include aminoglutethimide, aminoglycosides, oral sulfonylurea antidiabetes medication, antihistamines, barbiturates, phenytoin and related anti-seizure drugs, phenylbutazone, rifampin, antacids, aminosalicylic acid, cholestyramine, colestipol, anti-cancer combinations, kaolin-pectin mixtures, sucralfate, sulfasalazine, oral kanamycin, metoclopramide, and oral neomycin.

• Disopyramide may alter the effects of digoxin although the exact interaction is not well understood.

• Low blood-potassium—a common side effect of thiazide diuretics; furosemide; ethacrynic acid; and bumetanide will increase a digitalis glycoside's effect and increase the risk of developing side effects.

• Spironolactone may either increase or decrease the effect of a digitalis glycoside. Its effect is unpredictable.

• Spironolactone may increase or decrease the side effects of digitalis glycosides; amiloride may reduce the effect of a digitalis glycoside on the force of heart contraction.

• The effects of a digitalis glycoside on your heart may be additive to those of ephedrine, epinephrine and other stimulants, beta blockers, calcium salts, procainamide, and rauwolfia drugs.

• Thyroid drugs will change your digitalis glycoside requirement. Your doctor will have to adjust your digitalis glycoside dosage.

Food Interactions

Take each day's dose at the same time for consistency. Many people take their medication after their morning meal.

Usual Dose

Digitoxin
    Adult: Starting dosage—known as the digitalizing or loading dosage—is 2 mg over about 3 days or 0.4 mg a day for 4 days. Digitalization may also be accomplished with lower dosage over 10–14 days. Maintenance dosage—0.05–0.03 mg daily.
    Senior: Lower dosage is required because of increased sensitivity to adverse effects.
    Child: usually not recommended.

Digoxin
    Adult and Child (age 11 and over): Starting dosage—known as the digitalizing or loading dosage—is about 4–7 mcg per

lb. of body weight. Digitalization may also be accomplished with lower dosage over 7 days. Maintenance dosage—0.125–0.5 mg; it must be corrected for kidney function.

Senior: Lower dosage is required because of increased sensitivity to adverse effects.

Child (under age 11): starting dosage—5–30 mcg per lb. of body weight. Dosage does not vary directly with age because of variations in the way children react to this medication. For instance, children under age 2 receive 2–4 times more medication than those age 10. Daily maintenance dosage—20%–35% of the starting dosage. Careful measurement of your child's digoxin dosage is crucial to safe and effective treatment.

Overdosage

Adult: Symptoms of overdose are appetite loss, nausea, vomiting, diarrhea, headache, weakness, apathy, blurred vision, yellow or green spots or halos before the eyes, yellowing of the skin or whites of the eyes, or changes in heartbeat.

Senior: Vomiting, diarrhea, and eye trouble are frequently seen in seniors.

Child: An early sign of overdose in children is a change in heart rhythms.

Call your doctor immediately if any of these symptoms appear. Overdose victims must be taken to an emergency room for treatment. ALWAYS bring the prescription bottle or container with you.

Special Information

Do not stop taking a digitalis glycoside unless your doctor tells you to do so.

Lanoxicaps are better absorbed than tablet forms of digoxin. For this reason, each dose of lanoxicaps is slightly lower than the corresponding digoxin tablet.

Avoid over-the-counter diet and cold medication containing stimulants. Ask your pharmacist if you are not sure about which to avoid.

Call your doctor at once if you develop side effects.

There may by some variation between digitalis glycoside tablets from different manufacturers. Do not change drug brands without telling your doctor.

Check your pulse every day—your doctor will teach you how to do this—and call your doctor if it drops below 60 beats per minute.

If you forget to take a dose of a digitalis glycoside and remember at least 12 hours before your next dose, take it right away. If you do not remember until it is less than 12 hours before your next dose, skip the one you forgot and continue with your regular schedule. Do not take a double dose. Call your doctor if you forget to take a digitalis glycoside for 2 or more days.

Special Populations

Pregnancy/Breast-feeding

Digitalis glycosides cross into the fetal circulation, but they have not been found to cause birth defects. In fact, fetal heart disease has been treated by giving the mother digoxin. Nevertheless, women who are or might be pregnant should not take any digitalis glycoside without their doctor's approval. When this drug is considered crucial by your doctor, its potential benefits must be carefully weighed against its risks.

Small amounts of digoxin pass into breast milk, but it has caused no problems among breast-fed infants. It is not known if digitoxin passes into breast milk. You must consider the possible effect on the nursing infant if you are breast-feeding and taking a digitalis glycoside.

Seniors

Seniors are more sensitive to the effects of digitalis glycosides, especially appetite loss. Follow your doctor's directions and report any side effects at once.

Dilacor XR

*see **Diltiazem**, page 324*

Dilantin

*see **Phenytoin**, page 876*

Generic Name

Diltiazem (dil-TYE-uh-zem) Ⓖ

Brand Names

Cardizem	Dilacor
Cardizem CD	Dilacor XR
Cardizem SR	

Type of Drug

Calcium channel blocker.

Prescribed for

Angina pectoris, Raynaud's disease, prevention of second heart attacks, and tardive dyskinesia (severe side effects associated with antipsychotic and other drugs). Sustained-released diltiazem products may be used to treat hypertension (high blood pressure).

General Information

Diltiazem hydrochloride is one of many calcium channel blockers available in the U.S. These drugs block the passage of calcium, an essential factor in muscle contraction, into the heart and smooth muscles. Such blockage of calcium interferes with the contraction of these muscles, which in turn dilates (widens) the veins and vessels that supply blood to them. This action has several beneficial effects. Because arteries are dilated, they are less likely to spasm. In addition, because blood vessels are dilated, both blood pressure and the amount of oxygen used by the heart muscles is reduced. Diltiazem is therefore useful in treating not only hypertension but also angina pectoris (condition characterized by brief attacks of chest pain), a condition related to poor oxygen supply to the heart muscles. Other calcium channel blockers are prescribed for abnormal heart rhythm, heart failure, cardiomyopathy (loss of blood-pumping ability due to damaged heart muscle), and diseases that involve blood-vessel spasm, such as migraine and Raynaud's disease.

Diltiazem affects the movement of calcium only into muscle cells; it has no effect on calcium in the blood.

Cautions and Warnings

Diltiazem can slow your heart and interfere with normal

electrical conduction. For people with a condition called **sick sinus syndrome**, this can result in temporary heart stoppage; most people will not develop this effect.

Diltiazem should not be taken if you are having a **heart attack** or if you have **lung congestion**. Diltiazem should be taken with caution by people with **heart failure** because it can worsen that condition.

Low blood pressure may occur, especially in people also taking a beta blocker.

Diltiazem can cause severe **liver damage** and should be taken with caution if you have had hepatitis or any other liver condition.

Caution should also be exercised if you have a history of **kidney problems**, although no clear tendency toward causing kidney damage is seen with this drug.

Possible Side Effects

Diltiazem's side effects are generally mild and rarely cause people to stop taking it.

▼ Common: dizziness, light-headedness, weakness, headache, and fluid accumulation in the hands, legs, or feet.

▼ Less common: low blood pressure, fainting, increase or decrease in heart rate, abnormal heart rhythm, heart failure, nervousness, fatigue, nausea, rash, tingling in the hands or feet, hallucinations, temporary memory loss, difficulty sleeping, diarrhea, vomiting, constipation, upset stomach, itching, unusual sensitivity to sunlight, painful or stiff joints, liver inflammation, and increased urination, especially at night.

Drug Interactions

• Diltiazem taken with a beta-blocking drug for hypertension is usually well tolerated, but may lead to heart failure in people with already weakened hearts.

• Calcium channel blockers, including diltiazem, may add to the effects of digoxin. This effect is not observed with any consistency, however, and only affects people with a large amount of digoxin already in their systems.

• Cimetidine and ranitidine increase the amount of diltiazem in the bloodstream and may account for a slight increase in the drug's effect.

• Diltiazem may increase blood levels of cyclosporine, carbamazepine, encainide, and theophylline, and thus increase the chance of side effects from these drugs.

• Diltiazem may cause a decrease in blood lithium levels, possibly undermining lithium's antimanic effect.

Food Interactions

Diltiazem is best taken on an empty stomach, at least 1 hour before or 2 hours after meals.

Usual Dose

Immediate-release Products
30–60 mg 4 times a day.

Sustained-release Products
Cardizem SR—60–180 mg twice a day.
Cardizem CD—120–480 mg once a day.
Dilacor XR—240–480 mg once a day.

Overdosage

The major symptoms of diltiazem overdose are very low blood pressure and reduced heart rate. Overdose victims must be made to vomit with ipecac syrup—available at any pharmacy—within 30 minutes of taking the overdose. DO NOT INDUCE VOMITING IF THE VICTIM HAS FAINTED OR IS CONVULSING. If overdose symptoms have developed or more than 30 minutes have passed, vomiting is of little value. Take the victim to a hospital emergency room immediately. ALWAYS bring the prescription bottle or container with you.

Special Information

Call your doctor if you develop any of the following symptoms: swelling of the hands, legs, or feet; severe dizziness; constipation or nausea; or very low blood pressure.

Do not open, chew, or crush sustained-release capsules of Dilacor XR. They must be swallowed whole.

If you take your diltiazem 3 or 4 times a day and forget a dose, take it as soon as you remember. Space the remaining doses throughout the rest of the day. If you take diltiazem 1 or 2 times a day and forget to take a dose, take it as soon as you remember. If it is almost time for your next dose, skip the one you forgot and continue with your regular schedule. Never take a double dose.

Special Populations

Pregnancy/Breast-feeding

Animal studies with diltiazem at dosages greater than the usual human dosage have revealed a definite potential for harming a fetus. With increased dosages, adverse effects become more frequent and more severe. Diltiazem should not be taken by women who are or might be pregnant. When your doctor considers this drug crucial, its potential benefits must be carefully weighed against its risks.

Because diltiazem passes into breast milk, nursing mothers taking this drug should bottle-feed their infants. Diltiazem's safety in children has not been established.

Seniors

Seniors may be more sensitive to the effects of this drug because it takes longer to pass out of their bodies. Follow your doctor's directions and report any side effects at once.

Generic Name

Dimenhydrinate (dye-men-HYE-drih-nate) Ⓖ

Brand Names

Dimetabs   Nicovert

The information in this profile also applies to the following drugs:

Generic Ingredient: Meclizine Ⓖ

Antivert   Meni-D
Antivert 25   Ru-Vert-M
Antrizine

Type of Drug

Antihistamine and antiemetic (agent that prevents or relieves nausea and vomiting).

Prescribed for

Nausea, vomiting, and dizziness associated with motion sickness.

General Information

Dimenhydrinate is a mixture of diphenhydramine—an antihistamine believed to be the active ingredient—and another ingredient. While dimenhydrinate depresses middle-ear function, the way in which it actually prevents nausea, vomiting, and dizziness is not known. Meclizine is an antihistamine used to treat or prevent nausea, vomiting, and motion sickness. It takes a little longer to start working than dimenhydrinate but its effects last much longer. The way in which meclizine acts on the brain to prevent nausea and dizziness is not fully understood. In general, meclizine does a better job of preventing motion sickness than treating its symptoms. It takes 30 minutes to 1 hour to work and lasts for 12 to 24 hours.

Cautions and Warnings

People with a **prostate condition, stomach ulcer, bladder problems, difficulty urinating, glaucoma, asthma,** or **abnormal heart rhythms** should use dimenhydrinate only while under a doctor's care. **Newborn babies** and people who are **allergic or sensitive** to dimenhydrinate should not be given this drug.

Because it controls nausea and vomiting, dimenhydrinate may hide the symptoms of appendicitis and overdoses of other drugs. Your doctor may have difficulty reaching an accurate diagnosis in these conditions unless you tell your doctor that you are taking dimenhydrinate.

Possible Side Effects

▼ Most common: drowsiness.

▼ Less common: confusion; nervousness; excitation; restlessness; headache; sleeplessness, especially in children; tingling; heavy or weak hands; fainting; dizziness; tiredness; rapid heartbeat; low blood pressure; heart palpitations; blurred or double vision; difficult or painful urination; increased sensitivity to the sun; appetite loss; nausea; vomiting; diarrhea; upset stomach; constipation; nightmares; rash; drug reaction (symptoms include rash, itching, hives, and breathing difficulties); ringing or buzzing in the ears; dry mouth, nose, or throat; stuffy nose; wheezing; and increased chest phlegm or chest tightness.

Drug Interactions

• Taking dimenhydrinate with an alcoholic beverage, other

antihistamine, tranquilizer, or other nervous-system depressant may cause excessive dizziness, drowsiness, and/or other signs of nervous-system depression.

• Taking dimenhydrinate with a drug that causes dizziness or other ear-related side effects may mask early signs of these side effects, especially in infants and children.

Food Interactions

Take dimenhydrinate with food or milk if it upsets your stomach.

Usual Dose

Dimenhydrinate

Adult and Child (age 13 and over): 50–100 mg—1 or 2 tablets or 4–8 tsp.—every 4–6 hours; do not take more than 400 mg a day.

Child (age 6–12): 25–50 mg—½ or 1 tablet or 2–4 tsp.—every 6–8 hours; do not take more than 150 mg a day.

Child (age 2–5): up to 25 mg—½ tablet or 2 tsp.—every 6–8 hours; do not take more than 3 doses a day.

Child (under age 2): Consult your doctor.

Meclizine

Adult and Child (age 13 and over): 25–50 mg 1 hour before travel; repeat every 24 hours for duration of journey. Up to 100 mg may be needed to control dizziness from other causes.

Child: not recommended.

Overdosage

Symptoms of overdose include drowsiness, clumsiness, or unsteadiness. Feeling faint, facial flushing, and dry mouth, nose, or throat may also occur. Convulsions, coma, and breathing difficulties may develop after a massive overdose. Overdose victims should be taken to a hospital emergency room for treatment. ALWAYS bring the prescription bottle or container with you.

Special Information

For maximum effectiveness against motion sickness, take dimenhydrinate 1 to 2 hours before traveling; it may still be effective if taken 30 minutes before traveling.

Dimenhydrinate may cause dry mouth, nose, or throat.

Sugarless candy, gum, or ice chips can usually relieve these symptoms. Constant dry mouth may increase the likelihood of developing tooth decay or gum disease. Pay special attention to oral hygiene while you are taking dimenhydrinate, and contact your doctor if excessive mouth dryness lasts more than 2 weeks.

If you forget to take a dose of dimenhydrinate, take it as soon as you remember. If it is almost time for your next dose, skip the one you forgot and continue with your regular schedule. Do not take a double dose.

Special Populations

Pregnancy/Breast-feeding
Antihistamines have not been proven to cause birth defects in humans; animal studies, however, suggest that meclizine may cause birth defects. Do not take any antihistamine without your doctor's knowledge if you are or might be pregnant—especially during the last 3 months of pregnancy, because newborns may have severe reactions to antihistamines.

Small amounts of dimenhydrinate may pass into breast milk and affect a nursing infant. Dimenhydrinate may also slow milk production. Nursing mothers who must take dimenhydrinate should bottle-feed their infants.

Seniors
Seniors are more sensitive to antihistamine side effects and should take the lowest effective dose. Call your doctor if side effects are bothersome or unusual.

Generic Name

Diphenhydramine Hydrochloride

(dye-fen-HYE-druh-mene hye-droe-KLOR-ide) Ⓖ

Brand Names

Allegria-C	Dytuss
Allegria-CEN	Tusstat

Type of Drug

Antihistamine.

Prescribed for

Stuffy and runny nose, itchy eyes, and scratchy throat caused by seasonal allergy and for other symptoms of allergy such as itching, rash, and hives; also prescribed for motion sickness, insomnia because of its potent depressant effect, and Parkinson's disease.

General Information

Antihistamines generally work by blocking the release of histamine (chemical released by body tissue during an allergic reaction) from the cell at the H_1 histamine receptor site, drying up secretions of the nose, throat, and eyes. Diphenhydramine hydrochloride will also help you fall asleep at night.

Cautions and Warnings

Diphenhydramine hydrochloride should not be used if you are **allergic** to it. This drug should be avoided or used with extreme care if you have **narrow-angle glaucoma, stomach ulcer or other stomach problems, enlarged prostate,** or **problems passing urine.** It should not be used by people who have **deep-breathing problems such as asthma.** Use with care if you have a history of thyroid disease, heart disease, high blood pressure, or diabetes.

Possible Side Effects

▼ Common: itching, rash, sensitivity to bright light, perspiration, chills, lowering of blood pressure, headache, rapid heartbeat, sleeplessness, dizziness, disturbed coordination, confusion, restlessness, nervousness, irritability, euphoria (feeling high), tingling and weakness of the hands or feet, blurred or double vision, ringing in the ears, upset stomach, appetite loss, nausea, vomiting, constipation, diarrhea, urinary difficulties, thickening of lung secretions, tightness of the chest, wheezing, nasal stuffiness, and dry mouth, nose, or throat.

Drug Interactions

• Diphenhydramine hydrochloride should not be taken with a monoamine oxidase inhibitor (MAOI) antidepressant.

• The effects of tranquilizers, sedatives, and sleeping medication will be intensified when any of these drugs is com-

bined with diphenhydramine hydrochloride; it is extremely important that you discuss this with your doctor so that doses of these drugs can be properly adjusted.
• Diphenhydramine hydrochloride will increase the intoxicating and sedating effects of alcohol. Be careful with this combination.

Food Interactions

Take diphenhydramine hydrochloride with food if it upsets your stomach.

Usual Dose

Allergy
    Adult: 25–50 mg 3–4 times a day.
    Child (over 20 lbs.): 12.5–25 mg 3–4 times a day.

Nightime Sedation
    Adult: 25–50 mg at bedtime.

Overdosage

Symptoms of overdose include depression or stimulation— especially in children; dry mouth; fixed or dilated pupils; flushing of the skin; and upset stomach. Overdose victims should be made to vomit with ipecac syrup—available at any pharmacy. Follow the directions on the bottle or call your local poison control center. Take the overdose victim to a hospital emergency room immediately if you cannot induce vomiting. ALWAYS bring the prescription bottle or container with you.

Special Information

Diphenhydramine hydrochloride produces a depressant effect: Be extremely cautious when driving or operating heavy equipment.
    If you forget to take a dose of diphenhydramine hydrochloride, take it as soon as you remember. If it is almost time for your next dose, skip the one you forgot and continue with your regular schedule. Do not take a double dose.

Special Populations

Pregnancy/Breast-feeding

While antihistamines have not been proven to cause birth defects in humans, animal studies have shown that some antihistamines may cause birth defects. Do not take any antihistamine without your doctor's knowledge if you are or might be pregnant—especially during the last 3 months of pregnancy, because newborns may have severe reactions to antihistamines.

Small amounts of antihistamine pass into breast milk and may affect a nursing infant. Nursing mothers who must take diphenhydramine hydrochloride should bottle-feed their infants.

Seniors

Seniors are more sensitive to antihistamine side effects, especially confusion, difficult or painful urination, dizziness, drowsiness, feeling faint, nightmares, excitability, nervousness, restlessness, irritability, and dry mouth, nose, or throat.

Generic Name

Dipivefrin (dye-piv-EF-rin) G

Brand Name

AK-Pro   Propine

Type of Drug

Sympathomimetic.

Prescribed for

Glaucoma.

General Information

When applied to the eye, dipivefrin hydrochloride is converted to epinephrine, one of the cornerstone drugs of glaucoma treatment. It provides the same effect on glaucoma as epinephrine but has fewer side effects. Epinephrine decreases the production of the fluid inside the eye and opens the channels by which the eye fluid naturally drains. These two actions combine to reduce fluid pressure inside the eye. Dipivefrin may be used in combination with pilocarpine ophthalmic solution or a beta-blocker eyedrop to produce an even greater drop in eye pressure. The drug starts working about half an hour after it is applied and reaches maximum effect in about 1 hour.

Cautions and Warnings

Use this product with care if you have **reacted to dipivefrin** in the past. People who have reacted to epinephrine eyedrops in the past are not likely to react to dipivefrin and can probably use this product; this is because of the conversion step that must take place (see "General Information").

Dipivefrin eyedrops contain sulfite preservatives. If you are **sensitive to sulfites**, this drug might cause irritation or allergic reactions.

Possible Side Effects

▼ Common: burning or stinging upon applying the eyedrops.

▼ Rare: conjunctivitis, drug allergies, rapid heartbeat, abnormal heart rhythms, and high blood pressure.

Drug Interactions

• Dipivefrin eyedrops may be taken with other antiglaucoma eyedrops.

Usual Dose

1 drop in the affected eye every 12 hours.

Overdosage

Possible symptoms of overdose are rapid heartbeat, excitement, or sleeplessness. Call your local poison control center or hospital emergency room for more information.

Special Information

To administer eyedrops, lie down or tilt your head backward and look at the ceiling. Hold the dropper above your eye, hold out your lower lid to make a small pouch, and drop the medication inside while looking up. Release the lower lid and keep your eye open. Do not blink for about 30 seconds. Press gently on the bridge of your nose at the inside corner of your eye for about a minute to help circulate the medication around your eye. To prevent infection, do not touch the dropper tip to your finger or eyelid. Wait 5 minutes before using any other eyedrop or ointment.

If you forget a dose of dipivefrin, take it as soon as you remember. If it is almost time for your next dose, skip the dose you forgot and then go back to your regular schedule. Do not take a double dose.

Special Populations

Pregnancy/Breast-feeding

Pregnant women should not use dipivefrin unless its possible benefits have been carefully weighed against its risks.

It is not known if this drug passes into breast milk. No drug-related problems have been known to occur. Nursing mothers who use dipivefrin should exercise caution.

Seniors

Seniors may use dipivefrin without any special precautions. Some older adults may have weaker eyelid muscles. This creates a small reservoir for the eyedrops and may actually increase the drug's effect by keeping it in contact with the eye for a longer period. Your doctor may take this into account when determining the proper drug dosage.

Generic Name

Dirithromycin (dye-rith-roe-MYE-sin)

Brand Names

Dynabac

Type of Drug

Macrolide antibiotic.

Prescribed for

Infections caused by streptococcus, staphylococcus, and other bacteria against which penicillin or tetracycline antibiotics cannot be used.

General information

Dirithromycin is a member of the *macrolide* group of antibiotics. Drugs in this group also include erythromycin, azithromycin, and clarithromycin and are either bactericidal (bacteria-killing) or bacteriostatic (inhibiting bacterial growth) depending on the organism in question and the amount of antibiotic present.

Dirithromycin has been studied in bronchitis, sore throat, pneumonia, tonsillitis, and legionnaires' disease.

After you swallow a dirithromycin tablet, it must be converted in the intestine to an active antimicrobial form called erythromycylamine. Erythromycylamine is quickly distributed throughout the body into the blood and a variety of tissues. It is not broken down by the liver and passes out of the body through the stool.

Since the action of this antibiotic depends on its concentration in infected tissues, it is important for you to take this drug as directed by a doctor. The effectiveness of any antibiotic may be severely reduced if these instructions are not followed.

Cautions and Warnings

Do not take dirithromycin if you are **allergic** to it or any macrolide antibiotic.

Dirithromycin should not be taken for **serious blood infections** because too little of it reaches the bloodstream. It does not work for and should not be used for *Haemophilus influenzae*, a very contagious infection that often affects children in daycare centers and their families. No dosage changes are needed for people with mild **liver disease**, even though they may already have higher-than-normal levels of dirithromycin in their blood. This drug has not been studied in people with severe liver disease. No dosage change is required in people with kidney disease.

Colitis (bowel inflammation)—see "Possible Side Effects" for symptoms—has been associated with all antibiotics including dirithromycin.

Possible Side Effects

▼ Most common: abdominal pain, headache, nausea, and diarrhea.

▼ Less common: increased blood-platelet count, vomiting, upset stomach, increased blood potassium, dizziness, fainting, pain, weakness, stomach disorders, increasing cough, stomach gas, rash, breathing difficulties, itching, and sleeplessness. Some blood tests can also be affected.

▼ Rare: abnormal stools, allergic reaction, dim vision,

Possible Side Effects *(continued)*

appetite loss, anxiety, constipation, dehydration, depression, dry mouth, painful menstruation, flushing, swelling in the hands or feet, nosebleeds, eye disorders, fever, flu symptoms, stomach and intestinal irritation, vomiting blood, rapid breathing, not feeling well, mouth sores, muscle aches, neck pain, nervousness, heart palpitations, tingling in the hands or feet, tiredness, sweating, changes in sense of taste, thirst, ringing or buzzing in the ears, tremors, frequent urination, vaginal fungus infections, and vaginal irritation.

Drug Interactions

• When dirithromycin is taken immediately after an antacid or H_2-antagonist such as cimetidine, famotidine, nizatidine, or ranitidine—most of which can be found in over-the-counter products—the amount of dirithromycin absorbed is increased.

• Other macrolide antibiotics interfere with the elimination of theophylline from the body, but this does not seem to be the case with dirithromycin. Your doctor may want to check blood-theophylline levels when you start on this drug.

• Pimozide should not be taken with any macrolide antibiotic including dirithromycin. Two people died after combining a macrolide antibiotic and pimozide.

• Erythromycin and other macrolide antibiotics interact with terfenadine (a non-sedating antihistamine) to produce potentially fatal abnormal heart rhythms. Studies have not shown an interaction between dirithromycin and terfenadine but caution should be used when using this combination.

Food Interactions

Take with food or within 1 hour of having eaten. Food increases the amount of dirithromycin absorbed into the blood.

Usual Dose

Tablets

  Adult and Child (age 12 and older): 500 mg a day for 7–10 days.

  Child (under age 12): not recommended.

Overdosage

Dirithromycin overdose may result in nausea, vomiting,

stomach cramps, and diarrhea. Call your local poison control center or hospital emergency room for more information.

Special Information

Dirithromycin is a relatively safe antibiotic, but it is not the antibiotic of choice for severe infections.

Do not crush, cut, or chew dirithromycin tablets.

Call your doctor if you develop any of the following: nausea, vomiting, diarrhea, stomach cramps, severe abdominal pain, or other severe or persistent side effects.

If you forget a dose of dirithromycin, take it as soon as you remember. If you do not remember until the next day, skip the dose you forgot and go back to your regular schedule. Call your doctor if you forget more than 1 dose.

Remember to complete the full course of therapy prescribed by your doctor, even if you feel well after only a few days of dirithromycin use.

Special Populations

Pregnancy/Breast-feeding

Dirithromycin affected the fetus in animal studies, but there is no information on the use of this drug in pregnant women. When this drug is considered crucial by your doctor, its potential benefits must be carefully weighed against its risks.

Other macrolide antibiotics pass into breast milk, but it is not known if dirithromycin or erythromycylamine act similarly. Nursing mothers who must take this drug should bottle-feed their infants.

Seniors

Seniors may use dirithromycin without special restriction.

Generic Name

Disopyramide (die-soe-PIE-rah-mide)

Brand Names

Norpace   Norpace CR

Type of Drug

Antiarrhythmic.

Prescribed for

Abnormal heart rhythms.

General Information

Disopyramide phosphate slows the rate at which nerve impulses are carried through heart muscle, reducing the response of heart muscle to those impulses. It acts on the heart similarly to the more widely used antiarrhythmic medications—procainamide hydrochloride and quinidine sulfate. Disopyramide is often prescribed for people who do not respond to other antiarrhythmic drugs. It also may be prescribed for people who have had a myocardial infarction (heart attack) because it helps infarcted areas to respond to nerve impulses more like the adjacent healthy heart tissue.

Cautions and Warnings

This drug can worsen **heart failure** or trigger severely **low blood pressure**. It should be used in combination with another antiarrhythmic agent or beta blocker, such as propranolol hydrochloride, only when single-drug treatment has not been effective or the arrhythmia may be life-threatening.

In rare instances, disopyramide has caused a **reduction in blood-sugar levels**. Therefore, the drug should be used with caution by diabetics, older adults—who are more susceptible to this effect—and people with poor kidney or liver function. Blood-sugar levels should be measured periodically in people with heart failure or liver or kidney disease, those who are malnourished, and those taking a beta-blocking drug.

Because of its anticholinergic effects, disopyramide should be used with caution by people who have glaucoma, myasthenia gravis, or severe **difficulty urinating**—especially men with a severe prostate condition.

People with **liver or kidney disease** must take a reduced dose of disopyramide.

Possible Side Effects

▼ Most common: heart failure, low blood pressure, and urinary difficulty.

▼ Common: dry mouth, throat, or nose; constipation; and blurred vision.

Possible Side Effects *(continued)*

▼ Less common: urination, dizziness, fatigue, headache, nervousness, breathing difficulties, chest pain, nausea, stomach pain or bloating, gas, appetite loss, diarrhea, vomiting, itching, rashes, muscle weakness, generalized aches and pains, not feeling well, low blood-potassium levels, increases in blood-cholesterol and triglyceride levels, and dry eyes.

▼ Rare: male impotence, painful urination, reduced heart activity, anemia (condition characterized by a reduction in the number of red blood cells or amount of hemoglobin or blood), reduced white-blood-cell counts, sleeplessness, depression, psychotic reactions, liver inflammation, yellowing of the skin or whites of the eyes, numbness and tingling in the hands or feet, elevated blood urea nitrogen (BUN) and creatinine in tests of kidney function, low blood sugar, fever, swollen and painful male breasts, drug allergy, and glaucoma.

Drug Interactions

• Phenytoin and rifampin may increase the rate at which the body removes disopyramide from the blood. Your disopyramide dose may need alteration if this combination is used. Other drugs known to increase drug breakdown by the liver, such as barbiturates and primidone, may also have this effect.

• Other antiarrhythmic drugs, such as procainamide and quinidine, may increase the effect of disopyramide, making dosage reduction necessary. At the same time, disopyramide may reduce the effectiveness of quinidine.

• When disopyramide is combined with a beta-blocking drug, increased disopyramide effects, additive effects, or depression of heart function may result.

• Erythromycin may increase the amount of disopyramide in your blood, causing abnormal heart rhythms or other cardiac effects.

• Disopyramide may reduce the effectiveness of oral anticoagulant (blood-thinning) drugs. Your doctor should check your anticoagulant dosage to be sure you are getting the right amount.

• Disopyramide may increase the amount of digoxin in

your blood, though the amount of the increase is not likely to affect your heart.

Food Interactions

Disopyramide should be taken on an empty stomach at least 1 hour before or 2 hours after meals.

Usual Dose

Adult: 400 mg–600 mg a day, divided into 2 or 4 doses. In severe cases, 400 mg every 6 hours may be required. The sustained-release preparation is taken every 12 hours. People with reduced kidney function should receive a lower dosage, depending on the degree of kidney function present. People with liver failure should take 400 mg a day.

Child (age 13–18): 2.5–7 mg a day per lb. of body weight.
Child (age 5–12): 4.5–7 mg a day per lb. of body weight.
Child (age 1–4): 4.5–9 mg a day per lb. of body weight.
Child (under age 1): 4.5–13.5 mg a day per lb. of body weight.

Overdosage

Symptoms of overdose are breathing difficulties, abnormal heart rhythms, and unconsciousness. In severe cases, overdosage can lead to death. Overdose victims should be made to vomit with ipecac syrup—available at any pharmacy—to remove any remaining drug from the stomach. Call your doctor or poison control center before doing this. If you must go to a hospital emergency room, ALWAYS bring the prescription bottle or container with you. Prompt and vigorous treatment can mean the difference between life and death in severe overdosage.

Special Information

Disopyramide may cause symptoms of low blood sugar: anxiety, chills, cold sweats, drowsiness, excessive hunger, nausea, nervousness, rapid pulse, shakiness, unusual weakness, tiredness, or cool, pale skin. If this happens to you, eat some chocolate, candy, or other high-sugar food, and call your doctor at once.

Disopyramide can cause dry mouth, urinary difficulty, constipation, or blurred vision. Call your doctor if these symptoms become severe or intolerable, but do not stop taking the medication without your doctor's approval.

If disopyramide is required for a child and capsules are not

appropriate; your pharmacist can make a liquid product. Do
not do this at home: This medication requires special preparation. The liquid should be refrigerated and protected from
light and should be thrown away after 30 days.

If you forget to take a dose of disopyramide, take it as soon
as possible. However, if it is within 4 hours of your next dose,
skip the dose you forgot and go back to your regular schedule. Do not take a double dose.

Special Populations

Pregnancy/Breast-feeding
Do not take this drug if you are pregnant or planning to
become pregnant while using it, because it will pass into the
fetus and may affect its development. Also, disopyramide can
cause your uterus to contract if you are pregnant. When
disopyramide is considered crucial by your doctor, its potential benefits must carefully be weighed against its risks.

Nursing women should not take disopyramide because it
passes into breast milk. If you must take this medicine,
bottle-feed your baby.

Seniors
Seniors, especially those with liver or kidney disease, are more
sensitive to the effects of this drug; in particular, they more
frequently develop urinary difficulty and dry mouth. Follow
your doctor's directions and report any side effects at once.

Generic Name

Donepezil (don-EP-eh-zil)

Brand Name
Aricept

Type of Drug
Cholinesterase inhibitor.

Prescribed for
Alzheimer's disease.

General Information
Donepezil hydrochloride works by increasing the function of
certain receptors in the brain that are stimulated by a hor-

mone called acetylcholine. Donepezil accomplishes this by interfering with cholinesterase, the enzyme that breaks down acetylcholine. Tacrine, the only other drug available for Alzheimer's disease (a degenerative condition of the central nervous system), is also a cholinesterase inhibitor. There is no evidence that donepezil reverses the degenerative effects of Alzheimer's, but it may slow the rate at which the disease worsens.

Cautions and Warnings

Do not take this drug if you are **allergic** to it or to piperidine-type drugs.

Donepezil must be stopped in preparation for **surgery** because it will increase the effects of certain surgical anesthetic drugs.

Cholinesterase inhibitors like donepezil may **slow heart rate**. People with heart disease must be careful about using donepezil.

Donepezil has not been linked to other specific effects caused by cholinesterase inhibitors, such as an increase in the amount of **stomach acid** that may lead to ulcers or bleeding—alcohol and nonsteroidal anti-inflammatory drugs (NSAIDs) such as aspirin may worsen this effect. Use of cholinesterase inhibitors may also lead to **urinary blockage,** increase the risk of generalized **seizures,** and worsen **asthma** or other pulmonary disease.

Possible Side Effects

In clinical studies, people taking donepezil experienced side effects at about the same rate as those taking placebo (sugar pill).

▼ Most common: headache, pain, accidents, nausea, diarrhea, sleeplessness, and dizziness.

▼ Common: tiredness, vomiting, appetite loss, and muscle cramps.

▼ Less common: arthritis, depression, abnormal dreams, fainting, black-and-blue marks, and weight loss.

▼ Rare: Other effects may occur in virtually any body part or system.

Drug Interactions

• Donepezil interferes with the effects of anticholinergic drugs, often prescribed for stomach disorders.

• Donepezil can be expected to increase the effects of surgical anesthetic drugs and drugs that irritate the stomach and intestines, such as aspirin or other NSAIDs.

• Donepezil was found to have no interaction with furosemide, digoxin, warfarin, theophylline, or cimetidine.

• Ketoconazole and quinidine can slow the breakdown of donepezil in the liver. The importance of this interaction in people is not known.

Food Interactions

None known.

Usual Dose

Adult: 5 or 10 mg once a day.

Overdosage

Cholinesterase inhibitor overdose may be very serious. Symptoms include severe nausea, vomiting, salivation, sweating, slow heart rate, low blood pressure, slow breathing rate, convulsions, muscle weakness, and collapse. Overdose victims should be taken to a hospital emergency room at once. ALWAYS bring the prescription bottle or container with you.

Special Information

Take donepezil just before bedtime.

If you forget to take a dose, take it as soon as you remember. If it is almost time for your next dose, skip the dose you forgot and continue with your regular schedule. Never take a double dose.

Special Populations

Pregnancy/Breast-feeding

One animal study of donepezil indicated a small risk of birth defects. This drug should be taken during pregnancy only if it is absolutely necessary.

It is not known if donepezil passes into breast milk.

Seniors

Seniors may take this drug without special precaution.

Brand Name

Donnatal

Generic Ingredients:

Atropine Sulfate + Hyoscyamine Sulfate + Phenobarbital + Scopolamine Hydrobromide 🅖

Other Brand Names
Barbidonna	Spasmolin
Hyosophen	Susano
Malatal	

The information in this profile also applies to the following drugs:

Generic Ingredient: Hyoscyamine Sulfate
Donnamar

Generic Ingredients: Belladonna Alkaloids + Phenobarbital
Donnapine

Type of Drug

Anticholinergic combination.

Prescribed for

Stomach spasm and gastrointestinal (GI) cramps; also used to treat motion sickness.

General Information

Donnatal is a mild antispasmodic sedative. Its principal action is to counteract the effect of acetylcholine, an important neurohormone. Donnatal is used only to relieve symptoms, not to treat the underlying condition, and there is considerable doubt among medical experts that this drug lives up to its claims. In addition to the brand names listed above, there are about 50 other anticholinergic combinations with similar properties. All are used to relieve cramps, and all are about equally effective. Some have additional ingredients to reduce or absorb excess gas in the stomach, to coat the stomach, or to control diarrhea. Donnatal and products like it should not be used for more than the temporary relief of symptoms.

Cautions and Warnings

Donnatal should not be used by people with **glaucoma, rapid**

heartbeat, severe intestinal disease such as **ulcerative colitis, serious kidney or liver disease**, or a history of **allergy** to any of the ingredients of this drug.

Donnatal and other drugs of this class can reduce your ability to sweat and may lead to **heat exhaustion**. If you take this type of medication, avoid extended heavy exercise and limit your exposure to high summer temperatures.

Possible Side Effects

▼ Most common: blurred vision, dry mouth, urinary difficulties, flushing, and dry skin.

▼ Less common: rapid or unusual heartbeat, increased sensitivity to bright light, loss of the sense of taste, headache, nervousness, tiredness, weakness, dizziness, sleeplessness, nausea, vomiting, fever, stuffy nose, heartburn, loss of sex drive, decreased sweating, constipation, feeling bloated, and allergic reactions, such as fever and rash.

Drug Interactions

• Although Donnatal contains only a small amount of phenobarbital, it is wise to avoid alcohol or other sedative drugs. Although unlikely, phenobarbital interactions are possible with anticoagulants, adrenal corticosteroids, tranquilizers, narcotics, sleeping pills, digitalis or other cardiac glycosides, and antihistamines.

• Some phenothiazine drugs, tranquilizers, tricyclic antidepressants, and narcotics may increase the side effects of the atropine sulfate ingredient in Donnatal, causing dry mouth, urinary difficulties, and constipation.

Food Interactions

Take Donnatal 30 to 60 minutes before meals.

Usual Dose

Adult (age 13 and over): 1–2 tablets, capsules, or teaspoons 3–4 times a day.

Child (age 2–12): ½ the adult dosage.

Child (under age 2): not recommended.

Overdosage

Symptoms of overdose include dry mouth; difficulty swallowing; thirst; blurred vision; sensitivity to bright light; flushed, hot, or dry skin; rash; fever; abnormal heart rate; high blood pressure; urinary difficulties; restlessness; confusion; delirium; and breathing difficulties. The victim should be taken to a hospital emergency room immediately. ALWAYS bring the prescription bottle or container with you.

Special Information

Dry mouth from Donnatal usually can be relieved by chewing gum or sucking hard candy or ice chips. Constipation can be treated with a stool-softening laxative.

Donnatal may reduce the amount of saliva in your mouth, making it easier for bacteria to grow in your mouth. Pay special attention to dental hygiene while taking this medication to prevent cavities and/or gum disease from developing.

Donnatal may cause drowsiness and blurred vision. Be careful when driving or operating hazardous equipment.

If you forget to take a dose of Donnatal, take it as soon as you remember. If it is almost time for your next dose, skip the one you forgot and continue with your regular schedule. Do not take a double dose.

Special Populations

Pregnancy/Breast-feeding

Donnatal should be used with caution by pregnant women. Check with your doctor before taking it if you are or might be pregnant. Regular use of Donnatal during the last 3 months of pregnancy may lead to moderate drug dependency in the newborn. Donnatal use may also lead to prolonged labor, delayed delivery, and breathing problems in the newborn.

Donnatal may reduce the flow of breast milk and may cause tiredness, shortness of breath, and a slower than normal heartbeat in babies whose mothers are taking the drug. Nursing mothers who must take this medication should consider bottle-feeding their babies.

Seniors

Seniors are often more sensitive to the side effects of Donnatal, such as excitement, confusion, drowsiness, agitation, constipation, dry mouth, and urinary difficulties. Memory may be impaired and glaucoma worsened. Follow your doctor's directions and report any side effects at once.

Generic Name

Dorzolamide (door-ZOHL-ah-myde)

Brand Name

Trusopt

Type of Drug

Carbonic-anhydrase inhibitor.

Prescribed for

Glaucoma.

General Information

Dorzolamide hydrochloride is similar to acetazolamide, an oral carbonic-anhydrase inhibitor, except that it has been put in eyedrop form. Carbonic anhydrase is an enzyme found in many parts of the body, including the eye. Dorzolamide slows the formation of fluid in the eye, reducing eye pressure. In glaucoma, pressure inside the eye is higher than normal, and slowing fluid formation lowers that pressure.

Cautions and Warnings

Do not take dorzolamide if you are **sensitive or allergic** to it or to other sulfa drugs. Small amounts of any drug placed into your eye find their way into the bloodstream. Rarely, people using this eyedrop will experience **sulfa drug side effects** or allergies.

Dorzolamide has not been studied in people with very **poor kidney or liver function**. Since dorzolamide is released from the body through the kidney, another glaucoma drug should be used in people with impaired kidney function.

Possible Side Effects

▼ Most common: burning, stinging, or discomfort in the eye and a bitter taste immediately after use.

▼ Less common: allergic reactions, blurred vision, tearing, dryness of the eye, and unusual sensitivity to bright light.

Possible Side Effects *(continued)*

▼ Rare: headache, nausea, weakness, tiredness, skin rash, and kidney stones. The same types of side effects seen with other forms of sulfa drugs may also be seen with dorzolamide, but these are rare. Be sure to report anything unusual to your doctor at once.

Drug Interactions

• Make sure to wait at least 10 minutes before using any other eyedrops.

Usual Dose

Adult: One drop in the affected eye(s) 3 times a day.

Overdosage

Anyone who swallows dorzolamide should be taken to a hospital emergency room for treatment because of possible effects on potassium and other blood electrolytes. ALWAYS bring the prescription bottle or container with you.

Special Information

Dorzolamide is a sulfa drug; people allergic to sulfa drugs should avoid it. Report anything unusual to your doctor.

Call your doctor and stop using the eyedrops if you develop any unusual eye reaction or condition, including swollen eyelids or conjunctivitis (pinkeye).

If you wear soft contact lenses, take them out before using these eyedrops.

To administer eyedrops, lie down or tilt your head back. Hold the dropper above your eye, gently squeeze your lower lid to form a small pouch, and release the drop or drops of medication inside your lower lid while looking up. Release the lower lid, keeping your eye open. Do not blink for 40 seconds. Press gently on the bridge of your nose at the inside corner of your eye for 1 minute to help circulate the drug in your eye. Do not touch the dropper tip to your finger, eyelid, or any other surface. Wait at least 10 minutes before using another eyedrop or eye ointment.

If you forget to take a dose of dorzolamide eyedrops, take it as soon as you remember. If it is almost time for your next dose, skip the one you forgot and continue with your regular schedule. Do not take a double dose.

Special Populations

Pregnancy/Breast-feeding

At 31 times the human dose of dorzolamide, rabbit fetuses developed birth malformations. The chance of dorzolamide causing birth defects in humans is small, but pregnant women should not use this medication without first discussing it with their doctor.

In animal studies, dorzolamide was found to cause developmental problems at 94 times the human dose. It is not known if dorzolamide passes into breast milk, but nursing mothers should consult their doctors before using dorzolamide eyedrops.

Seniors

Seniors may be more sensitive to the side effects of this drug.

Generic Name

Doxazosin (dok-SAY-zoe-sin)

Brand Name

Cardura

Type of Drug

Antihypertensive.

Prescribed for

High blood pressure and benign prostatic hyperplasia (BPH); also used with digoxin and diuretic drugs to treat congestive heart failure.

General Information

Doxazosin mesylate is one of several alpha-adrenergic blocking agents, or alpha blockers, that work by opening blood vessels and reducing pressure in them. Other types of blood-pressure-lowering drugs block beta receptors, interfere with the movement of calcium in blood-vessel muscle cells, affect salt and electrolyte balance in the body, or interfere with the production of norepinephrine in the body. Alpha blockers like doxazosin block nerve endings known as alpha$_1$ receptors. The maximum blood-pressure-lowering effect of doxazosin is seen between 2 and 6 hours after taking a single dose. In BPH treatment, doxazosin works by relaxing smooth muscles in the prostate and neck of the bladder, which results from the blocking of alpha receptors in the affected muscles. Despite the fact that doxazosin reduces the symptoms of BPH, the drug's long-term effect on complications of BPH or the need for urinary surgery is not known. Response to doxazosin is not affected by age or race. Doxazosin's effect lasts for 24 hours. It is broken down in the liver; little passes out of the body via the kidneys.

Cautions and Warnings

Doxazosin may cause **dizziness** and **fainting**, especially the first few doses. This is known as a first-dose effect, which can be minimized by limiting the first dose to 1 mg at bedtime. First-dose effects occur in about 1% of people taking an alpha blocker and may recur if the drug is stopped for a few days and then restarted.

Doxazosin should be taken with caution if you have **liver disease**, because the drug is eliminated from your system almost exclusively via the liver.

People **allergic or sensitive** to any of the alpha blockers should avoid doxazosin because of the risk that they will react to it as well.

Doxazosin may slightly reduce cholesterol levels and increase the high density lipoprotein (HDL)/low density lipoprotein (LDL) ratio, a positive step for people with a blood-cholesterol problem. People who already have high blood-cholesterol levels should discuss this effect with their doctors.

In animals, doxazosin is toxic to the heart and causes loss of testicular function. These effects have not been seen in humans.

Red- and white-blood-cell counts may be slightly decreased in people taking doxazosin.

Possible Side Effects

▼ Most common: headache, dizziness, and weakness.

▼ Less common: heart palpitations, abnormal heart rhythms, chest pain, nausea, diarrhea, constipation, abdominal pain or discomfort, stomach gas, breathing difficulties, nosebleed, sore throat, runny nose, muscle or joint pain, visual disturbances, conjunctivitis (pinkeye),

Possible Side Effects *(continued)*

ringing in the ears, fainting, depression, decreased sex
drive or sexual function, tingling in the hands or feet,
nervousness, tiredness, anxiety, sleeplessness, poor
muscle coordination, muscle stiffness, poor bladder control, frequent urination, itching, rash, sweating, fluid
retention, facial swelling and flushing, and back, neck,
shoulder, arm, or leg pain.

▼ Rare: vomiting, dry mouth, sinus irritation, bronchitis, cold or flu symptoms, worsening of asthma, coughing, hair loss, weight gain, and fever.

Drug Interactions

• Doxazosin may interact with beta blockers to increase the
risk of dizziness or fainting after the first dose of doxazosin.

• The blood-pressure-lowering effect of doxazosin may be
reduced by indomethacin.

• When taken with other blood-pressure-lowering drugs,
doxazosin produces a severe reduction of blood pressure.

• The blood-pressure-lowering effect of clonidine may be
reduced by doxazosin.

• This drug does not affect the results of the prostate
specific antigen (PSA) test, often used to monitor the progress
of BPH.

Food Interactions

None known.

Usual Dose

1 mg at bedtime to start; may be increased to a total daily
dosage of 16 mg, taken once or twice a day.

Overdosage

Doxazosin overdose may produce drowsiness, poor reflexes,
and very low blood pressure. Overdose victims should be
taken to a hospital emergency room at once. ALWAYS bring
the prescription bottle or container with you.

Special Information

Take doxazosin exactly as prescribed. Do not stop taking it
unless directed to do so by your doctor. Avoid over-the-

counter drugs that contain stimulants because they may increase your blood pressure. Your pharmacist will be able to tell you what you can and cannot take.

Doxazosin may cause dizziness, headache, and drowsiness, especially 2 to 6 hours after you take your first dose, although these effects can persist after the first few doses.

Call your doctor if you develop severe dizziness, heart palpitations, or other bothersome or persistent side effects.

Wait 12 to 24 hours after taking your first dose of doxazosin before driving or doing anything that requires concentration. Take your dose at bedtime to minimize this problem.

If you forget to take a dose of doxazosin, take it as soon as you remember. If it is almost time for your next dose, skip the dose you forgot and continue with your regular schedule. Do not take a double dose.

Special Populations

Pregnancy/Breast-feeding

There have been no studies of doxazosin in pregnant women; its safety for use during pregnancy is not known.

Small amounts of doxazosin pass into breast milk. Nursing mothers who must take this drug should bottle-feed their babies.

Seniors

Seniors, especially those with liver disease, may be more sensitive to the effects and side effects of doxazosin. Report any unusual side effects to your doctor.

Generic Name

Dronabinol (droe-NAB-ih-nol)

Brand Name

Marinol

Type of Drug

Antinauseant.

Prescribed for

Nausea and vomiting associated with cancer chemotherapy

and appetite stimulation and weight loss prevention in people with AIDS.

General Information

Dronabinol is the first legal form of marijuana available to the American public. The psychoactive chemical ingredient in marijuana is also known as delta-9-THC. Dronabinol has all of the psychological effects of marijuana and is therefore considered to be a highly abusable drug. Its ability to cause personality changes, feelings of detachment, hallucinations, and euphoria (feeling high) has made dronabinol relatively unacceptable among older adults and those who feel they must be in control of their environment. Younger adults have reported a greater success rate with dronabinol, probably because they are better able to tolerate these effects.

Most people start on dronabinol while in the hospital because the doctor needs to monitor closely their response to the medication and possible adverse effects.

Dronabinol has been studied as a treatment for glaucoma.

Cautions and Warnings

Dronabinol **should not be used to treat nausea and vomiting caused by anything other than cancer chemotherapy**. It should not be used by people who are **allergic** to it, to **marijuana**, or to **sesame oil**. Dronabinol has a **profound effect on mental states**; it will impair your ability to operate complex equipment or engage in any activity that requires intense concentration, sound judgment, or coordination—such as driving a car.

Like other abusable drugs, dronabinol produces a definite set of **withdrawal symptoms** when the drug is stopped. Tolerance to the drug's effects develops after a month of use. Withdrawal symptoms may develop within 12 hours of the drug's discontinuation and include restlessness, sleeplessness, and irritability. Within a day after the drug has been stopped, stuffy nose, hot flashes, sweating, loose stools, hiccups, or appetite loss may occur. The symptoms usually subside within a few days.

Dronabinol should be used with caution by people with a **manic-depressive or schizophrenic history** because of the risk that it will aggravate the underlying disease.

In animal studies, dronabinol **reduced the number of sperm produced and the number of cells from which sperm are made**.

Possible Side Effects

▼ Most common: drowsiness, euphoria (feeling high), dizziness, anxiety, muddled thinking, perceptual difficulties, poor coordination, irritability, a weird feeling, depression, weakness, sluggishness, headache, hallucinations, memory lapses, loss of muscle coordination, unsteadiness, paranoia, depersonalization, disorientation, confusion, rapid heartbeat, and dizziness when rising from a sitting or lying position.

▼ Less common: difficulty talking or slurred speech, facial flushing, excessive perspiration, nightmares, ringing or buzzing in the ears, fainting, diarrhea, loss of ability to control bowel movement, and muscle pain.

Drug Interactions

• Dronabinol will increase the psychological effects of alcoholic beverages, tranquilizers, sleeping pills, sedatives, and other depressants. It will also enhance the effects of other psychoactive drugs including tricyclic antidepressants, amphetamines, cocaine, and other stimulants.

• Dronabinol may increase the effects of fluoxetine and disulfiram.

• The effects of theophylline drugs are reduced by dronabinol because it stimulates the liver to break down theophylline more quickly.

Food Interactions

This drug may be taken without regard to food or meals; as an appetite stimulant, it is often taken before meals.

Usual Dose

Antiemetic: 5–15 mg 1–3 hours before starting chemotherapy treatment and repeated every 2–4 hours after chemotherapy has been given, for a total of 4–6 doses a day. The dosage may be increased up to 30 mg a day if needed but psychiatric side effects increase greatly at higher dosages.

Appetite Stimulant: 2.5 mg before lunch and/or dinner or at bedtime. Dosage may be increased to 20 mg a day.

Overdosage

Overdose symptoms may occur at usual dosages or at higher

dosages if the drug is being abused. The primary symptoms of overdose are the psychological symptoms listed above (see "Possible Side Effects"). In some cases, overdose may lead to panic reactions or seizure. No deaths have been reported with either marijuana or dronabinol overdose. Dronabinol therapy may be restarted at lower dosages if other drugs are ineffective.

Special Information

Dronabinol may impair your ability to drive a car or perform complex tasks. Avoid alcohol and other nervous-system depressants while taking dronabinol.

Dronabinol may cause acute psychiatric or psychological effects. Call your doctor if any such side effects develop.

Dronabinol capsules must be stored in the refrigerator.

If you forget to take a dose of dronabinol, take it as soon as you remember. If it is almost time for your next dose, skip the one you forgot and continue with your regular schedule. Do not take a double dose.

Special Populations

Pregnancy/Breast-feeding

Dronabinol studies of pregnant animals taking dosages 10 to 400 times the human dose have shown no adverse effects on fetal development. However, dronabinol should not be taken by a pregnant woman unless it is absolutely necessary.

Dronabinol passes into breast milk and may affect a nursing infant. Nursing mothers who must take this drug should bottle-feed their infants.

Seniors

Seniors are more sensitive to this drug, especially its psychological effects. Follow your doctor's directions and report side effects at once.

Brand Name

Dyazide

Generic Ingredients

Hydrochlorothiazide + Triamterene [G]

Other Brand Names

Maxzide   Maxzide-25MG

The information in this profile also applies to the following drugs:

Generic Ingredients: Amiloride + Hydrochlorothiazide
Moduretic

Generic Ingredients: Spironolactone + Hydrochlorothiazide
Aldactazide

Type of Drug

Diuretic.

Prescribed for

Hypertension (high blood pressure) or any condition where it is desirable to eliminate excess water from the body.

General Information

A diuretic is an agent that increases urination. Dyazide is a combination of 2 diuretics—a thiazide diuretic and a potassium-sparing diuretic—and is a convenient, effective approach for the treatment of diseases where the elimination of excess water is required. One of the ingredients, triamterene, has the ability to hold potassium in the body while producing a diuretic effect. This balances the other ingredient, hydrochlorothiazide, which normally causes a loss of body potassium. Different brand-name and generic products contain differing concentrations of these 2 ingredients. Dyazide should be used only when you need the exact proportion of ingredients contained in this particular product and when you would benefit from the convenience of taking these 2 ingredients in a single pill.

Cautions and Warnings

Do not use Dyazide if you have **nonfunctioning kidneys**, are **allergic** to this drug or any sulfa drug, or have a history of **allergy** or **bronchial asthma**.

Do not take any **potassium supplement** with Dyazide unless specifically directed to do so by your doctor.

Possible Side Effects

▼ Most common: appetite loss, drowsiness, lethargy, headache, gastrointestinal upset, cramping, and diarrhea.

Possible Side Effects *(continued)*

▼ Less common: rash, mental confusion, fever, feeling unwell, inability to achieve or maintain an erection, bright red tongue, burning sensation in the tongue, tingling in the toes and fingers, restlessness, anemia or other effects on components of the blood, unusual sensitivity to sunlight, and dizziness when rising quickly from a sitting position. Dyazide may also produce muscle spasms, gout, weakness, and blurred vision.

Drug Interactions

• Dyazide increases the action of other blood-pressure-lowering drugs. This is a positive effect and is the reason why people with hypertension often take more than one medication.

• The possibility of developing imbalances in electrolytes (body fluids) is increased if you take medications such as digitalis drugs, amphotericin B, or adrenal corticosteroids while taking Dyazide. If you are taking insulin or an oral antidiabetic drug and begin taking Dyazide, the insulin or antidiabetic dosage may have to be modified.

• Combining Dyazide and allopurinol may increase the risk of experiencing allopurinol side effects.

• Dyazide may decrease the effects of oral anticoagulant (blood-thinning) drugs.

• Antigout drug dosage may have to be modified since Dyazide raises blood-uric-acid levels.

• Dyazide may prolong the effects of chemotherapy drugs on reducing white-blood-cell counts.

• Dyazide may increase the effects of diazoxide, which may lead to symptoms of diabetes.

• Dyazide should not be taken with loop diuretics because the combination can lead to an extreme diuretic effect and an extreme effect on blood-electrolyte (blood-salt) levels.

• Dyazide may increase the biological actions of vitamin D, which may cause high blood-calcium levels.

• Propantheline and other anticholinergics may increase the diuretic effect of Dyazide by increasing the amount of drug absorbed.

• Lithium carbonate taken with Dyazide should be monitored carefully by a doctor because there may be an increased risk of lithium side effects.

• Cholestyramine and colestipol bind Dyazide and prevent it from being absorbed into the blood. Dyazide should be taken at least 2 hours before taking cholestyramine or colestipol.

• Methenamine and other urinary agents may reduce the effect of Dyazide by reducing urinary acidity.

• Some nonsteroidal anti-inflammatory drugs (NSAIDs), particularly indomethacin, may reduce the effect of Dyazide. Sulindac, another NSAID, may increase the effect of Dyazide.

Food Interactions

Take this drug with food if it upsets your stomach.

Usual Dose

1–2 capsules or tablets a day.

Overdosage

Symptoms of overdose may include tingling in the arms or legs, weakness, fatigue, changes in heartbeat, a sickly feeling, dry mouth, restlessness, muscle pain or cramps, urinary difficulties, nausea, and vomiting. Take the overdose victim to a hospital emergency room immediately. ALWAYS bring the prescription bottle or container with you.

Special Information

Dyazide will cause excess urination at first, but that will subside after several weeks of taking the medication. Diuretics are usually taken early in the day to prevent excessive nighttime urination that may interfere with your sleep.

Dyazide may make you drowsy. Be careful when driving or operating hazardous machinery.

Call your doctor if you develop muscle pain, sudden joint pain, weakness, cramps, nausea, vomiting, restlessness, excessive thirst, tiredness, drowsiness, increased heart or pulse rate, diarrhea, dizziness, headache, or rash.

Diabetic patients may experience an increased blood-sugar level and a need for dosage adjustments of their antidiabetic medications.

Avoid other medications while taking Dyazide unless otherwise directed by your doctor. Avoid alcohol while taking Dyazide.

If you are taking Dyazide for the treatment of hypertension or congestive heart failure (CHF), avoid over-the-counter medications for the treatment of coughs, colds, or allergies; such medications may contain stimulants. If you are unsure about them, ask your pharmacist.

If you forget to take a dose of Dyazide, take it as soon as you remember. If it is almost time for your next dose, skip the dose you forgot and continue with your regular schedule. Do not take a double dose.

Take Dyazide exactly as prescribed. Be aware that all triamterene-hydrochlorothiazide products are not equal to each other and should not be freely substituted. Check with your doctor and pharmacist before switching brands.

Special Populations

Pregnancy/Breast-feeding

Dyazide may be used to treat specific conditions in pregnant women, but the decision to use this medication by pregnant women should be weighed carefully because the drug may cross the placental barrier into the blood of the fetus.

The thiazide diuretic in Dyazide passes into breast milk of nursing mothers. Be sure your baby's doctor knows you are taking Dyazide.

Seniors

Seniors are more sensitive to the effects of Dyazide. Closely follow your doctor's directions and report any side effects at once.

Generic Name

Econazole (ee-KON-uh-zole)

Brand Name

Spectazole

Type of Drug

Antifungal.

Prescribed for

Fungal infections of the skin, including athlete's foot, jock itch, and many common infections.

General Information

This drug is similar to another antifungal agent, miconazole nitrate. However, unlike miconazole, econazole nitrate is available only as a cream for application to the skin. Very small amounts of econazole are absorbed into the bloodstream, but quite a bit of the drug penetrates to the middle and inner layers of the skin, where it can kill fungal organisms that may have penetrated to deeper layers.

Cautions and Warnings

Do not use econazole if you have had an **allergic reaction** to it or any other ingredient in this product. Do not apply econazole cream in or near your eyes.

This product is generally safe, but it belongs to a family of drugs known to cause **liver damage**. Therefore, long-term application of this product to large areas of skin might produce an adverse effect on the liver.

Possible Side Effects

▼ Most common: burning, itching, stinging, and redness in the areas to which the cream has been applied.

Drug Interactions

None known.

Usual Dose

Apply enough of the cream to cover affected areas with a thin layer 1–2 times a day.

Overdosage

This cream should not be swallowed. If it is swallowed, the victim may become nauseous and have an upset stomach. Other possible effects are drowsiness and liver inflammation or damage. Little is known about econazole overdose; call your local poison control center for more information.

Special Information

Clean the affected areas before applying econazole cream unless otherwise directed by your doctor.

Call your doctor if the treated area burns, stings, or becomes red.

This product is quite effective and can be expected to relieve symptoms within a day or two after you begin using it. Follow your doctor's directions for the complete 2- to 4-week course of treatment to gain maximum benefit from the product. If treatment is stopped too soon, the drug may not have eliminated the fungus completely; this can lead to a relapse.

If you forget to take a dose of econazole, apply it as soon as you remember. If it is almost time for your next dose, skip the one you forgot and continue with your regular schedule. Do not apply a double dose.

Special Populations

Pregnancy/Breast-feeding

When given by mouth to pregnant animals in doses 10 to 40 times the amount normally applied to the skin, econazole was found to be toxic to the fetus. It should be strictly avoided during the first 3 months of pregnancy. During the last 6 months of pregnancy, it should be used only if absolutely necessary.

It is not known if econazole passes into breast milk. Animal studies show the drug and its by-products pass into breast milk. Nursing mothers should be cautious about using this medication.

Seniors

Seniors may take this drug without special restriction.

Effexor

see **Venlafaxine**, page 1150

Brand Name

EMLA

Generic Ingredients

Lidocaine + Prilocaine

Type of Drug

Topical anesthetic.

Prescribed for

Skin pain.

General Information

EMLA—which stands for Eutectic Mixture of Local Anesthetics—is a mixture of two anesthetics which, when mixed, turn to liquid on contact with the skin. The anesthetics penetrate all layers of skin, deadening nerve endings and providing an anesthetic effect that is as good as that achieved by injecting local anesthetics. EMLA is effective in preventing virtually any kind of pain associated with the skin. It may be used on people of almost any age and offers the advantage of preventing pain without injection. The cream must be applied under an occlusive bandage (one that prevents contact with air or water), which intensifies the contact between the skin and the anesthetic cream. It works after staying on the surface of the skin for at least 1 hour but may work more effectively if left on for 2 or 3 hours. The anesthetic effect remains for 2 hours after the cream has been removed from the surface of the skin. EMLA is also available in patch form.

EMLA cream has been studied for its effects on relieving the pain of intravenous catheter placement, minor plastic and skin surgery, shingles, and injections such as those used during vaccinations and blood donation.

Cautions and Warnings

Do not use EMLA cream if you are **allergic** to either of the anesthetics in the mixture. People with **methemoglobinemia** (a rare blood condition) should not use EMLA.

Do not apply EMLA cream beyond the area prescribed by your doctor. Excessive application of EMLA may put too much local anesthetic into your blood and expose you to the possibility of side effects. Do not put EMLA in your eyes or ears.

People with severe **liver disease** should use EMLA with caution because they may have difficulty removing the absorbed anesthetics from the bloodstream.

Possible Side Effects

▼ Most common: irritation, redness, and swelling of the area to which it is applied.

▼ Common: skin pallor, patches of white skin, itching, rash, and changes in how you sense skin temperature.

▼ Rare: severe allergic reaction (symptoms include

Possible Side Effects *(continued)*

breathing difficulties, rash, intense itching, and elevated pulse). In rare cases when EMLA is applied in excess, is used too often, or too much anesthetic is absorbed, the following reactions may occur: nervous system excitation; nervousness; apprehension; light-headedness; euphoria (feeling high); confusion; dizziness; drowsiness; ringing or buzzing in the ears; blurred or double vision; vomiting; feelings of warmth, coldness, or numbness; twitching; tremors; convulsions; unconsciousness; or a very slow breathing rate or cessation of breathing.

Drug Interactions

• Drugs associated with causing methemoglobinemia should not be taken with EMLA. This interaction is generally limited to children under 1 year. Some of these drugs are acetaminophen, sulfa drugs, oral antidiabetes drugs, thiazide diuretics, phenacetin, phenobarbital, phenytoin, primaquine, and quinine. Check with your doctor or pharmacist for more information about other methemoglobinemia-causing drugs.

Usual Dose

Cream

Adult and Child (age 1 month and over): Apply a thick layer—2½ g or ½ tsp.—and cover with the dressing provided in the package or some other occlusive bandage. Leave in place for at least 1–2 hours. The cream should be wiped away immediately before any surgical procedure or injection.

Senior: Avoid multiple uses over a short period of time because of the possibility of side effects.

Patch

Apply to designated area and leave in place for at least 1–2 hours before removing.

Overdosage

Accidental ingestion of EMLA may affect the heart by making it less efficient; this is directly attributable to the depressant effects of the local anesthetics in EMLA on the nerves within the heart. However, for this to happen someone would probably have to swallow an entire tube of EMLA. Call your local poison control center or hospital emergency room for more information. If you go for treatment, ALWAYS bring the prescription bottle or container with you.

Special Information

EMLA provides total loss of all feeling from the affected skin. Since there is no feeling in the skin, be careful not to accidentally scratch or burn yourself after the product has been applied.

When you apply the cream, place the entire dose in the center of the area you want to make pain-free. Then cover it with the occlusive dressing and allow the pressure of the dressing to spread the cream around.

Call your doctor if you develop severe, persistent, or unusually bothersome side effects from EMLA.

If you forget to apply EMLA, do so as soon as you can. But remember, it will be at least 1 hour after you apply the cream before your skin is numbed. Do not expect any pain relief before then.

Special Populations

Pregnancy/Breast-feeding

There is no evidence that EMLA cream interferes in any way with fetal development. Nevertheless, you should not use this drug during pregnancy unless you have first discussed it with your doctor.

The anesthetics in EMLA cream pass into breast milk. Watch your infant for side effects if you use EMLA cream while you are nursing.

Seniors

Seniors may be more sensitive to EMLA's side effects than are younger adults, especially if repeated applications are used.

Generic Name

Enalapril (uh-NAL-uh-pril)

Brand Name

Vasotec

Combination Products

Generic Ingredients: Enalapril + Hydrochlorothiazide
Vaseretic

Generic Ingredients: Enalapril + Felodipine
Lexxel (see page 587)

Type of Drug

Angiotensin-converting enzyme (ACE) inhibitor.

Prescribed for

Hypertension (high blood pressure) and congestive heart failure; also prescribed for diabetic kidney disease, childhood high blood pressure and high blood pressure related to scleroderma, and heart attack treatment when the function of the left ventricle has been affected.

General Information

Enalapril maleate belongs to the class of drugs known as ACE inhibitors. ACE inhibitors work by preventing the conversion of a hormone called angiotensin I to another hormone called angiotensin II, a potent blood-vessel constrictor. Preventing this conversion relaxes blood vessels, thus reducing blood pressure and relieving symptoms of heart failure by making it easier for a failing heart to pump blood through the body. Enalapril also affects the production of other hormones and enzymes that participate in the regulation of blood-vessel dilation; this action probably increases the drug's effectiveness. Enalapril begins working about 1 hour after you take it and continues to work for 24 hours.

Some people who start taking enalapril after they are already on a diuretic (agent that increases urination) experience a rapid drop in blood pressure after their first doses or when their dosage is increased. To prevent this from happening, your doctor may tell you to stop taking your diuretic 2 or 3 days before starting enalapril or to increase your salt intake during that time. The diuretic may then be restarted gradually. Heart failure patients generally have been on digoxin and a diuretic before beginning enalapril treatment.

Cautions and Warnings

Do not take enalapril if you are **allergic** to it.

Enalapril occasionally causes very **low blood pressure**.

Enalapril may affect your **kidney function**, especially if you have congestive **heart failure**. Your doctor should check your urine for protein content during the first few months of treatment. Dosage adjustment of enalapril is necessary if you have reduced kidney function.

Enalapril can affect **white-blood-cell counts,** possibly increasing your susceptibility to infection. Your doctor should monitor your blood counts periodically.

Possible Side Effects

▼ Most common: dizziness, fatigue, headache, nausea, and chronic cough. The cough usually goes away a few days after you stop taking the medication.

▼ Less common: chest tightness or pain, dizziness when rising from a sitting or lying position, fainting, abdominal pain, nausea, vomiting, diarrhea, bronchitis, urinary tract infection, breathing difficulties, weakness, and skin rash.

▼ Rare: itching; fever; heart attack; stroke; abdominal pain; abnormal heart rhythm; heart palpitations; difficulty sleeping; tingling in the hands or feet; appetite loss; odd taste perception; hepatitis and jaundice; blood in the stool; hair loss; unusual sensitivity to the sun; flushing; anxiety; nervousness; reduced sex drive; impotence; muscle cramps or weakness; muscle aches; arthritis; asthma; respiratory infections; sinus irritation; depression; not feeling well; sweating; kidney problems; anemia; blurred vision; swelling of the arms, legs, lips, tongue, face, and throat; upset stomach; and inflammation of the pancreas.

Drug Interactions

• The blood-pressure-lowering effect of enalapril is additive with diuretic drugs and beta blockers. Any other drug that causes a rapid drop in blood pressure should be used with caution if you are taking enalapril.

• Enalapril may increase blood-potassium levels, especially when taken with dyazide or other potassium-sparing diuretics.

• Enalapril may increase the effects of lithium; this combination should be used with caution.

• Antacids may reduce the amount of enalapril absorbed into the blood. Take these medications at least 2 hours apart.

• Capsaicin may trigger or aggravate the cough associated with enalapril therapy.

• Indomethacin may reduce the blood-pressure-lowering effects of enalapril.

• Phenothiazine tranquilizers and antiemetics may increase the effects of enalapril.

• Rifampin may reduce the effects of enalapril.

• The combination of allopurinol and enalapril increases the chance of side effects. Avoid this combination.

• Enalapril increases blood levels of digoxin, which may increase the chance of digoxin-related side effects.

Food Interactions

You may take enalapril with food if it upsets your stomach.

Usual Dose

2.5–40 mg once a day. Some people may take their daily dosage in 2 doses. People with poor kidney function need less medication to achieve reduced blood pressure.

Overdosage

The principal effect of enalapril overdose is a rapid drop in blood pressure, as evidenced by dizziness or fainting. Take the overdose victim to a hospital emergency room immediately. ALWAYS bring the prescription bottle or container with you.

Special Information

Enalapril can cause swelling of the face, lips, hands, or feet. This swelling can also affect the larynx (throat) or tongue and interfere with breathing. If this happens, go to a hospital emergency room at once. Call your doctor if you develop a sore throat, mouth sores, abnormal heartbeat, chest pain, persistent rash, or loss of taste perception.

You may get dizzy if you rise to your feet too quickly from a sitting or lying position. Avoid strenuous exercise and/or very hot weather because heavy sweating or dehydration can cause a rapid drop in blood pressure.

While taking enalapril, avoid over-the-counter diet pills, decongestants, and other stimulants that can raise blood pressure.

If you take enalapril once a day and forget to take a dose, take it as soon as you remember. If it is within 8 hours of your next dose, skip the one you forgot and continue with your regular schedule. If you take enalapril twice a day and miss a dose, take it right away. If it is within 4 hours of your next dose, take 1 dose immediately and another in 5 or 6 hours, then go back to your regular schedule. Never take a double dose.

Special Populations

Pregnancy/Breast-feeding
When taken during the last 6 months of pregnancy, ACE inhibitors have caused low blood pressure, kidney failure, slow skull formation, and death in fetuses. Women who are or might become pregnant should not take any ACE inhibitors. Sexually active women of childbearing age who must take enalapril must use an effective contraceptive method to prevent pregnancy. If you become pregnant, stop taking the medication and call your doctor immediately.

Relatively small amounts of enalapril pass into breast milk, and the effect on a nursing infant is likely to be minimal. However, nursing mothers who must take this drug should consider bottle-feeding: Infants, especially newborns, are more susceptible than adults to the drug's effects.

Seniors
Seniors may be more sensitive to the effects of this drug because of age-related losses in kidney or liver function. Dosage must be individualized to your needs.

Brand Name

Entex

Generic Ingredients
Guaifenesin + Phenylpropanolamine + Phenylephrine

Other Brand Names
Contuss   Despec

The information in this profile also applies to the following drugs:

Generic Ingredients: Guaifenesin + Phenylpropanolamine
Ami-Tex LA   Exgest LA
Dura-Vent   Guaipax
Entex LA   Guaitex LA

Partuss LA   ULR-LA
Phenylfenesin LA   Vanex-LA
Rymed-TR

Generic Ingredients: Guaifenesin + Pseudoephedrine
Guaifed   Histalet X
Guaimax-D

Generic Ingredients: Caramiphen Edisylate +
Phenylpropanolamine Hydrochloride Ⓖ
Ordrine AT   Tussogest
Rescaps-D S.R.   Tuss-Ornade Spansules
Tuss-Allergine Modified T.D.

Type of Drug

Decongestant-expectorant combination.

Prescribed for

Symptoms of a cold or allergy and for nasal congestion, stuffy nose, and runny nose associated with other upper respiratory conditions.

General Information

Entex and the other drugs listed in this section are only a few of the several hundred cold and allergy remedies available by prescription or over the counter. There are a variety of formulas used in these drugs such as the combination used in Entex. The decongestant ingredient, phenylpropanolamine, dramatically reduces congestion and stuffiness. The expectorant, guaifenesin, is supposed to help loosen thick mucus that may contribute to your feeling of chest congestion; the effectiveness of guaifenesin and other expectorant drugs has not been established. There are other drugs on the market using this same general formula—an expectorant plus a decongestant—but they use different decongestant ingredients or a combination of decongestants plus guaifenesin.

Entex should not be used over extended periods of time to treat persistent or chronic cough, especially one that may be caused by cigarette smoking, asthma, or emphysema. Information on other decongestant-expectorant combinations may be obtained from your pharmacist.

Since nothing cures a cold or allergy, the most that you may hope to achieve from taking this or any other cold or allergy remedy is symptom relief.

Cautions and Warnings

Entex may cause **anxiety** or **nervousness** or may **interfere with your sleep**.

Do not use Entex if you have **diabetes, heart disease, hypertension (high blood pressure), thyroid disease, glaucoma,** or a **prostate condition**.

Possible Side Effects

▼ Most common: fear, anxiety, restlessness, sleeplessness, tension, excitation, nervousness, dizziness, drowsiness, hallucinations, headache, psychological disturbances, tremor, and convulsions.

▼ Less common: nausea, vomiting, upset stomach, low blood pressure, heart palpitations, chest pain, rapid heartbeat, abnormal heart rhythms, irritability, euphoria (feeling high), eye irritation and tearing, hysterical reaction, appetite loss, urinary difficulties in men with a prostate condition, weakness, loss of facial color, and breathing difficulties.

Drug Interactions

• Entex should be avoided if you are taking a monoamine oxidase inhibitor (MAOI) antidepressant for depression or hypertension because the MAOI may cause a very rapid rise in blood pressure or increase side effects such as dry mouth or nose, blurred vision, and abnormal heart rhythms.

• The decongestant in Entex may interfere with the normal effects of blood-pressure-lowering medication. It may aggravate diabetes, heart disease, hyperthyroid disease, hypertension, a prostate condition, or stomach ulcer; it may also cause urinary blockage.

Food Interactions

Take Entex with food if it upsets your stomach.

Usual Dose

Capsules: 1 twice a day.

Liquid: 2 tsp. 4 times a day.

Overdosage

The main symptoms of overdose include sedation, sleepiness, increased sweating, and increased blood pressure. Hallucinations, convulsions, nervous-system depression, and breathing difficulties are particularly prominent in older adults. Most cases of overdose are not severe. Victims must be made to vomit with ipecac syrup—available at any pharmacy—to remove any remaining drug from the stomach. Call your doctor or poison control center before doing this. If you must go to a hospital emergency room, ALWAYS bring the prescription bottle or container.

Special Information

Call your doctor if your side effects are severe or gradually become intolerable.

If you forget to take a dose of Entex, take it as soon as you remember. If it is almost time for your next dose, skip the one you forgot and continue with your regular schedule. Do not take a double dose.

Special Populations

Pregnancy/Breast-feeding

Entex should be avoided by women who are or might be pregnant. Discuss the potential risks with your doctor.

Nursing mothers should use caution when taking Entex because the decongestant may pass into breast milk.

Seniors

Seniors are more sensitive to the effects of Entex. Follow your doctor's directions. Report side effects at once.

Brand Name

Equagesic

Generic Ingredients

Aspirin + Meprobamate G

Type of Drug

Analgesic combination.

Prescribed for

Pain from muscle spasms, sprains, strains, or bad backs.

General Information

Equagesic is one of several combination products containing a tranquilizer and an analgesic; it is used to relieve pain associated with muscle spasms. The meprobamate in this product can become habit-forming and possibly addictive, especially when taken with other tranquilizers or depressant drugs. Follow all of your doctor's instructions to help treat the basic problem.

Cautions and Warnings

Do not take this combination if you are **allergic** to any of its ingredients or to other salicylates or carisoprodol.

Aspirin can worsen **kidney function** in people who already have a kidney condition, and meprobamate should be used with caution by people with **liver or kidney disease**. Aspirin can irritate your stomach and should be avoided by people with **gastritis** or **ulcers**. Also, aspirin should be used with caution by people with mild **diabetes** or **bleeding tendencies**.

People taking meprobamate may become **dependent** on it. Avoid using this product for more than a few weeks at a time. Abruptly stopping this medicine can lead to drug withdrawal (symptoms include anxiety, appetite loss, insomnia, vomiting, tremors, muscle weakness or twitching, confusion, and hallucinations) or recurrence of symptoms. The dose should be gradually reduced over a period of 1 to 2 weeks.

Possible Side Effects

▼ Most common: nausea, vomiting, stomach upset, dizziness, and drowsiness.

▼ Less common: allergy, itching, rash, fever, swelling in the arms and/or legs, occasional fainting spells, and bronchial spasms leading to breathing difficulties.

▼ Rare: changes in blood components and blurred vision.

Drug Interactions

• Meprobamate can cause sleepiness, drowsiness, or difficulty breathing—in high doses. Avoid taking this medication with other nervous system depressants, including alcohol, barbiturates, narcotics, sleeping pills, tranquilizers, and some antihistamines.

• If you are taking an anticoagulant (blood-thinner) begin

taking an aspirin-meprobamate combination, your doctor may need to adjust your anticoagulant dosage because aspirin affects the ability of blood to clot.

Food Interactions

An aspirin-meprobamate combination may be taken with food if it upsets your stomach.

Usual Dose

Adult and Child (age 17 and over):1–2 tablets 3–4 times a day.
Child (under age 17): not recommended.

Overdosage

Overdoses are serious. Symptoms are drowsiness, light-headedness, sleepiness, nausea, and vomiting. Victims should be taken to a hospital emergency room immediately. ALWAYS bring the prescription bottle or container with you.

Special Information

Be careful when driving or performing complex tasks while taking this medication.

Call your doctor if drug side effects become bothersome or persistent.

If you forget a dose, take it as soon as you remember. If it is almost time for your next dose, skip the one you forgot and continue with your regular schedule. Do not take a double dose.

Special Populations

Pregnancy/Breast-feeding

These drugs cross into the fetal blood circulation. They have not caused birth defects, although meprobamate has been known to increase the chance of birth defects if taken during the first 3 months of pregnancy. When this medication is considered essential by your doctor, its potential benefits must be carefully weighed against its risks.

These drugs pass into breast milk. Nursing mothers taking this medication should consider bottle-feeding their babies.

Seniors

Seniors are more sensitive to the effects of this combination, especially drowsiness or sleepiness.

Generic Name

Ergoloid Mesylates

(ER-goe-loid MES-il-ates) G

Brand Names

Gerimal   Hydergine LC
Hydergine

Type of Drug

Psychotherapeutic agent.

Prescribed for

Age-related decline in mental capacity.

General Information

Ergoloid mesylates is used to treat decreased mental capacity that cannot be traced to known causes, in people over 60. This drug should not be used for any condition that is treatable with another drug or that may be reversible. People who respond to ergoloid mesylates are likely to have Alzheimer's disease or some other cause of dementia or age-related condition.

Nobody knows exactly how ergoloid mesylates produces its effect, but it improves the supply of blood to the brain in test animals, reduces heart rate, and improves muscle tone in blood vessels. Some studies show the drug to be very effective in relieving mild symptoms of mental impairment, while others find it to be only moderately effective. It is most beneficial in patients whose symptoms are due to the effects of high blood pressure in the brain. A 6-month period of treatment with ergoloid mesylates is recommended before your doctor can fully evaluate your response to the drug. Your doctor should periodically reevaluate your condition to determine if ergoloid mesylates is still needed and that it is working for you.

Cautions and Warnings

Ergoloid mesylates should not be taken if you are **allergic or sensitive** to it or if you have any psychotic symptoms or **psychosis**.

Possible Side Effects

▼ Common: Ergoloid mesylates does not produce serious side effects. When taken under the tongue, this drug may cause irritation, nausea, or stomach upset. Other side effects are drowsiness, slow heartbeat, and rash.

Drug Interactions

None known.

Food Interactions

Do not eat, drink, or smoke while you have an ergoloid mesylates pill under your tongue.

Usual Dose

1 mg 3 times a day. Do not exceed 12 mg a day.

Overdosage

Symptoms of overdose are blurred vision, dizziness, fainting, flushing, headache, appetite loss, nausea, vomiting, stomach cramps, and stuffy nose. Take the victim to a hospital emergency room for treatment. ALWAYS bring the prescription bottle or container with you.

Special Information

The effects of ergoloid mesylates are gradual and are frequently not seen for up to 6 months.

Dissolve sublingual tablets under the tongue. Do not chew or crush them; they are not effective if swallowed whole.

If you forget to take a dose of ergoloid mesylates, skip the dose you forgot and go back to your regular schedule. Do not take a double dose. Call your doctor if you forget to take 2 or more consecutive doses.

Special Populations

Pregnancy/Breast-feeding

Ergoloid mesylates may interfere with fetal development. Check with your doctor before taking it if you are or might be pregnant.

Nursing mothers who must take this drug should bottle-feed their babies.

Seniors
Seniors are more likely to develop side effects, especially hypothermia (low body temperature).

Ery-Tab

*see **Erythromycin**, page 377*

Generic Name

Erythromycin (eh-rith-roe-MYE-sin) [G]

Brand Names

A/T/S	Erymax
Akne-mycin	Ery-Tab
Benzamycin	Erythromycin Base Filmtab
E-Base	Ilotycin
Emgel	PCE Dispertab
E-Mycin	Robimycin Robitabs
Erycette	Staticin
EryDerm	Theramycin 2
Erygel	T-Stat 2

The information in this profile also applies to the following drugs:

Generic Ingredient: Erythromycin Estolate [G]

Ilosone	Ilosone Pulvules

Generic Ingredient: Erythromycin Ethylsuccinate [G]

E.E.S. 200	EryPed 200
E.E.S. 400	EryPed 400
EryPed	Erythromycin ES

Generic Ingredient: Erythromycin Stearate [G]

Eramycin	My-E
Erythrocin Stearate	Wyamycin S

Type of Drug

Macrolide antibiotic.

Prescribed for

Infections of virtually any part of the body: upper and lower respiratory tract infections; sexually transmitted diseases; urinary tract infections; infections of the mouth, gums, or teeth; and infections of the nose, ears, or sinuses. It is prescribed for acne and may be used for mild to moderate skin infections but is not considered the antibiotic of choice. Erythromycin is effective against diphtheria as well as amoeba infections in the intestinal tract that cause dysentery. Erythromycin eye ointment is used to prevent newborn gonococcal or chlamydial infections of the eye. It is also prescribed for legionnaires' disease, rheumatic fever, bacterial endocarditis, and a variety of other infections.

General Information

Erythromycin—also known as erythromycin base—erythromycin estolate, erythromycin ethylsuccinate, and erythromycin stearate are members of the group of antibiotics known as macrolides. Drugs in this group also include azithromycin, clarithromycin, and dirithromycin and are either bactericidal (bacteria-killing) or bacteriostatic (inhibiting bacterial growth) depending on the organism in question and the amount of antibiotic present.

Erythromycin is absorbed from the gastrointestinal tract but is deactivated by the acid content of the stomach. Because of this, the tablet form of this drug is formulated to bypass the stomach and dissolve in the intestine.

Since the action of this antibiotic depends on its concentration within the invading bacteria, it is crucial that you follow your doctor's directions regarding the spacing of doses as well as the number of days you should continue taking the medication. The effectiveness of this antibiotic may be severely reduced if these instructions are not followed.

Cautions and Warnings

Do not take erythromycin if you are **allergic** to it or to any macrolide antibiotic.

Erythromycin is excreted primarily through the liver. People with **liver disease or damage** should consult their doctors. Those on long-term therapy with erythromycin are advised to have periodic blood tests.

Erythromycin is available in a variety of types and formulations. Erythromycin estolate has occasionally produced **liver difficulties** (symptoms include fatigue, nausea, vomiting, abdominal cramps, and fever). If you are susceptible to

stomach problems, erythromycin may cause mild to moderate stomach upset; discontinuing the drug will reverse this condition. If you restart erythromycin after having experienced liver damage, it is likely that symptoms will recur within 48 hours.

A form of **colitis** (bowel inflammation)—see "Possible Side Effects" for symptoms—has been associated with all antibiotics, including erythromycin.

Possible Side Effects

Erythromycin should not be given to people with known sensitivity to this antibiotic. It may cause a yellowing of the skin or whites of the eyes. If this occurs, discontinue the drug and call your doctor immediately.

▼ Most common: nausea, vomiting, stomach cramps, and diarrhea. Colitis (symptoms include severe abdominal cramps and severe, persistent, and possibly bloody diarrhea) may develop after taking erythromycin.

▼ Less common: hairy tongue, itching, and irritation of the anal and/or vaginal region. If any of these symptoms appear, call your physician immediately.

▼ Rare: hearing loss—which reverses itself after the drug is stopped and occurs most often in people with liver and kidney problems—and abnormal heart rhythms.

Drug Interactions

• Erythromycin may slow the breakdown of carbamazepine (an anticonvulsant prescribed for seizures). Avoid this combination.

• Erythromycin may neutralize penicillin. It may also neutralize lincomycin and clindamycin (antibiotics). Avoid these combinations.

• Erythromycin interferes with the elimination of theophylline from the body, possibly leading to theophylline overdose. It may also increase the effects of caffeine, which is chemically related to theophylline.

• Erythromycin may increase blood levels of astemizole and terfenadine (non-sedating antihistamines). Combining these drugs may lead to serious cardiac side effects and should be avoided.

• Erythromycin may increase blood levels of alfentanil (an injectable pain reliever), bromocriptine, digoxin, disopyramide, ergotamine, cyclosporine, methylprednisolone (a corticosteroid), tacrolimus, and triazolam, resulting in an increase in side effects.

• Erythromycin estolate may increase the side effects of other drugs that affect the liver.

• Erythromycin may increase the anticoagulant (blood-thinning) effects of warfarin in people who take it regularly, especially older adults. People taking this combination should be tested regularly by their doctors.

Food Interactions

Food in the stomach will decrease the absorption rate of erythromycin and erythromycin stearate products. They are best taken on an empty stomach, or 1 hour before or 2 hours after meals but may be taken with food if they cause stomach upset. Other forms of erythromycin may be taken without regard to food or meals. Check with your pharmacist for specific directions.

Usual Dose

Tablet and Suspension
   Adult: 250–500 mg every 6 hours.
   Child: 50–200 mg per lb. of body weight a day in divided doses depending on age, weight, and severity of infection.

Eye Ointment
½ in. 2–3 times a day.

Topical Solution
Apply morning and night.

Doses of erythromycin ethylsuccinate are 60% higher due to differences in chemical composition.

Overdosage

Erythromycin overdose may cause severe side effects, especially nausea, vomiting, stomach cramps, and diarrhea. Mild hearing loss, ringing or buzzing in the ears, or fainting may also occur. Call your local poison control center or hospital emergency room for more information.

Special Information

Erythromycin is a relatively safe antibiotic. It is used instead of penicillin for mild to moderate infections in people who are allergic to penicillin. Erythromycin is not the antibiotic of choice for severe infections.

Erythromycin products should be stored at room temperature, except for oral and topical liquids, which should be kept in the refrigerator.

Take each dose of erythromycin with 6 to 8 oz. of water.

Call your doctor if you develop any of the following: nausea; vomiting; diarrhea; stomach cramps; severe abdominal pain; rash, itching, or redness; dark or amber-colored urine; yellowing of the skin or whites of the eyes; or other severe or persistent side effects.

If you forget a dose of oral erythromycin, take it as soon as you remember. If it is almost time for your next dose, space the next 2 doses over 4 to 6 hours, then continue with your regular schedule. Do not take a double dose.

Remember to complete the full course of therapy prescribed by your doctor, even if you feel well after only a few days of antibiotic treatment.

Special Populations

Pregnancy/Breast-feeding
Erythromycin passes into the circulation of the fetus. Erythromycin estolate has caused mild liver inflammation in about 10% of pregnant women who took it and should not be used if you are or might be pregnant. Other forms of erythromycin have been used safely without difficulty.

Erythromycin passes into breast milk. Nursing mothers who must take erythromycin should bottle-feed their infants.

Seniors
Seniors, except those with liver disease, may generally use this product without restriction.

Generic Name

Estazolam (es-TAZ-oe-lam)

Brand Name
ProSom

Type of Drug
Benzodiazepine sedative.

Prescribed for

Short-term treatment of insomnia or sleeplessness, difficulty falling asleep, frequent nighttime awakening, and waking too early in the morning.

General Information

Estazolam is a member of the group of drugs known as benzodiazepines. All have some activity as antianxiety agents, anticonvulsants, or sedatives. They work by a direct effect on the brain. Benzodiazepines make it easier to go to sleep and decrease the number of times you wake up during the night.

The principal difference among the various benzodiazepines lies in how long they work on your body. They all take about 2 hours to reach maximum blood level, but some remain in your body longer, so they work for a longer period of time. Estazolam is considered an intermediate-acting sedative and generally remains in your body long enough to give you a good night's sleep with minimal "hangover."

Sleeplessness may often signal an underlying disorder that this medication would not treat.

Cautions and Warnings

People with **respiratory disease** taking estazolam may experience **sleep apnea** (intermittent cessation of breathing during sleep).

People with **kidney or liver disease** should be carefully monitored while taking estazolam. Take the lowest possible dose to help you sleep.

Clinical **depression** may be increased by estazolam, which can depress the nervous system. Intentional overdose is more common among depressed people who take sleeping pills than among those who do not.

All benzodiazepines can be **addictive** if taken for long periods of time, and it is possible for a person taking a benzodiazepine to develop drug withdrawal symptoms if the drug is discontinued suddenly. Withdrawal symptoms include tremors, muscle cramps, insomnia, agitation, diarrhea, vomiting, sweating, and convulsions.

Possible Side Effects

▼ Common: drowsiness, headache, dizziness, talkativeness, nervousness, apprehension, poor muscle coor-

Possible Side Effects *(continued)*

dination, light-headedness, daytime tiredness, muscle weakness, slowness of movement, hangover, and euphoria (feeling high).

▼ Less common: nausea, vomiting, rapid heartbeat, confusion, temporary memory loss, upset stomach, stomach cramps and pain, depression, blurred or double vision and other visual disturbances, constipation, changes in sense of taste, appetite changes, stuffy nose, nosebleeds, common cold symptoms, asthma, sore throat, cough, breathing difficulties, diarrhea, dry mouth, allergic reaction, fainting, abnormal heart rhythm, itching, acne, dry skin, sensitivity to bright light or to the sun, rash, nightmares or strange dreams, sleeplessness, tingling in the hands or feet, ringing or buzzing in the ears, ear or eye pain, menstrual cramps, frequent urination and other urinary difficulties, blood in the urine, discharge from the penis or vagina, lower back and joint pain, muscle spasms and pain, fever, swollen breasts, and weight changes.

Drug Interactions

• As with all benzodiazepines, the effects of estazolam are enhanced if it is taken with an alcoholic beverage, antihistamine, tranquilizer, barbiturate, anticonvulsant medication, antidepressant, or monoamine oxidase inhibitor drug (MAOI). MAOIs are most often prescribed for severe depression.

• Oral contraceptives, cimetidine, disulfiram, and isoniazid may increase the effect of estazolam by interfering with the drug's breakdown in the liver. Probenecid also increases estazolam's effects.

• Cigarette smoking, rifampin, and theophylline may reduce the effect of estazolam.

• Levodopa's effectiveness may be decreased by estazolam.

• Estazolam may increase the amount of zidovudine (an AIDS drug—also known as AZT), phenytoin, or digoxin in your bloodstream, increasing the chances of side effects.

• The combination of clozapine and benzodiazepines has led to respiratory collapse in a few people. Estazolam should be stopped at least 1 week before starting clozapine treatment.

Food Interactions

Estazolam may be taken with food if it upsets your stomach.

Usual Dose

Adult (age 18 and older): 1–2 mg about 60 minutes before you want to go to sleep.

Senior: starting dose—0.5–1 mg. Dosage should be increased cautiously.

Child (under age 18): not recommended.

Overdosage

The most common symptoms of overdose are confusion, sleepiness, depression, loss of muscle coordination, and slurred speech. Coma may develop if the overdose is particularly large. Overdose symptoms can develop if a single dose of only 4 times the maximum daily dose is taken. Patients who take an overdose of this drug must be made to vomit with ipecac syrup—available at any pharmacy—to remove any remaining drug from the stomach: Call your doctor or a poison control center before doing this. If 30 minutes have passed since the overdose was taken or if symptoms have begun to develop, the victim must be taken immediately to a hospital emergency room for treatment. ALWAYS bring the prescription bottle or container with you.

Special Information

Never take more estazolam than your doctor has prescribed.

Avoid alcoholic beverages and other nervous system depressants while taking estazolam.

Exercise caution while performing tasks that require concentration and coordination; estazolam may make you tired, dizzy, or light-headed.

If you take estazolam daily for 3 or more weeks, you may experience some withdrawal symptoms when you stop taking the drug. Talk with your doctor about how best to discontinue the drug.

If you forget to take a dose of estazolam and remember within about 1 hour of your regular time, take it right away. If you do not remember until later, skip the dose you forgot and go back to your regular schedule. Do not take a double dose.

Special Populations

Pregnancy/Breast-feeding

Estazolam absolutely should not be used by pregnant women

or by women who may become pregnant. Animal studies have shown that estazolam passes easily into the fetal blood system and can affect fetal development.

Estazolam passes into breast milk and can affect a nursing infant. The drug should not be taken by nursing mothers.

Seniors
Seniors are more susceptible to the effects of estazolam and should take the lowest possible dosage.

Estrace

see Estrogens, page 385

Estraderm

see Estrogens, page 385

Type of Drug

Estrogens (ES-troe-jens)

Brand Names

Generic Ingredient: Chlorotrianisene
TACE

Generic Ingredients: Conjugated Estrogens
Premarin

*Generic Ingredients: Conjugated Estrogens +
Medroxyprogesterone*
Prempro   Premphase

Generic Ingredient: Dienestrol
Ortho Dienestrol

Generic Ingredient: Diethylstilbestrol
Diethylstilbestrol

Generic Ingredients: Esterified Estrogens
Estratab   Menest

Generic Ingredient: Estradiol

Climara   Estring
Estrace   Vivelle
Estraderm

Generic Ingredient: Estropipate

Ogen   Ortho-Est

Generic Ingredient: Ethinyl Estradiol

Estinyl

Generic Ingredient: Quinestrol

Estrovis

Prescribed for

Moderate to severe menopausal symptoms and postmenopausal osteoporosis; also prescribed for ovarian failure, breast
cancer in certain women and men, advanced cancer of the
prostate, osteoporosis, abnormal bleeding of the uterus,
vaginal irritation, female castration, Turner's syndrome, and
birth control.

General information

Six estrogenic substances have been identified in women but
only 3 are present in large amounts: estradiol, estrone, and
estriol. Estradiol is the most potent of the 3 and is the
principal estrogen produced by the ovaries. Estradiol is naturally modified to estrone, which is then turned into estriol, the
least potent of the 3. All forms of estrogen listed in this
section have the same actions and side effects when equal
doses are used, taking the different potencies of each into
account. More potent drugs require a smaller dosage to
produce the same effect.

Estrogen is a natural body substance with specific effects
including growth and maintenance of the female reproductive system and sex characteristics. Estrogen affects the
release of hormones from the pituitary gland (controller of
hormone production and regulator of basic bodily functions)
that control the opening of the capillaries (smallest blood
vessels), may cause fluid retention, affects protein breakdown in the body, prevents ovulation and breast engorgement in women after giving birth, and continues in the
shaping and maintenance of the skeleton through its influence on calcium in the body.

The differences between various products lie in the specific estrogenic substances they contain, dosage, and, in some cases, the fact that they affect one part of the body more than another. For the most part, however, estrogen products are interchangeable as long as differences in dosage are taken into account.

Diethylstilbestrol has been used as a "morning after" contraceptive but should only be used as an emergency treatment because of the damage it can cause the fetus if a pregnancy is not successfully prevented by the drug.

There is no evidence that estrogen works for nervousness or depression occurring during menopause. It should not be used to treat these conditions but should be used only to replace estrogen that is naturally absent after menopause.

Cautions and Warnings

Estrogen has been reported to increase by 5 to 10 times the risk of **endometrial cancer** in postmenopausal women taking it without progestin for prolonged periods of time; the risk depends upon the duration of treatment and the dosage of estrogen being taken. When long-term estrogen therapy is needed for the treatment of menopausal symptoms, taking a progestin product such as medroxyprogesterone reduces the risk of endometrial cancer and other problems. Or, your doctor may prescribe the combination product, Prempro. In women who have had a hysterectomy, there is no need for progestin treatment.

The estrogen diethylstilbestrol has been used as a **"morning-after" contraceptive**, primarily to prevent pregnancy in emergencies such as rape or incest. However, to be effective diethylstilbestrol must be taken no more than 72 hours after intercourse; if pregnancy is not prevented the drug may seriously harm the fetus. Combination oral contraceptives containing norgestrel and ethinyl estradiol are more commonly prescribed for this use.

Postmenopausal women taking estrogen have a 2 to 3 times greater risk of developing **gallbladder disease**.

If you are taking estrogen and experience **recurrent, abnormal, or persistent vaginal bleeding**, contact your doctor immediately.

If you have active **thrombophlebitis** or any **disorder associated with the formation of blood clots**, you probably should not take this drug. If you think that you have a disorder associated with blood clots and you are taking estrogen or a similar drug, contact your doctor immediately.

Estrogen should not be used to treat painful **breast engorgement with milk** that sometimes develops after giving birth. This condition usually responds to pain relievers and other treatments.

Animal studies show that prolonged continuous administration of estrogen may increase the frequency of **cancer of the breast, cervix, testes, uterus, vagina, kidney, and liver**. The question of whether estrogen increases the risk of breast cancer has not been answered. Some studies show an increased risk but others have not verified that result. Estrogen should be taken with caution by women with a strong **family history of breast cancer** and by those who have **breast nodules, fibrocystic disease of the breast,** or **abnormal mammograms**.

It is possible that women taking estrogen for extended periods of time may experience some of the same long-term side effects as women who have taken oral contraceptives for extended periods of time. These long-term problems may include the development of **blood-clotting disorders, liver cancer or other liver tumors, high blood pressure, glucose intolerance or worsening of the disease in diabetic patients, unusual sun sensitivity,** and **high blood levels of calcium**.

Vaginal estrogen cream may stimulate **bleeding of the uterus**. It may also cause **breast tenderness, vaginal discharge,** and **withdrawal bleeding**—if the product is suddenly stopped. Women with **endometriosis** may experience heavy vaginal bleeding.

Possible Side Effects

▼ Most common: breast enlargement or tenderness, ankle and leg swelling, appetite loss, weight changes, water retention, nausea, vomiting, abdominal cramps, and a feeling of bloatedness. The estrogen patch may cause rash, irritation, and redness at the patch site.

▼ Less common: bleeding gums, breakthrough vaginal bleeding, vaginal spotting, changes in menstrual flow, painful menstruation, premenstrual syndrome (PMS), absence of menstrual period during and after estrogen use, enlargement of uterine fibroids, vaginal infection with

Possible Side Effects *(continued)*

Candida, a cystitis-like syndrome, mild diarrhea, jaundice or yellowing of the skin or whites of the eyes, rash, loss of scalp hair, and development of new hairy areas. Lesions of the eye and contact-lens intolerance have also been associated with estrogen therapy. Migraine headache, mild dizziness, depression, increased sex drive in women, and decreased sex drive in men are also possible.

▼ Rare: stroke, blood-clot formation, dribbling or sudden passage of urine, loss of coordination, chest pain, leg pain, breathing difficulties, slurred speech, and changes in vision. Men who receive large estrogen dosages as part of the treatment of prostate cancer are at greater risk for heart attack, phlebitis, and blood clots in the lungs.

Drug Interactions

• Phenytoin, ethotoin, and mephenytoin may interfere with estrogen's effects. Estrogen may reduce the effect of oral anticoagulant (blood-thinning) drugs, an adjustment your doctor can make after a simple blood test.

• Estrogen increases the amount of calcium absorbed from the stomach. This interaction is used to help women with osteoporosis increase their calcium levels.

• Estrogen may increase the side effects of antidepressants and phenothiazine tranquilizers. Low estrogen dosages may increase phenothiazine's effectiveness.

• Estrogen may increase the levels of cyclosporine and corticosteroid drugs in your blood. Dosage adjustments of the non-estrogen drugs may be needed.

• Estrogen increases the toxic effects of other drugs on the liver, especially in women over age 35 and people with liver disease.

• Rifampin, barbiturates, and other drugs that stimulate the liver to break down drugs may reduce the amount of estrogen in the blood.

• Estrogen may interfere with the actions of tamoxifen and bromocriptine.

• Women, especially those over age 35, who smoke cigarettes and take estrogen have a much greater risk of developing stroke, hardening of the arteries, or blood clots in the lungs. The risk increases as age and tobacco use increase.

• Estrogen interferes with many diagnostic tests. Make sure your doctor knows you are taking estrogen before doing any blood tests or other diagnostic procedures.

Food Interactions

Estrogens may be taken with food to reduce nausea and upset stomach. Avoid drinking grapefruit juice if you are taking this drug.

Usual Dose

Estrogen dosage depends on the condition being treated and the individual's response. All of these products, including the transdermal skin patch, may be taken continuously or on a cyclic schedule of 3 weeks on, 1 week off.

Tablets
Chlorotrianisene: 12–200 mg.
  Conjugated estrogens: 0.3–7.5 mg.
  Diethylstilbestrol: 1–15 mg.
  Esterified estrogens: 0.3–30 mg.
  Estradiol: 1–60 mg.
  Estropipate: 0.625–7.5 mg.
  Ethinyl estradiol: 0.02–2.0 mg.
  Quinestrol: 100 mcg once a day for 7 days, then 100–200 mcg a week.

Transdermal Patch
Estradiol: 1 0.05–mg or 0.1–mg patch twice a week for 3 weeks; stop for 1 week, then start again. May be used continuously in some cases.

Vaginal Cream
Conjugated estrogens: 2–4 g a day for 3 weeks; stop for 1 week, then start again.
  Dienestrol: 1 applicatorful 1–2 times a day for 1–2 weeks, half the original dosage for another 1–2 weeks, then 1 applicatorful 1–3 times a week.
  Estradiol: 2–4 g a day for 2 weeks, half the starting dosage for another 2 weeks, then 1 g 1–3 times a week.
  Estropipate: 2–4 g a day for 3 weeks; stop for 1 week, then start again.

Use the lowest possible dosage. Your doctor should re-evaluate your need for estrogen vaginal cream every 3–6 months. Do not stop using the drug suddenly because this may increase your risk of developing unpredicted or break-through vaginal bleeding.

Overdosage

Overdose may cause nausea and withdrawal bleeding in adult women. Accidental overdose in children has not re-sulted in severe side effects. Call your local poison control center or hospital emergency room for information. ALWAYS bring the prescription bottle or container with you if you go to a hospital emergency room for treatment.

Special Information

Call your doctor if you develop breast pain or tenderness, swelling of the feet and lower legs, rapid weight gain, chest pain, breathing difficulties, pain in the groin or calves, un-usual vaginal bleeding, missed menstrual period, lumps in the breast, sudden severe headache, dizziness or fainting, disturbances in speech or vision, weakness or numbness in the arms or legs, abdominal pain, depression, yellowing of the skin or whites of the eyes, or jerky or involuntary muscle movement. Call your doctor if you are or might be pregnant.

Women using vaginal estrogen cream who develop breast tenderness, start to bleed, or have other vaginal discharge should contact their doctors at once.

Women who smoke cigarettes and take estrogen have a greater risk of cardiovascular side effects including stroke and blood clotting.

Estrogen skin patches should be applied to a clean, dry, non-oily, hairless area of intact skin, preferably on the abdo-men. Do not apply to your breasts or to your waist, or another area where tight-fitting clothes may loosen the patch from your skin. The application site should be rotated to prevent irritation and each site should have a patch-free period for 7 days.

It is important to maintain good dental hygiene while taking estrogen and to use extra care when using your toothbrush or dental floss because of the risk that estrogen will make you more susceptible to infection. Dental work should be com-pleted prior to starting estrogen.

Vaginal estrogen cream should be inserted high into the vagina, about ⅔ of the length of the applicator.

Some of these products contain tartrazine (a commonly used orange dye and food-coloring). Avoid tartrazine-containing products if you are allergic to tartrazine or have asthma. Check with your pharmacist to find out if your estrogen product contains tartrazine.

If you forget to take a dose of estrogen, take it as soon as you remember. If it is almost time for your next dose, skip the one you forgot and continue with your regular schedule. Do not take a double dose.

Special Populations

Pregnancy/Breast-feeding
Estrogen should not be used during pregnancy to prevent a possible miscarriage; it does not work for this purpose and is dangerous to the fetus.

Estrogen may reduce the flow of breast milk. The effects of estrogen on nursing infants are unpredictable. Either avoid estrogen while breast-feeding or bottle-feed your infant.

Seniors
Estrogen may be taken without special precaution by most seniors; the risk of certain side effects increases with age, especially if you smoke.

Generic Name

Etodolac (ee-TOE-doe-lak)

Brand Names

Lodine   Lodine XL

Type of Drug

Nonsteroidal anti-inflammatory drug (NSAID).

Prescribed for

Osteoarthritis; may also be used to treat rheumatoid arthritis, ankylosing spondylitis, mild to moderate pain, tendinitis, bursitis, painful shoulder, and gout.

General information

Etodolac is one of 16 NSAIDs, which are used to relieve pain and inflammation. We do not know exactly how NSAIDs work, but part of their action may be due to their ability to inhibit the body's production of a hormone called prostaglandin as well as the action of other body chemicals, including cyclooxygenase, lipoxygenase, leukotrienes, and lysosomal enzymes. NSAIDs are generally absorbed into the bloodstream quickly. Etodolac starts relieving pain in about 30 minutes and its effects last for 4 to 12 hours. Etodolac is broken down in the liver and eliminated through the kidneys.

Cautions and Warnings

People who are **allergic** to etodolac or any other NSAID and those with a history of **asthma** attacks brought on by an NSAID, iodides, or aspirin should not take etodolac.

Etodolac may cause **gastrointestinal (GI) bleeding, ulcers,** and **stomach perforation**. This can occur at any time, with or without warning, in people who take etodolac regularly. People with a history of **active GI bleeding** should be cautious about taking any NSAID. People who develop bleeding or ulcers and continue NSAID treatment should be aware of the possibility of developing more serious side effects.

Etodolac may affect platelets and **blood clotting** at high doses, and should be avoided by people with clotting problems and by those taking warfarin.

People with **heart problems** who use etodolac may experience swelling in their arms, legs, or feet.

Etodolac may cause severe toxic effects to the **kidney**. Report any unusual side effects to your doctor, who may need to periodically test your kidney function.

Etodolac may make you unusually sensitive to the effects of the sun.

Possible Side Effects

▼ Most common: diarrhea, nausea, vomiting, constipation, stomach gas, stomach upset or irritation, and appetite loss, especially during the first few days of treatment.

▼ Less common: stomach ulcers, GI bleeding, hepatitis, gallbladder attacks, painful urination, poor kidney function, kidney inflammation, blood and protein in the urine, dizziness, fainting, nervousness, depression, hallucinations, confusion, disorientation, tingling in the hands or feet, light-headedness, itching, increased sweating, dry nose and mouth, heart palpitations, chest pain, breathing difficulties, and muscle cramps.

Possible Side Effects *(continued)*

▼ Rare: severe allergic reactions including closing of the throat, fever and chills, changes in liver function, jaundice (yellowing of the skin or whites of the eyes), and kidney failure. People who experience such effects must be promptly treated in a hospital emergency room or doctor's office.

NSAIDs have caused severe skin reactions; if this happens to you, see your doctor immediately.

Drug Interactions

• Etodolac may increase the effects of oral anticoagulant (blood-thinning) drugs such as warfarin. You may take this combination, but your doctor might have to reduce your anticoagulant dose.

• Taking etodolac with cyclosporine may increase the kidney-related side effects of both drugs. Methotrexate side effects may be increased in people also taking etodolac.

• Etodolac may increase phenytoin blood levels, leading to increased side effects. Lithium blood levels may be increased in people taking etodolac.

• Etodolac blood levels may be affected by cimetidine.

• Probenecid may interfere with the elimination of etodolac from the body, increasing the chances for etodolac side effects.

• Aspirin and other salicylates may decrease the amount of etodolac in your blood. These drugs should never be combined with etodolac.

Food Interactions

Take etodolac with food or a magnesium-aluminum antacid if it upsets your stomach.

Usual Dose

200–400 mg every 6–8 hours, not to exceed 1200 mg a day. People weighing 132 lbs. or less should not take more than 20 mg for every 2.2 lbs. of body weight.

Overdosage

People have died from NSAID overdoses. The most common signs of overdose are drowsiness, nausea, vomiting, diarrhea, abdominal pain, rapid breathing, rapid heartbeat, increased sweating, ringing or buzzing in the ears, confusion, disorientation, stupor, and coma. Take the victim to a hospital emergency room at once. ALWAYS bring the prescription bottle or container with you.

Special Information

Take each dose with a full glass of water and do not lie down for 15 to 30 minutes afterward.

Etodolac can make you drowsy and/or tired: Be careful when driving or operating hazardous equipment. Do not take any over-the-counter products with acetaminophen or aspirin while taking etodolac. Avoid alcoholic beverages.

Contact your doctor if you develop skin rash or itching, visual disturbances, weight gain, breathing difficulties, fluid retention, hallucinations, black or tarry stools, persistent headache, or any unusual or intolerable side effect.

If you forget to take a dose of etodolac, take it as soon as you remember. If you take etodolac once a day and it is within 8 hours of your next dose, skip the dose you forgot and continue with your regular schedule. If you take several doses a day and it is within 4 hours of your next dose, skip the one you forgot and continue with your regular schedule. Never take a double dose.

Special Populations

Pregnancy/Breast-feeding

NSAIDs may cross into fetal blood circulation. They have not been found to cause birth defects, but may affect a developing fetal heart during the second half of pregnancy. Pregnant women should not take etodolac without their doctor's approval, particularly during the last 3 months of pregnancy. When the drug is considered crucial by your doctor, its potential benefits must be carefully weighed against its risks.

NSAIDs may pass into breast milk but have caused no problems in breast-fed infants, except for seizures in a baby whose mother was taking the NSAID indomethacin. There is a possibility that a nursing mother taking etodolac might affect her baby's heart or cardiovascular system. If you must take etodolac, bottle-feed your baby.

Seniors

Seniors may be more susceptible to etodolac side effects, especially ulcer disease.

Generic Name

Famciclovir (fam-SYE-kloe-vere)

Brand Name

Famvir

Type of Drug

Antiviral.

Prescribed for

Herpes zoster (shingles) and recurrent genital herpes.

General Information

Famciclovir was only the second antiviral drug used to treat
shingles, after acyclovir. Now acyclovir, famciclovir, and a
third drug—valacyclovir—are used for shingles and for herpes.

   After famciclovir is absorbed into the body, it is converted
to the anitviral penciclovir, the drug that actually works
against shingles by interfering with basic reproductive DNA
in the herpes virus. Penciclovir does not affect DNA in
uninfected body cells. Penciclovir is broken down by the liver
and eliminated from the body through the kidneys.

Cautions and Warnings

People **sensitive or allergic** to famciclovir should not take this
drug. Those with **reduced kidney function** should have their
dosage adjusted accordingly. **Severe liver disease** reduces
the maximum possible concentration of penciclovir in the
blood and increases the time it takes to reach this maximum
level; however, dosage adjustment is not normally required.

   Lab animals receiving 1½ times the maximum dose developed tumors and testicular toxicity (abnormal or reduced
numbers of sperm). The implication of this in humans is not
known.

Possible Side Effects

▼ Most common: headache, nausea, and diarrhea.

▼ Less common: fever, fatigue, pain, vomiting, constipation, appetite loss, dizziness, tingling in the hands or

---

Possible Side Effects *(continued)*

feet, sleepiness, sore throat, sinus irritation, itching, and signs of shingles.

▼ Rare: chills, abdominal pains, back or joint pain, and upset stomach.

Drug Interactions

• Probenecid, cimetidine, and theophylline interfere with the elimination of penciclovir from the body, possibly leading to higher levels of penciclovir in the blood.

• People who took famciclovir and digoxin together experienced increased digoxin in their blood.

Food Interactions

None known.

Usual Dose

Shingles

Adult (age 18 and over): 500 mg every 8 hours for 1 week. People with reduced kidney function may require a reduced dose taken as infrequently as once a day.

Child (under age 18): not recommended.

Genital Herpes

Adult (age 18 and over): 125 mg twice a day for 5 days. People with reduced kidney function take the same dose but less often, as infrequently as once every 2 days.

Child (under age 18): not recommended.

Overdosage

There is little information available on the effects of famciclovir overdose. Overdose victims should be taken to a hospital emergency room for treatment. ALWAYS bring the prescription bottle or container with you.

Special Information

Famciclovir treatment should be started as soon as shingles are diagnosed. For maximum benefit, be sure to complete the full week of treatment.

Famciclovir is not a cure for genital herpes and it is not known if it will prevent the transmission of the herpes virus to another person. Avoid sexual intercourse when herpes lesions are present even while taking famciclovir for genital herpes.

Begin taking famciclovir at the first sign of a herpes attack (symptoms include pain, tenderness, burning, itching, tingling, ulcers, or scabs). The effectiveness of starting famciclovir 6 hours or more after symptoms or lesions appear has not been established.

Call your doctor if you experience any unusual or intolerable side effects.

If you forget a dose of famciclovir, take it as soon as you remember. If it is almost time for your next dose, skip the dose you forgot. Do not take a double dose. Call your doctor if you forget more than 2 doses in a row.

Special Populations

Pregnancy/Breast-feeding
Famciclovir should only be taken by a pregnant woman if it is absolutely necessary and the possible benefits outweigh the risks to the fetus.

In animal studies, penciclovir (the active form of famciclovir) passed into breast milk in high concentrations but it is not known if this holds true for humans. Nursing mothers who must take this drug should bottle-feed their babies.

Seniors
Seniors clear penciclovir from the bloodstream more slowly than younger people and should have their dosage adjusted according to their level of kidney function.

Generic Name

Famotidine (fam-OE-tih-dine)

Brand Names

Pepcid   Pepcid AC

Type of Drug

Histamine H_2 antagonist.

Prescribed for

Ulcers of the stomach and duodenum (upper intestine); also

used to treat gastroesophageal reflux disease (GERD), stress ulcer, and other conditions characterized by the production of large amounts of gastric fluids; and to prevent stress ulcer, and stomach and upper intestinal bleeding. Famotidine may be prescribed when it is desirable to stop the production of stomach acid during surgery.

General Information

Famotidine works in the same way as the other histamine H_2 antagonists, by actually turning off the system that produces stomach acid and other secretions.

Famotidine is effective in treating the symptoms of ulcer and preventing complications of the disease, although an ulcer that does not respond to another histamine H_2 antagonist will probably not respond to famotidine because all these drugs work in exactly the same way. Histamine H_2 antagonists differ only in their potency. Cimetidine is the least potent; 1000 mg are roughly equal to 300 mg of either nizatidine or ranitidine, or 40 mg of famotidine. All these drugs have roughly equivalent success rates in treating ulcer disease and all carry comparable chances of side effects.

Cautions and Warnings

Do not take famotidine if you have ever had an **allergic** reaction to it or any histamine H_2 antagonist. People with **kidney or liver disease** should take famotidine with caution because ⅓ of each dose is broken down in the liver and the rest passes out of the body through the kidneys.

Possible Side Effects

▼ Most common: headache.

▼ Less common: dizziness, mild diarrhea, and constipation.

▼ Rare: drowsiness, dry mouth or skin, joint or muscle pain, appetite loss, depression, nausea or vomiting, abdominal discomfort, stomach pain, ringing or buzzing in the ears, rash or itching, temporary hair loss, changes in sense of taste, fever, swelling of the eyelids, chest tightness, rapid heartbeat, unusual bleeding or bruising, unusual tiredness or weakness, confusion, hallucination, anxiety, agitation, sleeplessness, reduced platelet counts, impotence, and reduced sex drive.

Drug Interactions

• Enteric-coated tablets should not be taken with famotidine. The change in stomach acidity that famotidine produces will cause the tablets to disintegrate prematurely in the stomach.

• Antacids, anticholinergics, and metoclopramide may slightly reduce the amount of famotidine absorbed into the blood. No special precaution is needed.

Food Interactions

Food may slightly increase the amount of drug absorbed, but this is of no consequence. Famotidine may be taken without regard to food or meals.

Usual Dose

Adult: 20–40 mg at bedtime, or 20 mg twice a day. Dosage should be reduced in people with severe kidney disease.

Overdosage

There is little information on famotidine overdose. Overdose victims might be expected to experience exaggerated side effects, but little else is known. Your local poison control center may advise giving the victim ipecac syrup—available at any pharmacy—to induce vomiting as soon as possible. This should remove any remaining drug from the stomach. Victims who have definite symptoms should be taken to a hospital emergency room for observation and possible treatment. ALWAYS bring the prescription bottle or container with you.

Special Information

You must take famotidine exactly as directed and follow your doctor's instructions regarding diet and other treatment in order to get the maximum benefit from the drug. Antacids may be taken together with famotidine if needed.

Cigarettes are known to be associated with stomach ulcers and may reverse the effect of famotidine on stomach acid.

Call your doctor at once if any unusual side effects develop, especially unusual bleeding or bruising, unusual tiredness, diarrhea, dizziness, or rash. Black, tarry stools or vomiting material that resembles coffee grounds may indicate your ulcer is bleeding.

If you forget to take a dose of famotidine, take it as soon as you remember. If it is almost time for your next dose, skip the one you forgot and continue with your regular schedule. Do not take a double dose.

Special Populations

Pregnancy/Breast-feeding
Although studies with laboratory animals reveal no damage to the fetus, famotidine should be avoided by women who are or might be pregnant. When this drug is considered crucial by your doctor, its possible benefits must be carefully weighed against its risks.

Famotidine may pass into breast milk. No problems have been identified in breast-fed babies, but nursing mothers must consider the risk of side effects in their babies.

Seniors
Seniors respond well to famotidine. They may need lower doses to achieve results, because the drug is eliminated through the kidneys and kidney function tends to decline with age. Seniors may be more susceptible to famotidine side effects.

Generic Name

Felbamate (FEL-bam-ate)

Brand Name
Felbatol

Type of Drug
Anticonvulsant.

Prescribed for
Partial seizure and Lennox-Gastaut syndrome in children.

General Information
Felbamate is related to the older tranquilizer-sedative meprobamate (Miltown). Exactly how felbamate works is not known, but it raises the seizure threshold and prevents the spread of the seizure in the brain, as do other anticonvulsant medications. Felbamate is well absorbed into the bloodstream. About half of each dose passes out of the body

through the kidneys; the other half is broken down and eliminated from the body by the liver. Because of the dangers associated with felbamate, this drug should only be used when other seizure medications have failed.

Cautions and Warnings

More than 20 cases—including 3 deaths—of **aplastic anemia** (severe reductions in white-blood-cell count) occurred in people taking felbamate for 5 weeks or more. Although this is a rare side effect, happening in only 2 to 5 per 1 million people, this drug should not be used unless it is essential for your treatment.

Dosages of felbamate should be only **gradually reduced** or replaced by other anticonvulsant medicines; this drug should never be suddenly stopped, because seizures may become more frequent.

People who are **allergic** to felbamate or related medications should not take this drug.

Felbamate may **increase your sensitivity to the sun**. Wear protective clothing and use sunscreen while taking this drug.

People with severe **liver or kidney disease** may require lower doses of felbamate.

Possible Side Effects

▼ Most common: sleeplessness, fatigue, headache, anxiety, dizziness, nervousness, tremors, depression, unusual walk, upset stomach, nausea, vomiting, diarrhea, constipation, weight loss, fever, liver inflammation, changes in sense of taste, appetite loss, hiccups, upper respiratory infection, runny nose, sore throat, coughing, double vision, middle ear infections, loss of urine control, black-and-blue marks, abnormal thinking, emotional instability, and pinpointed pupils.

▼ Less common: facial swelling, chest pain, generalized pain, tingling in the hands or feet, weakness, dry mouth, stupor, blurred or abnormal vision, sinus inflammation, bleeding between menstrual periods, urinary tract infections, muscle aches, and poor muscle control or coordination.

▼ Rare: weight gain and increased appetite, feeling unwell, flulike symptoms, drug allergy, heart palpitations, rapid heartbeat, euphoria (feeling high), suicidal tenden-

Possible Side Effects *(continued)*

cies, migraines, inflammation of the esophagus, swollen lymph glands, reduced levels of white blood cells and blood platelets, reduced body sodium and/or potassium, itching, rash, swollen skin eruptions, swelling of tissue inside the mouth, Stevens-Johnson syndrome, unusual muscle movements, and unusual sensitivity to the sun.

Drug Interactions

• Felbamate increases the breakdown of carbamazepine by the liver by as much as 40%. This increased breakdown becomes obvious within the first 2 to 4 weeks after you start taking felbamate. Carbamazepine dose adjustment is necessary. When this combination is taken together, the amount of felbamate in the blood is also reduced by almost 50% because the drug is cleared from the body more quickly.

• Felbamate decreases the rate at which phenytoin is broken down in the liver. Your daily phenytoin dosage may have to be reduced by as much as 30% to account for this effect. When this combination is taken together, the amount of felbamate in the blood is also reduced by almost 50% because the drug is cleared from the body more quickly.

• Felbamate increases the amount of valproic acid in the blood. Unlike other anticonvulsants, valproic acid does not affect felbamate.

Food Interactions

Felbamate is best taken on an empty stomach but may be taken with food if it upsets your stomach.

Usual Dose

Adult and Child (age 14 and over): 1200–3600 mg a day, divided into 3–4 doses.

Child (age 2–13): 6.8–20.5 mg per lb. a day, divided into 3–4 doses.

Overdosage

The only overdose effects that have been reported are upset stomach and increased heart rate. No serious effects have been seen, but one could expect to see felbamate side effects in overdose situations. Call your doctor, local poison control center, or hospital emergency room for more information. If you go to the emergency room for treatment, ALWAYS bring the prescription bottle or container with you.

Special Information

Do not take more felbamate than your doctor has prescribed.

Felbamate can cause drowsiness; be careful when driving or performing complicated tasks.

Avoid long exposure to the sun while taking felbamate.

Call your doctor if you develop any unusual or bothersome side effects.

It is important to maintain good dental hygiene while taking felbamate and to use extra care when using a toothbrush or dental floss because this drug can cause swollen gums. See your dentist regularly while taking this medication.

If you forget to take a dose of felbamate, take it as soon as you remember. If it is almost time for your next dose, take one dose right away and another in 3 or 4 hours, then go back to your regular schedule. Do not take a double dose.

Special Populations

Pregnancy/Breast-feeding

This drug may cross into the fetal blood circulation. When the drug is considered crucial by your doctor, its potential benefits must be carefully weighed against its risks.

Felbamate passes into breast milk, but its effect on nursing infants is not known. Consider bottle-feeding to avoid effects on the baby.

Seniors

Seniors, especially those with liver, kidney, or heart disease, may be more sensitive to the effects of this drug and should take doses in the low end of the range.

Generic Name

Felodipine (feh-LOE-dih-pene)

Brand Name

Plendil

Type of Drug

Calcium channel blocker.

Prescribed for

High blood pressure.

General Information

Felodipine is one of many calcium channel blockers available in the U.S. Its once-daily dosage schedule makes it particularly suited to treating high blood pressure. Felodipine blocks the passage of calcium, an essential factor in muscle contraction, into the heart and smooth muscles. Such blockage interferes with the contraction of these muscles, which in turn dilates (widens) the veins and vessels that supply blood to them. This action has several beneficial effects. Because arteries are dilated, they are less likely to spasm. In addition, because blood vessels are dilated, both blood pressure and the amount of oxygen used by the heart muscle are reduced. Felodipine is therefore useful in treating not only high blood pressure but also angina pectoris (brief attacks of chest pain), a condition related to poor oxygen supply to the heart muscles. Other calcium channel blockers are prescribed for abnormal heart rhythm, heart failure, cardiomyopathy (loss of blood-pumping ability due to damaged heart muscle), and diseases that involve blood-vessel spasm, such as migraine headache and Raynaud's syndrome.

Felodipine affects the movement of calcium only into muscle cells; it has no effect on calcium in the blood.

Cautions and Warnings

Felodipine should not be taken if you have had an **allergic reaction** to it in the past.

On rare occasions, felodipine may cause very **low blood pressure** that may lead to stimulation of the heart and rapid heartbeat and can worsen angina. This reaction may happen when treatment is first started, when dosage is increased, or if the drug is rapidly withdrawn; it may be avoided by reducing dosage gradually.

Studies have shown that people taking calcium channel blockers—usually those taken several times a day, not those taken only once daily—have a greater chance of having a **heart attack** than do people taking beta blockers or other medications for the same purposes. Discuss this with your doctor to be sure you are receiving the best possible treatment.

Patients taking a beta-blocking drug who begin taking felodipine may develop **heart failure** or increased **angina**.

People with **severe liver disease** break down felodipine much more slowly than people with mildly diseased or normal livers. Your doctor should take this factor into account when determining your felodipine dosage.

People taking felodipine who have had a **heart attack** and have lung congestion may experience worsened heart failure, since this drug can actually slow the force of each heartbeat.

Possible Side Effects

Side effects produced by calcium channel blockers are generally mild and rarely cause people to stop taking them. Side effects are more common with higher doses and in older patients.

▼ Most common: swelling in the ankles, feet, or legs; dizziness; light-headedness; muscle weakness or cramps; facial flushing; and headache.

▼ Less common: respiratory infections, cough, tingling in the hands or feet, upset stomach, abdominal pains, chest pains, nausea, constipation, diarrhea, heart palpitations, sore throat, runny nose, back pain, and rash.

▼ Rare: facial swelling and a feeling of warmth, rapid heartbeat, heart attack, very low blood pressure, fainting, angina, abnormal heart rhythm, vomiting, dry mouth, stomach gas, anemia, muscle and joint pain, bone pain, depression, anxiety, sleeplessness, irritability and nervousness, daytime tiredness, bronchitis, flulike symptoms, sinus irritation, breathing difficulties, nosebleeds, sneezing, itching, redness, bruising, sweating, blurred vision, ringing or buzzing in the ears, swelling of the gums, decreased sex drive, sexual difficulties, painful urination, and frequent and urgent urination.

Drug Interactions

• Felodipine may increase the amount of beta-blocking drugs in the bloodstream. This can lead to heart failure, very low blood pressure, or an increased incidence of angina. However, in many cases these drugs have been taken together with no problem.

• Felodipine increases the effects of other blood-pressure-lowering drugs. Such drug combinations are often used to treat hypertension.

• Cimetidine and ranitidine increase the amount of felo-dipine in the blood and may account for a slight increase in the drug's effect.

• Phenytoin and other hydantoin antiseizure medicines, carbamazepine, and barbiturate sleeping pills and sedatives may decrease the amount of felodipine in the blood, reducing its effect on the body.

• Erythromycin may increase the side effects of felodipine by slowing its release from the body.

• Felodipine may increase the effects of digoxin, theophyl-line (prescribed for asthma and other respiratory problems), and oral anticoagulant (blood-thinning) drugs.

• Felodipine may also interact with quinidine (prescribed for abnormal heart rhythm) to produce low blood pressure, very slow heart rate, abnormal heart rhythms, and swelling in the arms or legs.

Food Interactions

You may take felodipine with food if it upsets your stomach. Taking felodipine with concentrated grapefruit juice doubles the amount of the drug normally absorbed into the blood; avoid this combination.

Usual Dose

5–10 mg a day. No patient should take more than 20 mg a day.

Do not stop taking felodipine abruptly. The dosage should be reduced gradually over a period of time.

Overdosage

Felodipine overdose can cause low blood pressure. If you think you have taken an overdose of felodipine, call your doctor or go to a hospital emergency room. ALWAYS bring the prescription bottle or container with you.

Special Information

Call your doctor if you develop constipation, nausea, very low blood pressure, breathing difficulties, increased heart pain, dizziness, or light-headedness, or if other side effects are particularly bothersome or persistent.

Swelling of the hands or feet may develop within 2 or 3 weeks of starting felodipine. The chances of this happening depend both on your age and on the felodipine dosage. It occurs in less than 10% of people under age 50 taking 5 mg a day and in more than 30% of those over age 60 taking 20 mg a day.

Be sure to continue taking your medication and follow any instructions for diet restriction or other treatments to help maintain lower blood pressure. High blood pressure is a condition with few recognizable symptoms; it may seem to you that you are taking the drug for no good reason. Call your doctor or pharmacist if you have any questions.

Do not break or crush felodipine tablets.

It is important to maintain good dental hygiene while taking felodipine and to use extra care when using your toothbrush or dental floss because of the chance that the drug will make you more susceptible to certain infections.

If you forget to take a dose of felodipine, take it as soon as you remember. If it is almost time for your next dose, skip the dose you forgot and continue with your regular schedule. Do not take a double dose.

Special Populations

Pregnancy/Breast-feeding
Animal studies of felodipine have shown that it crosses into the fetal circulation and causes some birth defects. Women who are or who might become pregnant while taking this drug should not take it without their doctor's approval. The potential benefit of taking felodipine must be carefully weighed against its risks.

It is not known if felodipine passes into breast milk, but it has caused no problems among breast-fed infants. However, you must consider the drug's potential effect on the nursing infant.

Seniors
Seniors, especially those with liver disease, are more sensitive to the effects of this drug because it takes longer to pass out of their bodies. Follow your doctor's directions and report any side effects at once.

Generic Name

Fenoprofen (fen-oe-PROE-fen)

Brand Name
Nalfon

Type of Drug

Nonsteroidal anti-inflammatory drug (NSAID).

Prescribed for

Rheumatoid arthritis, juvenile rheumatoid arthritis, osteoarthritis, mild to moderate pain, sunburn, and migraine headache prevention and treatment.

General Information

Fenoprofen calcium is one of 16 NSAIDs, which are used to relieve pain and inflammation. We do not know exactly how NSAIDs work, but part of their action may be due to their ability to inhibit the body's production of a hormone called prostaglandin as well as the action of other body chemicals, including cyclooxygenase, lipoxygenase, leukotrienes, and lysosomal enzymes. NSAIDs are generally absorbed into the bloodstream quickly. Fenoprofen starts relieving pain within 24 hours, but its anti-inflammatory effect takes about 2 days to begin and 2 to 3 weeks to reach maximum effect. Fenoprofen is broken down in the liver and eliminated through the kidneys.

Cautions and Warnings

People **allergic** to fenoprofen or any other NSAID and those with a history of **asthma** attacks brought on by an NSAID, iodides, or aspirin should not take fenoprofen.

Fenoprofen may cause **gastrointestinal (GI) bleeding, ulcers,** and **stomach perforation**. This can occur at any time, with or without warning, in people who take fenoprofen regularly. People with a history of **active GI bleeding** should be cautious about taking any NSAID. People who develop bleeding or ulcers and continue NSAID treatment should be aware of the possibility of developing more serious side effects.

Fenoprofen can affect platelets and **blood clotting** at high doses, and should be avoided by people with clotting problems and by those taking warfarin.

People with **heart problems** who use fenoprofen may experience swelling in their arms, legs, or feet.

People with **impaired hearing** may be affected by fenoprofen and should have periodic hearing tests.

Fenoprofen may actually cause **headaches**. If this happens, you might have to stop taking the drug or switch to another NSAID.

Fenoprofen may cause severe toxic effects to the **kidney**. Report any unusual side effects to your doctor, who might need to periodically test your kidney function. People with kidney disease should not take fenoprofen.

Fenoprofen can make you unusually sensitive to the effects of the sun.

Possible Side Effects

▼ Most common: diarrhea, vomiting, nausea, constipation, stomach gas, stomach upset or irritation, and appetite loss, especially during the first few days of treatment.

▼ Less common: stomach ulcers, GI bleeding, hepatitis, gallbladder attacks, painful urination, poor kidney function, kidney inflammation, blood and protein in the urine, dizziness, fainting, nervousness, depression, hallucinations, confusion, disorientation, tingling in the hands or feet, light-headedness, heart palpitations, chest pain, itching, increased sweating, dry nose and mouth, breathing difficulties, and muscle cramps.

▼ Rare: severe allergic reactions including closing of the throat, fever and chills, changes in liver function, jaundice (yellowing of the skin or whites of the eyes), and kidney failure. People who experience such effects must be promptly treated in a hospital emergency room or doctor's office. NSAIDs have caused severe skin reactions; if this happens to you, see your doctor immediately.

Drug Interactions

• Fenoprofen may increase the effects of oral anticoagulant (blood-thinning) drugs such as warfarin. You may take this combination, but your doctor might have to reduce your anticoagulant dose.

• Combining fenoprofen with cyclosporine may increase the kidney-related side effects of both drugs. Methotrexate toxicity may be increased in people also taking fenoprofen.

• Fenoprofen may reduce the blood-pressure-lowering effect of beta blockers and loop diuretics.

• Fenoprofen may increase phenytoin blood levels, leading

to increased phenytoin side effects. Lithium blood levels may be increased in people taking fenoprofen.

• Fenoprofen blood levels may be affected by cimetidine.

• Probenecid may interfere with the elimination of fenoprofen from the body, increasing the chances for fenoprofen side effects.

• Aspirin and other salicylates may decrease the amount of fenoprofen in your blood. These drugs should never be combined with fenoprofen.

Food Interactions

Take fenoprofen with food or a magnesium-aluminum antacid if it upsets your stomach.

Usual Dose

Adult: mild to moderate pain—200 mg every 4–6 hours. Arthritis—300–600 mg 3–4 times a day to start, individualized to your needs. Total daily dosage not to exceed 3200 mg.

Child: not recommended.

Overdosage

People have died from NSAID overdoses. The most common signs of overdose are drowsiness, nausea, vomiting, diarrhea, abdominal pain, rapid breathing, rapid heartbeat, increased sweating, ringing or buzzing in the ears, confusion, disorientation, stupor, and coma. Take the victim to a hospital emergency room at once. ALWAYS bring the prescription bottle or container with you.

Special Information

Take each dose with a full glass of water and do not lie down for 15 to 30 minutes afterward.

Fenoprofen can make you drowsy and/or tired: Be careful when driving or operating hazardous equipment. Do not take any over-the-counter products containing acetaminophen or aspirin while taking fenoprofen.

Contact your doctor if you develop skin rash or itching, visual disturbances, weight gain, breathing difficulties, fluid retention, hallucinations, black or tarry stools, persistent headache, or any unusual or intolerable side effect.

If you forget to take a dose of fenoprofen, take it as soon as you remember. If you take fenoprofen once a day and it is within 8 hours of your next dose, skip the dose you forgot and continue with your regular schedule. If you take several doses a day and it is within 4 hours of your next dose, skip the dose you forgot and continue with your regular schedule. Never take a double dose.

Special Populations

Pregnancy/Breast-feeding

Fenoprofen may cross into the fetal bloodstream. It has not been found to cause birth defects, although animal studies indicate that it may affect a developing fetal heart during the second half of pregnancy. Pregnant women should not take fenoprofen without their doctor's approval, particularly during the last 3 months of pregnancy. When the drug is considered crucial by your doctor, its potential benefits must be carefully weighed against its risks.

Fenoprofen may pass into breast milk but has caused no problems in breast-fed infants. Other NSAIDs have caused problems in animal studies. There is a possibility that a nursing mother taking fenoprofen could affect her baby's heart or cardiovascular system. If you must take fenoprofen, talk to your doctor about bottle-feeding your baby.

Seniors

Seniors may be more susceptible to fenoprofen side effects, especially ulcer disease.

Generic Name

Finasteride (fin-AS-ter-ide)

Brand Names

Proscar   Propecia

Type of Drug

Alpha-reductase inhibitor.

Prescribed for

Benign prostatic hyperplasia (BPH) and male pattern baldness.

General Information

A gradual reduction in urine flow in men over age 50 is

usually associated with gradual enlargement of the prostate gland. This condition is known as BPH. The number of men with BPH increases with age. Finasteride works by interfering with the action of the enzyme alpha-reductase, which is essential to the process of converting testosterone into a much more potent substance called 5-dihydrotestosterone (DHT). A single 5-mg dose of finasteride produces a rapid drop in DHT levels, with the maximum reduction occurring 8 hours after taking the dose. DHT levels remain low for 24 hours and stay low as long as the drug is continued. You may need to take finasteride for 6 to 12 months before its effects can be assessed.

There is no way to predict who will and who will not respond to finasteride, but most people taking this drug have a dramatic reduction in the size of their prostate. Urine flow improves in about 60% of people taking finasteride and symptoms of BPH improve in about 30%. In one clinical study of finasteride, men experienced a significant regression in prostate size after 3 months and the reduction was maintained through the 12-month study period. Study subjects experienced a significant improvement in urine flow that could be maintained up to 36 months.

People who do not respond to finasteride may have another obstruction or problem causing BPH-like symptoms.

Finasteride has been studied as therapy following radical prostatectomy surgery and in the prevention of first-stage prostate cancer, male pattern baldness, acne, and unusual hairiness.

Studies of finasteride for hair loss on top of the scalp and back-middle of the scalp show that the drug stimulates new hair growth in 60% to 80% of men taking the drug continuously for 2 years. The drug must be taken for 3 months or more before it begins to have an effect and must be taken continuously for hair growth to be maintained. Once you stop taking this drug, any new hair you have grown while on it is likely to fall out in the next 12 months. Seventeen percent of men taking the drug continued to lose hair throughout the study period.

Cautions and Warnings

Do not take finasteride if you are **allergic** to any component of the product. This drug is **not to be used in women or children**.

Finasteride only works in BPH. Other conditions that may

mimic BPH such as infection, prostate cancer, bladder or nerve disorders, and physical obstruction of the urinary tubes, will not be improved by this medication.

Because it is broken down in the liver, finasteride must be used with caution by people with **liver disease**.

Animal studies have shown that finasteride may increase the risk of **testicular cancer** and **reduced male fertility**. Finasteride may mask **symptoms of prostate cancer** by causing a reduction in the level of prostate-specific antigen (PSA), an increasingly acknowledged indicator of prostate cancer. While a low PSA level does not necessarily exclude the possibility of prostate cancer, a higher one is cause for further investigation.

Possible Side Effects

Finasteride side effects are generally mild and well tolerated. Side effects often subside if you continue taking finasteride and always go away when you stop taking it.

▼ Most common: impotence, loss of sex drive, decreased amount of semen, breast tenderness and enlargement, and drug sensitivity reaction including lip swelling and rash.

Drug Interactions

• Finasteride increases the rate at which theophylline and aminophylline are broken down in the liver. These changes may not affect the amount of theophylline or aminophylline you need to control your asthma.

• Finasteride affects the PSA blood test used for prostate cancer screening. Be sure your doctor knows you are taking this drug if you have a PSA test done or are being tested for prostate cancer.

Food Interactions

You may take finasteride with food if it upsets your stomach.

Usual Dose

Benign Prostatic Hyperplasia
  Adult and Senior Men: 5 mg once a day.
  Woman and Child: Do not use.

Male Pattern Baldness
  Adult and Senior Men: 1 mg once a day.
  Woman and Child: Do not use.

Overdosage

People have taken single doses up to 400 mg and daily doses up to 80 mg for 3 months without any side effects. In animal studies, the drug was lethal at doses equal to 182 to 455 mg per lb. of body weight. Call your local poison control center or hospital emergency room for more information. If you go to a hospital for treatment, ALWAYS bring the prescription bottle or container with you.

Special Information

Crushed finasteride tablets should not be handled by women who are or might be pregnant because small amounts of the drug may be absorbed into the blood, possibly affecting the fetus.

If your sexual partner is or might be pregnant and you start taking finasteride, you must wear a condom to avoid directly exposing her to finasteride in the semen. Other options are to avoid sexual contact or stop taking the drug.

Semen volume may decrease while on finasteride but this should not interfere with normal sexual function. Impotence or reduced sex drive is a possibility.

If you forget a dose of finasteride, take it as soon as you remember. If it is almost time for your next dose, skip the one you forgot and continue with your regular schedule. Do not take a double dose. Call your doctor if you forget to take finasteride for 2 or more days.

Special Populations

Pregnancy/Breast-feeding

This drug is not intended for use by women. However, it is important to keep in mind that finasteride will harm the fetus if taken during pregnancy.

Seniors

Finasteride remains longer in the bodies of seniors, but dosage adjustment is not required nor is dosage adjustment needed in people with kidney disease.

Brand Name

Fioricet

Generic Ingredients

Acetaminophen + Butalbital + Caffeine G

Other Brand Names

Amaphen	Esgic Plus
Anoquan	Femcet
Butace	Medigesic
Endolor	Repan
Esgic	Two-Dyne

Type of Drug

Barbiturate-analgesic combination.

Prescribed for

Migraine and other types of pain.

General Information

Fioricet is one of many combination products containing a barbiturate—butalbital—and an analgesic—acetaminophen. Products of this kind often also contain a tranquilizer or a narcotic. Other analgesic combinations, such as Fiorinal, substitute aspirin for acetaminophen.

Cautions and Warnings

Do not take Fioricet if you are **allergic or sensitive** to it. Use this drug with extreme caution if you suffer from **asthma or other breathing problems** or if you have **kidney or liver disease** or a **viral infection of the liver**. Chronic (long-term) use of Fioricet may lead to **drug dependence or addiction**.

Butalbital is a respiratory depressant and affects the central nervous system (CNS), producing drowsiness, tiredness, or an inability to concentrate.

Possible Side Effects

▼ Most common: light-headedness, dizziness, sedation, nausea, vomiting, sweating, appetite loss, and mild stimulation.

▼ Less common: weakness, headache, upset stomach, sleeplessness, agitation, tremor, uncoordinated muscle movement, mild hallucinations, disorientation, visual disturbances, euphoria (feeling high), dry mouth, constipation, flushing of the face, changes in heart rate, palpitations, feeling faint, urinary difficulties, rash, itching, confusion, rapid breathing, and diarrhea.

Drug Interactions

• Combining Fioricet with alcohol, tranquilizers, barbiturates, sleeping pills, or other nervous-system depressants may cause tiredness, drowsiness, and trouble concentrating.

Food Interactions

Fioricet is best taken on an empty stomach but may be taken with food if it upsets your stomach.

Usual Dose

1–2 tablets or capsules every 4 hours or as needed; do not exceed 6 doses a day.

Overdosage

Overdose symptoms include breathing difficulties, nervousness progressing to stupor or coma, pinpointed pupils, cold and clammy skin and lowered heart rate or blood pressure, nausea, vomiting, dizziness, ringing in the ears, flushing, sweating, and thirst. The victim should be taken to a hospital emergency room immediately. ALWAYS bring the prescription bottle or container with you.

Special Information

Be careful if you are driving, operating hazardous machinery, or performing other functions requiring concentration. Alcohol may increase the risk of acetaminophen-related liver toxicity and butalbital-related drowsiness.

Call your doctor if you develop side effects that are unusual, persistent, or bothersome.

If you forget to take a dose of Fioricet, take it as soon as you remember. If it is almost time for your next dose, skip the one you forgot and continue with your regular schedule. Do not take a double dose.

Special Populations

Pregnancy/Breast-feeding

Fioricet should be avoided during pregnancy. There is an increased risk of birth defects associated with Fioricet. Regular use of Fioricet during the last 3 months of pregnancy may cause drug dependency in the newborn. Pregnant women using Fioricet may experience prolonged labor and delayed delivery; breathing problems may afflict the newborn. Alternative therapies should be used if you are pregnant.

Breast-feeding while using Fioricet may cause the baby to become tired, short of breath, or have a slow heartbeat. If you must take Fioricet, consider bottle-feeding your baby.

Seniors
The butalbital in Fioricet may have a greater depressant effect on seniors than on younger adults. Other effects that may be more prominent are light-headedness or dizziness, or fainting when rising suddenly from a sitting or lying position.

Brand Name
Fiorinal

Generic Ingredients
Aspirin + Butalbital + Caffeine G

Other Brand Names
Butalbital Compound	Lanorinal
Fiorgen PF	Marnal
Isollyl Improved	

Type of Drug
Barbiturate-analgesic combination.

Prescribed for
Migraine headache and other pain.

General Information
Pain relief products often combine an analgesic, or pain reliever, with a sedative. The analgesic ingredient in Fiorinal is aspirin; other brand-name products, such as Esgic and Fioricet, contain acetaminophen. The sedative ingredient in pain-relief combinations may be a barbiturate, narcotic, or other tranquilizer. Fiorinal contains the barbiturate butalbital. Fiorinal also contains caffeine, which is often used in analgesic combinations that treat headache because it enhances the pain-relieving effect of aspirin.

Cautions and Warnings
Do not take Fiorinal if you know you are **allergic or sensitive** to it or any of its ingredients, including aspirin, any salicylate, or any nonsteroidal anti-inflammatory drug (NSAID). Check

with your doctor or pharmacist if you are unsure of a drug allergy. Fiorinal and all other aspirin-containing products should not be taken by children under age 16. People with **liver damage** should avoid Fiorinal.

Use Fiorinal with extreme caution if you suffer from **asthma** or other breathing problems. Long-term use of this drug may cause drug dependence or **addiction**. Butalbital is a **respiratory depressant** and affects the central nervous system (CNS), producing drowsiness, tiredness, or inability to concentrate.

Alcoholic beverages may aggravate stomach irritation caused by aspirin. The risk of aspirin-related ulcers is increased by alcohol. Alcohol will also increase the nervous system depression caused by butalbital.

Do not take any aspirin-containing product if you develop **dizziness, hearing loss**, or **ringing or buzzing in your ears**. Aspirin may interfere with normal **blood coagulation** (clotting) and should be avoided for 1 week before surgery. Talk to your surgeon or dentist before taking an aspirin-containing product for pain after surgery.

Possible Side Effects

▼ Most common: light-headedness, dizziness, sedation, nausea, vomiting, sweating, stomach upset, appetite loss, and mild stimulation.

▼ Less common: weakness, headache, sleeplessness, agitation, tremor, uncoordinated muscle movements, mild hallucinations, disorientation, visual disturbances, euphoria (feeling high), dry mouth, constipation, flushing of the face, changes in heart rate, palpitations, faintness, urinary difficulties, rash, itching, confusion, rapid breathing, and diarrhea.

Drug Interactions

• Combining Fiorinal with alcohol, tranquilizers, barbiturates, sleeping pills, or other nervous system depressants may cause tiredness, drowsiness, and trouble concentrating.

• Combining Fiorinal with prednisone or other corticosteroids, phenylbutazone, or alcohol may irritate your stomach and increase the chance of developing an ulcer.

• Your anticoagulant (blood-thinning) dose will have to be changed if you begin taking Fiorinal, because Fiorinal contains aspirin.

• Fiorinal will counteract the effect of probenecid and sulfinpyrazone on the elimination of uric acid. Fiorinal may counteract the blood-pressure-lowering effects of angiotensin-converting enzyme (ACE) inhibitors and beta blockers.

• Fiorinal may counteract the effects of diuretics when given to people with severe liver disease.

• Fiorinal may increase blood levels of methotrexate or valproic acid when taken together, leading to increased chances of side effects.

• Combining Fiorinal and nitroglycerin tablets may lead to an unexpected drop in blood pressure.

• Do not take Fiorinal together with an NSAID. There is no benefit to the combination and the chance of side effects, especially stomach irritation, is vastly increased.

Food Interactions

Fiorinal is best taken on an empty stomach but may be taken with food if it upsets your stomach.

Usual Dose

1–2 tablets or capsules every 4 hours or as needed. Do not exceed 6 doses a day.

Overdosage

Overdose symptoms include breathing difficulties, nervousness progressing to stupor or coma, pinpointed pupils, cold and clammy skin, lowered heart rate or blood pressure, nausea, vomiting, dizziness, ringing in the ears, flushing, sweating, and thirst. Symptoms of mild overdose are rapid and deep breathing, nausea, vomiting, dizziness, ringing or buzzing in the ears, flushing, sweating, thirst, headache, drowsiness, diarrhea, and rapid heartbeat. Severe overdose may cause fever, excitement, confusion, convulsions, liver or kidney failure, coma, and bleeding. Any suspected overdose victim should be taken to a hospital emergency room immediately. ALWAYS bring the prescription bottle or container with you.

Special Information

Fiorinal may cause drowsiness, affecting your ability to drive a car or operate complicated machinery.

Call your doctor if you develop any unusual, persistent, or bothersome side effects.

If you forget to take a dose of Fiorinal, take it as soon as you remember. If it is almost time for your next dose, skip the dose you forgot and continue with your regular schedule. Do not take a double dose.

Special Populations

Pregnancy/Breast-feeding

Fiorinal should be avoided during pregnancy; alternative therapies should be used. Pregnant women taking Fiorinal may experience prolonged labor, delayed delivery, and bleeding problems. Fiorinal increases the chance of birth defects; it may cause breathing problems in newborns. Regular use of Fiorinal during the last 3 months of pregnancy may cause drug dependency in the newborn. If taken during the last 2 weeks of pregnancy, Fiorinal may cause bleeding problems in the newborn.

Breast-feeding while using Fiorinal may cause tiredness and shortness of breath or slowed heartbeat in the nursing baby. If you must take Fiorinal, consider bottle-feeding your baby.

Seniors

The butalbital in this combination product may have a more exaggerated depressant effect on seniors than on younger adults. Other Fiorinal side effects that may be more prominent are light-headedness and dizziness or fainting when rising suddenly from a sitting or lying position.

Brand Name

Fiorinal with Codeine

Generic Ingredients

Aspirin + Butalbital + Caffeine + Codeine Phosphate Ⓖ

Type of Drug

Barbiturate-narcotic-analgesic (pain reliever) combination.

Prescribed for

Migraine or other pain.

General Information

Fiorinal with Codeine is one of many combination products

containing a barbiturate, an analgesic, and a narcotic. In Fiorinal with Codeine, butalbital is the barbiturate, aspirin is the analgesic, and codeine is the narcotic. These products often also contain a tranquilizer, and acetaminophen may be substituted for aspirin.

Cautions and Warnings

Do not take Fiorinal with Codeine if you know you are **allergic or sensitive** to it. Use this drug with extreme caution if you suffer from **asthma or other breathing problems**. Long-term use of this drug may cause **drug dependence or addiction**. Fiorinal with Codeine is a **respiratory depressant** and affects the central nervous system (CNS), producing **sleepiness, tiredness,** or **inability to concentrate**.

Do not take this drug if you are **allergic** to aspirin, any salicylate, or any nonsteroidal anti-inflammatory drug (NSAID). Check with your doctor or pharmacist if you are not sure. This and all other aspirin-containing drugs **should not be taken by children under age 16**. People with **liver damage** should avoid all the active ingredients in this drug.

Alcohol may aggravate the stomach irritation caused by aspirin. The risk of aspirin-related ulcer is increased by alcohol. Alcohol will also increase the nervous-system depression caused by codeine and butalbital.

Do not use any aspirin-containing drug if you develop **dizziness, hearing loss,** or **ringing or buzzing in your ears**. Aspirin may interfere with normal **blood coagulation (clotting)** and should be avoided for 1 week before surgery for this reason. It would be wise to ask your surgeon or dentist for advice before taking an aspirin-containing drug for pain after surgery.

Possible Side Effects

▼ Most common: light-headedness, dizziness, sleepiness, nausea, vomiting, appetite loss, and sweating. If these occur, consider asking your doctor about lowering the dosage you are taking. Usually the side effects disappear if you simply lie down.

▼ Less common: euphoria (feeling high), breathing difficulties, weakness, sleepiness, headache, agitation, uncoordinated muscle movement, minor hallucinations, disorientation and visual disturbances, dry mouth, con-

Possible Side Effects *(continued)*

stipation, flushing of the face, rapid heartbeat, palpitations, feeling faint, urinary difficulties or hesitancy, reduced sex drive or potency, itching, rash, anemia, lowered blood sugar, and yellowing of the skin or whites of the eyes. Narcotic analgesics may aggravate convulsions in those who have had them in the past.

Drug Interactions

• Interaction with alcohol, tranquilizers, barbiturates, sleeping pills, or other drugs that produce depression may cause tiredness, drowsiness, and trouble concentrating.

• Combining this drug with prednisone or other corticosteroids, alcohol, or phenylbutazone may irritate your stomach.

• Your anticoagulant (blood-thinning) drug dosage will have to be changed if you begin taking Fiorinal with Codeine, which contains aspirin.

• This drug will counteract the uric acid-eliminating effects of probenecid and sulfinpyrazone.

• Fiorinal with Codeine may counteract the blood-pressure-lowering effects of angiotensin-converting enzyme (ACE) inhibitor and beta-blocker drugs.

• Fiorinal with Codeine may counteract the effects of diuretics (agents that increase urination) when given to people with severe liver disease.

• Combining this drug with methotrexate or valproic acid may increase blood levels of those drugs, increasing the risk of side effects.

• Combining Fiorinal with Codeine and nitroglycerin tablets may lead to an unexpected drop in blood pressure.

• Do not take this drug together with any NSAID drug. There is no benefit to the combination and the risk of side effects, especially stomach irritation, is significantly increased.

Food Interactions

Fiorinal with Codeine is best taken on an empty stomach but you may take it with food if it upsets your stomach.

Usual Dose

1–2 tablets or capsules every 4 hours or as needed; do not exceed the maximum of 6 doses a day.

Overdosage

Usual overdose symptoms include breathing difficulties, nervousness progressing to stupor or coma, pinpointed pupils, cold clammy skin and lowered heart rate or blood pressure, nausea, vomiting, dizziness, ringing in the ears, flushing, sweating, and thirst.

Symptoms of mild overdose include rapid and deep breathing, nausea, vomiting, dizziness, ringing or buzzing in the ears, flushing, sweating, thirst, headache, drowsiness, diarrhea, and rapid heartbeat.

Severe overdose may cause fever, excitement, confusion, convulsions, liver or kidney failure, coma, or bleeding. The suspected overdose victim should be taken to a hospital emergency room immediately. ALWAYS bring the prescription bottle or container.

Special Information

Fiorinal with Codeine may cause drowsiness, affecting your ability to drive a car or operate complicated machinery.

Call your doctor if you develop any side effects that are unusual, bothersome, or persistent.

If you forget to take a dose of Fiorinal with Codeine, take it as soon as you remember. If it is almost time for your next dose, skip the one you forgot and continue with your regular schedule. Do not take a double dose.

Special Populations

Pregnancy/Breast-feeding

Pregnant women should not take Fiorinal with Codeine because this drug carries an increased risk of birth defects. Regular use of Fiorinal with Codeine during the last 3 months of pregnancy may cause drug dependency of the newborn. Pregnant women using Fiorinal with Codeine may experience prolonged labor and delayed delivery, and breathing problems may afflict the newborn. If taken during the last 2 weeks of pregnancy, this drug may cause bleeding problems in an infant. Problems such as bleeding may also be experienced by the mother.

Breast-feeding while using Fiorinal with Codeine may cause increased tiredness, shortness of breath, or a slow heartbeat in the baby. If you must take this drug, consider bottle-feeding your infant.

Seniors
Both the codeine and butalbital in this drug may have a
greater depressant effect on seniors than on younger adults.
Other effects that may be more prominent are dizziness,
light-headedness, or fainting when rising suddenly from a
sitting or lying position.

Generic Name

Flecainide (FLEH-kan-ide)

Brand Name

Tambocor

Type of Drug

Antiarrhythmic.

Prescribed for

Abnormal heart rhythm.

General Information

Flecainide is prescribed in situations where the abnormal
rhythm is so severe as to be life-threatening and does not
respond to other drug treatments. Like other antiarrhythmic
drugs, flecainide works by affecting the movement of nervous impulses within the heart.

Flecainide's effects may not become apparent for 3 to 4
days after you start taking it. Since flecainide therapy is often
started while you are in the hospital, especially if you are
being switched from another antiarrhythmic drug to flecainide, your doctor will be able to closely monitor how well the
drug is working for you.

Cautions and Warnings

As with other antiarrhythmic drugs, there is no proof that
flecainide helps people live longer or avoid sudden death. Do
not take flecainide if you are **allergic** or **sensitive** to it or if you
have **heart block**, unless you have a cardiac pacemaker.

Flecainide causes **new arrhythmias** or worsens already
existing ones in 7% of people who take it; this risk increases
with certain kinds of underlying heart disease and higher
doses of the drug. Flecainide causes or worsens **heart failure**

in about 5% of people taking it because it tends to reduce the force and rate of each heartbeat.

Flecainide is extensively broken down in the liver. People with **poor liver function** should not take flecainide unless the benefits clearly outweigh the possible risks of side effects.

Possible Side Effects

▼ Most common: dizziness, fainting, light-headedness, unsteadiness, visual disturbances including blurred vision and seeing spots before the eyes, breathing difficulties, headache, nausea, fatigue, heart palpitations, chest pain, tremors, weakness, constipation, bloating, and abdominal pain.

▼ Less common: new or worsened heart arrhythmias or heart failure, heart block, slowed heart rate, vomiting, diarrhea, upset stomach, loss of appetite, stomach gas, a bad taste in your mouth, dry mouth, tingling in the hands or feet, partial or temporary paralysis, loss of muscle control, flushing, sweating, ringing or buzzing in the ears, anxiety, sleeplessness, depression, not feeling well, twitching, weakness, convulsions, speech disorders, stupor, memory loss, personality loss, nightmares, apathy, eye pain, unusual sensitivity to bright light, sagging eyelids, reduced white-blood-cell or blood-platelet counts, impotence, reduced sex drive, frequent urination, urinary difficulty, itching, rash, fever, muscle ache, closing of the throat, and swollen lips, tongue, or mouth.

Drug Interactions

• The combination of propranolol and flecainide may cause an exaggerated lowering in heart rate. Other drugs that slow the heart may also interact with flecainide to produce an excessive slowing of heart rate.

• The acidity of your urine affects the passing of flecainide out of your body. Less acidity increases the amount of drug released, and more acidity, such as can occur with megadoses of vitamin C, decreases the amount you release. Extreme increases in urine acid content may expose you to more side effects; extreme decreases may undermine the drug's effectiveness.

• The amount of flecainide in your blood and its effect on your heart may be increased if it is taken together with amiodarone, cimetidine, disopyramide, or verapamil.

• Cigarette smoking increases the rate at which flecainide is broken down in the liver. Smokers may need a larger dose than nonsmokers.

• Flecainide may increase the amount of digoxin in the bloodstream, increasing the chance of side effects.

Food Interactions

None known.

Usual Dose

Starting dose—50–100 mg every 12 hours. Your doctor can increase your dose by 50 mg every several days, if needed. The maximum dose of flecainide depends on your response to the drug, your kidney function, and the specific arrhythmia being treated, but may go up to 600 mg a day.

Overdosage

Flecainide overdose affects heart function, causing slower heart rate, low blood pressure, and possible death from respiratory failure. Victims of flecainide overdose should be taken to a hospital emergency room for treatment. ALWAYS bring the prescription bottle or container with you.

Special Information

Flecainide can make you dizzy, light-headed, or disoriented. Take care while driving or performing any complex tasks.

Call your doctor if you develop chest pains, an abnormal heartbeat, breathing difficulties, bloating in your feet or legs, tremors, fever, chills, sore throat, unusual bleeding or bruising, yellowing of the whites of your eyes, or any other intolerable side effect.

If you forget to take a dose of flecainide and remember within 6 hours, take it as soon as possible. If you do not remember until later, skip the dose you forgot and continue with your regular schedule. Do not take a double dose.

Special Populations

Pregnancy/Breast-feeding

Animal studies have shown that flecainide at 4 times the normal human dose damages a fetus, but it is not known if the drug passes into fetal blood circulation. When this drug is considered crucial by your doctor, its potential benefits must be weighed against its risks.

Flecainide passes into breast milk in concentrations about 2½ times that found in blood. Nursing mothers who must take this drug should bottle-feed their infants.

Seniors

Seniors with reduced kidney or liver function are more likely to develop side effects and require a lower dosage.

Flonase

see **Corticosteroids, Nasal**, page 266

Generic Name

Fluconazole (flue-KON-uh-zole)

Brand Name

Diflucan

Type of Drug

Antifungal.

Prescribed for

Infections of the blood, mouth, throat, vagina, or central nervous system due to *Candida*, a*spergillus*, or c*ryptococcus*.

General Information

Fluconazole is an antifungal agent that is effective against a variety of fungal organisms, including *aspergillus, cryptococcus*, and *Candida*. It works by inhibiting important enzyme systems in the organisms it attacks. Fluconazole's effectiveness against *Candida* and *cryptococcus* has made this drug an important contributor in the fight against the opportunistic fungal infections that inflict many people with AIDS.

Cautions and Warnings

Do not take fluconazole if you are **allergic** to it. People who are allergic to similar antifungals—ketoconazole, miconazole, and itraconazole—may also be allergic to fluconazole, but cross-reactions are not common and serious allergic reaction is rare.

Rarely, fluconazole causes **liver damage**. The drug should be used with caution in people with preexisting liver disease. In studies with laboratory animals, fluconazole caused an increase in liver tumors.

Skin rash may be an important sign of drug toxicity, especially in people with AIDS or others with compromised immune function. Report any skin rashes, especially ones that do not heal readily, to your doctor.

Possible Side Effects

Side effects are generally more common among AIDS patients, but they follow the same pattern for all people taking this drug.

▼ Most common: nausea, headache, skin rash, vomiting, abdominal pain, and diarrhea.

▼ Less common: liver toxicity, as measured by increases in specific lab tests. These changes in lab values are more common in people with AIDS or cancer, who are more likely to be taking several drugs, some of which may also be toxic to the liver; these include rifampin, phenytoin, isoniazid, valproic acid, and oral antidiabetes agents. People with AIDS or cancer who take fluconazole for fungal infections rarely develop severe liver or skin problems.

Drug Interactions

• Cimetidine and rifampin may reduce blood levels of fluconazole, but the importance of these interactions is not known.

• Fluconazole may increase the amount of the oral antidiabetes drugs tolbutamide, glyburide, and glipizide in the blood, causing low blood-sugar. Cyclosporine, phenytoin, theophylline, warfarin, and zidovudine (an AIDS drug—also known as AZT) are similarly affected. Dosage adjustments of these drugs may be required to offset the effect of fluconazole.

• Fluconazole may interfere with oral contraceptive drugs.

• Hydrochlorothiazide may increase blood levels of fluconazole up to 40%.

Food Interactions

None known.

Usual Dose

Adult and Child (age 14 and over): 100–400 mg once a day.
Child: 1.3–5.5 mg per lb. of body weight once a day; no more than 400 mg a day.

Overdosage

Symptoms of a very large fluconazole overdose may include breathing difficulties, lethargy, excess tearing, droopy eyelids, excess salivation, loss of bladder control, convulsions, and blue discoloration of the skin under the nails. Overdose victims should be taken to a hospital emergency room for treatment. ALWAYS bring the prescription bottle or container with you.

Special Information

Regular visits to your doctor are necessary to monitor your liver function and general progress.

Call your doctor if you develop reddening, loosening, blistering, or peeling of the skin; darkening of the urine; yellowing of the skin or whites of the eyes; loss of appetite; or abdominal pain, especially on the right side. Other symptoms need be reported only if they are bothersome or persistent.

If you forget to take a dose of fluconazole, take it as soon as you remember. If it is almost time for your next dose, skip the one you forgot and continue with your regular schedule. Do not take a double dose.

Special Populations

Pregnancy/Breast-feeding
Animal studies of fluconazole show very specific effects on the fetus that have not been seen in humans. Nevertheless, pregnant women should not use fluconazole unless the possible benefits clearly outweigh the risks.

Fluconazole passes into breast milk. Nursing mothers who must take this drug should bottle-feed their babies.

Seniors
Because seniors are more likely to have lost some kidney function, they may require a reduced dosage.

Generic Name

Flucytosine (floo-SYE-toe-sene)

Brand Name

Ancobon

Type of Drug

Antifungal.

Prescribed for

Serious blood-borne fungal infections.

General Information

Flucytosine is meant for fungal infections—*Candida*, *chromo-mycoses*, and *cryptococcus*—carried in the blood that affect the urinary tract, respiratory tract, central nervous system, heart, and other organs. It is not meant for fungal infections of the skin, such as common athlete's foot.

Cautions and Warnings

Do not take this drug if you are **allergic** to it. Flucytosine can worsen **bone-marrow depression** in people whose immune systems are already compromised. Liver and kidney function and blood composition should be monitored while you are taking this drug.

People with **kidney disease** should take this medication with extreme caution; they must be closely monitored by their doctors. Daily dosage must be reduced.

Possible Side Effects

▼ Most common: unusual tiredness or weakness, liver inflammation, yellowing of the eyes or skin, abdominal pain, diarrhea, loss of appetite, nausea, vomiting, skin rash, redness, itching, sore throat, fever, and unusual bleeding or bruising.

▼ Less common: chest pains, breathing difficulties, sensitivity to the sun or bright light, dry mouth, duodenal ulcers, severe bowel irritation, stomach bleeding, inter-ference with kidney function, kidney failure, reduced red-

---

Possible Side Effects *(continued)*

and white-blood-cell counts or other changes in blood
composition, headache, hearing loss, confusion, dizziness, weakness, shaking, sedation or tiredness, psychosis, hallucinations, heart attack, and low blood-sugar and
potassium levels.

Drug Interactions

• Amphotericin B increases flucytosine's effectiveness; this
combination is generally used to produce better results.
• Flucytosine may interfere with some routine blood tests.

Food Interactions

Take flucytosine with food if it upsets your stomach.

Usual Dose

22–66 mg per lb. a day, in divided doses.

Overdosage

There is little experience with flucytosine overdose, but it
would not be unusual for an overdose of flucytosine to cause
exaggerated drug side effects.

Special Information

Take the capsules a few at a time over 15 minutes to avoid
nausea and vomiting.

Call your doctor if any of the following symptoms develop:
unusual tiredness or weakness; yellowing of the skin or
whites of the eyes; skin rash, redness, or itching; sore throat
or fever; unusual bleeding or bruising; or any other persistent
or intolerable side effect.

It is important to maintain good dental hygiene while taking
flucytosine. Use extra care when using your toothbrush or
dental floss because of the chance that flucytosine will make
you more susceptible to some infections. Dental work should
be completed prior to starting on this drug.

If you forget a dose, take it as soon as you remember. If it
is almost time for your next dose, take one dose right away
and another in 3 or 4 hours, then go back to your regular
schedule. Do not take a double dose.

Special Populations

Pregnancy/Breast-feeding

Flucytosine causes birth defects in animals. It crosses the placenta, but no problems have occurred. However, flucytosine should be used by pregnant women only when its potential benefits clearly outweigh its risks.

It is not known if flucytosine passes into breast milk. Nursing mothers who must take this drug should bottle-feed their babies.

Seniors

Because seniors are likely to have some loss of kidney function, dosage adjustment may be required.

Type of Drug

Fluoroquinolone Anti-infectives

Brand Names

Generic Ingredient: Ciprofloxacin G
Ciloxan   Cipro

Generic Ingredient: Enoxacin
Penetrex

Generic Ingredient: Grepafloxacin
Raxar

Generic Ingredient: Levofloxacin
Levaquin

Generic Ingredient: Lomefloxacin
Maxaquin

Generic Ingredient: Norfloxacin
Chibroxin   Noroxin

Generic Ingredient: Ofloxacin
Floxin

Generic Ingredient: Sparfloxacin
Zagam

Generic Ingredient: Trovafloxacin
Trovan

Prescribed for

Lower respiratory, sinus, and urinary infections; also prescribed for sexually transmitted diseases, prostatitis, skin infections, abdominal infections, gynecologic infections, pelvic infections, bone and joint infections, infectious diarrhea, lung infections in people with cystic fibrosis, bronchitis, pneumonia, prostate infection, and traveler's diarrhea. Fluoroquinolone eyedrops are prescribed for ocular infections.

General Information

The fluoroquinolone anti-infectives are widely used and work against many organisms that traditional antibiotic treatments do not effectively kill. They do not work against the common cold, flu, or other viral infections. The fluoroquinolones are chemically related to an older antibacterial called nalidixic acid, but they work better against urinary infections. Some fluoroquinolone drugs, such as ciprofloxacin and trovafloxacin, are used to treat a wide variety of infections all over the body; others are used for more specific purposes. Trovafloxacin may be used prior to hysterectomy and colorectal surgery to prevent infection. In eyedrop form, fluoroquinolones are used to treat ocular infections.

Cautions and Warnings

Do not take a fluoroquinolone if you are **allergic** to it or another fluoroquinolone, or if you have had a reaction to a related medication such as **nalidixic acid**. Severe, possibly fatal, allergic reactions can occur even after the very first dose. Possible reactions include cardiovascular collapse, loss of consciousness, tingling, swelling of the face or throat, breathing difficulties, itching, and rash. If any of these symptoms appear, stop taking the drug and seek medical help at once.

Fluoroquinolone dose may need to be adjusted in the presence of **kidney failure** or **severe liver disease**.

Fluoroquinolones may cause increased pressure on parts of the brain, leading to **convulsions** and **psychotic reactions**. Other possible adverse effects include tremors, restlessness, light-headedness, confusion, and hallucinations. Fluoroquinolones should be used with caution in people with **seizure disorders** or other nervous system conditions.

People taking fluoroquinolone medications can be unusually **sensitive to sunlight**. Avoid the sun while taking this drug and for several days following therapy, *even if you are using a sunscreen.*

As with any other anti-infective, fluoroquinolones may trigger **colitis** ranging from mild to very serious. See your doctor if you develop diarrhea or cramps while taking this drug.

Prolonged fluoroquinolone use can lead to **fungal overgrowth**. Follow your doctor's directions exactly.

Possible Side Effects

Fluoroquinolone side effects are rarely serious enough to cause people to stop taking their medicine.

▼ Most common: ciprofloxacin—nausea. Enoxacin—vomiting. Oflaxacin—diarrhea.

▼ Less common: abdominal pain, headache, and liver inflammation.

▼ Rare: dry mouth; mouth pain; swallowing difficulty; upset stomach; constipation; gas; colitis; stomach bleeding; yellowing of the skin or whites of the eyes; fatigue; not feeling well; depression; sleeplessness; seizures; confusion; restlessness; psychotic reactions; tingling in the hands or feet; irritability; tremors; weakness; worsening of myasthenia gravis; appetite loss; flushing; hallucinations; nightmares; sensitivity to the sun; skin peeling; drug reactions; visual disturbances; eye pain; ringing or buzzing in the ears; uncontrolled rolling of the eyes; hearing loss; vaginal infection; high blood pressure; heart palpitations; angina pains; heart attack; blood clots in the lung or brain; general dizziness or dizziness when rising from a sitting or lying position; fainting; chills; fever; swelling in the ankles, legs, or arms; kidney damage; bronchial spasms; breathing difficulties; nose bleeds; vomiting blood; hiccups; swelling of the throat; fluid in the lungs; bad taste in the mouth; and oral infections. Other side effects can involve virtually any part of the body. Call your doctor if anything unusual develops.

Drug Interactions

• Antacids, didanosine, iron supplements, sucralfate, and zinc will decrease the amount of fluoroquinolone anti-infective absorbed into the bloodstream. If you must take any of these products, separate them from your fluoroquinolone dose by at least 2 hours.

• Probenecid cuts the amount of fluoroquinolone released

through your kidneys by half, and may increase the chance of side effects. Cimetidine may also increase fluoroquinolone blood levels.

• Fluoroquinolones may increase the effect of oral anticoagulant drugs such as warfarin. Your anticoagulant dose may have to be reduced.

• Fluoroquinolones may increase the toxic effects of cyclosporine—prescribed for organ transplants—on your kidneys.

• Fluoroquinolones may reduce the rate at which theophylline is released from your body, increasing the chance of theophylline-related side effects.

• Azlocillin may decrease the amount of ciprofloxacin released through your kidneys, and may increase the chance of side effects.

• Ciprofloxacin, enoxacin, and norfloxacin decrease the total body clearance of caffeine, possibly increasing its effect on your system.

• Anticancer drugs may decrease the amount of fluoroquinolones in your blood.

• Nitrofurantoin may antagonize norfloxacin's antibacterial effects. Do not take these drugs together.

• Ciprofloxacin may reduce blood levels of phenytoin—for seizures—requiring alteration of your daily dose.

Food Interactions

Grepafloxacin, levofloxacin, lomefloxacin, and trovafloxacin may be taken without regard to food or meals.

Enoxacin, ofloxacin, and norfloxacin must be separated from food. Take them 1 hour before or 2 hours after meals.

Ciprofloxacin is best taken 1 hour before or 2 hours after meals, but may be taken at any time. Dairy products interfere with the absorption of ciprofloxacin and should be avoided.

Usual Dose

Tablets
Ciprofloxacin: 250–750 mg twice a day.
   Enoxacin: 200–400 mg every 12 hours; a single dose of 400 mg for gonorrhea.
   Grepafloxacin: 400–600 mg once a day.
   Levofloxacin: 250–500 mg once a day.
   Lomefloxacin: 400 mg a day.
   Norfloxacin: 400 mg every 12 hours; a single dose of 800 mg for gonorrhea.

Ofloxacin: 200–400 mg every 12 hours.

Sparfloxacin: starting dose—400 mg tablets. Maintenance dose—200 mg a day.

Trovafloxacin: 100–200 mg once a day; a single dose of 200 mg for prevention of surgical infections; a single dose of 100 mg for gonorrhea.

Dosage is reduced in the presence of kidney failure.

Eyedrops
Ciprofloxacin and Norfloxacin: 1–2 drops in the affected eye several times a day.

Overdosage

One person experienced kidney failure when he took an overdose of a fluoroquinolone. Generally, the symptoms of fluoroquinolone overdose are the same as its side effects. Overdose victims should be taken to a hospital emergency room for treatment; ALWAYS bring the prescription bottle or container with you. Consult your local poison control center or hospital emergency room for specific instructions. You may be asked to induce vomiting with ipecac syrup—available at any pharmacy—to remove excess medication from the victim's stomach.

Special Information

Take each dose with a full glass of water. Be sure to drink at least 8 glasses of water per day while taking this medicine to promote removal of the drug from your system and to help avoid side effects.

If you are taking an antacid, didanosine, sucralfate, or an iron or zinc supplement while taking a fluoroquinolone, be sure to separate the doses by at least 2 hours to avoid a drug interaction.

Drug sensitivity reactions can develop after only one dose of this medication. Stop taking it and get immediate medical attention if you faint or if you develop itching, rash, facial swelling, breathing difficulties, convulsions, depression, visual disturbances, dizziness, headache, light-headedness, or any sign of a drug reaction.

Colitis can be caused by any anti-infective medication. If diarrhea develops after taking a fluoroquinolone, call your doctor at once.

Avoid excessive sunlight or exposure to a sunlamp while

taking fluoroquinolones. Call your doctor if you become unusually sensitive to the sun.

Follow your doctor's directions exactly. Do not stop taking it even if you begin to feel better after a few days, unless directed to do so by your doctor.

To use eyedrops, lie down or tilt your head backward and look at the ceiling. Hold the dropper above your eye, gently squeeze your lower lid to make a small pouch, and drop the medicine inside while looking up. Release the lower lid and keep your eye open. Do not blink for about 40 seconds. Press gently for about a minute on the bridge of your nose at the inside corner of your eye. This is to help circulate the drop around your eye. To avoid infection, do not touch the dropper tip to your finger or eyelid. Wait 5 minutes before using another eyedrop or ointment.

Call your doctor at once if your vision declines or if eye stinging, itching, burning, redness, irritation, swelling, or pain gets worse with the medication.

Since fluoroquinolones can cause visual changes, dizziness, drowsiness, or light-headedness, they can affect your ability to drive a car or perform other complex tasks.

If you forget to take a dose of fluoroquinolones, including eyedrops, take it as soon as you remember. If it is almost time for your next dose, skip the dose you forgot and continue with your regular schedule. Do not take a double dose.

Special Populations

Pregnancy/Breast-feeding

Pregnant women should not take fluoroquinolones unless the benefits clearly outweigh the risks. Animal studies have shown that fluoroquinolones may reduce your chances for a successful pregnancy or damage the fetus.

Nursing infants swallow small amounts of fluoroquinolones through breast milk. Mothers who must take fluoroquinolones should bottle-feed their babies. Be sure your doctor knows if you are breast-feeding.

Seniors

Studies in healthy seniors showed that most fluoroquinolones are released from older bodies more slowly because of natural decreases in kidney function. Dosage reductions may be made according to kidney function. Trovafloxacin is not affected by age or kidney function.

Seniors may use fluoroquinolone eyedrops without special

restriction. Some seniors may have weaker eyelid muscles; this creates a small reservoir for the eyedrops, which may actually increase the drug's effect by keeping it in contact with the eyes for a longer period. Your dosage may need to be adjusted.

Generic Name

Fluoxetine (flue-OX-eh-tene)

Brand Name

Prozac

Type of Drug

Selective serotonin reuptake inhibitor (SSRI).

Prescribed for

Depression, bulimic binge-eating and vomiting, and obsessive-compulsive disorder (OCD); also prescribed for obesity, alcoholism, anorexia, attention-deficit hyperactivity disorder (ADHD), bipolar affective disorder, borderline personality disorder, cataplexy and narcolepsy, kleptomania, migraine headache, chronic daily headache, tension headaches, post-traumatic stress disorder, schizophrenia, Tourette's syndrome, dyskinetic side effects of levodopa, and social phobias.

General Information

Fluoxetine and the other SSRI antidepressants—fluvoxamine, paroxetine, and sertraline—are chemically unrelated to the older tricyclic and tetracyclic antidepressant drugs. SSRIs work by preventing the movement of the neurohormone serotonin into nerve endings. This forces the serotonin to remain in the spaces surrounding nerve endings, where it works. Fluoxetine is effective in treating common symptoms of depression. It can help improve your mood and mental alertness, increase physical activity, and improve sleep patterns. In the years since its introduction, fluoxetine has been studied in a number of different disorders. Fluoxetine takes about 4 weeks to work and stays in the body for several weeks after you stop taking it. This fact may be important as your doctor considers when to start or stop treatment.

Cautions and Warnings

Do not take fluoxetine if you are **allergic** to it or other SSRI drugs. Some people have experienced serious drug reactions to fluoxetine. Allergies to non-SSRI antidepressants should not prevent you from taking fluoxetine because it is chemically different from other types of antidepressants.

Serious, potentially fatal reactions may occur if fluoxetine and a monoamine oxidase inhibitor **(MAOI)** antidepressant are taken together (see "Drug Interactions").

About 1 of every 25 people taking fluoxetine develop an **itching rash,** 1/3 of whom have to stop taking the medication. Other symptoms associated with the rash are fever, joint pain, swelling, wrist and hand pain, breathing difficulties, swollen lymph glands, and laboratory abnormalities. In most people, these symptoms go away when they stop taking fluoxetine and receive antihistamine or corticosteroid treatments.

People with severe **liver or kidney disease** should be cautious about taking fluoxetine and should be treated at below-normal doses.

As many as 1/3 of people taking an SSRI experience **anxiety, sleeplessness,** and **nervousness**.

Underweight depressed people who take fluoxetine may lose more weight. About 9% of people taking fluoxetine experience appetite loss, while 13% lose more than 5% of their body weight.

SSRIs may affect blood platelets, though their exact effect is not known. Some people have had abnormal **bleeding** while taking these drugs.

A few patients—less than 2 of every 1000—taking fluoxetine experience **seizures** or **convulsions**. This effect is similar to that seen with other antidepressants.

The possibility of **suicide** exists in severely depressed patients and may be present until the condition is significantly improved. Severely depressed people should be allowed to carry only small quantities of fluoxetine to limit the possibility of overdose.

Possible Side Effects

▼ Most common: headache, anxiety, nervousness, sleeplessness, drowsiness, tiredness, weakness, tremors, sweating, dizziness, light-headedness, dry mouth, upset

Possible Side Effects *(continued)*

or irritated stomach, appetite loss, nausea, vomiting, diarrhea, stomach gas, rash, and itching.

▼ Less common: changes in sex drive, abnormal ejaculation, impotence, abnormal dreams, difficulty concentrating, increased appetite, acne, hair loss, dry skin, chest pain, allergy, runny nose, bronchitis, abnormal heart rhythms, bleeding, blood pressure changes, dizziness or fainting when rising suddenly from a sitting position, bone pain, bursitis, twitching, breast pain, fibrocystic disease of the breast, cystitis, urinary pain, double vision, eye or ear pain, conjunctivitis, anemia, swelling, low blood sugar, and low thyroid activity.

▼ Rare: Side effects affecting virtually every body system have been reported by people taking fluoxetine. They affect only a small number of people. Be sure to report anything unusual to your doctor at once.

Drug Interactions

• At least 5 weeks should elapse between stopping fluoxetine treatment and starting an MAOI antidepressant. Two weeks should elapse between stopping an MAOI and starting fluoxetine. Taking these drugs too close together or at the same time may cause serious, life-threatening reactions.

• Fluoxetine blood levels may be increased if the drug is taken with a tricyclic antidepressant.

• Fluoxetine may increase blood levels of lithium, leading to lithium-related side effects. Your lithium dosage may need to be adjusted.

• The effects of fluoxetine may be reversed if it is taken together with cyproheptadine, an antihistamine.

• Hallucinations have occurred when people have combined fluoxetine with dextromethorphan, the most common cough suppressant ingredient in over-the-counter products. Do not take this combination.

• Combining fluoxetine with phenytoin can raise the level of phenytoin in the blood, leading to possible side effects.

• Fluoxetine can raise blood levels of the antipsychotic drugs clozapine—for schizophrenia—haloperidol, and pimozide; and of cyclosporine, an immune suppressant used in organ transplants.

• People who combine l-tryptophan and fluoxetine may develop agitation, restlessness, and upset stomach.

• Alcoholic beverages may increase tiredness and other depressant effects of fluoxetine on the nervous system.

• Fluoxetine may reduce the effectiveness of buspirone when these drugs are taken together, which has led to a worsening of OCD in people taking this combination to relieve OCD.

• Fluoxetine may raise blood levels of carbamazepine, increasing the chances of carbamazepine side effects.

• Fluoxetine may reduce the rate at which diazepam and other benzodiazepines are cleared from the body, increasing the effect of those drugs.

• People taking warfarin and fluoxetine may experience increased bleeding, although without testing differently for prothrombin time (a rate used to measure bleeding tendency).

Food Interactions

None known.

Usual Dose

20–80 mg a day. Seniors, people with kidney or liver disease, and people taking several different drugs may need a lower dosage.

Overdosage

Two people have died after taking a fluoxetine overdose and there have been at least 35 reported cases of non-fatal overdoses of fluoxetine alone or in combination with alcohol or other drugs. One person who took 3000 mg of fluoxetine had two grand mal seizures. Overdose symptoms may include seizures, nausea, vomiting, agitation, restlessness, and nervous system excitation. There is no specific antidote for fluoxetine overdose. Any person suspected of having taken a fluoxetine overdose should be taken to a hospital emergency room for treatment at once. ALWAYS bring the prescription bottle or container with you.

Special Information

Fluoxetine can make you dizzy or drowsy. Take care when driving or performing other tasks that require alertness and concentration. Avoid alcoholic beverages.

Be sure your doctor knows if you are pregnant, breast-feeding, or taking other drugs, including OTC drugs, while taking fluoxetine.

Call your doctor if you develop rash or hives, become excessively nervous or anxious, lose your appetite—especially if you are already underweight—or experience any unusual side effects while taking fluoxetine.

If you forget a dose of fluoxetine, take it as soon as you remember. If it is almost time for your next dose, skip the dose you forgot and continue with your regular schedule. Do not take a double dose.

Special Populations

Pregnancy/Breast-feeding

In one study, approximately 5% of women who took fluoxetine during pregnancy had babies with major abnormalities. In addition, women taking this drug were more likely to deliver prematurely. Do not take fluoxetine if you are or might be pregnant without first seeing your doctor and weighing its potential benefits against its risks.

Fluoxetine passes into breast milk. Nursing infants have not exhibited side effects; however, nursing mothers should be cautious about taking this drug.

Seniors

Fluoxetine has been studied in seniors. Several hundred seniors took the drug during its study phase without any unusual adverse effects. However, people with liver or kidney disease—more common among seniors—must receive a lower dose than an otherwise healthy person. Report any unusual side effects to your doctor.

Generic Name

Fluoxymesterone

(flue-OX-ee-MES-ter-one) Ⓖ

Brand Name

Halotestin

Type of Drug

Androgen (male hormone).

Prescribed for

Men: hormone replacement or augmentation and male menopause; also prescribed as safe, effective, and reversible male contraception for up to 12 months.

Women: breast pain and fullness in women who have given birth, and inoperable breast cancer.

General Information

Fluoxymesterone is an androgen. Other androgens are testosterone, methyltestosterone, calusterone, and dromostanolone propionate—the last two drugs are used primarily to treat breast cancer in women. Androgens are responsible for the normal growth and development of male sex organs and for maintaining secondary sex characteristics including growth of the prostate, penis and scrotum; beard and other hair distribution; vocal cord thickening; muscle development; fat distribution; and adolescent growth spurts.

Cautions and Warnings

Androgens have been used to improve **athletic performance** but they do not help; they do expose you to serious side effects.

Women taking any androgen should watch for deepening of the voice, oily skin, acne, hairiness, increased sex drive, menstrual irregularities, and effects related to the so-called virilizing (to cause or increase the development of male sex characteristics) effects of these hormones. **Virilization** is a sign that the drug is starting to produce changes in secondary sex characteristics. Androgens should be avoided if possible by young boys who have not gone through puberty.

Fluoxymesterone and other androgens will worsen **gynecomastia** (condition characterized by enlarged male breast tissue).

Men with unusually **high blood levels of calcium,** known or suspected **cancer of the prostate or prostate destruction,** or **breast cancer** should not use fluoxymesterone, nor should anyone with severe **liver, heart, or kidney disease.**

Long-term, high-dose androgen therapy may cause severe **liver disease**—including hepatitis and cancer, **reduced sperm count,** and **water retention. Blood cholesterol** may be altered by androgens.

Possible Side Effects

Men

▼ Most common: inhibition of testicle function, impotence, chronic erection, and painful enlargement of breast tissue.

Women

▼ Most common: unusual hairiness, baldness in a pattern similar to that seen in men, deepening of the voice, and enlargement of the clitoris. These changes are usually irreversible once they have occurred. Females also experience increases in blood calcium and menstrual irregularities.

Men and Women

▼ Most common: changes in sex drive, headache, anxiety, depression, a tingling feeling, sleep apnea (condition characterized by intermittent cessation of breathing during sleep), flushing of the skin, rash, acne, habituation, excitation, chills, sleeplessness, water retention, nausea, vomiting, diarrhea, hepatitis (symptoms include yellowing of the skin or whites of the eyes), liver inflammation, and liver cancer. Symptoms resembling a stomach ulcer may also develop.

Drug Interactions

• Fluoxymesterone may increase the effect of an oral anticoagulant (blood thinner); dosage of the anticoagulant may have to be reduced. It may also have an effect on the glucose-tolerance test, a blood test used to screen for diabetes. Androgens may interfere with some tests of thyroid function.

• Androgens given with imipramine or other tricyclic antidepressants may result in a severe paranoid reaction.

Food Interactions

Take fluoxymesterone with meals if it upsets your stomach.

Usual Dose

2.5–40 mg a day depending upon the disease being treated and response.

Overdosage

The acute (short-term) effects of androgen overdose are nausea, vomiting, and diarrhea. Call your local poison control center or hospital emergency room for additional information.

Special Information

Androgens are potent drugs. They must be taken only under the close supervision of your doctor and never used casually. The dosage and clinical effects of fluoxymesterone vary widely and require constant monitoring. Call your doctor if you develop nausea or vomiting, swelling of the legs or feet, yellowing of the skin or whites of the eyes, or a painful or persistent erection. Women should call their doctors immediately if they develop a deep or hoarse voice, acne, hairiness, male pattern baldness, or menstrual irregularities.

If you forget to take a dose of fluoxymesterone, take it as soon as you remember. If it is almost time for your next dose, skip the one you forgot and continue with your regular schedule. Do not take a double dose.

Special Populations

Pregnancy/Breast-feeding

Fluoxymesterone should never be taken by pregnant or nursing women. It may cause unwanted problems including the virilization of female infants.

Seniors

Seniors treated with fluoxymesterone run an increased risk of prostate enlargement or prostate cancer. A marked increase in sex drive may also occur.

Generic Name

Flurazepam (fluh-RAZ-uh-pam) Ⓖ

Brand Name

Dalmane

Type of Drug

Benzodiazepine sedative.

Prescribed for

Short-term treatment of insomnia or sleeplessness, difficulty falling asleep, frequent nighttime awakening, and waking too early in the morning.

General Information

Flurazepam is a member of the group of drugs known as benzodiazepines. All have some activity as antianxiety agents, anticonvulsants, or sedatives. Benzodiazepines work by a direct effect on the brain. They make it easier to go to sleep and decrease the number of times you wake up during the night.

The principal difference among the various benzodiazepines lies in how long they work in your body. They all take about 2 hours to reach maximum blood level, but some remain in your body longer, so they work for a longer period of time. Flurazepam and quazepam remain in your body the longest, thus resulting in the greatest incidence of morning "hangover."

Sleeplessness may often signal an underlying disorder that this medication will not treat.

Cautions and Warnings

People with **kidney or liver disease** should be carefully monitored while taking flurazepam. Take the lowest possible dose to help you sleep.

People with **respiratory disease** may experience **sleep apnea** (intermittent cessation breathing during sleep) while taking flurazepam.

Clinical **depression** may be increased by flurazepam, which can depress the nervous system. Intentional overdose is more common among depressed people who take sleeping pills than among those who do not.

All benzodiazepines can be **addictive** if taken for long periods of time, and it is possible for a person taking a benzodiazepine to develop drug withdrawal symptoms if the drug is discontinued suddenly. Withdrawal symptoms include tremors, muscle cramps, insomnia, agitation, diarrhea, vomiting, sweating, and convulsions.

Possible Side Effects

▼ Common: drowsiness, headache, dizziness, talkativeness, nervousness, apprehension, poor muscle coor-

Possible Side Effects *(continued)*

dination, light-headedness, daytime tiredness, muscle
weakness, slowness of movement, hangover, and euphoria (feeling high).

▼ Less common: nausea, vomiting, rapid heartbeat,
confusion, temporary memory loss, upset stomach,
stomach cramps and pain, depression, blurred or double
vision and other visual disturbances, constipation, changes
in sense of taste, appetite changes, stuffy nose, nosebleeds, common cold symptoms, asthma, sore throat,
cough, breathing difficulties, diarrhea, dry mouth, allergic
reaction, fainting, abnormal heart rhythm, itching, rash,
acne, dry skin, sensitivity to the sun, nightmares or
strange dreams, sleeplessness, tingling in the hands or
feet, ringing or buzzing in the ears, ear or eye pain,
menstrual cramps, frequent urination and other urinary
difficulties, blood in the urine, discharge from the penis
or vagina, lower back and other pain, muscle spasms and
pain, fever, swollen breasts, and weight changes.

Drug Interactions

• As with all benzodiazepines, the effects of flurazepam are
enhanced if it is taken with an alcoholic beverage, antihistamine, tranquilizer, barbiturate, anticonvulsant medication,
antidepressant, or monoamine oxidase inhibitor (MAOI).
MAOIs are most often prescribed for severe depression.

• Oral contraceptives, cimetidine, disulfiram, and isoniazid
may increase the effect of flurazepam by reducing the drug's
breakdown in the liver. Probenecid also increases Flurazepam's effects.

• Cigarette smoking, rifampin, and theophylline may reduce the effect of flurazepam on your body by increasing the
rate at which it is broken down by the liver.

• Levodopa's effectiveness may be decreased by flurazepam.

• Flurazepam may increase the amount of zidovudine (an
AIDS drug—also known as AZT), phenytoin, or digoxin in
your bloodstream, increasing the chances of side effects.

• The combination of clozapine and benzodiazepines has
led to respiratory collapse in a few people. Flurazepam
should be stopped at least 1 week before starting clozapine
treatment.

Food Interactions

Flurazepam may be taken with food if it upsets your stomach.

Usual Dose

Adult and Child (age 15 and over): 15–30 mg at bedtime. Dosage must be individualized for maximum benefit.
Senior: starting dose—15 mg at bedtime.
Child (under age 15): not recommended.

Overdosage

The most common symptoms of overdose are confusion, sleepiness, depression, loss of muscle coordination, and slurred speech. Coma may develop if the overdose is particularly large. Overdose symptoms can develop if a single dose of only 4 times the maximum daily dose is taken. Patients who overdose on this drug must be made to vomit with ipecac syrup—available at any pharmacy—to remove any remaining drug from the stomach: Call your doctor or a poison control center before doing this. If 30 minutes have passed since the overdose was taken or if symptoms have begun to develop, do not make the victim vomit. Immediately take him or her to a hospital emergency room for treatment. ALWAYS bring the prescription bottle or container with you.

Special Information

Never take more flurazepam than your doctor has prescribed.

Avoid alcoholic beverages and other nervous system depressants while taking flurazepam.

Exercise caution while performing tasks that require concentration and coordination. Flurazepam may make you tired, dizzy, or light-headed.

If you take flurazepam daily for 3 or more weeks, you may experience some withdrawal symptoms when you stop taking the drug. Talk with your doctor about how best to discontinue the drug.

If you forget a dose and remember within 1 hour, take it as soon as you remember. If you do not remember until later, skip the dose you forgot and go back to your regular schedule. Do not take a double dose.

Special Populations

Pregnancy/Breast-feeding

Flurazepam absolutely should not be used by pregnant women

or by women who may become pregnant. Animal studies have shown that flurazepam passes easily into the fetal blood system and can affect fetal development.

Flurazepam passes into breast milk and can affect a nursing infant. The drug should not be taken by nursing mothers.

Seniors
Seniors are more susceptible to the effects of flurazepam and should take the lowest possible dosage.

Generic Name

Flurbiprofen (flur-bih-PROE-fen)

Brand Names

Ansaid   Ocufen

Type of Drug

Nonsteroidal anti-inflammatory drug (NSAID).

Prescribed for

Rheumatoid arthritis, osteoarthritis, ankylosing spondylitis, mild to moderate pain, menstrual pain, tendinitis, bursitis, painful shoulder, gout, sunburn, and migraine headache. Flurbiprofen eyedrops are used to prevent movement of the eye muscles during surgery.

General Information

Flurbiprofen sodium is one of 16 NSAIDs, which are used to relieve pain and inflammation. We do not know exactly how NSAIDs work, but part of their action may be due to their ability to inhibit the body's production of a hormone called prostaglandin as well as the action of other body chemicals, including cyclooxygenase, lipoxygenase, leukotrienes, and lysosomal enzymes. NSAIDs are generally absorbed into the bloodstream quickly. Pain relief comes within 1 hour after taking the first dose of flurbiprofen, but its anti-inflammatory effect generally takes several days to 2 weeks to become apparent and may take a month or more to reach maximum effect. Flurbiprofen is broken down in the liver and eliminated through the kidneys. Along with flurbiprofen, other NSAIDs are also used in eyedrop form; for example, diclofenac is prescribed for inflammation following cataract extraction, ketorolac for itching and redness due to seasonal allergies.

Cautions and Warnings

People **allergic** to flurbiprofen or any other NSAID and those with a history of **asthma** attacks brought on by an NSAID, iodides, or aspirin should not take flurbiprofen.

Flurbiprofen may cause **gastrointestinal (GI) bleeding, ulcers,** and **stomach perforation**. This can occur at any time, with or without warning, in people who take flurbiprofen regularly. People with a history of **active GI bleeding** should be cautious about taking any NSAID. People who develop bleeding or ulcers and continue NSAID treatment should be aware of the possibility of developing more serious side effects.

Flurbiprofen may affect platelets and **blood clotting** at high doses, and should be avoided by people with clotting problems and by those taking warfarin.

People with **heart problems** who use flurbiprofen may experience swelling in their arms, legs, or feet.

Flurbiprofen may cause toxic effects to the **kidneys**. Report any unusual side effects to your doctor, who might need to periodically test your kidney function.

Flurbiprofen may make you unusually sensitive to the effects of the sun.

Possible Side Effects

Tablets

▼ Most common: diarrhea, nausea, vomiting, constipation, stomach gas, stomach upset or irritation, and appetite loss, especially during the first few days of treatment.

▼ Less common: stomach ulcers, GI bleeding, hepatitis, gallbladder attacks, painful urination, poor kidney function, kidney inflammation, blood and protein in the urine, dizziness, fainting, nervousness, depression, hallucinations, confusion, disorientation, tingling in the hands or feet, light-headedness, itching, increased sweating, dry nose and mouth, heart palpitations, chest pain, breathing difficulties, and muscle cramps.

▼ Rare: severe allergic reactions including closing of

Possible Side Effects *(continued)*

the throat, fever and chills, changes in liver function, jaundice (yellowing of the skin or whites of the eyes), and kidney failure. People who experience such effects must be promptly treated in a hospital emergency room or doctor's office. NSAIDs have caused severe skin reactions; if this happens, see your doctor immediately.

Eyedrops
▼ Most common: temporary burning, stinging, or other minor eye irritation.

▼ Less common: nausea, vomiting, viral infections, and eye allergies including redness, burning, itching, or tearing. The risk of developing bleeding problems or other systemic (whole-body) side effects with flurbiprofen eyedrops is low because only a small amount of the drug is absorbed into the bloodstream.

Drug Interactions

Tablets
• Flurbiprofen may increase the effects of oral anticoagulant (blood-thinning) drugs such as warfarin. You may take this combination, but your doctor might have to reduce your anticoagulant dose.

• Combining flurbiprofen with cyclosporine may increase the kidney-related side effects of both drugs. Methotrexate side effects may be increased in people also taking flurbiprofen.

• Flurbiprofen may reduce the blood-pressure-lowering effect of beta blockers and loop diuretics.

• Flurbiprofen may increase phenytoin blood levels, leading to increased phenytoin side effects. Lithium blood levels may be increased in people taking flurbiprofen.

• Flurbiprofen blood levels may be affected by cimetidine.

• Probenecid may interfere with the elimination of flurbiprofen from the body, increasing the chances for flurbiprofen side effects.

• Aspirin and other salicylates may decrease the amount of flurbiprofen in your blood. These drugs should never be combined with flurbiprofen.

Eyedrops
* Flurbiprofen eyedrops may inactivate acetylcholine or carbachol eyedrops.

Food Interactions

Take flurbiprofen with food or a magnesium-aluminum antacid if it upsets your stomach.

Usual Dose

Tablets: 200–300 mg a day. Seniors and people with kidney problems should start with a lower dose.

Eyedrops: 1 drop every ½ hour for 2 hours before eye surgery.

Overdosage

People have died from NSAID overdoses. The most common signs of overdose are drowsiness, nausea, vomiting, diarrhea, abdominal pain, rapid breathing, rapid heartbeat, increased sweating, ringing or buzzing in the ears, confusion, disorientation, stupor, and coma. Take the victim to a hospital emergency room at once. ALWAYS bring the prescription bottle or container with you.

Special Information

Tablets: Take each dose with a full glass of water and do not lie down for 15 to 30 minutes afterward.

Flurbiprofen can make you drowsy and/or tired: Be careful when driving or operating hazardous equipment. Do not take any over-the-counter products containing acetaminophen or aspirin while taking flurbiprofen. Avoid alcoholic beverages.

Contact your doctor if you develop skin rash or itching, visual disturbances, weight gain, breathing difficulties, fluid retention, hallucinations, black or tarry stools, persistent headache, or any unusual or intolerable side effect.

If you forget to take a dose of flurbiprofen, take it as soon as you remember. If you take flurbiprofen once a day and it is within 8 hours of your next dose, skip the dose you forgot and continue with your regular schedule. If you take several doses a day and it is within 4 hours of your next dose, skip the one you forgot and continue with your regular schedule. Never take a double dose.

Eyedrops: To self-administer the eyedrops, lie down or tilt your head backward. Hold the dropper above your eye and drop the medication inside your lower lid while looking up. To prevent possible infection, do not allow the dropper to touch your fingers, eyelids, or any surface. Release the lower lid, keeping your eye open. Do not blink for 30 seconds. Press gently on the bridge of your nose at the inside corner of your eye for 1 minute; this will help circulate the medicine in your eye. Wait at least 5 minutes before using any other eyedrops.

If you forget to take your eyedrops, take them as soon as you remember. If it is almost time for your next dose, skip the dose you forgot and continue with your regular schedule. Do not take a double dose.

Special Populations

Pregnancy/Breast-feeding

NSAIDs may cross into the fetal bloodstream. They have not been found to cause birth defects, but may affect the developing fetal heart during the second half of pregnancy. Pregnant women should not take flurbiprofen without their doctor's approval, especially during the last 3 months of pregnancy. When the drug is considered crucial by your doctor, its potential benefits must be carefully weighed against its risks.

NSAIDs may pass into breast milk but have caused no problems in breast-fed infants, except for seizures in a baby whose mother was taking the NSAID indomethacin. Other NSAIDs have caused problems in animal studies. There is a possibility that a nursing mother taking flurbiprofen could affect her baby's heart or cardiovascular system. If you must take flurbiprofen, consider bottle-feeding your baby.

Seniors

Seniors may be more susceptible to flurbiprofen side effects, especially ulcer disease.

Generic Name

Flutamide (FLUE-tuh-mide)

Brand Name

Eulexin

Type of Drug

Antiandrogen.

Prescribed for

Prostate cancer, both local and metastatic (cancer that has spread).

General Information

Flutamide, an antiandrogen, works by slowing the uptake of androgen (male) hormone or by interfering with the binding of androgen to body tissues. Prostatic cancer is sensitive to anything that removes the source of androgen. It is always prescribed together with a luteinizing hormone-releasing hormone (LHRH) drug. People taking flutamide often also receive radiation treatments.

Cautions and Warnings

Do not take flutamide if you are **allergic** to it.

One breakdown product of flutamide is a form of aniline. This may lead to toxic effects including **jaundice** and a severe blood condition called **hemolytic anemia**. Severe **liver toxicity** may occur with flutamide; your doctor should check your liver function.

Two men taking this drug have developed **breast cancer**. Flutamide may **reduce sperm counts**.

Possible Side Effects

▼ Most common: diarrhea, cystitis, and bleeding from the rectum.

▼ Common: rectal irritation, blood in the urine, hot flashes, nausea, skin rash, and swollen breasts.

▼ Less common: drowsiness, confusion, depression, anxiety, nervousness, appetite loss, stomach problems, anemia, low white-blood-cell and blood-platelet counts, arm or leg swelling, urinary and muscle problems, and high blood pressure.

▼ Rare: hepatitis, jaundice, and lung problems.

Food and Drug Interactions

None known.

Usual Dose

Adult: 250 mg (2 capsules) every 8 hours, 3 times a day.

Overdosage

Overdose symptoms may include tiredness or low activity

levels, slow breathing, weakness, tearing, appetite loss, vomiting, swollen and tender breasts, and liver inflammation. Overdose victims should be taken to a hospital emergency room where vomiting may be induced with ipecac syrup—available at any pharmacy—if the victim is still alert. ALWAYS bring the prescription bottle or container with you.

Special Information

Report anything unusual to your doctor, especially severe itching, dark urine, persistent appetite loss, yellowing of the skin or whites of the eyes, unexplained flu symptoms, and unexplained abdominal pain. These may be signs of severe liver toxicity.

Flutamide can turn your urine amber or yellow-green and can cause unusual sun sensitivity. Use a sunscreen and wear long-sleeved protective clothing while you are taking flutamide.

Flutamide must be taken exactly as prescribed. Call your doctor if you miss any doses of this drug.

Special Populations

Seniors
Seniors may take this drug without special precaution.

Generic Name

Fluvastatin (flue-vuh-STAT-in)

Brand Name

Lescol

Type of Drug

Cholesterol-lowering agent (HMG-CoA reductase inhibitor).

Prescribed for

High blood-cholesterol, LDL-cholesterol, and triglyceride levels, in conjunction with a low-cholesterol diet program. It is also prescribed to slow the progression of atherosclerosis (hardening of the arteries) reduce the risk of death in people with heart disease, and treat inherited blood-lipid problems or lipid problems associated with diabetes or kidney disease.

General Information

Fluvastatin is one of several cholesterol-lowering drugs that work by inhibiting an enzyme called HMG-CoA reductase. They interfere with the natural process for manufacturing cholesterol in your body, altering that process in order to produce a harmless by-product. Studies have closely related high blood-fat levels—total cholesterol, LDL cholesterol, and triglycerides—to heart and blood-vessel disease. Drugs that reduce levels of any of these blood fats and increase HDL cholesterol—"good" cholesterol—have been assumed for several years to reduce the risk of death and heart attack. Recently, medication in this class has been proven to slow the formation of blood-vessel plaque—associated with atherosclerosis—and reduce the risk of heart attack and death related to heart disease.

Fluvastatin reduces total triglyceride, cholesterol, and LDL-cholesterol counts while increasing HDL cholesterol. A very small amount of the drug actually reaches the body's circulation. Most is broken down and eliminated by the liver; 10% to 20% of the drug is released from the body through the kidneys. A significant blood-fat-lowering response is seen after 1 to 2 weeks of treatment. Blood-fat levels are lowest within 4 to 6 weeks after taking fluvastatin and remain at or close to that level as long as you continue to take the drug. The effect lasts for 4 to 6 weeks after you stop taking it.

Fluvastatin generally does not benefit anyone under age 30, so it is not usually recommended for children. It may, under special circumstances, be prescribed for teenagers in the same dose as adults.

Cautions and Warnings

Do not take fluvastatin if you are **allergic** to it or to any other HMG-CoA reductase inhibitor.

People with a history of **liver disease** and **those who drink large amounts of alcohol** should avoid drugs in this group because they may aggravate or cause liver disease. Your doctor should take a blood sample to test your liver function every month or so during the first year of treatment.

These drugs cause **muscle aches** and/or **muscle weakness** in a small number of people, which may be signs of a more serious condition.

At doses between 50 and more than 100 times the maximum human dose, HMG-CoA reductase inhibitors have caused central nervous system lesions, liver tumors, and male infertility in lab animals. The importance of this information for humans is not known.

Possible Side Effects

Most people who take fluvastatin tolerate it quite well; about 1% of people stop taking it because of drug side effects.

▼ Most common: upper respiratory infection, flu symptoms, headache, back pain, and upset stomach.

▼ Common: nausea, vomiting, diarrhea, abdominal cramps or pain, constipation, stomach gas, dental problems, muscle aches, arthritis, joint aches, dizziness, sleeplessness, runny nose, cough, sore throat, sinus irritation, itching, rash, tiredness, and allergy.

▼ Rare: Effects may occur in virtually any part of the body. Report anything unusual to your doctor.

Drug Interactions

• Drinking alcohol after a meal and within 1 hour of taking fluvastatin increases the amount of medication in the blood by 30% to 40%.

• The cholesterol-lowering effects of fluvastatin and colestipol or cholestyramine are additive when the drugs are taken together. Take fluvastatin 1 hour before or 4 hours after colestipol or cholestyramine.

• Fluvastatin may increase the effects of warfarin or digoxin. If you take either of these drugs with fluvastatin you should be periodically checked by your doctor.

• Digoxin, propranolol, and niacin (nicotinic acid) may reduce the amount of fluvastatin absorbed by the blood, reducing its effect. Avoid these combinations.

• The combination of cyclosporine, erythromycin, gemfibrozil, or niacin with fluvastatin may cause severe muscle aches or degeneration and other muscle problems. These combinations should be avoided.

• The effect of fluvastatin may be reduced by combining it with isradipine.

• Itraconazole may increase HMG-CoA reductase inhibitor levels by 20 times. Avoid this combination by temporarily stopping lovastatin if you take itraconazole.

• Combining rifampin with fluvastatin may cause a reduction in the amount of fluvastatin absorbed by the blood.

Food Interactions

None known. Continue your low-cholesterol diet while taking this medicine.

Usual Dose

20–80 mg at bedtime. Your fluvastatin dosage may be adjusted monthly, based on your doctor's assessment of how well the drug is working to reduce your blood cholesterol.

Overdosage

There are only a few reports of fluvastatin poisoning, including one involving 2 children; all victims recovered. The effects of fluvastatin overdose are not well understood. A person suspected of having taken a fluvastatin overdose should be taken to a hospital emergency room. ALWAYS bring the prescription bottle or container with you.

Special Information

Call your doctor if you develop blurred vision or muscle aches, pain, tenderness, or weakness, especially if you are also feverish or feel sick.

Drugs in this group are always prescribed in combination with a low-fat diet. Be sure to follow your doctor's dietary instructions, since both diet and medication are necessary to treat your condition.

Do not take more cholesterol-lowering medication than your doctor has prescribed or stop taking the medication without your doctor's knowledge.

Fluvastatin may cause unusual sensitivity to the sun. Use sunscreen and wear protective clothing while in the sun until you determine if you are affected.

If you forget to take a dose of fluvastatin, take it as soon as you remember. If it is almost time for your next dose, skip the one you forgot and continue with your regular schedule. Do not take a double dose.

Special Populations

Pregnancy/Breast-feeding

Pregnant women and those who might become pregnant absolutely must not take fluvastatin. Cholesterol is essential to the health and development of a fetus. Anything that interferes with that process will damage the developing brain and nervous system. Since hardening of the arteries is a long-term process, you should be able to stop this medication during pregnancy without developing atherosclerosis. If you become pregnant while taking fluvastatin, stop the drug immediately and call your doctor.

Fluvastatin passes into breast milk in concentrations twice as high as blood concentrations. Women taking fluvastatin should bottle-feed their infants to avoid possible interference with the baby's development.

Seniors

People over age 65 have shown a greater cholesterol-lowering response to fluvastatin than have people under age 65 and may require less medicine than younger adults. Be sure to report any side effects to your doctor.

Generic Name

Fluvoxamine (flue-VOX-uh-mene)

Brand Name

Luvox

Type of Drug

Selective serotonin reuptake inhibitor (SSRI).

Prescribed for

Obsessive-compulsive disorder (OCD); may also be prescribed for depression.

General Information

Fluvoxamine and the other SSRI antidepressants—fluoxetine, paroxetine, and sertraline—are chemically unrelated to the older tricyclic and tetracyclic antidepressant drugs. SSRIs work by preventing the movement of the neurohormone serotonin into nerve endings. This forces the serotonin to remain in the spaces surrounding nerve endings, where it works. Fluvoxamine is effective in treating common symptoms of OCD and allowing people to function without having to devote time and effort to compulsive behaviors. The drug takes several weeks to work and stays in the body for several weeks after you stop taking it. This fact may be important as your doctor considers when to start or stop treatment.

Cautions and Warnings

Do not take fluvoxamine if you are **allergic** to it or other SSRI drugs. Some people have experienced serious drug reactions to fluvoxamine. Allergies to non-SSRI antidepressants should not prevent you from taking fluvoxamine, since it is chemically different from other types of antidepressants.

Serious, potentially fatal reactions may occur if fluvoxamine and a monoamine oxidase inhibitor (**MAOI**) antidepressant are taken together (see "Drug Interactions").

SSRIs may affect blood platelets, though their exact effect is not known. Some people have had abnormal **bleeding** while taking these drugs.

People with severe **liver disease** should be cautious about taking fluvoxamine and should be treated at lower doses.

Possible Side Effects

▼ Most common: headache, weakness, sleeplessness, tiredness, nervousness, dizziness, nausea, upset stomach, diarrhea, dry mouth, and constipation.

▼ Common: anxiety, tremors, respiratory infection, stomach gas, appetite loss, vomiting, and excessive sweating.

▼ Less common: allergy or allergic reactions, flu-like symptoms, chills, palpitations, flushing, dizziness when rising from a sitting or lying position, high blood pressure, fainting, rapid heartbeat, depression, reduced sex drive or function, muscle twitching, agitation, muscle stiffness, nervous system stimulation, fatigue, not feeling well, memory loss, emotional upset, apathy, mood changes, manic or psychotic reaction, swelling, weight changes, stomach irritation, cavities or other teeth disorders, swallowing difficulties, liver inflammation, cough, sinus irritation, breathing difficulties, bronchitis, and yawning.

▼ Rare: Side effects affecting virtually every body system have been reported by people taking fluvoxamine. They are considered infrequent or rare and affect only a small number of people. Report anything unusual to your doctor at once.

Drug Interactions

• At least 5 weeks should elapse between stopping fluvoxamine treatment and starting an MAOI antidepressant. Two weeks should elapse between stopping an MAOI and starting fluvoxamine. Taking these drugs too close together or at the same time may cause serious, life-threatening reactions.

• Fluvoxamine blood levels may be increased if taken together with a tricyclic antidepressant.

• Lithium may increase blood levels of fluvoxamine, leading to fluvoxamine side effects. Your dosage may need to be adjusted.

• People who combine l-tryptophan and fluvoxamine may develop agitation, restlessness, and upset stomach.

• Alcoholic beverages may increase the tiredness and other depressant effects of fluvoxamine on the nervous system.

• Fluvoxamine may raise blood levels of clozapine, diltiazem, methadone, sumatriptan carbamazepine, or theophylline, increasing the chances of side effects from these drugs. Dosage adjustment may be needed.

• Fluvoxamine may raise blood levels of the beta-blocking drugs propranolol and metoprolol, increasing their effects. Blood levels of the beta blocker atenolol were not affected by fluvoxamine.

• Cigarette smoking may increase the speed at which the body breaks down fluvoxamine by 25%.

• Blood levels of the non-sedating antihistamines astemizole and terfenadine may be increased if taken with fluvoxamine, which increases the risk of potentially fatal cardiac reactions to those drugs. Haloperidol blood levels may also be increased, which can affect memory.

• Fluvoxamine may reduce the rate at which diazepam and other benzodiazepines are cleared from the body, increasing the effect of those drugs.

• People taking warfarin may experience an increase in its effect if they start taking fluvoxamine; your doctor should reevaluate your warfarin dosage.

Food Interactions

None known.

Usual Dose

50–300 mg at bedtime. Seniors, people with liver disease, and people taking several different drugs should start with a lower dosage.

Overdosage

Of more than 350 people who took a fluvoxamine overdose, 19 died. Symptoms of overdose may include drowsiness, diarrhea, vomiting, and dizziness. Other signs are coma, change in heart rate, low blood pressure, convulsions, and liver or cardiac abnormalities. There is no specific antidote for fluvoxamine. Fluvoxamine overdose victims should be taken to a hospital emergency room at once. ALWAYS bring the prescription bottle or container with you.

Special Information

Fluvoxamine can make you dizzy or drowsy. Take care when driving or doing other tasks that require alertness and concentration. Avoid alcoholic beverages.

Be sure your doctor knows if you are pregnant, breast-feeding, or taking other drugs, including over-the-counter drugs, while taking fluvoxamine.

Call your doctor if you develop rash or hives, become excessively nervous or anxious, or lose your appetite—especially if you are already underweight—or experience any unusual side effect while taking fluvoxamine.

If you forget a dose of fluvoxamine take it as soon as you remember. If it is almost time for your next dose, skip the dose you forgot and continue with your regular schedule. Do not take a double dose.

Special Populations

Pregnancy/Breast-feeding

Animal studies indicate that fluvoxamine may affect the fetus. If you are or might be pregnant, do not take this drug without first weighing its potential benefits against its risks with your doctor.

Fluvoxamine passes into breast milk; nursing mothers should be cautious about taking this drug.

Seniors

Older adults clear fluvoxamine twice as slowly as younger adults. Seniors should begin with a 25-mg dose, to be increased as needed every 4 to 7 days. Be sure to report any unusual side effects to your doctor.

Fosamax

*see **Alendronate**, page 29*

Generic Name

Fosfomycin (fos-foe-MYE-sin)

Brand Name

Monurol Granules

Type of Drug

Urinary anti-infective.

Prescribed for

Uncomplicated urinary infections.

General Information

Fosfomycin kills a wide variety of bacteria. It works by helping to prevent bacteria from sticking to the wall of the urinary tract and by interfering with the bacteria's process of making a new cell wall when it divides. The drug is absorbed rapidly into the blood and converted to free fosfomycin, the form in which it is active in the body. Generally, bacteria that are resistant to other antibiotics are not resistant to fosfomycin; thus your doctor may prescribe fosfomycin for a urinary infection that did not respond to another medication.

Cautions and Warnings

Do not take fosfomycin if you are **allergic** to it. Fosfomycin is meant to be taken once, in a single dose. **Taking more than one packet** of fosfomycin for a urinary infection only increases side effects; it does not improve the drug's effectiveness.

Possible Side Effects

▼ Less common: diarrhea, vaginal irritation, runny nose, nausea, and headache.

Possible Side Effects *(continued)*

▼ Rare: back pain, painful menstruation and other menstrual problems, sore throat, abdominal pain, rash, dizziness, upset stomach, weakness, tiredness, abnormal stools, appetite loss, constipation, dry mouth, painful urination, fever, stomach gas, flu symptoms, blood in the urine, infection, sleeplessness, swollen lymph glands, migraines, muscle aches, nervousness, tingling in the hands or feet, itching, liver irritation, vomiting, worsening of asthma, yellow discoloration of the skin or whites of the eyes, and aplastic anemia (symptoms include pale skin, sore throat and fever, unusual bleeding or bruising, and unusual tiredness or weakness).

Drug Interactions

• Combining metoclopramide and fosfomycin results in lower fosfomycin blood levels.

Food Interactions

Food may slightly reduce the rate at which fosfomycin is absorbed, but it does not affect the total amount absorbed. You may take fosfomycin with or without food.

Usual Dose

Adult: 1 packet.
Child (under age 18): not recommended.

Overdosage

Animal studies using single doses 50 to 125 times the normal human dose produced only minor side effects, such as diarrhea and loss of appetite. There have been no cases of fosfomycin overdose. Call your local poison control center or a hospital emergency room for more information.

Special Information

Do not take fosfomycin powder in its dry form. Always mix the contents of the packet with 3 to 4 oz. of cool or cold water and mix it until it dissolves. Drink the solution immediately after the powder is dissolved.

Call you doctor if your infection does not improve within 2 or 3 days after you take a dose of fosfomycin. Another medication may be needed.

Special Populations

Pregnancy/Breast-feeding
There is no information on the effect of taking fosfomycin during pregnancy. Pregnant women should only take fosfomycin after the possible risks and benefits have been discussed with their doctors.

It is not known if fosfomycin passes into breast milk. Nursing mothers who must take fosfomycin should bottle-feed their babies.

Seniors
Seniors may take fosfomycin without any special restrictions.

Generic Name

Fosinopril (fos-IN-oe-pril)

Brand Name
Monopril

Type of Drug
Angiotensin-converting enzyme (ACE) inhibitor.

Prescribed for
High blood pressure.

General Information
Fosinopril sodium belongs to the class of drugs known as ACE inhibitors. The ACE inhibitors work by preventing the conversion of a hormone called angiotensin I to another hormone called angiotensin II, a potent blood-vessel constrictor. Preventing this conversion relaxes blood vessels, thus reducing blood pressure and relieving the symptoms of heart failure by making it easier for a failing heart to pump blood through the body. Fosinopril affects the production of other hormones and enzymes that participate in the regulation of blood vessel dilation; this action probably increases the drug's effectiveness. Fosinopril begins working 2 to 6 hours after you take it.

Some people who start taking an ACE inhibitor after they are already on a diuretic (agent that increases urination) experience a rapid drop in blood pressure after their first doses or when the dosage is increased. To prevent this from happening, you may be told to stop taking the diuretic 2 or 3 days before starting the ACE inhibitor or to increase your salt intake during that time. The diuretic may then be restarted gradually.

Cautions and Warnings

Do not take fosinopril if you have had an **allergic reaction** to it in the past. Fosinopril occasionally causes very **low blood pressure** or affects your **kidneys**. Your doctor should check your urine for changes during the first few months of treatment.

ACE inhibitors can affect **white-blood-cell count**, possibly increasing your susceptibility to infection. Blood counts should be checked periodically.

Possible Side Effects

▼ Most common: headache and chronic cough. The cough usually goes away a few days after you stop taking the medicine.

▼ Less common: chest pain; low blood pressure; dizziness, especially when rising from a sitting or lying position; fatigue; diarrhea; vomiting; and nausea.

▼ Rare: angina, low blood pressure, stroke, abnormal heart rhythm, heart palpitations, difficulty sleeping, tingling in the hands or feet, confusion, fainting, abdominal pain, constipation, dry mouth, hepatitis, pancreatitis, asthma, sinusitis, sweating, flushing, itching, rash, unusual sensitivity to the sun, reduced sex drive, muscle cramps or aches, joint pain, and ringing in the ears.

Drug Interactions

• The blood-pressure-lowering effect of fosinopril is additive with diuretic drugs and beta blockers. Any other drug that causes a rapid drop in blood pressure should be used with caution if you are taking an ACE inhibitor.

• Fosinopril may increase potassium levels in your blood, especially when taken with dyazide or other potassium-sparing diuretics.

• Fosinopril may increase the effects of lithium; this combination should be used with caution.

• Antacids may reduce the amount of fosinopril absorbed

into the blood. Separate doses of these medications by at least 2 hours.

• Capsaicin may trigger or aggravate the cough associated with fosinopril therapy.

• Indomethacin may reduce the blood-pressure-lowering effects of fosinopril.

• Phenothiazine tranquilizers and antivomiting drugs may increase the effects of fosinopril.

• The combination of allopurinol and fosinopril increases the chance of side effects.

• ACE inhibitors increase blood levels of digoxin, possibly increasing the chance of digoxin-related side effects.

Food Interactions

You may take fosinopril with food if it upsets your stomach.

Usual Dose

10–80 mg once a day. People with liver disease may require lower dosages. No adjustment is required for kidney disease.

Overdosage

The principal effect of ACE inhibitor overdose is a rapid drop in blood pressure, as evidenced by dizziness or fainting. Take the overdose victim to a hospital emergency room immediately. ALWAYS bring the prescription bottle or container with you.

Special Information

Call your doctor if you develop swelling of the face or throat, if you have sudden difficulty in breathing, or if you develop a sore throat, mouth sores, abnormal heartbeat, chest pain, persistent rash, or loss of taste perception.

Unexplained swelling of the face, lips, hands, and feet can also affect the larynx (throat) and tongue and interfere with breathing. If this happens, the victim should be taken to a hospital emergency room at once.

You may get dizzy if you rise to your feet quickly from a sitting or lying position.

Avoid strenuous exercise and/or very hot weather, because heavy sweating or dehydration can cause a rapid decrease in blood pressure.

Avoid over-the-counter diet pills, decongestants, and other stimulants that can raise blood pressure.

If you forget to take a dose of fosinopril, take it as soon as you remember. If it is within 8 hours of your next dose, skip the one you forgot and continue with your regular schedule. Do not take a double dose.

Special Populations

Pregnancy/Breast-feeding
ACE inhibitors have caused low blood pressure, kidney failure, slow formation of the skull, and death in fetuses when taken during the last 6 months of pregnancy. Women who are pregnant should not take ACE inhibitors; women who may become pregnant should use an effective contraceptive method while taking an ACE inhibitor and stop taking the drug if they do become pregnant.

Because large amounts of fosinopril pass into breast milk, this drug should not be taken by nursing mothers. Nursing mothers who must take this drug should consider bottle-feeding. Infants, especially newborns, are more susceptible than adults to the drug's effects.

Seniors
Seniors are generally given the same fosinopril dosage as younger adults, but may be more sensitive to the effects of fosinopril.

Generic Name

Ganciclovir (gan-SYE-kloe-vere)

Brand Names

Cytovene   Vitrasert

Type of Drug

Antiviral.

Prescribed for

Cytomegalovirus (CMV) infections of the eye and CMV infections in other parts of the body, in people with compromised immune systems.

General Information

Ganciclovir works by preventing reproduction of the virus

CMV. Unlike other antiviral drugs, it works only against this virus and no others. Because viral resistance develops more quickly to the capsules, the capsule form of ganciclovir is restricted to follow-up treatment in people who have received intravenous treatment for CMV infections. Only 5% to 9% of the drug in each capsule is actually absorbed into your blood. Ganciclovir must be converted to an active form in the body before it can work. The drug is eliminated through the kidneys.

Intravenous ganciclovir has been given to a small number of children under age 12 with mixed results. Side effects were similar to those experienced by adults taking the drug. Studies of ganciclovir in African Americans, Hispanics, and Caucasians showed a trend toward higher blood levels among Caucasians than other groups.

Though most often used for CMV retinitis (eye infection), ganciclovir has also been used for CMV infections of the urine, blood, throat, and semen. It is also used in the prevention of CMV infection. In heart or bone marrow transplant patients, ganciclovir was helpful in controlling CMV infection.

Cautions and Warnings

Ganciclovir causes **anemia**, **reduced white-blood-cell count**, and **blood platelet loss**. Regular monitoring of blood and platelet counts is recommended while taking this drug.

Oral ganciclovir is linked to a faster progression of CMV eye infection than the intravenous form of the drug. The **risk of rapid progression of eye infection** should be balanced against the benefits of taking oral CMV.

People **allergic** to acyclovir or ganciclovir should not take ganciclovir.

Ganciclovir is intended only for people who are immuno-compromised. It is not intended to treat or prevent CMV infections in **newborns**.

Detachment of the retina has been noted in people taking ganciclovir, as well as in people with CMV who have not taken the drug. The relationship between ganciclovir and this effect is not well known.

In animal studies, ganciclovir causes **cancer**, **birth defects**, and **reduced sperm production**.

Ganciclovir causes unusual **sensitivity to the sun**; use a sunscreen and/or wear protective clothes when you go outside.

Possible Side Effects

▼ Most common: fever, diarrhea, abdominal pain, reduced white-blood-cell counts, anemia, rash, sweating, nausea, vomiting, and appetite loss.

▼ Common: infection; chills; stomach gas; low platelet counts (symptoms include bleeding or oozing blood); tingling; burning; numbness or pain in the hands, arms, legs, or feet; itching; pneumonia; weakness; and headache.

▼ Less common: Other reactions may affect almost any part of the body. Report any unusual side effect to your doctor.

Drug Interactions

• Dapsone, pentamidine, flucytosine, vincristine, vinblastine, adriamycin, amphotericin B, trimethoprim-sulfamethoxazole, and other antiviral drugs may increase the toxic effects of ganciclovir and should be used together only if absolutely necessary, and only if the potential benefits outweigh the risks.

• People taking imipenem-cilastatin together with ganciclovir have experienced generalized seizures. Avoid this combination.

• Mixing ganciclovir with other drugs that can be damaging to the kidneys may increase the rate and extent of kidney damage.

• Probenecid interferes with ganciclovir release through the kidneys and substantially increases blood levels of ganciclovir.

• Mixing ganciclovir with the anti-HIV drugs didanosine or zidovudine (AZT) may increase didanosine or AZT levels and reduce ganciclovir levels. Because AZT and ganciclovir both cause anemia and low white-blood-cell counts, many people cannot tolerate this combination.

Food Interactions

High-fat, high-calorie meals can increase the amount of ganciclovir absorbed into the blood. Take this drug with food.

Usual Dose

Adult and Child (age 13 and over): 3000 mg a day, divided

into 3 or 6 equal doses. People with reduced kidney function will need to have their dosage reduced accordingly, to as little as 500 mg 3 times a week.

Child (under age 13): not recommended.

Overdosage

No overdoses have been reported with ganciclovir capsules. As much as 6000 mg a day has been taken with only passing lowering of white-blood-cell count. Call your hospital emergency room for instructions in case of accidental ganciclovir overdose.

Special Information

Ganciclovir does not cure CMV eye infection, and immuno-compromised people taking this drug may find their disease worsening. Dosage reductions or discontinuation of the drug may be necessary if white-blood-cell or platelet counts get too low.

Ganciclovir may cause infertility in both men and women. Pregnant women taking this drug should use effective contraception. Men should use a condom while taking the drug and for at least 90 days afterward to avoid passing the drug to their partners.

Good dental hygiene is important while taking ganciclovir to minimize the chances of infection. If you have dental work done while taking this drug, expect the healing process to take longer.

Regular blood tests are necessary to watch for white-blood-cell or platelet-level alterations.

It is very important to take ganciclovir exactly as directed. If you forget a dose, take it as soon as you remember and continue with your regular schedule. If you take ganciclovir 3 times a day and it is almost time for your next dose, take one dose immediately, another in 6 hours, and then continue with your regular schedule. If you take it 6 times a day and it is almost time for your next dose, skip the dose you forgot and continue with your regular schedule.

Special Populations

Pregnancy/Breast-feeding

In animal studies, ganciclovir has been shown to be toxic to the fetus. There is no reliable information about its effect in pregnant women, but it should be taken only when the possible benefits outweigh the risks. Women who are likely to become pregnant while taking this drug should use reliable contraception.

It is not known if ganciclovir passes into breast milk, but the possible toxic effects of this drug on a nursing infant should be kept in mind. Nursing mothers who must take this drug should bottle-feed their babies.

Seniors
Seniors often have reduced kidney function; dosage adjustments may be needed.

Generic Name

Gemfibrozil (jem-FYE-broe-zil) Ⓖ

Brand Name
Lopid

Type of Drug
Anti-hyperlipidemic (blood-fat reducer).

Prescribed for
High levels of blood triglycerides.

General Information
Gemfibrozil consistently reduces blood-triglyceride levels and may reduce the risk of heart disease in people with high levels of triglycerides, low levels of high-density lipoprotein (HDL) cholesterol, and high levels of low-density lipoprotein (LDL) cholesterol. It is usually prescribed only for people with very high blood-fat levels who have not responded to dietary changes or other therapies. Normal triglyceride levels range between 50 and 200 mg. People with very high levels—1000 to 2000 mg—are likely to have severe abdominal pain and pancreatic inflammation. Gemfibrozil usually has little effect on blood-cholesterol levels, although it may reduce blood cholesterol in some people.

Gemfibrozil works by affecting the breakdown of body fats and by reducing the amount of triglyceride manufactured by the liver. It is not known if these 2 mechanisms are solely responsible for the drug's effect on triglyceride levels.

Cautions and Warnings

Gemfibrozil should not be taken by people with severe **liver or kidney disease**—some people taking gemfibrozil have experienced **worsening of kidney function**—or by those who have had **allergic reactions** to it in the past. Gemfibrozil users may have an increased chance of developing **gallbladder disease**. People taking gemfibrozil may develop **muscle aches** and **inflammation**. Make sure to tell your doctor about any new muscle tenderness or weakness.

Long-term studies in which male rats were given between 1 and 10 times the maximum human dosage showed an increase in **liver tumors**, both cancerous and noncancerous. Other studies of male rats, in which 3 to 10 times the human dosage was given for 10 weeks, showed that the drug reduced **reduced sperm activity**, although this effect has not been reported in humans.

Estrogens may cause massive increases in triglyceride levels and may have to be discontinued when using gemfibrozil. Other diseases such as **thyroid disease** and **diabetes** should also be considered as causes of high blood triglycerides.

Gemfibrozil may cause a moderate rise in blood sugar and mild decreases in white-blood-cell counts.

Possible Side Effects

▼ Most common: abdominal and stomach pain, gas, diarrhea, nausea, and vomiting.

▼ Less common: rash, itching, dizziness, blurred vision, anemia, reduced levels of certain white blood cells, increased blood sugar, and muscle pain—especially in the arms or legs.

▼ Rare: dry mouth, constipation, appetite loss, upset stomach, sleeplessness, tingling in the hands or feet, ringing or buzzing in the ears, back pain, painful muscles or joints, swollen joints, fatigue, feeling unwell, reduction in blood potassium, and abnormal liver function.

Drug Interactions

• Gemfibrozil increases the effects of oral anticoagulant (blood-thinning) drugs; your doctor will have to reduce your anticoagulant dosage when gemfibrozil treatment is started.

• Combining gemfibrozil with a "statin-type" of blood-fat

reducer such as lovastatin or simvastatin has led to the destruction of skeletal muscles. This effect may begin as early as 3 weeks after you start taking the combination or may not appear for months.

Food Interactions

Gemfibrozil is best taken on an empty stomach 30 minutes before meals but may be taken with food if it upsets your stomach. It is important that you follow your doctor's dietary instructions.

Usual Dose

1200 mg a day divided in 2 doses taken 30 minutes before breakfast and dinner.

Overdosage

There are no reports of gemfibrozil overdose. Victims may develop severe side effects. Overdose victims must be made to vomit with ipecac syrup—available at any pharmacy—to remove any remaining drug from the stomach. Call your doctor or poison control center before doing this. If you go to a hospital emergency room, ALWAYS bring the prescription bottle or container with you.

Special Information

Your doctor should perform periodic blood counts during the first year of gemfibrozil treatment to check for anemia or other blood effects. Liver-function tests are also necessary. Blood-sugar levels should be checked periodically while you are taking gemfibrozil, especially if you are diabetic or have a family history of diabetes.

Gemfibrozil may cause dizziness or blurred vision. Use caution while driving or doing anything else that requires concentration or alertness.

Call your doctor if side effects become severe or intolerable, especially diarrhea, nausea, vomiting, or stomach pain or gas. These may disappear if your doctor reduces the dosage.

If you forget to take a dose of gemfibrozil, take it as soon as you remember. If it is almost time for your next dose, skip the one you forgot and continue with your regular schedule. Do not take a double dose.

Special Populations

Pregnancy/Breast-feeding
There have been no gemfibrozil studies involving pregnant
women. However, this drug should be avoided if you are or
might be pregnant. When gemfibrozil is considered crucial by
your doctor, its potential benefits must be carefully weighed
against its risks.

Because of the tumor-stimulating effect of gemfibrozil,
nursing mothers who must take this drug should bottle-feed
their infants.

Seniors
Seniors may be more likely to develop side effects because
the drug primarily passes out of the body through the
kidneys, and kidney function declines with age.

Generic Name

Glatiramer (glah-TYE-ram-er)

Brand Name
Copaxone

Type of Drug
Anti-multiple-sclerosis agent.

Prescribed for
Relapsing-remitting multiple sclerosis (MS).

General Information
Glatiramer is a random mixture of several amino acids. It is
thought to work by modifying the immune processes responsible for MS, though no one knows specifically how it works.
In studies with glatiramer, people who took the drug over a
period of a year were twice as likely to be relapse-free as
people who took an inactive placebo (56% vs. 28%).

Cautions and Warnings
Do not use this drug if you are **allergic** to it or to mannitol.

About 10% of people who self-administer glatiramer injections experience a post-injection reaction with symptoms
that include **flushing, chest pain, heart palpitations, anxiety,**

breathing difficulties, closing of the throat, and **an itching rash**. These symptoms usually go away on their own and do not require special treatment. This reaction generally does not begin until after several months of glatiramer use, though it may occur earlier in treatment.

About half of the people who took glatiramer in drug studies had **chest pains**, but the exact relationship of these pains to glatiramer use could not be determined. Report any chest pain to your doctor at once.

Glatiramer may interfere with your normal **immune response**, increasing your sensitivity to infections and tumors that would normally be taken care of by your immune system. People using glatiramer may develop unusual immune responses, including the deposition of immune complexes in the kidney that can interfere with its function.

Possible Side Effects

In drug studies, groups taking glatiramer and groups taking an inactive placebo reported very similar side effects: rash, itching, sweating, nausea, and diarrhea.

▼ Most common: infections, weakness, pain, chest pain, flu symptoms, back pain, flushing, heart palpitations, anxiety, muscle stiffness or spasticity, feeling a need to urinate, swollen lymph glands, injection site reactions (including pain, inflammation, itching, an unknown mass at the injection site, welts, skin marks, and bleeding), breathing difficulties, runny nose, and joint pain.

▼ Common: fever, neck pain, facial swelling, bacterial infection, migraines, fever, rapid heartbeat, tremors, fainting, appetite loss, vomiting, general stomach disorders, vaginal infection, painful menstruation, black-and-blue marks, swelling in the arms or legs, bronchial irritation, spasm of the larynx, and ear pain.

▼ Less common: chills, cysts, agitation, foot drop, nervousness, rolling eyeballs, confusion, speech problems, cold sores, redness, itching rash, skin nodule, stomach pains and irritation, weight gain, and eye disorders.

▼ Rare: Other side effects associated with glatiramer can affect virtually any body system. Report any unusual reaction to your doctor.

Food and Drug Interactions

None known.

Usual Dose

Adults (age 18 and older): 20 mg per day, by injection under the skin.

Child: not recommended.

Overdosage

No information is available. Call your poison control center or hospital emergency room for instructions if an overdose occurs.

Special Information

Mix each vial of glatiramer only with the diluent supplied by the manufacturer.

Suggested injection sites are the arms, abdomen, hips, and thighs. Be sure to rotate injection sites.

Be sure to tell your doctor if you become pregnant while using glatiramer. If you are nursing, consult your doctor about bottle-feeding your baby while taking glatiramer.

If you forget your regular daily glatiramer injection, take it as soon as you remember. If it is almost time for your next dose, skip the dose you forgot and continue with your regular schedule. Do not take a double dose. Call your doctor if you miss more than 2 doses in a row.

Special Populations

Pregnancy/Breast-feeding

There is no information about the use of glatiramer during pregnancy. Pregnant women should discuss the possible risks and benefits of glatiramer with their doctor before taking it.

It is not known if glatiramer passes into breast milk. Nursing mothers who must take glatiramer should consider bottle-feeding their babies.

Seniors

Seniors may use glatiramer without special precaution.

Glucophage

see **Metformin**, *page 670*

Glucotrol XL

*see **Antidiabetes Drugs**, page 60*

Generic Name

Granisetron (gran-IS-eh-tron)

Brand Name

Kytril

Type of Drug

Antiemetic.

Prescribed for

Prevention of nausea and vomiting due to certain cancer chemotherapy treatments.

General Information

Granisetron hydrochloride, like ondansetron, produces its effect in a unique way. It antagonizes the receptor for a special form of the neurohormone serotonin, 5HT3. Receptors of this type are found in both the part of the brain that controls vomiting—the chemoreceptor trigger zone—and the vagus nerve in the stomach and intestines.

Women absorb granisetron faster than men, and they clear the drug more slowly from their bodies. This means that women will have more granisetron in their blood than men after taking the same dose, but this difference is not reflected in drug response.

Granisetron is extremely effective in preventing nausea and vomiting and works in many situations in which older antiemetics are ineffective.

Cautions and Warnings

Do not take granisetron if you are **allergic** or **sensitive** to it. People with **liver failure** break the drug down about half as quickly as others, but dosage adjustment is generally not required.

Possible Side Effects

▼ Most common: headache, nausea, weakness, and constipation.

▼ Less common: abdominal pains, liver inflammation, vomiting, diarrhea, high blood pressure, dizziness, sleeplessness, anxiety, tiredness, fever, appetite reduction, anemia, low white-blood-cell and platelet counts, and hair loss.

▼ Rare: low blood pressure, angina pain, fainting, rapid heartbeat, breathing difficulties, skin rash, intense itching, and shock.

Drug Interactions

None known.

Food Interactions

Food slightly decreases the amount of granisetron absorbed but does not affect your granisetron dose.

Usual Dose

Adult and Child (age 12 and older): 1 mg 2 times a day, given 1 hour before chemotherapy and then 12 hours later.

Child (under age 12): not recommended.

Overdosage

Little is known about granisetron overdose. Call your local poison control center or hospital emergency room for more information. If you go to the hospital for treatment, ALWAYS bring the prescription bottle or container with you.

Special Information

Call your doctor if you begin to have chest tightness, wheezing, trouble breathing, chest pains, or other unusual or severe side effects.

If you forget to take a dose of granisetron, take it as soon as you remember. If it is almost time for your next dose, skip the dose you forgot and continue with your regular schedule. Forgetting more than 1 dose may increase your chances of vomiting.

Special Populations

Pregnancy/Breast-feeding

Animal studies of granisetron have revealed no potential for birth defects. Nevertheless, when your doctor considers this drug crucial, its potential benefits must be weighed against its risks.

It is not known if granisetron passes into breast milk. Nursing mothers who take this drug should carefully observe their infants for possible side effects.

Seniors

Seniors may take this drug without restriction.

Generic Name

Guanabenz (GWAN-uh-benz) [G]

Brand Name

Wytensin

Type of Drug

Antihypertensive.

Prescribed for

High blood pressure.

General Information

Guanabenz acetate works by stimulating certain central nervous system receptors, which results in a general reduction of the level at which the nervous system is stimulated by the brain. Initially, guanabenz reduces blood pressure without a major effect on blood vessels; however, long-term chronic use of guanabenz may result in widening of blood vessels and a slight slowing of pulse rate. Guanabenz may be taken alone or together with a thiazide diuretic.

Cautions and Warnings

Do not take guanabenz if you are sensitive or **allergic** to it. People with severe **kidney or liver disease** should take this drug with caution.

Possible Side Effects

Side effects become more common and severe as your dose of guanabenz increases.

▼ Most common: drowsiness, sedation, dry mouth, dizziness, weakness, and headache.

▼ Less common: chest pain; swelling in the hands, legs, or feet; heart palpitations or abnormal heart rhythms; stomach or abdominal pain or discomfort; nausea; diarrhea; vomiting; constipation; anxiety; poor muscle control; depression; difficulty sleeping; stuffy nose; blurred vision; muscle aches and pains; breathing difficulties; frequent urination; impotence; unusual taste in the mouth; and swollen and painful breasts in men.

Drug Interactions

• The effect of guanabenz is increased by taking it together with other blood-pressure-lowering agents.

• The sedating effects of guanabenz are increased by combining it with tranquilizers, sleeping pills, or other nervous system depressants, including alcohol.

• People taking this drug for high blood pressure should avoid over-the-counter drugs that might aggravate their condition, including decongestants, cold and allergy remedies, and diet pills—all of which may contain stimulants. If you are unsure about which medications to avoid, ask your pharmacist.

Food Interactions

This drug is best taken on an empty stomach, but it may be taken with food if it upsets your stomach.

Usual Dose

4 mg twice a day to start; increased gradually to a maximum dose of 32 mg twice a day—although doses this large are rarely needed.

Overdosage

Guanabenz overdose causes sleepiness, lethargy, low blood pressure, irritability, pinpoint pupils, and reduced heart rate. Overdose victims should be made to vomit with ipecac syrup—available at any pharmacy—to remove any drug remaining in the stomach, but call your doctor or poison control center before inducing vomiting. If you must go to a hospital emergency room, ALWAYS bring the prescription bottle or container with you.

Special Information

Take guanabenz exactly as prescribed for maximum benefit. If any side effects become severe or intolerable, contact your doctor, who may need to reduce your dosage.

Guanabenz often causes tiredness or dizziness; avoid alcohol when taking this drug because alcohol tends to increase these effects. Take care when driving or doing anything else that requires concentration.

Do not stop taking guanabenz without your doctor's approval. Suddenly stopping this drug may cause a rapid increase—rebound—in blood pressure. Dosage must be gradually reduced by your doctor.

If you forget to take a dose of guanabenz, take it as soon as you remember. If it is almost time for your next dose, skip the one you forgot and continue with your regular schedule. Do not take a double dose. Call your doctor if you miss 2 or more consecutive doses.

Special Populations

Pregnancy/Breast-feeding

Reports of the effects of guanabenz in pregnant women have yielded are conflicting results. Because it may adversely affect the fetus, guanabenz should be avoided by women who are or might be pregnant. When guanabenz is considered crucial by your doctor, its potential benefits must be carefully weighed against itsits risks.

Nursing mothers should bottle-feed their babies if they must take guanabenz.

Seniors

Seniors are more sensitive to the sedating and blood-pressure-lowering effects of guanabenz. Follow your doctor's directions, and report any side effects at once.

Generic Name

Guanfacine (GWAWN-fuh-sene) Ⓖ

Brand Name

Tenex

Type of Drug

Antihypertensive.

Prescribed for

High blood pressure, heroin withdrawal, migraine headache, nausea, and vomiting.

General Information

Guanfacine hydrochloride works by stimulating a particular portion of the nervous system that dilates (widens) blood vessels. Because the studies of guanfacine were conducted only in people also taking a thiazide diuretic, it is recommended for use only in combination with a thiazide. Guanfacine's effect is long acting; it can be taken only once a day. Because drowsiness is a common side effect of guanfacine, it is usually taken at bedtime.

Cautions and Warnings

Do not use guanfacine if you are **allergic** to it. Guanfacine should be used with caution if you have **severe coronary insufficiency**, a **recent history of heart attack, blood vessel disease of the brain**, or **kidney or liver failure**. People with kidney disease should have their dosage adjusted because the drug passes out of the body primarily through the kidneys.

Guanfacine causes **sedation**, especially when it is first taken. Sedation increases with larger doses and is intensified by other nervous system depressants, including phenothiazine antipsychotic drugs, benzodiazepine sedatives and sleeping pills, and barbiturate sedatives and sleeping pills.

Abruptly stopping guanfacine may result in a rebound reaction consisting of anxiety, nervousness, and occasional increases in blood pressure. When rebound reactions occur with guanfacine, they happen 2 to 4 days after the drug is stopped. This is consistent with the fact that it takes longer for guanfacine to leave the body than clonidine or other similar drugs.

Possible Side Effects

Guanfacine may cause sedation, especially when treatment is first started. The frequency with which drowsiness occurs tends to increase with increased dosage, but this effect often becomes less severe as you continue to take the drug.

▼ Most common: drowsiness.

▼ Less common: heart palpitations, chest pain, slow heartbeat, abdominal pain, diarrhea, upset stomach, difficulty swallowing, nausea, memory loss, confusion, depression, loss of sex drive, runny nose, changes in sense of taste, ringing or buzzing in the ears, conjunctivitis (pinkeye), eye irritation, blurring and other visual disturbances, leg cramps, unusually slow movements, breathing difficulties, itching, rash, skin redness, sweating, testicle disorders, poor urinary control, feeling unwell, and tingling in the hands or feet.

▼ Rare: dry mouth, weakness, dizziness, headache, constipation, and sleeplessness.

Drug Interactions

• Alcohol or any other nervous system depressant will increase the sedative effects of guanfacine.

• Indomethacin, ibuprofen, and other nonsteroidal antiinflammatory drugs (NSAIDs) may decrease guanfacine's effectiveness. Stimulants, including those used in over-the-counter decongestants and diet pills, may counteract guanfacine's effect.

• Estrogen drugs may cause fluid retention, which increases blood pressure.

• Any drug that lowers blood pressure will increase the blood-pressure-lowering effect of guanfacine.

Food Interactions

Guanfacine may be taken with food if it upsets your stomach.

Usual Dose

Adult and Child (age 12 and over): 1–3 mg a day, taken at

bedtime. Doses above 3 mg a day are rarely used because side effects increase, whereas effectiveness does not.

Child (under age 12): not recommended.

Overdosage

Symptoms of guanfacine overdose are likely to be drowsiness, slow heartbeat, low blood pressure, and weakness. Overdose victims should be taken to a hospital emergency room. ALWAYS bring the prescription bottle or container with you.

Special Information

High blood pressure is usually a symptomless condition. Be sure to continue taking your medication even if you feel perfectly healthy. If the drug causes problems, do not stop taking it without your doctor's advice. Abruptly stopping guanfacine treatment may result in a rebound increase in blood pressure within 2 to 4 days.

Call your doctor if you develop breathing difficulties; slow heartbeat; extreme dizziness; dry mouth that lasts more than 2 weeks and is not relieved by gum, candy, or saliva substitutes; dry, itchy, or burning eyes; loss of sex drive; headache; nausea or vomiting; sleeping difficulties; unusual tiredness or weakness during the daytime; or any other persistent or intolerable side effect.

Be careful when performing tasks requiring concentration and coordination, because guanfacine may make you tired, dizzy, or light-headed.

Visit your doctor regularly to check on your progress and be sure to follow your doctor's directions for diet, salt restriction, and other lifestyle approaches.

Pay extra attention to dental hygiene while taking guanfacine. The dry mouth caused by the drug may make it easier for you to develop cavities and gum disease.

Guanfacine is generally taken at bedtime. If you forget to take a dose at night, you may take it the following morning, although it may make you tired during the day. If you do not remember until it is almost time for your next dose, skip the dose you forgot and continue with your regular schedule. Do not take a double dose. Call your doctor if you miss 2 or more consecutive doses.

Special Populations

Pregnancy/Breast-feeding

Animal studies indicate that high doses of guanfacine may be toxic to the fetus. This drug is not recommended to treat high blood pressure during pregnancy. Consult your doctor.

Guanfacine passes into animal breast milk, but it is not known if this is also true in humans. Nursing mothers who must take guanfacine should exercise caution.

Seniors

Seniors may be more sensitive to the sedative and blood-pressure-lowering effects of guanfacine because of age-related losses of kidney function. This factor should be taken into account by your doctor when determining your daily dosage of guanfacine.

Generic Name

Haloperidol (hal-oe-PER-ih-dol) G

Brand Name

Haldol

Type of Drug

Butyrophenone antipsychotic.

Prescribed for

Psychotic disorders, including Tourette's syndrome, for which it is sometimes combined with nicotine gum; severe behavioral problems in children; short-term treatment of hyperactive children; chronic schizophrenia; vomiting; treatment of acute psychiatric situations; and phencyclidine psychosis.

General Information

Haloperidol is one of many nonphenothiazine agents used in the treatment of psychosis. These drugs are equally effective when given in therapeutically equivalent doses. The major differences are in type and severity of side effects. Some people may respond well to one and not at all to another; this variability is not easily explained and is thought to result from inborn biochemical differences.

Haloperidol acts on a portion of the brain called the hypothalamus. It affects parts of the hypothalamus that control metabolism, body temperature, alertness, muscle tone, hormone balance, and vomiting and may be used to treat problems related to any of these functions. Haloperidol is available in liquid form for those who have trouble swallowing tablets.

Cautions and Warnings

Haloperidol should not be used by people who are **allergic** to it.

People with very **low blood pressure, Parkinson's disease**, or **blood, liver, or kidney disease** should avoid this drug.

If you have **glaucoma, epilepsy, ulcers,** or **difficulty urinating,** haloperidol should be used with caution and under strict supervision of your doctor.

Avoid **exposure to extreme heat** because this drug can upset your body's temperature-regulating mechanism.

Possible Side Effects

▼ Most common: drowsiness, especially during the first or second week of therapy. If the drowsiness becomes troublesome, contact your doctor.

▼ Less common: jaundice (yellowing of the whites of the eyes or skin), which may occur in the first 2 to 4 weeks. The jaundice usually goes away when the drug is discontinued, but there have been cases in which it did not. If you notice this effect, develop fever, or generally feel unwell, contact your doctor immediately. Other less common side effects are changes in components of the blood, including anemias; raised or lowered blood pressure; abnormal heartbeat; heart attack; and feeling faint or dizzy.

▼ Rare: neurological effects such as spasms of the neck muscles, severe stiffness of the back muscles, rolling back of the eyes, convulsions, difficulty in swallowing, and symptoms associated with Parkinson's disease. These effects seem very serious but disappear after the drug has been withdrawn; however, symptoms of the face, tongue, or jaw may persist for years, especially in seniors with a long history of brain disease. If you experience any of these effects, contact your doctor immediately. Haloperidol may cause an unusual increase in psychotic symptoms or may cause paranoid reactions, tiredness, restlessness, hyperactivity, confusion at night, bizarre dreams, inability to sleep, depression, euphoria

Possible Side Effects *(continued)*

(feeling high), itching, swelling, unusual sensitivity to bright light, red skin or rash, dry mouth, stuffy nose, headache, nausea, vomiting, appetite loss, change in body temperature, loss of facial color, excessive salivation, excessive perspiration, constipation, diarrhea, changes in urine and bowel habits, worsening of glaucoma, blurred vision, weakening of eyelid muscles, spasms of bronchial and other muscles, increased appetite, excessive thirst, and skin discoloration, particularly in sun-exposed areas. There have been cases of breast enlargement, false-positive pregnancy tests, changes in menstrual flow in females, and impotence and changes in sex drive in males.

Drug Interactions

• Be cautious about taking haloperidol with barbiturates, sleeping pills, narcotics or other tranquilizers, alcohol, or any other medication that may produce a depressive effect.

• Anticholinergic drugs may reduce the effectiveness of haloperidol and increase the risk of side effects.

• The blood-pressure-lowering effect of guanethidine may be counteracted by haloperidol.

• Taking lithium together with haloperidol may lead to disorientation or loss of consciousness. This combination may also cause uncontrolled muscle movements.

• Combining propranolol and haloperidol may lead to unusually low blood pressure.

• Blood concentrations of tricyclic antidepressant drugs may increase if they are taken together with haloperidol. This can lead to antidepressant side effects.

Food Interactions

Haloperidol is best taken on an empty stomach, but you may take it with food if it upsets your stomach.

Usual Dose

Adult: starting dose—0.5–2 mg 2 or 3 times a day. Your doctor may later increase your dose up to 100 mg a day, according to your needs. Seniors generally need smaller doses.

Child (age 3–12 or 33–88 lbs.): starting dose—0.5 mg a day. Dosage may be increased in 0.5-mg steps every 5–7 days until a satisfactory effect is realized.

Child (under age 3): not recommended.

Overdosage

Symptoms of overdose are depression, extreme weakness, tiredness, desire to sleep, coma, lowered blood pressure, uncontrolled muscle spasms, agitation, restlessness, convulsions, fever, dry mouth, and abnormal heart rhythm. The victim should be taken to a hospital emergency room immediately. ALWAYS bring the prescription bottle or container with you.

Special Information

This medication may cause drowsiness. Use caution when driving or operating hazardous equipment; also, avoid alcoholic beverages while taking it.

Haloperidol may cause unusual sensitivity to the sun. It may also turn your urine reddish-brown or pink.

If dizziness occurs, avoid sudden changes in posture and avoid climbing stairs. Use caution in hot weather. This medication may make you more prone to heat stroke.

If you forget to take a dose of haloperidol, take it as soon as you remember. Take the rest of the day's doses evenly spaced throughout the day. Do not take a double dose.

Special Populations

Pregnancy/Breast-feeding

Serious problems have been seen in pregnant animals given large amounts of haloperidol. Although haloperidol has not been studied in pregnant women, you should avoid this drug if you are or might be pregnant.

Haloperidol passes into breast milk. Nursing mothers who must use this medication should bottle-feed their babies to avoid the risk of side effects in their infants.

Seniors

Seniors are more sensitive to the effects of this medication and usually require ½ to ¼ the usual adult dose to achieve the desired results. Seniors are also more likely to develop side effects.

Brand Name

Helidac

Generic Ingredients

Bismuth Subsalicylate + Metronidazole + Tetracycline

Type of Drug

Antibacterial combination.

Prescribed for

Duodenal ulcers.

General Information

Revolutionary research into the causes of ulcers has shown that the bacteria known as *Helicobacter pylori* is nearly always present in ulcer disease and some forms of gastritis. This discovery has led to a major change in the treatment of these diseases. Drugs to treat the *H. pylori* infection are now prescribed along with a drug that alleviates ulcer symptoms by blocking stomach acid. Doctors have developed a variety of approaches to treating ulcers by using combinations of various antibiotic and acid-blocking drugs. Helidac combines 3 different drugs with antibacterial or antibiotic action, and it is generally prescribed together with ranitidine, cimetidine, or another acid blocker. Other treatments use other combinations of drugs.

Bismuth works against *H. pylori* by disrupting the bacteria's cell wall. Bismuth is also thought to prevent the bacteria from sticking to cells in the stomach lining. It may also prevent the bacteria from becoming resistant to some antibiotic therapies. The bismuth compound in Helidac is the same one found in the over-the-counter product Pepto-Bismol.

Metronidazole works well against certain kinds of bacteria that can survive with little or no oxygen. Inside a bacterial cell, metronidazole interferes with DNA duplication and prevents the bacteria from multiplying. The exact way it works against *H. pylori* is not known.

Tetracycline works by interfering with the bacteria's internal protein-manufacturing systems and it is effective in an acidic environment; it is very active against *H. pylori*.

Cautions and Warnings

Do not take Helidac if you are **sensitive** or **allergic** to any of its ingredients.

Bismuth has rarely caused severe **nervous-system toxicity**. Symptoms go away after the drug is stopped. Bismuth subsalicylate can cause **dark stools** or **darkening of the tongue**. This darkening of the stools is not dangerous; however, be aware that blood in the stool often manifests as blackening of the stool.

Children or teenagers who have or are recovering from chickenpox should not use Helidac because it contains a small amount of salicylate, which is related to aspirin. **Children or teenagers who take aspirin or a salicylate may develop Reye's syndrome,** symptoms of which include nausea and vomiting.

Metronidazole can cause **convulsive seizures** and nervous system effects—including **numbness or tingling in the arms, legs, hands, or feet.** The chance of developing these effects increases with the size of the dose and the length of time you take metronidazole. Call your doctor at once if you experience any of these effects while taking Helidac.

Metronidazole should be taken with caution by people who have had **blood diseases**. *Candida* infections may worsen while you are taking metronidazole. If this happens, your doctor may prescribe another medicine specifically for the *Candida*. People with **liver disease** break down metronidazole more slowly than other people and may require smaller doses.

Tetracycline should be avoided by people with severe **kidney disease**. Other infections, called **superinfections**, can develop while you are taking tetracycline. If this happens, your doctor will have you stop taking Helidac and prescribe a different drug to treat your *H. pylori*, as well as another drug to treat the superinfection. People taking tetracycline can develop pseudotumor cerebri (pressure inside the brain), the symptoms of which are usually headache and **blurred vision**. Symptoms usually go away when the drug is stopped, but permanent damage can result. Tetracycline may make you **unusually sensitive to the sun**. Use sunscreen and wear protective clothing while taking Helidac.

Possible Side Effects

For more information on possible side effects, see "Metronidazole" and "Tetracycline."

▼ Most common: nausea and diarrhea.

▼ Less common: abdominal pain, blood in the stool, anal discomfort, appetite loss, dizziness, tingling in the hands or feet, vomiting, muscle weakness, constipation, sleeplessness, pain, and respiratory infections.

Drug Interactions

• Tetracycline antibiotics, which are bacteriostatic, may interfere with the action of bactericidal (bacteria-killing) agents such as penicillin. You should not take both kinds of antibiotics for the same infection.

• Antacids, mineral supplements, and multivitamins containing bismuth, calcium, zinc, magnesium, and iron can reduce the effectiveness of tetracycline by interfering with its absorption into the bloodstream. Separate doses of your antacid, mineral supplement, vitamin with minerals, or sodium bicarbonate and Helidac by at least 2 hours—although the effect of this interaction is questionable in Helidac's case because the importance of an antibiotic's absorption into the blood in treating *H. pylori* is not known.

• Tetracycline and metronidazole may each increase the effect of anticoagulant (blood-thinning) drugs such as warfarin. Consult your doctor because an adjustment in the anticoagulant dosage may be required.

• Cimetidine, ranitidine, and other H_2 antagonists may reduce the amount of tetracycline absorbed into the bloodstream, thereby decreasing its effectiveness. The importance of this interaction is questionable because the importance of an antibiotic's absorption into the blood in treating *H. pylori* is not known.

• Cimetidine can interfere with the liver's ability to break down metronidazole, causing increased metronidazole levels in your blood. Your metronidazole dosage may be reduced if you are also taking cimetidine.

• Tetracycline may increase blood levels of digoxin in a small number of people, leading to possible digoxin side effects. In some people this interaction with digoxin can occur for months after tetracycline has been stopped. If you are taking this combination, watch carefully for digoxin side effects and call your doctor if any develop.

• Tetracycline may reduce diabetic insulin requirements. If you are using this combination, be sure to carefully monitor your blood-sugar level.

• Tetracycline may increase or decrease lithium blood levels. Metronidazole raises lithium blood levels, effects, and toxicity.

• Avoid alcoholic beverages: Interaction with metronidazole may cause abdominal cramps, nausea, vomiting, headaches, and flushing. Modification of the taste of alcoholic beverages has also been reported. Metronidazole should not be used if you are taking disulfiram (a drug used to maintain alcohol abstinence) because the combination can cause confusion and psychotic reactions.

• Phenobarbital and other barbiturates can increase the rate at which metronidazole is broken down, compromising its effectiveness.

• Drugs that cause nervous system toxicity, such as mexiletine, ethambutol, isoniazid, lincomycin, lithium, pemoline, quinacrine, and long-term high-dose pyridoxine (vitamin B_6) should not be taken with metronidazole because of the increased risk of nervous system side effects.

• Metronidazole may increase blood levels of phenytoin by interfering with its breakdown in the liver. This could increase the risk of phenytoin side effects; your doctor may need to adjust your phenytoin dosage.

Food Interactions

Do not take this drug with milk or milk products. Helidac should be taken with meals and at bedtime.

Usual Dose

Adult: Each dose consists of 4 pills. Take all 4 pills, 4 times a day for 14 days. Take your acid blocker according to your doctor's directions.

Child: not recommended.

Overdosage

All three ingredients in Helidac can be dangerous if taken in overdose, but salicylate poisoning is the most threatening. Symptoms of salicylate toxicity are rapid or heavy breathing, nausea, vomiting, ringing or buzzing in the ears, high fever, lethargy, rapid heartbeat, and confusion. Other more serious symptoms may develop. Overdose victims should be taken to a hospital emergency room at once for treatment. ALWAYS bring the prescription bottle or container with you.

Special Information

Each Helidac dose consists of 2 pink, round, chewable tablets (bismuth subsalicylate); 1 white tablet (metronidazole); and 1 pale orange and white capsule (tetracycline). Chew the 2 bismuth tablets and then swallow the other 2 pills with a full glass (8 oz.) of water. Take the acid blocker according to your doctor's directions.

Tetracycline can reduce the effectiveness of oral contraceptive drugs and you should use backup contraception while taking Helidac. Breakthrough bleeding is also possible.

Bismuth can cause a temporary darkening of your tongue or stool. This is a harmless effect. Stool darkening should not be confused with blood in the stool, which turns it black.

Avoid alcoholic beverages while you are taking any metronidazole product and for 1 day after you stop taking the drug.

Call your doctor if you develop ringing in the ears. This can be a sign of salicylate toxicity from the bismuth subsalicylate.

If you forget to take a dose of Helidac, take it as soon as you remember. If it is almost time for your next dose, skip the dose you forgot and continue with your regular schedule. Never take a double dose. If you have any doses left after 14 days, continue to take them at your regular times until you have used up all the medication. Call your doctor if you forget more than 4 doses in 14 days.

Special Populations

Pregnancy/Breast-feeding
Tetracycline affects bone and tooth development in the fetus. Helidac should not be taken by pregnant women.

Seniors
Seniors may take this medicine without special restriction.

Humulin 70/30

see **Insulin Injection**, page 516

Humulin N

see *Insulin Injection, page 516*

Humulin R

see *Insulin Injection, page 516*

Generic Name

Hydralazine (hye-DRAL-uh-zene) Ⓖ

Brand Names

Apresoline

Type of Drug

Antihypertensive.

Prescribed for

High blood pressure, aortic insufficiency after heart valve replacement, and congestive heart failure.

General Information

Although its mechanism of action is not completely understood, hydralazine hydrochloride is believed to lower blood pressure by enlarging blood vessels throughout the body. This also helps to improve heart function and blood flow to the kidneys and brain.

Cautions and Warnings

Long-term administration of more than 200 mg a day of hydralazine may produce the arthritis-like syndrome, **lupus erythematosus** (chronic condition affecting the body's connective tissue). Symptoms include muscle and joint pain, skin reactions, fever, and anemia, although they usually disappear when the drug is discontinued. Report any fever, chest pain, feelings of ill health, or other unexplained symptoms to your doctor. The chances of developing lupus increase with increased dosage; 10% to 20% of people taking 400 mg a day of hydralazine develop lupus.

Hydralazine may actually improve kidney blood flow and kidney function in people who have below-normal function. It should be used with caution in people with advanced **kidney damage**.

Hydralazine may worsen specific heart problems and should be used with care in people with a history of **heart disease**. It can cause angina pain and has been thought to cause heart attacks.

Tingling in the hands or feet caused by hydralazine may be relieved by taking pyridoxine (vitamin B_6).

People taking hydralazine may develop **reduced hemoglobin and red-blood-cell counts. Reduced white-blood-cell and platelet counts** may also occur. Periodic blood counts are recommended while taking hydralazine.

Possible Side Effects

▼ Most common: headache, appetite loss, nausea, vomiting, diarrhea, rapid heartbeat, and chest pain.

▼ Less common: stuffy nose, flushing, tearing of the eyes, itching or redness of the eyes, numbness or tingling in the hands or feet, dizziness, tremors, muscle cramps, depression, disorientation, anxiety, itching, rash, fever, chills, occasional hepatitis (symptoms include yellowing of the skin or whites of the eyes), constipation, urinary difficulties, and adverse effects on normal blood composition.

Drug Interactions

• Taking hydralazine with the beta blockers metoprolol or propranolol may result in increased blood levels of both hydralazine and the beta blocker.

• Indomethacin may reduce the effects of hydralazine.

• Do not use over-the-counter cough, cold, or allergy medications. These products often contain stimulant ingredients that can increase blood pressure.

Food Interactions

Take hydralazine with food.

Hydralazine may counteract the benefits of vitamin B_6, which can result in peripheral neuropathy (symptoms include tremors and tingling and numbness of the fingers, toes, or extremities). If these symptoms occur, your doctor may consider pyridoxine supplements.

Usual Dose

Adult: 40 mg a day for the first few days; increased to 100 mg a day for the rest of the first week. Dose then is increaseed until the maximum effect is seen. As with other antihypertensive drugs, dosage must be tailored to your individual needs.

Child: 0.34 mg per lb. of body weight a day; increased up to 200 mg a day.

Overdosage

If symptoms of extreme lowering of blood pressure, rapid heartbeat, headache, generalized skin flushing, chest pains, or poor heart rhythms develop, contact your doctor immediately. If you go to a hospital emergency room for treatment, ALWAYS bring the prescription bottle or container with you.

Special Information

Take hydralazine exactly as prescribed.

Call your doctor if you experience a prolonged period of unexplained tiredness, fever, muscle or joint aching, or chest pains while taking this drug.

If you forget to take a dose of hydralazine, take it as soon as you remember. If it is almost time for your next dose, skip the one you forgot and continue with your regular schedule. Do not take a double dose.

Special Populations

Pregnancy/Breast-feeding

Animal studies with high doses of hydralazine show that it causes birth defects, although they have not been reported in humans. Blood-related problems have been seen in newborns whose mothers took hydralazine during pregnancy. These problems got better on their own in 1 to 3 weeks. Women who are or might be pregnant should not take hydralazine unless its possible benefits have been carefully weighed against its risks.

Hydralazine passes into breast milk but has caused no problems in breast-fed infants.

Seniors

Seniors are more sensitive to the blood-pressure-lowering effects of hydralazine and to its side effects, especially low body temperature. Follow your doctor's directions and report any side effects at once.

Generic Name

Hydroxyzine (hye-DROK-suh-zene) Ⓖ

Brand Names

Anxanil	Hydroxyzine Pamoate
Atarax	Vistaril Ⓢ

Type of Drug

Antihistamine.

Prescribed for

Nausea, vomiting, anxiety, tension, agitation, itching caused by allergy, and sedation before or after general anesthetic; also prescribed in injectable form for acute adult psychiatric emergency including acute alcoholism, surgical sedation, and sedation before or after delivery.

General Information

Hydroxyzine is an antihistamine with muscle-relaxing, anti-emetic (preventing or alleviating nausea and vomiting), bronchial-dilation, pain-relieving, and antispasmodic properties. As such, hydroxyzine has been used to treat a variety of problems including stress related to dental or other minor surgical procedures, acute emotional problems, anxiety associated with stomach and digestive disorders, skin problems, and behavior difficulties in children. It is a relatively old drug and has been passed by for newer medications by most doctors, but it still works in a wide variety of situations.

Cautions and Warnings

Hydroxyzine should not be used if you are **sensitive** or **allergic** to it.

Possible Side Effects

Wheezing, chest tightness, and breathing difficulties are signs of a drug-sensitivity reaction.

Possible Side Effects *(continued)*

▼ Most common: dry mouth and drowsiness. These usually disappear after a few days of continuous use or when the dose is reduced.

▼ Rare: occasional tremors or convulsions at higher doses.

Drug Interactions

• Hydroxyzine has a depressive effect on the nervous system, producing drowsiness and sleepiness. It should not be used with alcohol, sedatives, tranquilizers, or other antihistamines or depressants. When hydroxyzine is taken with one of these drugs, the dose of the latter should be cut in half.

Food Interactions

Take hydroxyzine with food if it upsets your stomach.

Usual Dose

Adult: 25–100 mg 3–4 times a day.
Child (age 6 and over): 5–25 mg 3–4 times a day.
Child (under age 6): 5–10 mg 3–4 times a day.

Overdosage

The most common sign of overdose is sleepiness. Overdose victims should be taken to a hospital emergency room for treatment. ALWAYS bring the prescription bottle or container with you.

Special Information

Be aware of the depressive effect of hydroxyzine: Be careful when driving, operating hazardous machinery, or doing anything that requires concentration.

The dry mouth associated with taking hydroxyzine may increase your risk of dental cavities and decay. Pay attention to dental hygiene while taking this drug.

If you develop a drug-sensitivity reaction to hydroxyzine (see "Possible Side Effects"), call your doctor.

If you forget a dose of hydroxyzine, take it as soon as you remember. If it is almost time for your next dose, skip the one you forgot and continue with your regular schedule. Do not take a double dose.

Special Populations

Pregnancy/Breast-feeding

Antihistamines have not been proven to cause birth defects in humans. Animal studies have shown that regular treatment with hydroxyzine may cause birth defects during the first few months of pregnancy. Do not take any antihistamine without your doctor's knowledge if you are or might be pregnant. This is especially important during the last 3 months of pregnancy, because newborns may have severe reactions to antihistamines.

Hydroxyzine may reduce the amount of breast milk you produce. Small amounts of hydroxyzine may pass into breast milk and sedate a nursing infant. Nursing mothers who must take hydroxyzine should bottle-feed their infants.

Seniors

Seniors are more sensitive to side effects, such as confusion, difficult or painful urination, drowsiness, dizziness, feeling faint, nightmares or excitability, nervousness, restlessness, irritability, and dry mouth, nose, or throat.

Hytrin

see *Terazosin*, page 1049

Generic Name

Ibuprofen (EYE-bue-PROE-fen) G

Brand Names

Advil	Midol-IB
Arthritis Foundation	Motrin
Bayer Select Pain Relief Formula	Motrin Caplets
	Motrin IB
Children's Advil	Nuprin
Children's Motrin	Pediaprofen
IBU	Saleto

Type of Drug

Nonsteroidal anti-inflammatory drug (NSAID).

Prescribed for

Rheumatoid arthritis, osteoarthritis, mild to moderate pain, juvenile rheumatoid arthritis, sunburn, menstrual pain, and fever.

General Information

NSAIDs relieve pain and inflammation. We do not know exactly how they work, but part of their action may be due to their ability to inhibit the body's production of a hormone called prostaglandin as well as the action of other body chemicals, including cyclooxygenase, lipoxygenase, leukotrienes, and lysosomal enzymes. Most NSAIDs are broken down in the liver and eliminated through the kidneys. NSAIDs are absorbed into the bloodstream rapidly, but some work more quickly than others. Over-the-counter (OTC) doses of ibuprofen provide pain relief within 1 hour; however, significant anti-inflammatory effects are not usually seen at OTC dosage levels. Ibuprofen's anti-inflammatory effects occur with doses in the prescription range — 400 or more mg per dose — and take a week or more to manifest.

Cautions and Warnings

People **allergic** to ibuprofen or any other NSAID and those with a history of **asthma** attacks brought on by an NSAID, iodides, or aspirin should not take ibuprofen.

Ibuprofen may cause **gastrointestinal (GI) tract bleeding, ulcers,** and **perforation**. This can occur at any time, with or without warning, in people who take ibuprofen regularly. People with a history of **active GI bleeding** should be cautious about taking any NSAID. People who develop these symptoms and continue NSAID treatment should be aware of the possibility of developing more serious side effects.

Ibuprofen can affect platelets and **blood clotting** at high doses, and should be avoided by people with clotting problems and those taking warfarin.

People with **heart problems** who use ibuprofen may experience swelling in their arms, legs, or feet.

People taking ibuprofen, especially those with a **collagen disease** such as **systemic lupus erythematosus,** may experience an unusually severe drug-sensitivity reaction. Report any unusual symptoms to your doctor at once.

Ibuprofen may cause severe toxic effects to the **kidney**.

Report any unusual side effects to your doctor, who might need to periodically test your kidney function.

Ibuprofen may make you unusually sensitive to the effects of the sun.

Possible Side Effects

▼ Common: diarrhea; nausea; vomiting; constipation; minor stomach upset, distress, or gas, especially during the first few days of treatment.

▼ Less common: stomach ulcers, GI bleeding, appetite loss, hepatitis, gallbladder attacks, painful urination, poor kidney function, kidney inflammation, blood and protein in the urine, dizziness, fainting, nervousness, depression, hallucinations, confusion, disorientation, tingling in the hands or feet, light-headedness, itching, sweating, dry nose and mouth, heart palpitations, chest pain, breathing difficulties, and muscle cramps.

▼ Rare: severe allergic reactions including closing of the throat, fever and chills, changes in liver function, jaundice (yellowing of the skin and whites of the eyes), and kidney failure. These people must be treated in a hospital emergency room or doctor's office. NSAIDs have caused severe skin reactions; if this happens to you, see your doctor immediately.

Drug Interactions

• Ibuprofen may increase the effects of oral anticoagulant (blood-thinning) drugs such as warfarin. You may take this combination, but your doctor might have to adjust your anticoagulant dose.

• Ibuprofen may reduce the blood-pressure-lowering effect of beta blocker drugs.

• Combining ibuprofen with cyclosporine may increase the kidney-related side effects of both drugs.

• Ibuprofen may increase digoxin blood levels.

• Ibuprofen may increase phenytoin blood levels, leading to increased phenytoin side effects.

• Lithium blood levels may be increased in people taking ibuprofen.

• Methotrexate side effects may be increased in people also taking ibuprofen.

• Ibuprofen blood levels may be affected by cimetidine.

• Probenecid may interfere with the elimination of ibuprofen from the body, increasing the chances for NSAID side effect.

• Aspirin and other salicylates may decrease the amount of ibuprofen in your blood. These drugs should never be combined with ibuprofen.

Food Interactions

Take ibuprofen with food or a magnesium/aluminum antacid if it upsets your stomach.

Usual Dose

Adult: 200–800 mg 4 times a day depending on the condition being treated; follow your doctor's directions. 200 mg every 4–6 hours is appropriate for mild to moderate pain.

Child: juvenile arthritis — 9–18 mg per lb. of body weight a day, divided into several doses.

Overdosage

People have died from NSAID overdoses. The most common signs of overdose are drowsiness, nausea, vomiting, diarrhea, abdominal pain, rapid breathing, rapid heartbeat, sweating, ringing or buzzing in the ears, confusion, disorientation, stupor, and coma. Take the victim to a hospital emergency room at once for treatment. ALWAYS bring the prescription bottle or container with you.

Special Information

Take each dose with a full glass of water and do not lie down for 15 to 30 minutes afterward.

Ibuprofen may make you drowsy and/or tired: Be careful when driving or operating hazardous equipment. Do not take OTC products containing acetaminophen or aspirin while taking ibuprofen. Avoid alcoholic beverages.

Contact your doctor if you develop skin rash, itching, visual disturbances, weight gain, breathing difficulties, fluid retention, hallucinations, black stools, persistent headache, or any unusual or intolerable side effect.

If you forget to take a dose of ibuprofen, take it as soon as you remember. If you take several doses a day and it is within 4 hours of your next dose, skip the dose you forgot and continue with your regular schedule. Do not take a double dose.

Special Populations

Pregnancy/Breast-feeding

NSAIDs may cross into the blood circulation of the fetus. They have not been found to cause birth defects, but animal studies indicate that NSAIDs may affect a developing fetal heart during the last half of pregnancy. Women who are or might become pregnant should not take ibuprofen without their doctor's approval. When the drug is considered crucial by your doctor, its potential benefits must be carefully weighed against its risks.

NSAIDs may pass into breast milk but have caused no problems in breast-fed infants, except for seizures in a baby whose mother was taking the NSAID indomethacin. Other NSAIDs have caused problems in animal studies. There is a possibility that a nursing mother taking ibuprofen could affect her baby's heart or cardiovascular system. If you must take ibuprofen, bottle-feed your baby.

Seniors

Seniors, especially those with poor kidney or liver function, may be more susceptible to NSAID side effects.

Imdur

see *Isosorbide Dinitrate*, page 534

Generic Name

Imiquimod (ih-MIH-kwih-mod)

Brand Name

Aldara

Type of Drug

Immune modifier.

Prescribed for

Genital warts, perianal warts, and condyloma acuminata.

General Information

Imiquimod has no direct antiviral activity. Animal studies suggest that imiquimod stimulates the skin to produce cyto-kines, potent natural chemicals that fight the warts, but its actual effect on genital warts and condyloma is not known. Only minimal amounts of imiquimod are absorbed into the blood after it is applied to the skin. In studies of the drug, 50% of people who used it had complete clearance of their warts. But imiquimod is not a cure for genital warts — new ones may develop while others are being treated.

Cautions and Warnings

Do not use this product if you are **sensitive or allergic** to it.

Imiquimod has not been studied in other viral diseases of the skin, such as papilloma virus, and should not be used to treat them, since its effect is unknown.

Do not apply imiquimod to any area until it has healed from any previous drug or surgery. Imiquimod can worsen skin that is already inflamed.

Possible Side Effects

▼ Most common: redness, itching, erosion of the skin, burning, flaking, abrasions, swelling, and fungal infections in women.

▼ Common: pain, marks on the skin, ulcers, skin scabbing, and headache.

▼ Less common: skin soreness, flu-like symptoms, skin discoloration, muscle aches, fungal infections in men, and diarrhea.

Drug Interactions

• Do not apply imiqumod with other drugs that may cause irritation.

Usual Dose

Adult: Apply a thin layer of the cream to external warts and rub it in until the cream disappears. Leave on the skin for 6–10 hours, then remove the cream with mild soap and water. Do this 3 times a week — for example, Monday, Wednesday, and Friday. Continue treatment for up to 16 weeks or until the warts go away.

Child (under age 18): not recommended.

Overdosage

Overdose is not likely because such a small amount of imiquimod is absorbed through the skin. The most serious effect of swallowing imiquimod is low blood pressure. Anyone who has swallowed imiquimod should be taken to a hospital emergency room. ALWAYS bring the prescription bottle or container with you.

Special Information

Wash your hands before each application of imiquimod.

Most skin reactions are mild. If you develop a severe skin reaction to imiquimod, call your doctor and remove the cream with a mild soap and water. You can resume treatment with imiquimod after the reaction has completely subsided.

Imiquimod may weaken condoms and vaginal diaphragms. These birth control methods may prove undependable while you are using imiquimod cream. Avoid sexual contact while the cream is on your skin.

Uncircumcised men who use imiquimod to treat warts under the foreskin should retract the foreskin and cleanse the area every day.

Imiquimod is meant to be applied to the skin only. Do not let it get into your eyes, mouth, nose, or other mucous membranes.

Special Populations

Pregnancy/Breast-feeding

There is no information on the effect of imiquimod on pregnant women or nursing mothers. It is not known if imiquimod passes into breast milk. Do not use imiquimod without first discussing the possible risks and benefits with your doctor.

Seniors

Seniors may use this product without special precaution.

Imitrex

see **Sumatriptin**, page 1028

Generic Name

Indinavir (in-DIN-uh-vere)

Brand Name

Crixivan

Type of Drug

Protease inhibitor.

Prescribed for

Human immunodeficiency virus (HIV) infection.

General Information

Part of the multidrug cocktail responsible for the most important gains in the fight against acquired immunodeficiency
syndrome (AIDS), indinavir sulfate belongs to a group of
anti-HIV drugs called protease inhibitors. Triple-drug cocktails
are considered responsible for the first overall reduction in
the AIDS death rate, recorded in 1996. Protease inhibitors
work in a unique way but are not a cure for HIV infection or
AIDS. When the HIV virus attacks a cell, it must be converted
into viral DNA. Older drugs, known as reverse transcriptase
inhibitors, interfere with this step, but they need help in
fighting HIV. Protease inhibitors work at the end of the HIV
reproduction process, when proteins are "cut" into strands of
exactly the right size to duplicate HIV. The protein is cut by a
protease enzyme. Protease inhibitors prevent the mature HIV
virus from being formed by interfering with this cutting
process. Proteins that are cut to the wrong length or that
remain uncut are inactive.

Protease inhibitors are always taken with one or two
nucleoside antiviral drugs such as AZT, ddI, ddC, or 3TC.
Protease inhibitors revolutionized HIV treatment because,
when taken in combination, they reduce the amount of HIV
virus in the bloodstream to levels that are often undetectable
by current methods — CD_4 cell (immune system cell) counts
and viral load (amount of virus in the blood) measurements.
Multiple drug therapy has changed the current view of HIV
from a fatal disease to a manageable chronic illness.

People taking a protease inhibitor may still develop infections or other conditions associated with HIV disease. Be-

cause of this, it is very important for you to remain under the care of a doctor or other health care provider. The long-term effects of indinavir are not known. You may be able to pass the HIV virus to others even if you are on triple-drug therapy.

Cautions and Warnings

Do not take indinavir if you are **allergic** to it. People with mild or moderate **liver disease** or **cirrhosis** break down indinavir more slowly than those with normal liver function and may be more likely to develop side effects. People with cirrhosis should receive a reduced dose of indinavir.

About 4 of every 100 people taking indinavir can develop a **kidney stone,** indicated by pain in the middle to lower abdomen or back, or painful urination. Drinking at least 6 full glasses of liquid—48 oz.—a day will reduce your risk of developing a stone.

Indinavir may raise your blood sugar, worsen your **diabetes,** or bring out latent diabetes. Diabetics who take indinavir may have to have the dose of their antidiabetes medication adjusted against this effect.

Indinavir interferes with the liver's ability to break down terfenadine, astemizole, cisapride, triazolam, and midazolam. Do not combine indinavir with any of these drugs, as severe side effects may result.

Possible Side Effects

▼ Most common: nausea, abdominal pain, and headache.

▼ Common: weakness or fatigue, pain in the side, diarrhea, vomiting, changes in sense of taste, acid regurgitation, and sleeplessness.

▼ Less common: dizziness, drowsiness, and back pain.

▼ Rare: heart palpitations, chest pain, dizziness, chills, fever, anxiety, teeth grinding, excitement, rash, itching, body odor, flushing, sweats, appetite loss, mouth ulcers, bleeding gums, frequent urination, urinary infection or other problems, muscle pain, stiffness, coughing, bad breath, breathing difficulties, and visual difficulties.

Drug Interactions

• Rifampin stimulates the enzymes that break down indinavir, reducing the amount of indinavir in the blood. Do not combine these drugs.

• Indinavir interferes with the liver's ability to break down terfenadine, astemizole, cisapride, triazolam, and midazolam. Do not combine indinavir with any of these drugs, as severe side effects may result.

• Combining indinavir with clarithromycin or with zidovudine increases the amount of each drug in the blood. Combining indinavir with isoniazid increases the amount of isoniazid in the blood.

• Combining indinavir with rifabutin can reduce the amount of indinavir absorbed into the blood by ⅓ and double the amount of rifabutin absorbed.

• Didanosine (ddI) interferes with the absorption of indinavir into the body. If you need both of these medications, take them at least 1 hour apart.

• Combining fluconazole with indinavir reduces the amount of indinavir in the blood by about 20%.

• Combining indinavir with ketoconazole increases the amount of indinavir in the blood by about 65%.

• Combining indinavir with quinidine raises indinavir levels by about 10%.

• Taking indinavir with zidovudine and lamivudine results in ⅓ more zidovudine in the blood and small decreases in lamivudine blood levels.

• Indinavir raises the amount of stavudine absorbed into the blood by 25% and the amount of trimethoprim by about 20%.

• Combining indinavir with oral contraceptives can result in higher blood hormone levels. This may lead to an excess of hormone-related side effects. If this happens to you, your doctor may be able to lower the dose of your contraceptive pills.

Food Interactions

Indinavir is best taken with water — or liquids such as skim milk, juice, coffee — at least 1 hour before or 2 hours after a meal. Taking indinavir with a high-calorie, high-fat, and high-protein meal may interfere with indinavir's absorption into the blood. Because of this, you should not eat meals that are high in calories, fat, and protein from 1 hour before to 2 hours after taking indinavir. You may take indinavir with a light meal, such as: 1) unbuttered toast with jelly, apple juice, and coffee with or without skim milk and sugar, or 2) corn flakes with skim milk and sugar. What you eat at other times will not influence how indinavir is absorbed into the blood.

Usual Dose

Adult: 800 mg every 8 hours, around the clock. People with cirrhosis should take 600 mg every 8 hours.

Child: not recommended.

Overdosage

The consequences of an indinavir overdose other than severe drug side effects are not known. Take overdose victims to a hospital emergency room at once. ALWAYS bring the pre-scription bottle or container with you.

Special Information

Indinavir does not cure HIV. It will not prevent you from transmitting HIV to another person; you must still practice safe sex.

It is imperative to take your HIV medication exactly as prescribed. Missing doses of indinavir makes you more likely to become resistant to the drug and to lose the benefits of therapy.

Call your doctor if you develop pains in the middle to lower abdomen, back pain, or painful urination, because these may be signs of a kidney stone. Drink at least 48 oz. of liquid each day—for example, 6 8-oz. glasses a day. This may help prevent you from developing kidney pain or a kidney stone.

Stay in close touch with your doctor while taking indinavir and report anything unusual.

If you forget a dose of indinavir, take it as soon as you remember. If it is almost time for your next dose, skip the dose you forgot and continue with your regular schedule. Do not take a double dose.

Special Populations

Pregnancy/Breast-feeding

If you are or become pregnant while taking indinavir, talk to your doctor. There is little information on how indinavir affects pregnant women and their fetuses.

Nursing mothers who must take indinavir should bottle-feed their babies. In any case, nursing mothers who are HIV positive should bottle-feed their babies to avoid transmitting the virus through their milk. Because you must continue to take indinavir regularly for it to be effective, talk to your doctor or health care provider first.

Seniors
Seniors may take indinavir without special restriction.

Generic Name

Indomethacin (IN-doe-METH-uh-sin)

Brand Names

Indochron E-R   Indocin SR
Indocin

Type of Drug

Nonsteroidal anti-inflammatory drug (NSAID).

Prescribed for

Rheumatoid arthritis; osteoarthritis; ankylosing spondylitis; menstrual pain; tendinitis; bursitis; painful shoulder; gout — except Indocin SR; sunburn prevention and treatment; and migraine and cluster headache prevention — except Indocin SR. Indomethacin has been used to prevent premature labor, although prolonged use of this drug may affect development of the fetal heart and should be avoided. Indomethacin is also used in place of surgery to treat a rare condition in premature infants called patent ductus arteriosus, in which the heart is not fully formed. Topical indomethacin has been used in eyedrop form to treat a severe and unusual inflammation in the retina.

General Information

Indomethacin is one of 16 NSAIDs, which are used to relieve pain and inflammation. We do not know exactly how NSAIDs work, but part of their action may be due to their ability to inhibit the body's production of a hormone called prostaglandin as well as the action of other body chemicals, including cyclooxygenase, lipoxygenase, leukotrienes, and lysosomal enzymes. Indomethacin is absorbed into the bloodstream quickly. Pain relief comes about 30 minutes after taking the first dose of indomethacin and lasts for 4 to 6 hours, but its anti-inflammatory effect takes a week to become apparent and may take 2 weeks to reach maximum effect. Indomethacin is broken down in the liver and eliminated through the kidneys.

Cautions and Warnings

People **allergic** to indomethacin or any other NSAID and those with a history of **asthma** attacks brought on by an NSAID, iodides, or aspirin should not take indomethacin.

Indomethacin may cause **gastrointestinal (GI) bleeding, ulcers,** and **stomach perforation,** which can occur at any time, with or without warning, in people who take indomethacin regularly. People with a history of **active GI bleeding** should be cautious about taking any NSAID. People who develop bleeding or ulcers and continue NSAID treatment may develop more serious side effects.

Indomethacin may affect platelets and **blood clotting** at high doses, and should be avoided by people with clotting problems and by those taking warfarin.

People with **heart problems** who use indomethacin may experience swelling in their arms, legs, or feet.

Indomethacin should not be used by people who have had **ulcers** or other stomach lesions.

Indomethacin may worsen **depression** or other **psychiatric disorders, epilepsy,** and **parkinsonism**.

Indomethacin should never be used as "first therapy" for any disorder, with the possible exception of ankylosing spondylitis, because of the severe side effects associated with this drug.

Indomethacin may cause severe toxic effects to the **kidney**. Report any unusual side effects to your doctor, who might need to periodically test your kidney function.

Indomethacin may make you unusually sensitive to the effects of the sun.

Possible Side Effects

▼ Most common: diarrhea, nausea, vomiting, constipation, stomach gas, stomach upset or irritation, and appetite loss, especially during the first few days of treatment.

▼ Less common: stomach ulcers, GI bleeding, hepatitis, gallbladder attacks, painful urination, poor kidney function, kidney inflammation, blood and protein in the urine, dizziness, fainting, nervousness, depression, hallucinations, confusion, disorientation, tingling in the hands or feet, light-headedness, itching, increased sweating, dry

---

Possible Side Effects *(continued)*

nose and mouth, heart palpitations, chest pain, breathing difficulties, and muscle cramps.

▼ Rare: severe allergic reactions including closing of the throat, fever and chills, changes in liver function, jaundice (yellowing of the skin or whites of the eyes), and kidney failure. People who experience such effects must be promptly treated in a hospital emergency room or doctor's office. NSAIDs have caused severe skin reactions; if this happens to you, see your doctor immediately.

Drug Interactions

• Indomethacin may increase the effects of oral anticoagulant (blood-thinning) drugs such as warfarin. You may take this combination, but your doctor might have to reduce your anticoagulant dose.

• When combined with a thiazide diuretic, indomethacin may reduce the effect of the diuretic.

• Diflunisal increases the amount of indomethacin in your blood; this combination has resulted in fatal GI hemorrhage.

• Indomethacin may reduce the blood-pressure-lowering effect of beta blockers, angiotensin-converting enzyme (ACE) inhibitor drugs, and loop diuretics.

• Taking indomethacin with cyclosporine may increase the kidney-related side effects of both drugs. Methotrexate side effects may be increased in people also taking indomethacin.

• Indomethacin may increase digoxin levels in the blood.

• Combining indomethacin with phenylpropanolamine — found in many over-the-counter (OTC) drug products — may cause an increase in blood pressure.

• Combining indomethacin and dipyridamole may increase water retention.

• Indomethacin may increase phenytoin blood levels, leading to increased side effects. Lithium blood levels may be increased in people taking indomethacin.

• Indomethacin blood levels may be affected by cimetidine.

• Probenecid may interfere with indomethacin's elimination from the body, increasing the chances for indomethacin side effects.

• Aspirin and other salicylates may decrease the amount of indomethacin in your blood. These drugs should never be combined with indomethacin.

Food Interactions

Take indomethacin with a glass of water, food, or a magnesium/aluminum antacid to avoid an upset stomach.

Usual Dose

Adult and Child (age 15 and over): 50–200 mg a day, individualized to your needs.

Child (under age 15): not recommended.

Overdosage.

People have died from NSAID overdoses. The most common signs of overdose are drowsiness, nausea, vomiting, diarrhea, abdominal pain, rapid breathing, rapid heartbeat, increased sweating, ringing or buzzing in the ears, confusion, disorientation, stupor, and coma. Take the victim to a hospital emergency room at once. ALWAYS bring the prescription bottle or container with you.

Special Information

Take each dose with a full glass of water and do not lie down for 15 to 30 minutes afterward.

Indomethacin can make you drowsy and/or tired: Be careful when driving or operating hazardous equipment. Do not take any OTC products containing acetaminophen or aspirin while taking indomethacin. Avoid alcoholic beverages.

Contact your doctor if you develop skin rash or itching, visual disturbances, weight gain, breathing difficulties, fluid retention, hallucinations, black or tarry stools, persistent headache, or any unusual or intolerable side effect.

If you forget to take a dose of indomethacin, take it as soon as you remember. If you take indomethacin once a day and it is within 8 hours of your next dose, skip the dose you forgot and continue with your regular schedule. If you take several doses a day and it is within 4 hours of your next dose, skip the one you forgot and continue with your regular schedule. Never take a double dose.

Special Populations

Pregnancy/Breast-feeding

Indomethacin may cross into fetal blood circulation. It does not cause birth defects, but does affect the developing fetal heart if used during the second half of pregnancy. Pregnant women should not take indomethacin without their doctor's approval. When the drug is considered crucial by your doctor, its potential benefits must be carefully weighed against its risks.

Indomethacin may pass into breast milk but has caused few problems in breast-fed infants, except for seizures in a baby whose mother was taking it. There is a possibility that the heart of a nursing baby could be affected by indomethacin received in breast milk. Nursing mothers who must take indomethacin should bottle-feed their babies.

Seniors

Seniors may be more susceptible to indomethacin side effects, especially ulcer disease.

Generic Name

Insulin Injection (IN-suh-lin)

Most Common Brand Names

Humulin N (NPH insulin)	Humulin 70/30 (NPH +
Humulin R (regular insulin)	regular insulin)

Type of Drug

Antidiabetic.

Prescribed for

Type I (insulin-dependent) diabetes mellitus and type II (non-insulin-dependent) diabetes mellitus that cannot be controlled by diet. Insulin may also be used in a hospital, together with glucose injection, to treat hyperkalemia (high blood-potassium levels). It is also used for severe complications of diabetes, including ketoacidosis (diabetic coma).

General Information

Insulin is a complex hormone normally produced by the pancreas. Diabetes develops when the body does not make enough insulin or when the insulin does not work. At one time, most of the insulin used as a drug was obtained from animals. Today, human insulin manufactured by biosynthetic techniques is most often used. Animal insulin used for injection is the unmodified material derived from an animal source, usually beef or pork.

Insulin derived from pork is closer in chemical structure to our own insulin than that derived from beef, and causes fewer allergic reactions. Synthetic human insulin, however, is identical in structure to the insulin we make in our bodies. Human insulin may act more quickly and last a shorter time than pork insulin in some people. Human insulins may also be produced by semisynthetic processes, but these semisynthetic insulins start with an animal product and may contain some of the same impurities. People whose diabetes is well controlled by insulin derived from an animal source should not automatically be switched to a human insulin product, but new diabetics are usually treated with highly purified synthetic human insulin. Human insulin is the product of choice for (1) people allergic to other insulin products, (2) all pregnant diabetic women, (3) people who need insulin only during surgery or for short periods of time, and (4) all newly diagnosed diabetics.

Regular insulin starts to work quickly and lasts only 6 to 8 hours. People using only insulin injection must take several injections per day. Pharmaceutical scientists have been able to add other chemical structures onto the insulin molecule to extend the time over which the drug works. Prompt Insulin Zinc Suspension — also called Semilente Insulin — like insulin for injection, is considered rapid-acting. It starts to work in 30 to 60 minutes and lasts 12 to 16 hours.

The intermediate-acting insulins — NPH or Isophane Insulin and Lente or Insulin Zinc Suspension — start working 1 to 2 ½ hours after injection and continue to work for 24 hours. Long-acting insulins — PZI or Protamine Zinc Insulin Suspension and Ultralente or Extended Insulin Zinc Suspension — begin working 4 to 8 hours after injection and last for 36 hours or more. Other factors that have a definite influence on insulin response include diet, exercise, and other drugs being used.

Insulin products derived from natural sources contain a number of normal contaminants. In the 1970s, processes were developed to remove many of these contaminants. The first process resulted in single-peak insulin, making the action of the drug more predictable and safer. Today, all insulin sold in the U.S. is single-peak, and most of that is identical to natural human insulin. The second refinement resulted in purified insulin, which produces fewer reactions at the injection site than single-peak insulin.

Cautions and Warnings

Be sure to take the **exact dose** of insulin your doctor prescribed. Too much insulin will excessively lower blood sugar, and too little will not control the diabetes. **Do not change insulin brands** or types unless you are under direct medical supervision. Diabetics taking insulin must **follow the prescribed diet** and should **avoid alcoholic beverages**.

Low blood sugar (see "Overdosage" for symptoms) can result from taking too much insulin, doing excess physical work or exercise without eating, not absorbing food normally because meals are postponed or skipped, or because of illness with vomiting, fever, or diarrhea. Often, you can correct the situation by consuming sugar, food with sugar, or a commercial 40% glucose product. The **symptoms of low blood sugar** are less pronounced if you are taking human insulin rather than an animal insulin, but the possible consequences are just as dire.

Possible Side Effects

▼ Most common: allergic reactions, breakdown of fat tissue at the site of injection causing a depression in the skin, and accumulation of fat under the skin from using the same site for many insulin injections.

Drug Interactions

• Your insulin dosage may need to be raised if you are taking drugs that increase blood-sugar levels. These include corticosteroids, oral contraceptives, dextrothyroxine, diltiazem, dobutamine, epinephrine, cigarettes, thiazide-type diuretics, thyroid hormones, estrogens, furosemide, molindone, phenytoin, and ethacrynic acid.

• Other drugs can lower blood sugar and may require a reduced insulin dosage. These include alcohol, anabolic steroids, beta-blocking drugs, clofibrate, fenfluramine, phenylbutazone, sulfinpyrazone, tetracycline, guanethidine, monoamine oxidase inhibitor (MAOI) antidepressants, and large doses of aspirin.

• Oral antidiabetes drugs also lower blood sugar and should be taken with insulin only under the direct supervision of a doctor. Nonsteroidal anti-inflammatory drugs (NSAIDs) may also increase the blood-sugar-lowering effect of insulin, but by a different mechanism.

• Beta-blocking drugs can mask the symptoms of low blood sugar and thus increase the risk of taking insulin.

• Quitting smoking, using a nicotine patch or gum, or taking other smoking deterrents can also lower blood sugar by increasing the amount of insulin that is absorbed after injection under the skin. Lowering insulin dose may be necessary if you stop smoking.

• Insulin may affect blood-potassium levels and can affect digitalis drugs.

Food Interactions

Follow your doctor's directions for diet restrictions. Diet is a key element in controlling your disease.

Usual Dose

The dose and kind of insulin must be individualized to your specific need. Insulin is generally injected a half hour before meals; the longer-acting forms are taken a half hour before breakfast. Since insulin can be given only by injection, diabetics must learn to give themselves their insulin subcutaneously (under the skin) or have a family member or friend give them injections. Hospitalized patients may receive insulin injection directly into a vein.

One manufacturer has developed a device to aid in injecting insulin. The device looks like a pen and is easily used. Another type of injection convenience device is the insulin-infusion pump. The pump automatically administers a predetermined amount of regular insulin. Consult your doctor or pharmacist for complete details on either of these devices.

Overdosage

If swallowed, insulin has little or no effect, because it is not absorbed into the blood. Injecting too much insulin will cause an insulin reaction or low blood sugar. Symptoms come suddenly and include weakness, fatigue, nervousness, confusion, headache, double vision, convulsions, dizziness, psychoses, unconsciousness, rapid shallow breathing, numbness or tingling around the mouth, hunger, nausea, loss of skin color, dry skin, and pulse changes. Overdose victims should eat chocolate, candy, or another sugar source at once to raise blood-sugar levels.

The symptoms of an insulin reaction are different from those of ketoacidosis coma. Insulin coma comes on in hours or days; the symptoms are drowsiness, dim vision, a feeling that you cannot get enough air, thirst, nausea, vomiting, breath that smells like acetone (nail polish remover), abdominal pains, loss of appetite, dry and red skin, and rapid pulse. Call your doctor immediately if either of these groups of symptoms occur.

Special Information

Use the same brand and strength of insulin and insulin syringes or administration devices to avoid dosage errors. Rotate injection sites to prevent fat loss at the site.

Combine insulins according to your doctor's directions; do not change the mixing method or the mixing order.

You may develop low blood sugar if you take too much insulin, work or exercise more strenuously than usual, skip a meal, take insulin too long before a meal, or vomit before a meal. Signs of low blood sugar may be fatigue, headache, drowsiness, nausea, tremulous feeling, sweating, or nervousness. If you develop any of these signs while taking insulin, your blood sugar may be too low. The usual treatment for low blood sugar is eating a candy bar or lump of sugar, which diabetics should carry with them at all times. If the signs of low blood sugar do not clear up within 30 minutes, call your doctor. You may need further treatment.

Your insulin requirements may change if you get sick, especially if you vomit or have a fever.

If your insulin is in suspension form, you must evenly distribute the particles throughout the liquid before taking the dose out. Do this by gently rotating the vial and turning it over several times. Do not shake the vial.

Diabetics must pay special attention to dental hygiene because of their increased chance of developing oral infections. Also, your dentist may detect other signs of advancing diabetes during an examination. Be sure your dentist knows you have diabetes.

Have your eyes checked regularly. One of the primary complications of diabetes—blood-vessel disease—may be seen by an eye doctor during a routine eye examination.

Read and follow all patient information provided with the

insulin products you are using. Monitor your blood and urine regularly for sugar and ketones, using over-the-counter testing products.

Insulin products are generally stable at room temperature for about 2 years. They must be kept away from direct sunlight and extreme temperatures. Most manufacturers, however, still recommend that insulin be stored in a refrigerator or another cool place whenever possible. Insulin should not be put in a freezer or exposed to very high temperatures; this can affect its stability. Partly used vials of insulin should be thrown away after several weeks if not used. Do not use any insulin that looks lumpy or grainy or that sticks to the bottle. Regular insulin should be clear and colorless; do not use it if it is thick or cloudy.

Some insulin products can be mixed. Mix 2 or more different insulins only if you have been so directed by your doctor. Your pharmacist may also mix your insulins to ensure accuracy. Insulin for injection may be mixed with Isophane Insulin Suspension and Protamine Zinc Insulin in any proportion. Insulin Zinc Suspension, Insulin Zinc Suspension (Prompt), and Insulin Zinc Suspension (Extended) may also be mixed in any proportion. Insulin for injection and Insulin Zinc Suspension must be mixed immediately before using.

If you forget a dose of insulin, take it as soon as you remember. If it is almost time for your next dose, or if you completely forget one or more doses, call your doctor for exact instructions.

Special Populations

Pregnancy/Breast-feeding
Insulin is the preferred method for controlling diabetes in pregnant women, though pregnancy usually complicates the process. Pregnant diabetic women must follow their doctor's directions for insulin use exactly, because insulin requirements normally decrease during the first half of pregnancy and then increase to more than normal requirements during the second half. Pregnant women who must take insulin injections should use human insulin.

Insulin does not pass into breast milk. Breast-feeding can reduce your insulin needs, despite the need for more calories. Your doctor should closely monitor your insulin dosage during this period.

Seniors
Seniors may use insulin without special restriction. Follow your doctor's directions for medication and diet.

Generic Name

Interferon Beta (in-ter-FEER-on bay-tuh)

Brand Names

Avonex   Betaseron

Type of Drug

Multiple sclerosis (MS) therapy.

Prescribed for

MS.

General Information

MS is an inflammatory disease in which protective central-nervous-system myelin sheaths are broken down by immune-system abnormalities. This leads to gradual and progressive loss of muscle tone and function, progressive weakness, and paralysis. Exacerbations—episodes of MS in which the disease worsens—develop slowly and may not recede for weeks or months. Interferon beta drugs are used to treat patients with the relapsing-remitting form of the disease. About 66% of MS sufferers have the relapsing-remitting form, in which stable periods are followed by periods of worsening. Until now, MS treatment has been aimed at controlling symptoms of the disease. Interferon beta is a biotechnological product that has been found to help reduce the number and severity of MS flare-ups. It shares anti-tumor, antiviral, and other actions with other interferons but has a greater effect on the immune system.

Interferon beta is the first drug to be approved for any form of MS. Studies will continue to investigate whether interferon beta may slow or prevent the worsening of MS. Nobody knows how this drug produces its effect.

Interferon beta is also being studied for AIDS, AIDS-related Kaposi's sarcoma, metastatic renal-cell cancer, herpes of the lips or genitals, malignant melanoma, skin cancer, and acute non-A, non-B hepatitis.

Avonex contains interferon beta-1a. Betaseron contains interferon beta-1b.

Cautions and Warnings

Do not take interferon beta if you are **allergic** to either form of the drug or to human albumin.

The safety and benefit of interferon beta in chronic progressive MS is unproven.

People taking interferon beta in drug studies have had potentially severe **depression and suicidal tendencies**. But depressive feelings or tendencies are generally more common among people with MS, and those not taking interferon beta in the studies also experienced depression, so the drug was judged not to be the cause of depression. Report depression or other other psychological symptoms to your doctor.

People with **seizure disorders** may be more likely to develop a seizure while taking interferon beta.

Up to 75% of people who take interferon beta are likely to develop flu-like symptoms including fever, chills, muscle aches, sweating, and feeling unwell. These symptoms may prove stressful to people with **heart disease**.

Interferon beta may cause **sensitivity to the sun**. Wear protective clothing and use sunscreen.

Possible Side Effects

In general, interferon beta-1a has fewer side effects than interferon beta-1b. The risk of experiencing a side effect is also less with the beta-1a form.

Interferon Beta-1a

▼ Most common: respiratory infection, sinusitis, headache, fever, weakness, chills, dizziness, muscle aches, abdominal pain, flu-like symptoms, painful menstruation, diarrhea, nausea, upset stomach, and sleeping difficulties.

▼ Less common: swelling, pelvic pain, cyst, thyroid goiter, heart palpitations, bleeding, laryngitis, breathing difficulties, joint pain, stiffness, tiredness, speech problems, convulsions, uncontrolled movements, hair loss, urinary urgency, and cystitis. Pain, burning, or stinging at the injection site may also occur.

▼ Rare: Other effects may occur in virtually any part of the body. Report these reactions to your doctor.

Interferon Beta-1b

▼ Most common: pain, burning, or stinging at the injection site, sinusitis, headache, migraine, fever, weakness, chills, muscle ache, abdominal pain, flu-like

Possible Side Effects *(continued)*

symptoms, menstrual disorders, painful menstruation, constipation, vomiting, liver inflammation, sweating, and reduced white-blood-cell count.

▼ Less common: itching, swelling, pelvic pain, cyst, thyroid goiter, heart palpitations, high blood pressure, rapid heartbeat, bleeding, laryngitis, breathing difficulties, muscle weakness, stiffness, tiredness, speech problems, convulsions, uncontrolled movements, visual disturbances or conjunctivitis (pinkeye), urinary urgency, cystitis, breast pain, cystic breast disease, beast cancer, and weight changes.

▼ Rare: Other effects may occur in virtually any part of the body. Report these reactions to your doctor.

Food and Drug Interactions

None known.

Usual Dose

Interferon Beta-1a: 30 mcg once a week by intramuscular injection.

Interferon Beta-1b: 8 million units—250 mcg—every other day by subcutaneous injection.

This drug may be self-administered at home in much the same way as are insulin injections.

Overdosage

Interferon Beta-1b: The effects of interferon beta-1b overdose are unknown. Symptoms are most likely to be exaggerated side effects. Call your doctor or poison control center for more information.

Special Information

Interferon Beta-1a: Interferon beta-1a may be associated with severe depression. Mood swings or changes, lack of interest in daily activities, excessive sleep, and other possible signs of depression should be reported to your doctor at once.

Interferon beta-1a injections should be taken at the same time each week to establish them as part of your normal routine. If you forget a dose of interferon beta-1a, take it as soon as you remember. If it is almost time for your next dose, skip the one you forgot and continue with your regular schedule. Do not take a double dose.

Interferon Beta-1b: Interferon beta-1b may be associated with sever depression. Mood swings or changes, lack of interest in daily activities, excessive sleep, and other possible signs of depression should be reported to your doctor at once.

Interferon beta-1b injections should be taken at the same time each day to establish them as part of your daily routine. If you forget to take a dose of interferon beta-1b, take it as soon as you remember. If it is almost time for your next dose, skip the one you forgot and continue with your regular schedule. Do not take a double dose.

Special Populations

Pregnancy/Breast-feeding
Though animal studies show that either type of interferon beta may cause abortion, the effect of interferon beta on humans is unknown. Do not take interferon beta if you are or might be pregnant.

It is not known if interferon beta passes into breast milk. Nursing mothers should consider bottle-feeding their babies. Exercise caution with all medication.

Seniors
Seniors may use this medication without special restriction.

Generic Name

Ipratropium (ipe-ruh-TROE-pee-um)

Brand Name
Atrovent

Type of Drug
Anticholinergic.

Prescribed for
Bronchospasm that is part of chronic lung diseases, such as bronchitis and emphysema; also prescribed for runny nose from allergies or the common cold.

General Information

Ipratropium bromide is chemically related to atropine sulfate, another anticholinergic drug. After ipratropium is inhaled, it works against acetylcholine in the bronchial muscles, causing them to dilate. Ipratropium works principally on the bronchial muscles and has little effect on other parts of the body, an advantageous characteristic that reduces the risk of side effects. Much of each inhaled dose is swallowed and passes out of the body in the stool. Like all anticholinergic drugs, ipratropium has a drying effect; the nasal spray provides relief from runny nose.

Cautions and Warnings

Do not use ipratropium if you are **allergic** to atropine or to any related product. It should be used with caution if you have **glaucoma, prostate disease,** or **bladder obstruction**.

Ipratropium is not meant for the treatment of acute bronchospasm where rapid response is needed. This drug should be used only to prevent bronchospasm associated with chronic lung diseases.

Possible Side Effects

Generally, ipratropium side effects are infrequent and mild.

Inhalation

▼ Most common: nervousness, dizziness, headache, nausea, upset stomach, blurred vision, sensitivity to bright light, dry mouth, throat irritation, cough, worsening of symptoms, heart palpitations, rash, and mouth irritation.

▼ Less common: rapid heartbeat, urinary difficulties, tingling in the hands or feet, poor coordination, itching, hives, flushing, loss of hair, constipation, tremors, fatigue or sleeplessness, and hoarseness.

▼ Rare: worsening of glaucoma, eye pain, low blood pressure, and severe skin reactions.

Nasal Spray

▼ Most common: nosebleeds and nasal dryness.

▼ Less common: dry mouth or throat and stuffed nose.

▼ Rare: changes in sense of taste, nasal burning, red

> **Possible Side Effects** *(continued)*
>
> and itchy eyes, coughing, dizziness, hoarseness, heart palpitations, rapid heartbeat, thirst, ringing or buzzing in the ears, blurred vision, and difficulty urinating.

Drug Interactions

None known.

Food Interactions

Do not inhale a dose of ipratropium if you have any food in your mouth.

Usual Dose

Inhalation
   Adult and Child (age 12 and over): 2 inhalations — 36 mcg — 4 times a day; no more than 12 inhalations every 24 hours.
   Child (under age 12): not recommended.

Nasal Spray:
   Adult and Child (age 12 and over): 2 sprays of 0.03% solution per nostril 2–3 times a day or 2 sprays of 0.06% solution per nostril 3–4 times a day.
   Child (under age 12): not recommended.

Overdosage

The risk of overdose is small because very little ipratropium is absorbed into the bloodstream. Ipratropium accidentally sprayed into the eye will cause blurred vision. ALWAYS bring the prescription bottle or container with you if you go to an emergency room for treatment.

Special Information

Use this product according to your doctor's instructions. Since the long-term use of ipratropium may reduce the number of bronchial attacks you experience, you may feel that you have gotten better and no longer need the drug. Do not stop taking ipratropium without your doctor's approval.
   Call your doctor if you develop rash or hives, sores on the mouth or lips, blurred vision, or other side effects that are bothersome or persistent.
   Call your doctor if you stop responding to your usual dose

of ipratropium: This may be a sign that your condition has worsened and requires reevaluation.

Prolonged use of ipratropium may decrease or stop the flow of saliva produced in your mouth. This can expose you to an increased chance of cavities, gum disease, oral infections, and other problems. Dry mouth can be relieved with hard candies or regular fluids. Increased attention to dental hygiene is important.

If, in addition to ipratropium, you take a corticosteroid inhaler or cromolyn sodium for your lung disease, use the ipratropium about 5 minutes before the other inhaler.

If you take ipratropium and albuterol, metaproterenol, or another beta-stimulating aerosol product for your bronchial disease, use the beta stimulator about 5 minutes before ipratropium, unless otherwise instructed by your doctor. Ipratropium solution for inhalation can be mixed with albuterol or metaproterenol for inhalation so long as the mixture is used within 1 hour.

The first use of the ipratropium nasal pump requires 7 pumps to prime the spray. Regular use of the spray should prevent the need to prime the pump again. If you do not use the spray for a day, you will have to pump twice to prime the spray. If you do not use the spray for a week, you will have to prime the spray with 7 pumps.

If you forget to take a dose of ipratropium, take it as soon as you remember. If it is almost time for your next dose, skip the one you forgot and continue with your regular schedule. Do not take a double dose.

Store this product at room temperature—59 to 86°F—and avoid freezing. Unused vials of the solution for inhalation should be stored in their foil wrapper.

Special Populations

Pregnancy/Breast-feeding

Massive oral doses of ipratropium have caused birth defects in animals, but there is no information to indicate that the drug would have the same effect if used by pregnant women. Ipratropium should be used during pregnancy only if clearly needed.

It is not known if ipratropium passes into breast milk, but it is unlikely that enough ipratropium would be absorbed to affect a nursing infant. Nevertheless, nursing mothers who take this drug should observe their infants for side effects.

Seniors
Seniors, especially those with prostate disease, may be more sensitive to the side effects of this drug and may require a dosage adjustment.

Generic Name

Irbesartan (er-bih-SAR-tan)

Brand Name

Avapro

Type of Drug

Angiotensin II-receptor (A-II) antagonist.

The information in this profile also applies to the following drug:

Generic Ingredient: Eprosartan
Teveten

Prescribed for

Hypertension (high blood pressure).

General Information

Irbesartan is a member of a relatively new class of drug products for hypertension called A-II antagonists. These drugs work by interfering with special sites in blood vessels and other tissue where angiotensin II, a potent hormone that normally works as part of the body's system for maintaining blood pressure, exerts its effect. The effect of irbesartan is improved by taking it with a thiazide-type diuretic (agent that increases urination) but may be combined with other antihypertensives as well. A fixed combination of irbesartan and hydrochlorthiazide, a diuretic, was approved at the same time as was irbesartan but has not yet been marketed. Do not confuse A-II antagonists with the many angiotensin-converting enzyme (ACE) inhibitors that are in use today; they interrupt the body's production of angiotensin II.

Cautions and Warnings

Do not take irbesartan if you are **sensitive or allergic** to it.

People who are **dehydrated** or who suffer from salt depletion should receive a lower dosage of irbesartan.

Possible Side Effects

In studies the risk of experiencing side effects was less in people taking irbesartan than in those taking a placebo (sugar pill).

▼ Less common: diarrhea, upset stomach or heartburn, muscle pain, tiredness, upper respiratory infection, abdominal pain, anxiety or nervousness, chest pain, swelling, dizziness, headache, sore throat, runny nose, nausea, vomiting, rash, rapid heartbeat, and urinary infection.

▼ Rare: low blood pressure and fainting. Other effects may occur in almost any part of the body.

Drug Interactions

• Irbesartan may interfere with the breakdown of certain drugs in the liver. Studies of irbesartan have shown no important interactions with hydrochlorothiazide, digoxin, warfarin, or nifedipine.

Food Interactions

You may take irbesartan without regard to food or meals.

Usual Dose

Adult: starting dosage—150 mg once a day. Dosage may be increased to 300 mg once a day if necessary. A lower dosage of 75 mg may be prescribed for people who are dehydrated or who suffer from salt depletion.

Child: Irbesartan has not been studied in children under age 18 and should not be given to young children.

Overdosage

Little is known about irbesartan overdose. Dosages of 900 mg a day for 8 weeks have been well tolerated. Lethal animal dosages of this drug are 25 to 50 times the maximum human dosage. Symptoms of irbesartan overdose may include very low blood pressure and rapid heartbeat; very slow heartbeat may also occur. Overdose victims should be taken to a hospital emergency room for evaluation and treatment. ALWAYS bring the prescription bottle or container with you.

Special Information

If you become dizzy or faint while taking irbesartan, lie down face up and call your doctor at once.

The effect of irbesartan is the same in men and women and in African American and Caucasian patients.

No dosage adjustments are needed for people who have kidney or liver disease.

Avoid strenuous exercise or very hot weather because excessive sweating or dehydration may cause a rapid drop in blood pressure.

Avoid over-the-counter diet pills, decongestants, and stimulants that may raise blood pressure.

If you forget to take a dose of irbesartan, take it as soon as you remember. If it is almost time for your next dose, skip the one you forgot and continue with your regular schedule. Do not take a double dose.

Special Populations

Pregnancy/Breast-feeding

A-II antagonists including irbesartan should not be taken during the last 6 months of pregnancy because they may cause fetal injury. This does not appear to happen if irbesartan or another A-II antagonist is taken during the first 3 months of pregnancy. If you are pregnant, you should take a different antihypertensive.

In animal studies, small amounts of irbesartan have passed into breast milk but it is not known if this occurs in humans. Nursing mothers who must take irbesartan should bottle-feed their infants.

Seniors

Seniors may take irbesartan without special precautions.

Type of Drug

Iron Supplements G

Brand Names

Generic Ingredient: Ferrous Fumarate, 33% Iron
Nephro-Fer

Generic Ingredient: Polysaccharide Iron Complex

Hytinic	Nu-Iron V
Niferex Forte	Nu-Iron Plus $
Niferex PN Forte	

Prescribed for

Iron-deficiency anemia.

General Information

Iron supplements are used to treat anemias that result from iron deficiency; they are of no value in treating other kinds of anemias. They work by being incorporated into red blood cells, where oxygen is carried throughout the body. Iron is absorbed only in a small section of the gastrointestinal (GI) tract called the duodenum, the upper part of the small intestine. Sustained-release preparations of iron should be used only to help minimize the stomach discomfort that iron supplements can cause, as some of the drug in these forms may pass the duodenum and therefore cannot be absorbed.

Other products combining iron with other vitamins or with special extracts may be used to treat iron-deficiency anemia. Many iron supplements are available over the counter including ferrous sulfate (20% iron) and ferrous gluconate (11.6% iron) supplements.

Cautions and Warnings

Do not take an iron supplement if you have **hemochromatosis, hemosiderosis,** or a **hemolytic anemia.**

Do not take iron supplements if you have a history **of stomach problems, peptic ulcer,** or **ulcerative colitis.** People with normal iron balance in their bodies should not take any iron product on a regular basis.

Possible Side Effects

▼ Common: stomach upset or irritation, nausea, diarrhea, constipation, appetite loss, and darkened stools.

Drug Interactions

• Iron and tetracycline each interfere with the other's absorption into the blood. Separate doses of these medications by at least 2 hours.

• Iron interferes with the absorption of levodopa, methyldopa, penicillamine, and quinolone antibacterials into the bloodstream.

• Antacids and cimetidine will interfere with the absorption of iron.

• Ascorbic acid (vitamin C) and chloramphenicol increase the amount of iron absorbed into the bloodstream.

Food Interactions

Iron salts and iron-containing products are best taken on an empty stomach, but if they upset your stomach, take them with food. Be aware that eggs and milk interfere with iron absorption. Coffee or tea taken with a meal or within an hour after will interfere with the absorption of iron from your food. Do not take iron products together with calcium supplements and food: This combination may reduce the amount of iron absorbed by 1/3.

Usual Dose

Iron dosage is the same regardless of the type of iron you take. In order to figure out how much iron you are receiving, you may consult the percentage-of-iron-content list above or read the iron content in mg directly from the product's label.

Adult and Child (age 13 and over): 0.9–1 1/3 mg per lb. of body weight a day.

Pregnant Women: 30 mg of iron daily. Do not take with food or meals.

Child (age 3–12): 1 1/3 mg per lb. of body weight a day.

Child (age 6 months–2 years): up to 2 3/4 mg per lb. of body weight a day.

Child (under age 2): 10–25 mg a day.

Overdosage

Overdose symptoms usually appear after 30 minutes to several hours; they include tiredness, vomiting, diarrhea, stomach upset, weak and rapid pulse, and lowered blood pressure—or, after massive doses, shock, black and tarry stools due to massive bleeding in the stomach or intestine, and pneumonia. Be sure to call a doctor before inducing vomiting. Quickly induce vomiting by giving ipecac syrup— available in any pharmacy—and feed the victim eggs and milk until he or she can be taken to a hospital. Emergency treatment must begin as soon as possible: Stomach pumping should not be performed after the first hour of iron ingestion because of the risk of perforation of the stomach wall. In the hospital emergency room, measures to treat shock, loss of water, loss of blood, and respiratory failure may be necessary. ALWAYS bring the prescription bottle or container with you.

Special Information

Iron often causes black discoloration of stools and is slightly constipating. However, stools that are black or tarry in consistency may indicate some bleeding in the stomach or intestine. If you experience this symptom, discuss it with your doctor at once.

Do not chew or crush extended-release iron products. Liquid iron products may stain your teeth. Drink lots of water or juice with them and sip the iron through a straw to prevent tooth contact.

If you forget to take a dose of iron, take it as soon as you remember. If it is almost time for your next dose, skip the one you forgot and continue with your regular schedule. Do not take a double dose.

Special Populations

Pregnancy/Breast-feeding

This drug has been found to be safe for use during pregnancy and breast-feeding and is frequently prescribed for pregnant and nursing women. If you are pregnant, however, you should check with your doctor before taking any medication.

Seniors

Seniors may require larger doses to correct an iron deficiency because the ability to absorb iron decreases with age.

Generic Name

Isosorbide Dinitrate

(eye-soe-SORE-bide dih-NYE-trate) G

Brand Names

Dilatrate-SR	Isordil Titradose
Isordil Tembids	Sorbitrate

The information in this profile also applies to the following drugs:

Generic Ingredient: Isosorbide Mononitrate

Imdur	Monoket
ISMO	

Type of Drug

Antianginal agent.

Prescribed for

Heart or chest pain associated with angina pectoris; also prescribed in congestive heart failure and similar conditions to prevent the recurrence of chest or heart pain and to reduce stress on the heart.

General Information

Isosorbide dinitrate belongs to the class of drugs known as nitrates, which are used to treat pain associated with heart problems. The exact nature of their action is not fully understood. However, they are believed to relax muscles in veins and arteries. Isosorbide dinitrate sublingual tablets begin working in 2 to 5 minutes and last for 1 to 3 hours. The regular tablets begin working in 20 to 40 minutes and continue for 4 to 6 hours. Sustained-release isosorbide dinitrate may take up to 4 hours to begin working and lasts for 6 to 8 hours. Isosorbide mononitrate begins working in 30 to 60 minutes and lasts for an undetermined period of time.

Cautions and Warnings

If you know that you are **allergic or sensitive** to this drug or other drugs for heart pain, such as nitroglycerin, do not use isosorbide dinitrate.

Anyone who currently has or recently had a **head injury** should use this drug with caution.

Other conditions in which the use of isosorbide dinitrate may be inappropriate are severe **anemia, glaucoma,** severe **liver disease, overactive thyroid, cardiomyopathy** (loss of blood-pumping ability due to damaged heart muscle), **low blood pressure, recent heart attack,** severe **kidney problems,** and **overactive gastrointestinal tract**.

Possible Side Effects

▼ Common: headache and flushing of the skin, which should disappear after your body gets used to the drug. You may experience dizziness and weakness in the process. There is a possibility of blurred vision and dry

---

Possible Side Effects *(continued)*

mouth; if this happens, stop taking the drug and call your doctor.

▼ Less common: nausea, vomiting, weakness, sweating, and rash with itching, redness, and peeling. If these symptoms appear, discontinue the medication and consult your physician.

Drug Interactions

• If you take isosorbide dinitrate, do not self-medicate with over-the-counter cough and cold remedies, since many of them contain ingredients that may aggravate heart disease.

• Taking this drug with large amounts of alcoholic beverages may rapidly lower blood pressure, resulting in weakness, dizziness, and fainting.

• Nitrates raise the amount of dihydroergotamine absorbed into the blood, which may raise blood pressure or inhibit the effects of isosorbide.

• Aspirin and calcium channel blockers can lead to higher isosorbide dinitrate blood levels and increased side effects.

Food Interactions

Take isosorbide dinitrate on an empty stomach with a glass of water unless you get a persistent headache. If this occurs, the drug can be taken with meals.

Usual Dose

Isosorbide Dinitrate: 10–20 mg, 4 times a day. If needed, the drug may be given in doses from 5–40 mg. Sustained-release dosage is 40–80 mg every 8–12 hours.

Isosorbide Mononitrate: 20 mg twice a day, with the 2 doses taken 7 hours apart. Usually, the first dose is taken upon waking and the second dose is taken 7 hours later.

Overdosage

Isosorbide dinitrate overdose can result in low blood pressure; very rapid heartbeat; flushing; perspiration followed by cold, bluish, and clammy skin; headache; heart palpitations; blurred vision and other visual disturbances; dizziness; nausea; vomiting; difficult, slow breathing; slow pulse; confusion; moderate fever; and paralysis. Overdose victims should be taken to a hospital emergency room at once for treatment. ALWAYS bring the prescription bottle or container with you.

Special Information

If you take this drug sublingually (under the tongue), be sure the tablet is fully dissolved before you swallow the drug. Do not crush or chew sustained-release capsules or tablets.

Avoid alcoholic beverages while taking any of these drugs.

Do not switch brands of isosorbide dinitrate without consulting your doctor or pharmacist. All brands of isosorbide dinitrate may not be equivalent.

Call your doctor if you develop a persistent headache, dizziness, facial flushing, blurred vision, or dry mouth.

If you take regular isosorbide dinitrate and forget to take a dose, take it as soon as you remember, unless it is within 2 hours of your next dose. If that happens, skip the dose you forgot and continue with your regular schedule.

If you take long-acting isosorbide dinitrate and miss a dose, take it as soon as you remember, unless it is within 6 hours of your next dose. In that case, skip the dose you forgot and continue with your regular schedule. Do not take a double dose.

Special Populations

Pregnancy/Breast-feeding

This drug crosses into the fetal circulation but has not been found to cause birth defects. Nevertheless, women who are or might become pregnant should not take isosorbide dinitrate without their doctor's approval. When the drug is considered crucial by your doctor, its potential benefits must be carefully weighed against its risks.

This drug passes into breast milk but has caused no problems among breast-fed infants.

Seniors

Seniors may take isosorbide dinitrate without special restriction. Be sure to follow your doctor's directions and to report any side effects.

Generic Name

Isotretinoin (EYE-soe-TRET-ih-noin)

Brand Name

Accutane

Type of Drug

Anti-acne.

Prescribed for

Severe cystic acne that has not responded to other treatment, including antibiotics and medication applied to the skin. Isotretinoin has been used experimentally to treat a variety of other skin disorders such as keratinization (hardening of skin cells) and mycosis fungoides — a condition that begins in the skin and may develop into leukemia. Isotretinoin in relatively high doses is usually successful for the latter 2 conditions.

General Information

Isotretinoin was one of the first specialized products of vitamin research to be prescribed by doctors. Researchers have long known that several vitamins, including A and D, have properties that make them attractive treatments for certain conditions. However, the vitamins themselves are not appropriate treatments for these conditions because of the side effects that would develop if a patient took the amount needed to produce the desired effect.

It is not known exactly how isotretinoin works in cases of severe cystic acne. It reduces the amount of sebum (the skin's natural oily lubricant), shrinks the skin glands that produce sebum, and inhibits keratinization (hardening of the skin cells) — key to the problem of severe acne because it leads to the buildup of sebum within skin follicles and causes the formation of closed comedones (whiteheads). Sebum production may be permanently reduced after isotretinoin treatment.

Cautions and Warnings

People **allergic or sensitive to vitamin A** (or any vitamin A product) or to paraben preservatives — used in isotretinoin — should not use isotretinoin.

Isotretinoin has been associated with **pseudotumor cerebri (increased pressure in the brain)**. The symptoms of this condition include severe headaches, nausea, vomiting, and visual disturbances.

Diabetics taking this drug may have their diabetes drugs reevaluated by their doctors. Some new cases of diabetes were found in people taking isotretinoin, but no direct relationship to drug therapy has been found.

Isotretinoin may cause temporary opaque spots on the cornea of your eye, causing **visual disturbances**. These usually are gone by 2 months after the drug is stopped.

Difficulty seeing at night or in the dark can develop suddenly while taking isotretinoin.

Several cases of **severe bowel inflammation** (symptoms include abdominal discomfort and pain, severe diarrhea, or bleeding from the rectum) have developed in people taking isotretinoin.

About 25% of people who take isotretinoin develop **high blood-triglyceride levels**. Fifteen percent have lower high-density lipoprotein (HDL)—"good" cholesterol—and 7% have higher total cholesterol.

Several cases of **hepatitis** have been linked to this drug. Fifteen percent of people who take it develop signs of **liver inflammation**.

Occasionally, cystic acne lesions crust while healing. Acne may seem worse when isotretinoin treatment is first started.

Possible Side Effects

Side effects increase with dosage; the most severe effects occur at daily doses above 0.45 mg per lb. of body weight.

▼ Most common: dry, chapped, or inflamed lips; dry mouth; dry nose; nosebleeds; eye irritation; conjunctivitis (pinkeye); dry or flaky skin; rash; itching; peeling skin on the face, palms, or soles; unusual sensitivity to the sun; temporary skin discoloration; brittle nails; inflammation of the nailbed or bone under toes or fingernails; temporary hair thinning; nausea; vomiting; abdominal pain; tiredness; lethargy; sleeplessness; headache; tingling in the hands or feet; dizziness; protein, blood, or white blood cells in the urine; urinary difficulties, blurred vision; bone and joint aches or pains; and muscle pain or

Possible Side Effects *(continued)*

stiffness. Isotretinoin causes extreme elevations of blood-triglyceride levels and milder elevations of other blood-fat levels including cholesterol. It also can raise blood-sugar or uric-acid levels and can increase liver-function-test values.

▼ Less common: wound crusting caused by an exaggerated healing response stimulated by the drug, hair problems other than thinning, appetite loss, upset stomach or intestinal discomfort, severe bowel inflammation, stomach or intestinal bleeding, weight loss, visual disturbances, contact lens intolerance, *pseudotumor cerebri* (symptoms include severe headaches, nausea, vomiting, and visual disturbances), mild bleeding or easy bruising, fluid retention, and lung or respiratory system infection. Several people taking isotretinoin have developed widespread herpes simplex infections.

Drug Interactions

• Vitamin A supplements increase isotretinoin's side effects and must be avoided while taking this drug. Avoid alcohol because this combination can severely raise blood-triglyceride levels.

• People taking isotretinoin who have developed pseudotumor cerebri have usually also been taking a tetracycline antibiotic. Though this link. has not been definitely established, avoid tetracycline antibiotics while taking isotretinoin.

• Isotretinoin may reduce the amount of carbamazepine (an anticonvulsant) in the blood.

Food Interactions

Isotretinoin should be taken with food or meals. Avoid eating beef or chicken liver while taking isotretinoin, because liver contains very large amounts of vitamin A. Limit your intake of foods containing moderate to large amounts of vitamin A such as apricots, broccoli, cantaloupe, carrots, endive, persimmons, pumpkin, spinach, and winter squash.

Usual Dose

0.22–0.9 mg per lb. of body weight a day in 2 divided doses for 15–20 weeks. Lower doses may be effective, but relapses are more common. Isotretinoin, like vitamin A, dissolves in body fat. People weighing more than 155 lbs. may need doses at the high end of the usual range.

If the total acne lesion count drops by 70% in 15–20 weeks, the drug may be discontinued. Stop taking isotretinoin for 2 months after 15–20 weeks of treatment. A second course of treatment may be needed if the acne does not clear.

Overdosage

Isotretinoin overdose is likely to cause nausea, vomiting, lethargy, and other common drug side effects. Overdose victims must be made to vomit with ipecac syrup—available at any pharmacy—to remove any remaining drug from the stomach. Call your doctor or poison control center before doing this. If you must go to a hospital emergency room, ALWAYS bring the prescription bottle or container.

Special Information

Women of childbearing age should not take isotretinoin unless their severe, disfiguring acne has not responded to any other treatment, they are using effective contraception, and they have had a negative pregnancy test during the 2 weeks before taking isotretinoin. You should start taking isotretinoin on day 2 or 3 of your next period. Be sure your doctor knows if you plan to become pregnant while taking isotretinoin, are breast-feeding, diabetic, taking a vitamin A supplement—as a multivitamin or vitamin A alone—or if you or any family member has a history of high blood-triglyceride levels.

Your skin may become unusually sensitive to the sun while you are taking this drug. Use sunscreen and wear protective clothing until your doctor can determine if you are likely to develop this effect.

Call your doctor if you develop any severe or unusual side effects, such as abdominal pain; bleeding from the rectum; severe diarrhea; headache, nausea, or vomiting; visual difficulties; severe muscle, bone, or joint aches or pains; or unusual sensitivity to sunlight or to ultraviolet light.

Your acne may worsen when isotretinoin treatment begins, but then it should improve. Do not be alarmed if this happens, but tell your doctor.

Do not donate blood during isotretinoin treatment—or for at least 30 days after you have stopped—because of the risk to the fetus of a pregnant woman who may receive the blood.

If you forget a dose of isotretinoin, take it as soon as you remember. If it is almost time for your next dose, skip the one you forgot and continue with your regular schedule. Do not take a double dose.

Special Populations

Pregnancy/Breast-feeding

Pregnant women should NEVER take isotretinoin because it injures the fetus. Isotretinoin causes fetal head, brain, eye, ear, and hearing abnormalities. Taking isotretinoin for even a short time affects the fetus. Several cases of spontaneous abortion have been linked to this drug.

You must confirm that you are not pregnant before starting isotretinoin. You must also be absolutely certain that you are using effective birth control starting 1 month before treatment and continued at least 1 month after isotretinoin is stopped. Accidental pregnancy during isotretinoin therapy may be grounds for an abortion due to the severe effects of this drug on the fetus. Call your doctor immediately.

It is not known if isotretinoin passes into breast milk. Nursing mothers should not take isotretinoin because of the possibility that it will affect the nursing infant.

Seniors

Seniors may take this medication without special restriction. Follow your doctor's directions and report any side effects at once.

Generic Name

Isradipine (is-RAD-ih-pene)

Brand Names

DynaCirc   CynaCirc CR

Type of Drug

Calcium channel blocker.

Prescribed for

High blood pressure; also prescribed for chronic stable angina pectoris.

General Information

Isradipine is one of many calcium channel blockers available in the U.S. These drugs block the passage of calcium, an essential factor in muscle contraction, into the heart and smooth muscles. Such blockage of calcium interferes with contraction of these muscles, which in turn dilates (widens) the veins and vessels that supply blood to them. This action has several beneficial effects. Because arteries are dilated, they are less likely to spasm. In addition, because blood vessels are dilated, both blood pressure and the amount of oxygen used by the heart muscle are reduced. Isradipine is therefore useful in treating not only high blood pressure but also angina pectoris (brief attacks of chest pain), a condition related to poor oxygen supply to the heart muscle. Other calcium channel blockers are prescribed for abnormal heart rhythm, heart failure, cardiomyopathy (loss of blood-pumping ability due to damaged heart muscle), and diseases that involve blood-vessel spasm, such as migraine headache and Raynaud's syndrome.

Isradipine affects the movement of calcium into muscle cells only; it has no effect on calcium in the blood.

Cautions and Warnings

Do not take this drug if you have had an **allergic reaction** to it.

Abruptly stopping this medication can cause increased **chest pain**. If you must stop, the drug dose should be gradually reduced.

Use isradipine with caution if you have **heart failure**, since the drug may slow heart rate and thereby worsen this condition.

On rare occasions, isradipine may cause very **low blood pressure**. This may lead to stimulation of the heart and rapid heartbeat and can worsen angina in some people.

Isradipine may cause angina when treatment is first started, when dosage is increased, or if the drug is rapidly withdrawn. This can be avoided by reducing dosage gradually.

Studies have shown that people taking calcium channel blockers—usually those taken several times a day, not those taken only once daily—have a greater chance of having a **heart attack** than do people taking beta blockers or other medication for the same purposes. Discuss this with your doctor to be sure you are receiving the best possible treatment.

People with severe **liver disease** break down isradipine much more slowly than people with mildly diseased or normal livers. Your doctor should take this into account when determining your isradipine dosage.

Possible Side Effects

Isradipine side effects are generally mild and self-limiting.

▼ Most common: headache.

▼ Less common: low blood pressure, chest pain, rapid heartbeat, dizziness, diarrhea, a feeling of warmth, nausea, light-headedness, fatigue and lethargy, itching, rash, flushing, changes in certain blood-cell components, and swelling of the legs, ankles, or feet.

▼ Rare: fainting, heart failure, heart attack, abnormal heart rhythm, stroke, numbness, drowsiness, nervousness, depression, paranoia, memory loss, hallucinations, psychoses, visual disturbances, sleeplessness, tingling in the hands or feet, heart palpitations, constipation, stomach upset and cramps, vomiting, dry mouth, sweating, reduced sex drive or sexual difficulties, leg and foot cramps, muscle cramps and inflammation, joint pain, sore throat, cough, increases in certain blood enzyme tests, and frequent urination, especially at night.

Drug Interactions

• Isradipine may interact with beta-blocking drugs to cause heart failure, very low blood pressure, or an increased incidence of angina pain. However, in many cases these drugs have been taken together with no problem.

• Combining isradipine with fentanyl (a narcotic pain reliever) can result in very low blood pressure.

Food Interactions

Taking isradipine with food has a minor effect on the absorption of the drug. You may take it with food if it upsets your stomach. Avoid drinking grapefruit juice if you are taking this medication.

Usual Dose

5–20 mg a day in 2 doses. Do not stop taking the drug abruptly. The dosage should be reduced gradually over a period of time.

Overdosage

Overdose of isradipine can cause nausea, dizziness, weakness, drowsiness, confusion, slurred speech, very low blood pressure, reduced heart efficiency, and unusual heart rhythms. Victims of an isradipine overdose should be taken to a hospital emergency room. ALWAYS bring the prescription bottle or container with you.

Special Information

Call your doctor if you develop swelling in the arms or legs, breathing difficulties, abnormal heartbeat, increased heart pains, dizziness, constipation, nausea, light-headedness, or very low blood pressure.

If you forget to take a dose of isradipine, take it as soon as you remember. If it is almost time for your next dose, skip the dose you forgot and continue with your regular schedule. Do not take a double dose.

Special Populations

Pregnancy/Breast-feeding

Isradipine affects the development of animal fetuses in laboratory studies, but has not been found to cause human birth defects. Nevertheless, women who are or might be pregnant should not take isradipine without their doctor's approval. When the drug is considered crucial by your doctor, its potential benefits must be carefully weighed against its risks.

It is not known if isradipine passes into breast milk. Women who must take isradipine should consider the possible effect of the drug on their infants before breast-feeding.

Seniors

Seniors may absorb more isradipine than younger adults and may release the drug more slowly from their bodies. Follow your doctor's directions and report any side effects at once.

Generic Name

Itraconazole (ih-trah-KON-uh-zole)

Brand Name

Sporanox

Type of Drug

Antifungal.

Prescribed for

Fungal infections — blastomycosis and histoplasmosis — of the blood and infections of the skin and nails in normal and immunodeficient people. Itraconazole also works against a number of other common fungal infections that do not respond to other drugs.

General Information

Itraconazole is effective against a variety of fungal organisms. The broad range of its effectiveness may make it an important therapy for people with AIDS or cancer whose immune systems are compromised. It works by inhibiting important enzyme systems in the organisms it attacks. Drug treatment must be continued for at least 3 months until the fungal infection subsides. Itraconazole is broken down in the liver, but the effect of liver disease on it is not known.

Cautions and Warnings

The combination of itraconazole and either astemizole or terfenadine, non-sedating antihistamines, can cause severe **cardiac side effects** and should be avoided.

Do not take itraconazole if you have had an **allergic** reaction to it. People who are allergic to similar antifungals — ketoconazole, miconazole, and fluconazole — may also be allergic to itraconazole, although cross-reactions are uncommon.

On rare occasions, itraconazole causes **reversible liver damage**. It should be used with caution by people who already have liver disease. In studies with laboratory animals, itraconazole caused an increase in lung tumors.

Possible Side Effects

▼ Most common: nausea, vomiting, and rash.

▼ Less common: diarrhea, abdominal pain, appetite loss, swelling in the legs or feet, fatigue, fever, feeling unwell, itching, headache, dizziness, reduced sex drive, tiredness, high blood pressure, liver or kidney function abnormalities, low blood potassium, and impotence.

Possible Side Effects *(continued)*

▼ Rare: stomach gas, sleeplessness, depression, ringing or buzzing in the ears, and swollen or painful breasts in men or women.

Drug Interactions

• People who have taken terfenadine or astemizole with itraconazole have experienced severe cardiac side effects. DO NOT TAKE THESE COMBINATIONS.

• Itraconazole increases the amounts of cisapride, digoxin, sulfonylurea-type antidiabetes drugs, phenytoin, quinidine, tacrolimus, and warfarin in the blood, leading to possible side effects. Your doctor should evaluate your dosage of these drugs if you start taking itraconazole: important adjustments may be required.

• People taking itraconazole with the calcium channel blockers amlodipine and nifedipine can retain fluid. These combinations should be avoided.

• On rare occasions, people who combine itraconazole with a blood-fat-lowering drug of the HMG-CoA-inhibitor type — lovastatin and simvastatin — experience muscle pain and destruction. Some people who have experienced this interaction were also taking cyclosporine, the dose of which should be lowered if it is being taken with itraconazole and an HMG-CoA-inhibitor type drug.

• Cimetidine, ranitidine, famotidine, nizatidine, isoniazid, phenytoin, and rifampin may reduce the amount of itraconazole in your blood, possibly interfering with its effectiveness.

Food Interactions

Itraconazole should be taken with or after a full meal.

Usual Dose

Adult: 200–600 mg once a day.

Child (age 3–16): 100 mg a day has been prescribed, but the long-term effects of itraconazole in children are not known.

Overdosage

Symptoms of itraconazole overdose may include any of the drug's side effects; liver toxicity is especially important. Call your doctor, local poison control center, or hospital emergency room for more information. ALWAYS take the prescription bottle or container with you if you seek treatment.

Special Information

Itraconazole must be taken for at least 3 months to determine its effectiveness. Taking this medication for less than the prescribed time may lead to recurrence of the original infection.

Call your doctor if you develop unusual fatigue, yellowing of the skin or whites of the eyes, nausea or vomiting, appetite loss, dark urine or pale stools, or if you develop unusually bothersome or persistent side effects.

If you forget to take a dose of itraconazole, take it as soon as you remember. If it is almost time for your next dose, skip the one you forgot and continue with your regular schedule. Do not take a double dose.

Special Populations

Pregnancy/Breast-feeding

Animal studies have shown that doses of itraconazole 5 to 20 times the human dose cause damage to the fetus. The drug's effect in humans is not known. Pregnant women should not use itraconazole unless the possible benefits have been carefully weighed against the risks.

Itraconazole passes into breast milk. Nursing mothers should bottle-feed their babies if they must take this drug.

Seniors

Seniors may use this drug without special restriction. Report any side effects to the doctor at once.

Generic Name

Ivermectin (EYE-ver-MEK-tin)

Brand Name

Stromectol

Type of Drug

Anthelmintic.

Prescribed for

Strongyloidiasis and onchocerciasis (worm infections).

General Information

Ivermectin has been used to fight rare human and animal worm infections for many years. The drug works by interfering with nerve and muscle cells in the worm. Ivermectin does not affect human nerve and muscle systems in the same way because our nerve and muscle cells do not contain the sites that ivermectin binds to in worm cells. Ivermectin is broken down in the liver and passes out of the body through the stool. A single dose of ivermectin usually eliminates strongyloides; however, repeated doses are usually necessary to kill the adult onchocerca.

Cautions and Warnings

Do not take this drug if you are **sensitive or allergic** to it.

People being treated with anthelmintic drugs may develop skin and eye reactions because of the body's reaction to the death of the infecting worms. These reactions are likely if you are being treated for onchocerciasis but unlikely if you are being treated for strongyloidiasis.

Possible Side Effects

▼ Most common: itching, swelling, rashes, and lymph gland enlargement and tenderness.

▼ Common: joint pain.

▼ Less common: dizziness, diarrhea, nausea, eye problems, rapid heartbeat, swelling in the arms or legs, facial swelling, dizziness or fainting when standing up, and liver irritation.

▼ Rare: weakness, tiredness, abdominal pain, appetite loss, constipation, vomiting, headache, muscle ache, and worsening of asthma.

Drug Interactions

None known.

Food Interactions

Take ivermectin with water.

Usual Dose

Adult and Child (age 6 and over): a single dose of 0.07–0.09 mg per lb. of body weight. People with onchocerciasis may need a second dose in 3 months.

Child (under age 6): Ivermectin has not been studied in children this young.

Overdosage

Overdose symptoms include weakness, diarrhea, dizziness, swelling, headache, nausea, rash, vomiting, abdominal pain, poor muscle coordination, breathing difficulties, tingling in the hands or feet, seizures, and itching rashes. Overdose victims should be taken to a hospital emergency room for treatment. ALWAYS bring the prescription bottle or container with you.

Special Information

Remember to take ivermectin with water.

If you have strongyloides infection, you need to check your stool to make sure that the infection has been eliminated by the ivermectin.

If you have onchocerca infection, be sure to stay in touch with your doctor. Another dose of ivermectin is usually needed to eliminate the infection.

Special Populations

Pregnancy/Breast-feeding

Ivermectin causes birth defects in animal studies at doses up to 8 times the maximum human dose. Pregnant women should not take ivermectin.

Ivermectin passes into breast milk. Nursing mothers should talk to their doctor, and only take ivermectin if its possible benefits outweigh its risks.

Seniors

Seniors may take this drug without special precaution.

K-Dur

see **Potassium Replacements**, page 900

Generic Name

Ketoconazole (kee-toe-KON-uh-zole)

Brand Name

Nizoral

Type of Drug

Antifungal.

Prescribed for

Thrush and other systemic fungal infections, including candidiasis, histoplasmosis, and blastomycosis. Ketoconazole may also be prescribed for fungal infections of the skin, fingernails, and vagina. High-dose ketoconazole may be effective in treating fungal infections of the brain. The drug has been studied for the treatment of advanced prostate cancer and Cushing's syndrome. Ketoconazole shampoo is used to treat dandruff.

General Information

This drug is effective against a wide variety of fungal organisms. It works by disrupting the membrane of a fungus cell, ultimately destroying the cell.

Cautions and Warnings

At least 1 of every 10,000 people who take ketoconazole develop **liver inflammation** and damage. In most cases, the inflammation subsides when the drug is discontinued.

Do not take ketoconazole if you have had an **allergic** reaction to it.

Ketoconazole should not be used to treat **fungal infections of the nervous system** because only small amounts of the drug enter that body system.

Ketoconazole reduces **testosterone levels** and the amount of **corticosteroid hormone** produced by the body.

In studies of ketoconazole in **prostate cancer,** 11 people died within 2 weeks of starting high-dose ketoconazole treatment. The reasons for these deaths are not known but may be related to the fact that the medication can suppress the body's natural production of adrenal corticosteroid hormones.

On rare occasions, people taking ketoconazole for the first

time experience serious, **life-threatening reactions including itching, rash, and breathing difficulties**. Victims of this rare reaction must receive emergency treatment at once.

Possible Side Effects

▼ Common: nausea, vomiting, upset stomach, abdominal pain or discomfort, itching, and swollen breasts in men. Most of these side effects are mild, and only a small number of people—1.5%—have to stop taking the drug because of severe side effects.

▼ Less common: headache, dizziness, drowsiness or tiredness, fever, chills, unusual sensitivity to bright light, diarrhea, impotence, and reduced levels of blood platelets. Reduced sperm counts have been associated with ketoconazole, but only at dosages above 400 mg a day.

Drug Interactions

• Antacids, histamine H_2 antagonists including cimetidine and ranitidine, and other drugs that reduce stomach acid will counteract the effects of ketoconazole by preventing it from being absorbed. Ketoconazole requires an acid environment to pass into the blood.

• When ketoconazole is taken together with rifampin, the effects of both drugs may be reduced.

• The combination of isoniazid and ketoconazole causes a neutralization of ketoconazole's effects. This interaction occurs even when doses of the 2 drugs are separated by 12 hours.

• Ketoconazole increases the amount of cyclosporine in the bloodstream and the chances for kidney damage caused by cyclosporine. It also increases the effect of oral anticoagulant (blood-thinning) drugs. Ketoconazole increases the blood levels of cisapride and of the antihistamines terfenadine and astemizole, which leads to an increased chance of developing serious cardiac side effects from those drugs.

• Combining ketoconazole and phenytoin may affect blood levels of both drugs, increasing or decreasing either's effect.

• Ketoconazole may decrease blood levels of theophylline, possibly precipitating an asthmatic attack. Your doctor may adjust your theophylline dose.

• Ketoconazole may increase the amount of oral corticosteroid drugs absorbed into the bloodstream while slowing their removal from the body, possibly leading to increased corticosteroid side effects.

Food Interactions

Food stimulates acid release; ketoconazole is absorbed much more efficiently when acid is present in the stomach. Take ketoconazole with food or at meals to improve absorption and to avoid stomach upset.

Usual Dose

Tablets
   Adult: 200–400 mg once a day. Treatment may continue for several months, depending on the type of infection being treated.
   Child (age 2 and over): 1.5–3 mg per lb. of body weight once a day.
   Child (under age 2): not recommended.

Cream
Apply to affected and immediately surrounding areas 1–2 times a day for 14 days.

Overdosage

The most likely effects of ketoconazole overdose are liver damage and exaggerated side effects. Victims of overdose should immediately be given bicarbonate of soda or any other antacid to reduce the amount of ketoconazole absorbed into the blood. Call your local poison control center for more information. If you take the victim to a hospital emergency room for treatment, ALWAYS bring the prescription bottle or container with you.

Special Information

If you must take antacids or other ulcer treatments, separate doses of these medications from ketoconazole by at least 2 hours. Anything that reduces stomach-acid levels will reduce the amount of ketoconazole absorbed into the blood.
   Ketoconazole may cause headaches, dizziness, and drowsiness. Use caution while doing anything that requires intense concentration, like driving or operating machinery.
   Call your doctor if you develop pains in the stomach or abdomen, severe diarrhea, high fever, unusual tiredness, appetite loss, nausea, vomiting, yellowing of the skin or whites of the eyes, pale stools, or dark urine.

If you forget to take a dose of ketoconazole, take it as soon as you remember. If it is almost time for your next dose, take 1 dose immediately and the next dose in 10 to 12 hours. Then go back to your regular schedule. Do not take a double dose.

Special Populations

Pregnancy/Breast-feeding
In doses larger than the maximum human dose, ketoconazole causes damage in animal fetuses. Ketoconazole should be not be taken by women who are or might be pregnant unless the risks of the have been carefully weighed against the potential benefits.

Nursing mothers who must take ketoconazole should bottle-feed their infants because the drug passes into breast milk.

Seniors
Seniors may take this medication without special restriction. Follow your doctor's directions and report any side effects at once.

Generic Name

Ketoprofen (KEE-toe-PROE-fen)

Brand Names

Orudis   Oruvail Extended-Release

Type of Drug

Nonsteroidal anti-inflammatory drug (NSAID).

Prescribed for

Rheumatoid arthritis, juvenile rheumatoid arthritis, osteoarthritis, mild to moderate pain, menstrual pain, menstrual headache, sunburn, and migraine prevention. Controlled-release ketoprofen is prescribed only for various forms of arthritis.

General Information

Ketoprofen is one of 16 NSAIDs, which are used to relieve pain and inflammation. We do not know exactly how NSAIDs work, but part of their action may be due to their ability to inhibit the body's production of a hormone called prostaglandin as well as the action of other body chemicals, including cyclooxygenase, lipoxygenase, leukotrienes, and lysosomal enzymes. NSAIDs are generally absorbed into the bloodstream quickly. Pain relief comes within 1 hour after taking the first dose of ketoprofen, but its anti-inflammatory effect generally takes several days to 2 weeks to become apparent and may take a month or more to reach maximum effect. Controlled-release ketoprofen is not recommended for acute pain relief because it can take up to 7 hours to reach its maximum concentration in the blood. Ketoprofen is broken down in the liver and eliminated from the body through the kidneys.

Cautions and Warnings

People **allergic** to ketoprofen or any other NSAID and those with a history of **asthma** attacks brought on by an NSAID, iodides, or aspirin should not take ketoprofen.

Ketoprofen may cause **gastrointestinal (GI) bleeding, ulcers,** and **stomach perforation.** This can occur at any time, with or without warning, in people who take ketoprofen regularly. People with a history of **active GI bleeding** should be cautious about taking any NSAID. People who develop bleeding or ulcers and continue taking ketoprofen should be aware of the chances of developing more serious side effects.

Ketoprofen may affect platelets and **blood clotting** at high doses, and should be avoided by people with clotting problems and by those taking warfarin.

People with **heart problems** who use ketoprofen may experience swelling in their arms, legs, or feet.

Ketoprofen may cause severe toxic effects to the **kidney.** Report any unusual side effects to your doctor, who might need to periodically test your kidney function.

Ketoprofen may make you unusually sensitive to the effects of the sun.

Possible Side Effects

▼ Most common: diarrhea; nausea; vomiting; constipation; minor stomach upset, distress or gas; and appetite loss; especially during the first few days of treatment.

▼ Less common: stomach ulcers, GI bleeding, hepatitis, gallbladder attacks, painful urination, poor kidney

Possible Side Effects *(continued)*

function, kidney inflammation, blood and protein in the urine, dizziness, fainting, nervousness, depression, hallucinations, confusion, disorientation, light-headedness, tingling in the hands or feet, itching, increased sweating, dry nose and mouth, heart palpitations, chest pain, breathing difficulties, and muscle cramps.

▼ Rare: severe allergic reactions including closing of the throat, fever and chills, changes in liver function, jaundice (yellowing of the skin or whites of the eyes), and kidney failure. People who experience such effects must be promptly treated in a hospital emergency room or doctor's office. NSAIDs have caused severe skin reactions; if this happens to you, see your doctor immediately.

Drug Interactions

• Ketoprofen may increase the effects of oral anticoagulant (blood-thinning) drugs such as warfarin. You may take this combination, but your doctor might have to reduce your anticoagulant dose.

• Mixing ketoprofen with cyclosporine may increase the kidney-related side effects of both drugs. Methotrexate side effects may be increased in people also taking ketoprofen.

• Ketoprofen may reduce the blood-pressure-lowering effect of beta blockers and loop diuretics.

• Ketoprofen may increase phenytoin blood levels, leading to increased phenytoin side effects. Lithium blood levels may be increased in people taking ketoprofen.

• Ketoprofen blood levels may be affected by cimetidine.

• Probenecid may interfere with the elimination of ketoprofen from the body, increasing the chances for ketoprofen side effects.

• Aspirin and other salicylates may decrease the amount of ketoprofen in your blood. These drugs should never be combined with ketoprofen.

Food Interactions

Take ketoprofen with food or a magnesium/aluminum antacid if it upsets your stomach.

Usual Dose

Capsules
  Adult: 50–75 mg 3–4 times a day. Do not exceed 300 mg a day. Seniors and people with kidney problems should start with ⅓ to ½ of the usual dose.

Controlled-Release Capsules
  Adult and Senior: 200 mg once a day.

Overdosage

People have died from NSAID overdoses. The most common signs of overdose are drowsiness, nausea, vomiting, diarrhea, abdominal pain, rapid breathing, rapid heartbeat, increased sweating, ringing or buzzing in the ears, confusion, disorientation, stupor, and coma. Take the victim to a hospital emergency room at once. ALWAYS bring the prescription bottle or container with you.

Special Information

Take each dose with a full glass of water and do not lie down for 15 to 30 minutes afterward.

Ketoprofen can make you drowsy and/or tired: Be careful when driving or operating hazardous equipment. Do not take any over-the-counter products containing acetaminophen or aspirin while taking ketoprofen. Avoid alcoholic beverages.

Contact your doctor if you develop skin rash or itching, visual disturbances, weight gain, breathing difficulties, fluid retention, hallucinations, black or tarry stools, persistent headache, or any unusual or intolerable side effect.

If you forget to take a dose of ketoprofen, take it as soon as you remember. If you take ketoprofen once a day and it is within 8 hours of your next dose, skip the dose you forgot and continue with your regular schedule. If you take several doses a day and it is within 4 hours of your next dose, skip the one you forgot and continue with your regular schedule. Never take a double dose.

Special Populations

Pregnancy/Breast-feeding

NSAIDs may cross into fetal blood circulation. They have not been found to cause birth defects, but animal studies indicate that they may affect a developing fetal heart during the second half of pregnancy. Pregnant women should not take ketoprofen without their doctor's approval, especially during the last 3 months of pregnancy. When the drug is considered crucial by your doctor, its potential benefits must be carefully weighed against its risks.

NSAIDs may pass into breast milk but have caused no problems in breast-fed infants, except for seizures in a baby whose mother was taking the NSAID indomethacin. Other NSAIDs have caused problems in animal studies. There is a possibility that a nursing mother taking ketoprofen could affect her baby's heart or cardiovascular system. If you must take ketoprofen, bottle-feed your baby.

Seniors

Seniors may be more susceptible to ketoprofen side effects, especially ulcer disease.

Generic Name

Ketorolac (kee-TOE-roe-lak)

Brand Names

Acular Eyedrops　　　　　　　　Toradol

Type of Drug

Nonsteroidal anti-inflammatory drug (NSAID).

Prescribed for

Short-term treatment of moderately severe pain that has required narcotic pain-relievers. Ketorolac eyedrops are prescribed for eye redness and inflammation caused by seasonal allergies and for inflammation following cataract surgery.

General Information

Ketorolac tromethamine is one of 16 NSAIDs, which are used to relieve pain and inflammation. We do not know exactly how NSAIDs work, but part of their action may be due to their ability to inhibit the body's production of a hormone called prostaglandin as well as the action of other body chemicals, including cyclooxygenase, lipoxygenase, leukotrienes, and lysosomal enzymes. Ketorolac is absorbed into the blood-stream quickly. Pain relief comes within 1 hour after taking the first dose. Unlike the others in this group, ketorolac is a potent drug with serious risks (see "Cautions and Warnings"). Taking more ketorolac than is prescribed only increases risk; it does not offer better results. Ketorolac tablets should only be taken by people who have first been treated with ketorolac injection. Total treatment with injectable and oral ketoroladc should not exceed 5 days.

NSAID eyedrops may be used during eye surgery to prevent movement of the eye muscles. In addition to ketorolac, other NSAID eyedrops — including diclofenac, flurbiprofen, and suprofen — are also used in eye surgery, for inflammation following cataract extraction, and for itching and redness caused by seasonal allergies.

Cautions and Warnings

People **allergic** to ketorolac or any other NSAID and those with a history of **asthma** attacks brought on by an NSAID, iodides, or aspirin should not take ketorolac.

Ketorolac may cause **gastrointestinal (GI) bleeding, ulcers,** and **stomach perforation**. This can occur at any time, with or without warning, in people who take ketorolac regularly. People with a history of **active GI bleeding** should be cautious about taking any NSAID. People who develop bleeding or ulcers and continue NSAID treatment should be aware of the possibility of developing more serious side effects.

Ketorolac may affect platelets and **blood clotting** at high doses, and should be avoided by people with clotting problems and by those taking warfarin.

People with **heart problems** who use ketorolac may experience swelling in their arms, legs, or feet.

Ketorolac may actually cause **headaches**. If this happens, you might have to stop taking this drug or switch to another NSAID.

Ketorolac may cause severe toxic effects to the **kidney**. Report any unusual side effects to your doctor, who might need to periodically test your kidney function.

People taking ketorolac on a regular basis should have their **liver function** checked periodically.

Ketorolac may make you unusually sensitive to the effects of the sun.

Possible Side Effects

Injection and Tablets

▼ Most common: diarrhea; nausea; vomiting; constipation; minor stomach upset, distress, or gas; and appetite loss; especially during the first few days of treatment.

▼ Less common: stomach ulcers, GI bleeding, hepatitis, gallbladder attacks, painful urination, poor kidney function, kidney inflammation, blood and protein in the urine, dizziness, fainting, nervousness, depression, hallucinations, confusion, disorientation, tingling in the hands or feet, light-headedness, itching, increased sweating, dry nose and mouth, heart palpitations, chest pain, breathing difficulties, and muscle cramps.

▼ Rare: severe allergic reactions including closing of the throat, fever and chills, changes in liver function, jaundice (yellowing of the skin or whites of the eyes), and kidney failure. People who experience such effects must be promptly treated in a hospital emergency room or doctor's office. NSAIDs have caused severe skin reactions; if this happens to you, see your doctor immediately.

Eyedrops

▼ Most common: temporary burning, stinging, or other minor eye irritation.

▼ Less common: nausea, vomiting, viral infections, and eye reactions including persistent redness, burning, itching, or tearing. The risk of developing bleeding problems or other systemic (whole-body) side effects with ketorolac eyedrops is low because only a small amount of the drug is absorbed into the blood.

Drug Interactions

Injection and Tablets

• Ketorolac may increase the effects of oral anticoagulant (blood-thinning) drugs such as warfarin. You may take this combination; however, your doctor might have to reduce your anticoagulant dose.

• Taking ketorolac with cyclosporine may increase the kidney-related side effects of both drugs. Methotrexate side effects may be increased in people also taking ketorolac.

• Ketorolac may reduce the blood-pressure-lowering effect of beta blockers and loop diuretics.

• Ketorolac may raise phenytoin blood levels, leading to increased phenytoin side effects. Lithium blood levels may be raised in people taking ketorolac.

• Ketorolac blood levels may be affected by cimetidine.

• Probenecid may interfere with the body's elimination of ketorolac, increasing the chances for ketorolac side effects.

• Aspirin and other salicylates may decrease the amount of ketorolac in your blood. These drugs should never be combined with ketorolac.

Eyedrops
None known.

Food Interactions

Take ketorolac with food or a magnesium/aluminum antacid if it upsets your stomach.

Usual Dose

Tablets: Up to 40 mg a day, for no more than 5 consecutive days.

Eyedrops: 1 drop 4 times a day for itching and irritation due to seasonal allergies.

Overdosage

People have died from NSAID overdoses. The most common signs of overdose are drowsiness, nausea, vomiting, diarrhea, abdominal pain, rapid breathing, rapid heartbeat, increased sweating, ringing or buzzing in the ears, confusion, disorientation, stupor, and coma. Take the victim to a hospital emergency room at once. ALWAYS bring the prescription bottle or container with you.

Special Information

Injection and Tablets: Take each dose with a full glass of water, and do not lie down for 15 to 30 minutes afterward.

Ketorolac can make you drowsy and/or tired: Be careful when driving or operating hazardous equipment. Do not take any over-the-counter products containing acetaminophen or aspirin while taking ketorolac. Avoid alcoholic beverages.

Contact your doctor if you develop skin rash or itching, visual disturbances, weight gain, breathing difficulties, fluid retention, hallucinations, black or tarry stools, persistent headache, or any unusual or intolerable side effect.

If you forget to take a dose of ketorolac tablets, take it as soon as you remember. If you take ketorolac once a day and it is within 8 hours of your next dose, skip the dose you forgot and continue with your regular schedule. If you take several doses a day and it is within 4 hours of your next dose, skip the one you forgot and continue with your regular schedule. Never take a double dose.

Eyedrops: To self-administer the eyedrops, lie down or tilt your head back. Hold the dropper above your eye and drop the medication inside your lower lid while looking up. To prevent possible infection, do not allow the dropper to touch your fingers, eyelids, or any surface. Release the lower lid, keeping your eye open. Do not blink for 30 seconds. Press gently on the bridge of your nose at the inside corner of your eye for 1 minute to help circulate the medication in your eye. Wait at least 5 minutes before using any other eyedrops.

If you forget a dose of ketorolac eyedrops, take it as soon as you remember. If it is almost time for your next dose, skip the dose you forgot and continue with your regular schedule. Do not take a double dose.

Special Populations

Pregnancy/Breast-feeding
Ketorolac should not be taken by pregnant women because it may affect fetal blood circulation and prevent normal labor.

There is a possibility that a nursing mother taking ketorolac could affect her baby's heart or cardiovascular system. If you must take ketorolac, bottle-feed your baby.

Seniors
Seniors may be more susceptible to ketorolac side effects, especially ulcer disease.

Klonopin

see *Clonazepam,* page 219

Generic Name

Labetalol (luh-BET-uh-lol)

Brand Names

Normodyne   Trandate

Type of Drug

Adrenergic blocker and antihypertensive.

Prescribed for

Hypertension (high blood pressure).

General Information

Labetalol hydrochloride, first studied for its effect as a beta blocker, is a unique antihypertensive drug because it selectively blocks both alpha- and beta-adrenergic impulses. This combination of actions contributes to its ability to reduce blood pressure. Other drugs can increase or decrease heart rate; labetalol may be better than other beta blockers because it rarely affects heart rate.

Cautions and Warnings

People with **asthma, severe heart failure, reduced heart rate,** and **heart block** (disruption of the electrical impulses that control heart rate) should not take labetalol. People with **angina** who take labetalol for hypertension risk aggravating their angina if they suddenly stop taking the drug. These people should have their dosage reduced gradually over 1 to 2 weeks. Labetalol should be used with caution if you have **liver disease** because your ability to eliminate the drug from your body may be impaired.

Possible Side Effects

Labetalol side effects develop early in the course of treatment and increase with larger doses.

▼ Most common: dizziness, tingling of the scalp, nausea, vomiting, upset stomach, distortion in the sense of taste, fatigue, sweating, impotence, urinary difficulties, diarrhea, bile-duct blockage, bronchial spasm, breathing

---

Possible Side Effects *(continued)*

difficulties, muscle weakness, cramps, dry eyes, blurred vision, rash, facial swelling, and hair loss.

▼ Less common: aggravation of lupus erythematosus (chronic condition affecting the body's connective tissue), stuffy nose, depression, confusion, disorientation, loss of short-term memory, emotional instability, colitis, drug allergy (symptoms include fever, sore throat, and breathing difficulties), and reduction in the levels of white blood cells and blood platelets.

Drug Interactions

• Labetalol may suppress normal signs of low blood sugar and may also interfere with the action of oral antidiabetes drugs.

• Combining labetalol and a tricyclic antidepressant may cause tremor.

• Labetalol may interfere with the effect of some anti-asthma drugs, especially ephedrine, isoproterenol, and other beta stimulants.

• Cimetidine increases the amount of labetalol absorbed into the bloodstream from oral tablets.

• Glutethimide decreases the amount of labetalol in the blood by increasing the rate at which it is broken down by your liver.

• Labetalol may increase the blood-pressure-lowering effect of nitroglycerin.

Food Interactions

This drug may be taken with food if it upsets your stomach. In fact, food increases the amount of labetalol absorbed into the blood.

Usual Dose

Starting dosage — 100 mg twice a day; may be increased gradually to as much as 1200 mg twice a day. Maintenance dosage — 200–400 mg twice a day.

Overdosage

Labetalol overdose slows heart rate and causes an excessive drop in blood pressure. The possible consequences of these effects can be treated only in a hospital emergency room. ALWAYS bring the prescription bottle or container with you.

Special Information

You may experience scalp tingling, especially when you first start taking labetalol.

Labetalol is meant to be taken on a continuing basis. Do not stop this drug unless instructed to do so by your doctor.

Weakness; swelling of your ankles, feet, or legs; breathing difficulties; or other side effects should be reported to your doctor as soon as possible. Most side effects are not serious, but a small number of people — about 7% — have to switch to another drug because of side effects.

If you forget to take a dose of labetalol, take it as soon as possible. However, if it is within 8 hours of your next dose, skip the dose you forgot and go back to your regular schedule. Do not take a double dose.

Special Populations

Pregnancy/Breast-feeding

Labetalol crosses into the fetal circulation. It has not been found to cause birth defects. However, women who are or might be pregnant should not take this drug without their doctor's approval. When the drug is considered crucial by your doctor, its possible benefits must be carefully weighed against its risks.

This drug passes into breast milk but has caused no problems among breast-fed infants. Nursing mothers who must take labetalol may want to bottle-feed their babies.

Seniors

Seniors may be more sensitive to the effects of labetalol. Your dosage must be individually adjusted by your doctor, especially if you have liver disease. Seniors may be more likely to suffer from cold hands and feet, reduced body temperature, chest pain, feeling unwell, sudden breathing difficulties, sweating, or changes in heartbeat.

Generic Name

Lamivudine (lam-IV-ue-dene)

Brand Name

Epivir

Combination Products

Generic Ingredients: Lamivudine + Zidovudine
Combivir

Type of Drug

Antiviral.

Prescribed for

Human immunodeficiency virus (HIV) infection, in combination with other anti-HIV drugs.

General Information

Lamivudine, also known as 3-TC, is a nucleoside-type antiviral that works on the HIV virus in the same way as zalcitibine, zidovidudine (AZT), stavudine, and other drugs of this type. It is generally given in combination with AZT and a protease inhibitor to people who do not respond to single-drug treatment. Lamivudine is rapidly absorbed into the blood. Most of it passes out of the body in the urine.

Cautions and Warnings

Do not take lamivudine if you are **sensitive** or **allergic** to it. People with **kidney disease** need less lamivudine than people with normal kidney function.

Possible Side Effects

Because this drug is always taken with AZT, the listed side effects are those of the drugs in combination. The long-term effects of lamivudine are not known.

▼ Most common: headache, not feeling well, fever, chills, skin rash, nausea, vomiting, diarrhea, appetite loss, abdominal pain or cramps, nervous system problems including tingling and poor coordination, sleeplessness, dizziness, depression, stuffy or runny nose, cough, and muscle pain.

▼ Common: upset stomach, joint pain, and tingling in the hands or feet in children. Lamivudine may affect the results of a variety of blood tests.

▼ Rare: pancreas irritation, more often seen in children than adults.

Drug Interactions

• Lamivudine increases maximum blood levels of AZT by 39%, which is helpful in fighting the HIV virus.

• Trimethoprim-sulfamethoxazole, taken for opportunistic AIDS-related infections, increases the amount of lamivudine in the blood.

Food Interactions

Lamivudine is absorbed more slowly when taken with food, but not enough to affect the total amount of drug that reaches the blood.

Usual Dose

Lamivudine

Adult and Child (age 12 and over): 150 mg twice a day. Adults who weigh less than 110 lbs. should receive about 1 mg per lb. of body weight twice a day. Dosage is reduced as kidney function decreases.

Child (3 months–12 years): about 2 mg per lb. of body weight twice a day, no more than 150 mg per dose.

Lamivudine-zidovudine

Adult and Child: 1 tablet — lamivudine 150 mg plus zidovudine 300 mg — twice a day. Poor kidney function requires reducing the dosage of both drugs. In this situation, it is preferable to take the individual drugs separately so that you retain maximum dosage flexibility.

Overdosage

There has been only one reported case of lamivudine overdose; no side effects were noted. Call your local poison control center for more information.

Special Information

Lamivudine does not cure AIDS. It will not prevent you from transmitting the HIV virus to another person; you must still practice safe sex. People taking this drug will still develop opportunistic infections and other complications of AIDS.

It is very important to take lamivudine exactly as prescribed. If you forget a dose, take it as soon as you remember. If it is almost time for your next dose, skip the dose you forgot and continue with your regular schedule. Call your doctor if you forget 2 or more doses in a row.

Call your doctor at once if your child develops signs of pancreas inflammation while taking lamivudine. Symptoms include very severe abdominal pain, tense abdominal muscles, sweating, feeling very ill, shallow and rapid breathing, fever, and possible fainting.

Special Populations

Pregnancy/Breast-feeding

Lamivudine passes into the blood circulation of the fetus. Some animal studies of lamivudine indicate that it may be dangerous to the fetus, but others showed no effect. There is no information about the effect of lamivudine in pregnant women. Like all drugs, lamivudine should be taken during pregnancy only if absolutely necessary. A registry has been established to record the effects of lamivudine in pregnant women, and doctors are encouraged to register their patients who qualify.

It is not known if lamivudine passes into breast milk. Nursing mothers who must take lamivudine should bottle-feed their babies. In any case, nursing mothers who are HIV positive should bottle-feed their babies to avoid transmitting the virus through their milk.

Seniors

Seniors may require a smaller dose of lamivudine, depending on their kidney function. Otherwise, seniors may take this drug without special restriction.

Generic Name

Lamotrigine (lam-OE-trih-jene)

Brand Name

Lamictal

Type of Drug

Anticonvulsant.

Prescribed for

Adult epilepsy and partial seizure; also prescribed for tonic-clonic, absence, and myoclonic seizures and for infants and children with Lennox-Gastaut syndrome.

General Information

Much like phenytoin and carbamazepine, lamotrigine works on voltage-dependent channels in the brain to stabilize them and to prevent the release of chemicals that would stimulate the nervous system, leading to seizure. Lamotrigine is one of the first new anti-seizure drugs available in more than 10 years.

Lamotrigine is absorbed rapidly into the bloodstream after you take it, reaching maximum blood concentration in 1½ to 5 hours. Lamotrigine is eliminated from the body by the liver, but the process can be affected by other drugs (see "Drug Interactions").

Cautions and Warnings

Severe and possibly life-threatening **rashes** may occur in people taking lamotrigine, nearly always within 2 to 8 weeks of the time they start taking it. **Minor rashes** also occur with this medication, but it is not possible to tell which ones may become life threatening. If you develop a rash while taking this drug, call your doctor at once.

Twenty sudden and **unexplained deaths** occurred in people taking lamotrigine before it was approved for general use. It is thought that these deaths were unrelated to taking lamotrigine.

Five people who were taking lamotrigine died from acute **liver failure** or **multi-organ failure** before the drug was approved for general use. Although all the people affected were taking lamotrigine, it is not known if the drug played a role in these deaths.

Lamotrigine is not recommended for general use in children under age 16.

Lamotrigine binds to melanin, a body hormone commonly found in the skin and eyes. The long-term effects of lamotrigine on the eyes are not known.

When you stop taking lamotrigine, the dose should be reduced gradually over a period of 2 weeks or more to prevent **withdrawal seizures.**

Status epilepticus, a severe seizure disorder, and **worsening of existing seizure disorders** may develop in a small number of people taking lamotrigine.

People with **heart disease, severe kidney disease** or **liver disease** should use this drug with caution.

Lamotrigine may make you **unusually sensitive to the sun.**

Always wear protective clothing and use a sunscreen while taking this drug.

Possible Side Effects

▼ Most common: headache, dizziness, nausea, weakness, tiredness, runny nose, double vision, and blurred vision.

▼ Common: accidental injury, flu-like symptoms, abdominal pain, vomiting, infection, neck pain, feeling unwell, worsening of seizure, diarrhea, upset stomach, constipation, dental problems, loss of coordination, sleeplessness, tremors, depression, anxiety, convulsions, irritability, itching, visual difficulties, painful menstruation, and vaginal irritation.

▼ Less common: chills, hot flashes, heart palpitations, appetite loss, dry mouth, joint ache, muscle weakness, speech disorders, sore throat, coughing, tongue speech muscle problems, memory loss, confusion, loss of concentration, sleep disorders, emotional upset, fainting, racing thoughts, rolling of the eyes, muscle spasm, breathing difficulties, hair loss, acne, ear pain, ringing or buzzing in the ears, and missed periods.

▼ Rare: facial swelling, bad breath, enlarged abdomen, unusual sensitivity to the sun, attempted suicide, flushing, migraines, dizziness, rapid heartbeat, angina, bleeding, vein irritations, high blood pressure, heart attack, dizziness when rising quickly, dry skin, eczema, hairiness, sweating, herpes infections, difficulty in swallowing, gum infections and bleeding, gum overgrowth, increased appetite, increased salivation, mouth ulcers, excessive thirst, stomach noises, stomach bleeding or irritation, tongue swelling, liver disease, overactive thyroid, anemia, black-and-blue marks, swollen lymph glands, allergic reactions, weight loss, arthritis, bursitis, leg cramps, broken bones, hiccoughs, pneumonia, bronchial spasm, red-eye, dry eyes, changes in or loss of sense of taste, and deafness.

Drug Interactions

• When lamotrigine and sodium valproate are mixed, lamotrigine concentrations in the blood are doubled and valproate is reduced by ¼. Your doctor will adjust your drug dosage to take these effects into account. Also, skin rash may be more common in people taking both lamotrigine and sodium valproate.

- Combining carbamazepine and lamotrigine increases the amount of carbamazepine in the blood, possibly leading to side effects, and reduces the amount of lamotrigine in the blood by 40%.
- Acetaminophen and lamotrigine are broken down by the same system in the liver. Taking acetaminophen at the same time as lamotrigine can slightly increase the rate at which lamotrigine is broken down, but occasional use of the two drugs together is not likely to be a problem. Regular acetaminophen users may need more lamotrigine.
- Unlike other medications for seizure control, lamotrigine does not seem to interact with oral contraceptives.
- Anti-folate drugs — often used in cancer treatment — can increase the effects of lamotrigine.
- Phenobarbital and primidone may reduce the effects of lamotrigine.
- Mixing phenytoin with lamotrigine reduces the amount of lamotrigine in the blood by about ¼.

Food Interactions

None known.

Usual Dose

Adult and Child (age 16 and over): Starting dose — 25 or 50 mg a day. Increase gradually to a maximum daily dose of 500 mg. Lamotrigine is usually taken twice a day; be sure to take your doses 12 hours apart.

Child (under age 16): not recommended.

Overdosage

There have been reports of overdoses of 4000 mg leading to coma. Other overdose symptoms are dizziness, headache, and sleepiness. Overdose victims should be taken to a hospital emergency room at once for treatment. ALWAYS bring the prescription bottle or container with you.

Special Information

Once you start taking lamotrigine, your liver may actually increase the rate at which it breaks down the drug, which may increase your dosage requirement. Your doctor will have to check your lamotrigine blood levels periodically to see if any dosage changes are needed.

Call your doctor at once if you develop a rash, but do not change your lamotrigine dosage or stop taking it on your own.

Lamotrigine may cause drowsiness, dizziness, or blurred vision, effects that are increased by alcoholic beverages. Be careful while driving or engaging in any other activity requiring intense concentration, alertness, and coordination.

If you take acetaminophen while you are taking lamotrigine, especially for a lamotrigine headache, do not take more acetaminophen than is directed on the package.

If you take lamotrigine once a day and forget to take a dose, take it as soon as you remember. If it is within 8 hours of your next dose, skip the one you forgot and continue with your regular schedule. Do not take a double dose.

After the first 2 weeks of treatment, most people take lamotrigine twice a day. If you take it twice a day, be sure to take your medication every 12 hours. If you take lamotrigine twice a day and forget a dose, take it as soon as you remember. If it is within 4 hours of your next dose, take one dose as soon as you remember and another in 5 or 6 hours, then go back to your regular schedule.

Special Populations

Pregnancy/Breast-feeding

Animal studies of up to 500 mg a day show some evidence of injury to the fetus. Lamotrigine reduces the amount of folate in the fetus, an effect that is associated with birth defects, but no cases of birth defects have been seen in infants born to mothers who take lamotrigine. A higher incidence of birth malformations has generally been noted among women with seizure disorders. A pregnant woman should take lamotrigine only if the possible risks and benefits have been discussed with her doctor. The drug's manufacturer has established a special registry for pregnant women taking lamotrigine to keep track of possible drug effects during pregnancy.

Lamotrigine passes into breast milk, but the effect of the drug on a nursing infant is not known. Nevertheless, nursing mothers taking lamotrigine should bottle-feed their babies.

Seniors

Seniors may take lamotrigine without special restriction.

Lanoxin

*see **Digitalis Glycosides**, page 319*

Generic Name

Lansoprazole (lan-SOPE-ruh-zole)

Brand Name

Prevacid

Type of Drug

Proton-pump inhibitor.

Prescribed for

Duodenal (upper intestinal) ulcer, esophagitis, and Zollinger-Ellison syndrome.

General Information

Lansoprazole, like the related drug omeprazole, interferes with the "proton pump" in the mucous lining of the stomach, at the last stage of acid production. As a result, lansoprazole can turn off stomach acid production within 1 hour after it is taken. Lansoprazole is accepted in the U.S. for short-term treatment of duodenal ulcers plus longer-term — up to a year — maintenance of healed ulcers. It is also used for treatment, lasting up to 16 weeks, of erosive esophagitis, a condition in which stomach contents flow backward into the esophagus (pipe connecting the throat and stomach), resulting in erosion of the esophagus by stomach acid. Lansoprazole is also approved for other conditions in which stomach acid plays a key role or in which excess stomach acid is produced as a part of the condition; Zollinger-Ellison syndrome is the most common of these. Lansoprazole has not yet been accepted for treatment of stomach ulcer, although omeprazole is widely prescribed for that purpose.

Cautions and Warnings

Do not take this drug if you are **sensitive or allergic** to it. People with **severe liver disease** should receive lower doses of this drug. Animal studies indicate that long-term use of this medication can be related to an increase in **stomach tumors**, but it is not known if this is also a problem for humans. Lansoprazole relieves symptoms very quickly, but this may not mean that the underlying problem has been solved.

Possible Side Effects

Generally, lansoprazole causes relatively few side effects.
▼ Most common: diarrhea.
▼ Less common: nausea, abdominal pain, and headache.
▼ Rare: Other side effects reported by people taking lansoprazole affect virtually any body system. However, these rare side effects occurred in fewer than 1 of every 100 people taking the medication.

Drug Interactions

• Lansoprazole reduces the absorption of drugs into the bloodstream that depend on having acid present in the stomach, such as ampicillin, digoxin, iron, and ketoconazole.

• Lansoprazole slightly increases the rate at which theophylline is released from the body, but this is not likely to affect most people taking theophylline for asthma.

• Sucralfate interferes with the absorption of lansoprazole into the blood. If you take both drugs, take the lansoprazole at least 30 minutes before you take the sucralfate.

Food Interactions

Lansoprazole should be taken before a meal, preferably breakfast. Taking it after meals seriously interferes with the absorption of lansoprazole into the blood.

Usual Dose

Adult: 15–30 mg a day. In some cases, 120 mg or more a day may be prescribed. People with severe liver disease may need lower doses.
Child (under age 18): not recommended.

Overdosage

In one case of a 600-mg overdose, there were no adverse effects. Call your local poison control center or hospital emergency room for information if you suspect a lansoprazole overdose. If you go to an emergency room for treatment, ALWAYS bring the prescription bottle or container with you.

Special Information

Lansoprazole capsules should be swallowed whole. Do not open or crush them.

If you forget to take a dose of lansoprazole, take it as soon as you remember. If it is almost time for your next dose, skip the dose you forgot and continue with your regular schedule. Do not take a double dose.

Special Populations

Pregnancy/Breast-feeding

There is no information about the effect of taking lansoprazole during pregnancy. This drug should not be taken during pregnancy unless absolutely necessary.

It is not known if this drug passes into human breast milk. Nursing mothers who must take lansoprazole should consider bottle-feeding their babies because of the chance that the drug could affect the nursing infant.

Seniors

Seniors clear this drug from their bodies more slowly than do younger adults. Daily doses greater than 30 mg should not be taken unless specifically necessary to control symptoms.

Lasix

see **Loop Diuretics**, page 600

Generic Name

Latanoprost (lah-TAN-oe-prost)

Brand Name

Xalatan

Type of Drug

Anti-glaucoma.

Prescribed for

Open-angle glaucoma and ocular hypertension (high pressure inside the eye).

General Information

Latanoprost is believed to reduce pressure inside the eye by increasing the natural outflow of fluid from inside the eye. After you put the drops in your eye, latanoprost is absorbed through the cornea, where it is transformed into its active form. Maximum concentrations are reached within 2 hours. Maximum pressure-lowering effect is seen in 8 to 12 hours. Studies have shown that the 0.005% concentration of latanoprost is equivalent to 0.5% of timolol in its ability to reduce pressure inside the eye.

Cautions and Warnings

Do not use latanoprost eyedrops if you are **allergic or sensitive** to them.

Latanoprost may change your eye color because it increases the number of pigment granules in the cornea, which in turn increases the brown pigment in the iris. This color change occurs gradually over a period of months or years. Typically, the brown color around the pupil spreads slowly to the outer part of the iris. This change is more noticeable in people with green-brown, blue/gray-brown or yellow-brown eye color. The long-term effect of latanoprost on eye pigment granules is not known; your doctor may tell you to stop using these eyedrops if the color change persists or is especially noticeable.

The effect of latanoprost on the cornea, where it is transformed to its active form, is not known.

Possible Side Effects

▼ Most common: blurred vision; stinging, burning, and redness of the eyes; a sensation of something in the eye; itching; and brownish eye coloration.

▼ Less common: dry eye, excessive tearing, swelling or redness of the eyelid, eyelid discomfort or pain, and unusual sensitivity to bright light.

▼ Rare: blood clot in the artery supplying the retina, detachment of the retina, and bleeding inside the eye.

Possible Side Effects *(continued)*

General side effects from traces of latanoprost passing into the blood can include colds, flu, or other respiratory infections; muscle, joint, or back pain; chest pain; angina pain; and skin rash or allergic reactions.

Drug Interactions

• If you use other eyedrops that contain a thimerosal preservative, separate the administration of each eyedrop by at least 5 minutes. Ask your pharmacist if you're not sure if other eyedrops you may be using contain thimerosal.

Usual Dose

Adult: One drop — 1.5 mcg — in affected eye(s) once a day in the evening.
Child: not recommended.

Overdosage

The most common effects of latanoprost overdose are eye irritation and redness. Severe overdosage may also cause abdominal pains, dizziness, fatigue, flushing, nausea, and sweating. Overdose victims may require emergency room care. Call your emergency room or local poison control center for more information.

Special Information

Call your doctor if you develop eye irritation or any other side effect of the eyes.

If you use any eyedrops in addition to latanoprost, wait 5 minutes between each application.

To self-administer eyedrops, lie down or tilt your head backward and look at the ceiling. Hold the dropper above your eye and drop the medicine inside your lower lid while looking up. To prevent infection, keep the dropper from touching your fingers, eyelids, or any surface: Eye infection can develop from eyedrop containers that are contaminated by improper usage. Release the lower lid, keeping your eye open. Do not blink for 30 seconds. Press gently on the bridge of your nose at the inside corner of your eye for 1 minute. This will help circulate the medicine around your eye.

If you wear contact lenses, take them out before putting

latanoprost eyedrops into your eyes. Latanoprost contains a benzalkonium preservative that can be absorbed by the contacts.

Do not take more latanoprost than prescribed. Taking it more often may actually reduce its effectiveness. If you forget a dose of latanoprost eyedrops, administer it as soon as you remember. If it is almost time for your next dose, skip the one you forgot and continue with your regular schedule. Do not take a double dose.

Store unopened bottles of latanoprost in the refrigerator. Once opened, the eyedrops can be kept at room temperature — up to 77°F — for 6 weeks.

Special Populations

Pregnancy/Breast-feeding
Animal studies have shown that at doses equal to 80 times the maximum human dose, latanoprost can be harmful to the fetus. There is no information on the effect of latanoprost in pregnant women. Pregnant women should not use these eyedrops unless the possible benefits outweigh the risks.

Many drugs pass into breast milk, but there is no information on this aspect of latanoprost. Nursing mothers should be cautious about using latanoprost eyedrops because of possible effects on the nursing infant.

Seniors
Seniors may use latanoprost without special precaution.

Lescol

see **Fluvastatin**, page 456

Generic Name

Levamisole (lee-VAM-ih-sole)

Brand Name
Ergamisol

Type of Drug
Immune-system modulator.

Prescribed for

Duke's stage-C colon cancer, together with fluorouracil; also prescribed for malignant melanoma after surgery in people in whom the disease has not spread.

General Information

Levamisole hydrocbloride, used to cure worm infection in animals, was found to restore depressed immune function in people. It stimulates the formulation of antibodies to various agents, enhances T-cell response by stimulating and activating these important immune-system cells, and stimulates the functions of various white-blood-cell types — including their infection-fighting capabilities. The exact way that it works in concert with fluorouracil is not known. In one clinical study of levamisole, the survival rate of Duke's stage-C colon cancer patients was improved by 27% for levamisole plus fluorouracil and 28% for levamisole alone. The reduced recurrence rate for the disease was 36% for the drug combination and 28% for levamisole alone. Another study showed 33% improved survival and 41% reduction in disease recurrence for the 2 drugs. The drug is broken down in the liver and passes out of the body through the kidneys.

Cautions and Warnings

Do not take levamisole if you are **allergic** to it.

People taking levamisole may develop **agranulocytosis (condition characterized by a reduction in the number of white blood cells)**. Common symptoms of agranulocytosis are fever, chills, and flu-like symptoms; agranulocytosis may develop suddenly and without warning. Regular blood monitoring is necessary while you are on levamisole: Your doctor may suddenly stop treatment if blood tests indicate the development of this problem, which may reverse when you stop the drug.

Possible Side Effects

Virtually all people taking fluorouracil and levamisole experience side effects. Often side effects are due to either one or both of the drugs; the actual source of certain side effects may not be distinguishable. In levamisole studies, the most common reasons for people stop-

Possible Side Effects (continued)

ping drug treatment were rash, joint and muscle aches, fever, white-blood-cell depression, urinary infection, and cough.

▼ Most common: nausea, vomiting, diarrhea, mouth sores, appetite loss, abdominal pain, constipation, a metallic taste, joint and muscle aches, dizziness, headache, tingling in the hands or feet, white-blood-cell reduction, rash, hair loss, fatigue, sleepiness, fever, chills, and infection.

▼ Less common: reduced platelet levels, itching, upset stomach, stomach gas, changes in sense of smell, depression, nervousness, sleeplessness, anxiety, blurred vision, and red eyes.

▼ Rare: peeling rash, swelling around the eyes, vaginal bleeding, severe allergic reaction (symptoms include breathing difficulties, rash, intense itching, and elevated pulse), confusion, convulsions, hallucinations, loss of concentration, and kidney failure.

Drug Interactions

• People taking levamisole who drink alcoholic beverages may experience severe side effects. Avoid this combination.

• People taking phenytoin who also take combined therapy with fluorouracil and levamisole may have higher-than-usual levels of phenytoin in their blood, increasing the risk of side effects.

Food Interactions

None known.

Usual Dose

Colon Cancer: 50 mg every 8 hours for 3 days starting 7–30 days after surgery; then 50 mg every 8 hours for 3 days every 2 weeks.

Malignant Melanoma: 2½ mg once daily for 2 consecutive days each week.

Overdosage

A levamisole dosage was fatal in a child who took the equivalent of 6.8 mg per lb. of body weight. An adult died after taking 14.5 mg per lb. — 0.5–1 mg per lb. is the usual adult dosage. The most likely symptoms of overdose are severe side effects including those that affect the blood system, stomach, and intestines. Overdose victims should be taken to a hospital emergency room at once. ALWAYS bring the prescription bottle or container with you.

Special Information

Call your doctor if you develop any side effects, especially fever, chills, or flu-like symptoms. Taking more than the recommended dosage of levamisole increases side-effect risk without improving the drug's effectiveness. Carefully follow your doctor's directions.

If you forget to take a dose of levamisole, do not take the dose you forgot and do not take a double dose. Call your doctor for more information.

Special Populations

Pregnancy/Breast-feeding

While there is no direct information on pregnancy in humans, animal studies indicate that levamisole may injure the fetus. When this drug is considered crucial by your doctor, its potential benefits must be weighed against its risks. Use effective contraceptive measures to be sure that you do not become pregnant while taking levamisole and fluorouracil.

Levamisole may pass into breast milk. Nursing mothers who must take levamisole should bottle-feed their infants.

Seniors

Seniors may take this drug without special restriction. Report any side effects to your doctor.

Generic Name

Levocabastine (LEE-voe-kuh-BAS-tene)

Brand Name

Livostin

Type of Drug

Antihistamine.

Prescribed for

Allergic conjunctivitis (pinkeye).

General Information

Levocabastine hydrochloride is an antihistamine eyedrop
that is used to relieve the tearing and itching that accompany
seasonal allergy.

Cautions and Warnings

People who wear **soft contact lenses** should take them out
before using levocabastine.

Possible Side Effects

▼ Most common: temporary eye burning, stinging,
discomfort, and headache.

▼ Less common: visual disturbances, eye pain, dry
eye, swelling of the eyelid, dry mouth, fatigue, sore
throat, conjunctivitis, tearing or other eye discharge,
cough, nausea, rash or redness, and breathing difficulties.

Drug Interactions

• Do not use other eyedrops together with levocabastine.

Usual Dose

Adult and Child (age 12 and over): 1 drop in the affected eye
4 times a day for up to 2 weeks.

Child (age 11 and under): not recommended.

Overdosage

Accidental ingestion of levocabastine may cause any of the
side effects listed above (see "Possible Side Effects"). Call
your local poison control center or emergency room for more
information.

Special Information

Shake the eyedrop bottle well before using. Protect the bottle
from freezing.

To administer eyedrops, lie down or tilt your head back.
Hold the dropper above your eye, gently squeeze your lower
lid to form a small pouch, and release the drop or drops of

medication inside your lower lid while looking up. Release the lower lid, keeping your eye open. Do not blink for 40 seconds. Press gently on the bridge of your nose at the inside corner of your eye for 1 minute to help circulate the drug in your eye. To avoid infection, do not touch the dropper tip to your finger, eyelid, or any other surface. Wait at least 5 minutes before using another eyedrop or eye ointment.

Call your doctor at once if eye stinging, itching, burning, redness, irritation, swelling, or pain worsens or if you have trouble seeing.

If you forget a dose of levocabastine, administer it as soon as you remember. If it is almost time for your next dose, skip the dose you forgot and continue with your regular schedule. Do not take a double dose.

Special Populations

Pregnancy/Breast-feeding

Antihistamines have not been proven to cause birth defects in humans. In animal studies, large doses of levocabastine have caused birth defects. Do not take any antihistamine without your doctor's knowledge if you are or might be pregnant — especially during the last 3 months of pregnancy, because newborns may have severe reactions to antihistamines. When levocabastine is considered crucial by your doctor, its potential benefits must be carefully weighed against its risks.

Small amounts of levocabastine pass into breast milk after the drug is put into the eye. Nursing mothers who must use levocabastine should bottle-feed their infants.

Seniors

Seniors may use levocabastine without special restriction.

Generic Name

Levodopa (lee-voe-DOE-puh) G

Brand Names

Dopar   Larodopa

Type of Drug

Antiparkinsonian.

Prescribed for

Parkinson's disease, restless legs syndrome, and herpes zoster (shingles).

General Information

Parkinson's disease can develop as a result of changes in the brain's use of dopamine; it may also develop from central nervous system damage caused by carbon monoxide or manganese poisoning. It usually develops in older adults because of hardening of the arteries, but in many cases the cause is not known. When levodopa — also known as L-dopa — enters the brain, it is converted to dopamine, a chemical found naturally in the central nervous system and deficient in people with Parkinson's disease. Some people who take levodopa develop the "on-off" phenomenon, in which they may suddenly lose all drug effect and then regain it minutes or hours later. About 15% to 40% of people with Parkinson's disease will develop this phenomenon after 2 to 3 years of levodopa treatment. The on-off effect becomes more frequent after 5 years, and levodopa patients may experience a gradual decline in drug effect.

Cautions and Warnings

People with a history of **heart attacks,** severe **heart or lung disease, glaucoma, asthma,** or **kidney, liver, or hormone disease** should be cautious about using this drug. Do not take it if you have a history of **stomach ulcer.** People with a **psychotic history** must be treated with extreme care; this drug can cause **depression with suicidal tendencies.** Levodopa may activate an existing **malignant melanoma:** People with a family history of melanoma or suspicious skin lesions should not take this drug.

Possible Side Effects

▼ Most common: muscle spasms or inability to control arm, leg, or facial muscles; loss of appetite; nausea; vomiting, with or without stomach pain; dry mouth; drooling; difficulty eating due to poor muscle control; tiredness; hand tremors; headache; dizziness; numbness; weakness or a faint feeling; confusion; sleeplessness; grinding of the teeth; nightmares; euphoria (feeling high), hallucina-

---

Possible Side Effects *(continued)*

tions; delusions; agitation; anxiousness; and feeling unwell.

▼ Less common: heart irregularities or palpitations; dizziness when standing or arising, particularly in the morning; mental changes, including depression with or without suicidal tendencies, paranoia, and loss of intellectual function; difficulty urinating; muscle twitching; burning of the tongue; bitter taste; diarrhea; constipation; unusual breathing patterns; blurred or double vision; hot flashes; weight gain or loss; darkening of the urine; and increased perspiration.

▼ Rare: stomach bleeding, ulcer, high blood pressure, convulsions, adverse effects on the blood, difficulty controlling the eye muscles, feeling of being stimulated, hiccups, loss of hair, hoarseness, decreasing size of male genitalia, and retention of fluids.

Drug Interactions

• Levodopa's effect is decreased when it is mixed with an anticholinergic drug, such as trihexyphenidyl. Other drugs that may interfere with levodopa are benzodiazepine-type tranquilizers and sedatives, phenothiazine antipsychotic medication, phenytoin, methionine, papaverine, pyridoxine, and tricyclic antidepressants.

• Antacids may increase the effects of levodopa.

• Metoclopramide may increase the amount of levodopa absorbed into the bloodstream; levodopa may reduce metoclopramide's effects on the stomach. Levodopa may interact with drugs for high blood pressure to further reduce pressure. Dosage adjustments in the high-blood-pressure medication may be required. Methyldopa (an antihypertensive) may increase the effects of levodopa.

• People taking monoamine oxidase inhibitor (MAOI) antidepressants should stop taking them at least 2 weeks before starting to take levodopa.

Food Interactions

Do not take vitamin preparations that contain vitamin B_6 (pyridoxine), which will decrease the effectiveness of levodopa.

Since levodopa may upset your stomach, take each dose with food. A low-protein diet may help to minimize variations in drug response that occur in some people.

Usual Dose

0.5–8 g a day. Dosage must be individualized to your needs.

Overdosage

People taking an overdose of levodopa must be treated in a hospital emergency room immediately. ALWAYS bring the prescription bottle or container with you.

Special Information

Be careful while driving or operating any complex or hazardous equipment.

Call your doctor immediately if any of the following occur: fainting, dizziness, or light-headedness; abnormal results in diabetic urine tests; uncontrollable movements of the face, eyelids, mouth, tongue, neck, arms, hands, or legs; mood changes; palpitations or irregular heartbeats; difficulty urinating; or severe nausea or vomiting.

If you forget to take a dose of levodopa, take it as soon as possible. However, if it is within 2 hours of your next dose, skip the dose you forgot and go back to your regular schedule. Do not take a double dose.

Special Populations

Pregnancy/Breast-feeding

Levodopa has not been studied in humans, but animal studies indicate that it may interfere with fetal development. Pregnant women should take this drug only if it is absolutely necessary.

Nursing mothers taking this drug should bottle-feed their infants.

Seniors

Seniors may require smaller dosages because the body enzyme that breaks down the drug decreases with age. Seniors are also more likely than younger adults to experience side effects.

Seniors who respond to levodopa treatments, especially those with osteoporosis, should resume activity gradually. Sudden increases in mobility may increase the risk of broken bones.

Seniors, especially those with heart disease, are more likely to develop abnormal heart rhythm and other cardiac side effects. Regular monitoring by your doctor is essential.

Levoxyl

see **Thyroid Hormone Replacements**, page 1079

Brand Name

Lexxel

Generic Ingredients

Enalapril + Felodipine

Type of Drug

Antihypertensive combination.

Prescribed for

Hypertension (high blood pressure).

General Information

Lexxel is a fixed-dose combination of 5 mg of felodipine, a calcium channel blocker, and 5 mg of enalapril, an angiotensin-converting enzyme (ACE) inhibitor. In other words, if your needs change, your doctor may have to prescribe the 2 ingredients separately in the necessary dosages. The 2 drugs in this combination belong to 2 widely prescribed groups of hypertension medication. Lexxel is not meant for the initial treatment of hypertension. In general, people taking this product have taken one of the ingredients as a separate pill and need more medication to control their blood pressure. Felodipine works by blocking the passage of calcium into heart and smooth-muscle tissue, especially the smooth muscle found in arteries. Since calcium is an essential factor in muscle contraction, any drug that affects calcium in this way will interfere with the contraction of these muscles. This causes the veins to dilate (open), reducing blood pressure. Also, the amount of oxygen used by the muscles is reduced.

ACE inhibitors such as enalapril work by preventing the

conversion of a hormone called angiotensin I to another hormone called angiotensin II, a potent blood-vessel constrictor. Preventing this conversion relaxes blood vessels and helps to reduce blood pressure and relieve the symptoms of heart failure by making it easier for a failing heart to pump blood through the body. The production of other hormones and enzymes that participate in the regulation of blood-vessel dilation is also affected by enalapril and probably plays a role in the effectiveness of this medication. Enalapril begins working about 1 hour after you take it and continues to work for 24 hours.

Cautions and Warnings

Do not take Lexxel if you are **sensitive or allergic** to either of its ingredients. Rarely, it may cause **very low blood pressure**. It may also affect your **kidneys**, especially if you have **congestive heart failure** (CHF). Your doctor should check your urine for protein content during the first few months of treatment.

Enalapril may affect **white-blood-cell counts**, possibly increasing your **susceptibility to infection**. Your doctor should monitor your blood counts periodically.

Patients taking a beta-blocking drug who begin taking felodipine may develop **heart failure** or increased **angina pain**. Angina pain may also increase if your felodipine dosage is increased. People with severe **liver disease** break down felodipine much more slowly than do people with less severe disease or normal livers.

A sudden, painless swelling in the hands, face, feet, lips, tongue, or throat may develop while you are taking any ACE inhibitor including enalapril. If this happens you must call your doctor and stop taking the medication at once. This condition usually goes away on its own though antihistamines may also prove helpful.

Possible Side Effects

Calcium-channel-blocker side effects are generally mild and rarely cause people to stop taking them. Side effects are more common with higher dosages and increasing age.

▼ Most common: swelling in the ankles, feet, and legs; dizziness; light-headedness; muscle weakness or cramps;

Possible Side Effects *(continued)*

facial flushing; headache; fatigue; nausea; and chronic (long-term) cough. The cough usually goes away a few days after you stop taking the medication.

▼ Less common: respiratory infection, cough, tingling in the hands or feet, upset stomach, abdominal pain, chest pain, nausea, constipation, diarrhea, heart palpitations, sore throat, runny nose, back pain, rash, angina (condition characterized by brief attacks of chest pain), dizziness when rising from a sitting or lying position, fainting, vomiting, bronchitis, urinary tract infection, breathing difficulties, and weakness.

▼ Rare: facial swelling and a feeling of warmth; rapid heartbeat; heart attack; very low blood pressure; angina pain; abnormal heart rhythms; vomiting; dry mouth; stomach gas; anemia; muscle joint and bone pain; depression; anxiety; sleeplessness; irritability; nervousness; bronchitis; flu-like symptoms; sinus irritation; nosebleeds; sneezing; itching; redness; bruising; sweating; blurred vision; ringing or buzzing in the ears; swelling of the gums; decreased sex drive; loss of sexual ability; painful urination; frequent and urgent urination; fever; stroke; difficulty sleeping; tingling in the hands or feet; appetite loss; odd taste perception; hepatitis or jaundice (symptoms of either condition include yellowing of the skin or whites of the eyes); blood in the stool; hair loss; unusual skin sensitivity to the sun; flushing; anxiety; muscle aches; arthritis; asthma; feeling unwell; sweating; kidney problems; blurred vision; swelling of the arms, lips, tongue, face, and throat; and inflammation of the pancreas.

Drug Interactions

• The blood-pressure-lowering effect of Lexxel is additive with that of diuretic (agent that increases urination) drugs or beta blockers. Any other drug that causes a rapid blood-pressure drop should be used with caution if you are taking Lexxel.

• Lexxel may raise blood-potassium levels, especially when taken with dyazide or other potassium-sparing diuretics.

• Lexxel may increase the effects of lithium; this combination should be used with caution.

• Capsaicin may cause or aggravate the cough associated with Lexxel therapy.

• Indomethacin may reduce the blood-pressure-lowering effect of Lexxel.

• Phenothiazine tranquilizers and antiemetics may increase the effects of Lexxel.

• Rifampin may reduce the effects of Lexxel.

• Combining allopurinol with Lexxel increases the risk of experiencing an adverse drug reaction. Avoid this combination.

• Cimetidine and ranitidine increase the amount of felodipine in the blood, causing a slight increase in the drug's effect.

• Phenytoin and other hydantoin anti-seizure drugs, carbamazepine, and barbiturate sleeping pills and sedatives may decrease the amount of felodipine in the blood, reducing its effect.

• Erythromycin may increase the side effects of felodipine by slowing its release from the body.

• Felodipine may increase the effects of theophylline (a drug used to treat asthma and other respiratory problems) and oral anticoagulant (blood-thinning) drugs.

• Felodipine may also interact with quinidine (an antiarrhythmic) to produce low blood pressure, very slow heart rate, abnormal heart rhythms, and swelling in the arms or legs.

Food Interactions

Lexxel may be taken without regard to food or meals; you may take it with food if it upsets your stomach. Avoid grapefruit juice while you are on Lexxel. It doubles the amount of felodipine normally absorbed into the blood.

Usual Dose

1 tablet a day. If your medication needs change, you may have to take each ingredient as a separate pill.

Overdosage

Lexxel overdose may cause low blood pressure. If you think you have taken an overdose of this medication, call your doctor or go to a hospital emergency room. ALWAYS bring the prescription bottle or container with you.

Special Information

Call your doctor if you develop a sore throat, mouth sores, abnormal heartbeat, chest pain, a persistent rash, loss of taste perception, constipation, nausea, very low blood pressure, breathing difficulties, increased heart pain, dizziness, or light-headedness or if other side effects are particularly bothersome or persistent.

Be sure to continue taking your medication and follow any instructions for diet restriction or other treatments to help maintain lower blood pressure. Hypertension is a condition with few recognizable symptoms; it may seem to you that you are taking medication that you do not need. Call your doctor or pharmacist if you have any questions.

Do not break or crush Lexxel tablets.

It is important to maintain good dental hygiene while taking Lexxel and to use extra care when using your toothbrush or dental floss because of the risk that the drug will make you more susceptible to infection.

Avoid over-the-counter diet pills, decongestants, and stimulants while taking Lexxel; they may raise blood pressure.

If you forget to take a dose of Lexxel, take it as soon as you remember. If it is almost time for your next dose, skip the dose you forgot and continue with your regular schedule. Do not take a double dose.

Special Populations

Pregnancy/Breast-feeding

Women who are or might be pregnant should not take Lexxel. ACE inhibitors have caused low blood pressure, kidney failure, slow skull formation, and death in the fetus when taken during the last 6 months of pregnancy. Women who are or might be pregnant should not take any ACE inhibitor. Sexually active women of childbearing age who must take Lexxel must use an effective contraceptive method to prevent pregnancy or use a different drug. If you become pregnant, stop taking the medication and call your doctor immediately.

Relatively small amounts of enalapril pass into breast milk; the effect on a nursing infant is likely to be minimal. However, nursing mothers who must take Lexxel should consider bottle-feeding because infants, especially newborns, are more susceptible to enalapril's effects than are adults. The effects of felodipine on newborns is likely to be minimal.

Seniors

Seniors, especially those with liver disease, may be more sensitive to the effects of this drug because it takes longer to pass out of their bodies. Follow your doctor's directions and report any side effects at once.

Generic Name

Lisinopril (lye-SIN-oe-pril)

Brand Names

Prinivil   Zestril

Combination Products

Generic Ingredients: Lisinopril + Hydrochlorothiazide
Zestoretic

Type of Drug

Angiotensin-converting-enzyme (ACE) inhibitor.

Prescribed for

Hypertension (high blood pressure), congestive heart failure, and improving survival after a heart attack.

General Information

ACE inhibitors work by preventing the conversion of a hormone called angiotensin I to another hormone called angiotensin II, a potent blood-vessel constrictor. Preventing this conversion relaxes blood vessels, thus reducing blood pressure and relieving the symptoms of heart failure by making it easier for a failing heart to pump blood through the body. Lisinopril also affects the production of other hormones and enzymes that participate in the regulation of blood vessel dilation; this action probably increases the drug's effectiveness. Lisinopril begins working about 1 hour after you take it and lasts for a full 24 hours.

Some people who start taking an ACE inhibitor after they are already on a diuretic (agent that increases urination) experience a rapid drop in blood pressure after their first doses or when the dosage is increased. To prevent this from happening, you may be told to stop taking the diuretic 2 or 3 days before starting the ACE inhibitor or to increase your salt intake during that time. The diuretic may then be restarted gradually. Heart failure patients generally have been on digoxin and a diuretic before beginning treatment with an ACE Inhibitor.

Cautions and Warnings

Do not take lisinopril if you have had an **allergic reaction** to it in the past. Occasionally, severe allergic reactions have occurred in people undergoing desensitization treatments or certain kinds of kidney dialysis.

Lisinopril occasionally causes very **low blood pressure.**

Lisinopril may affect your kidneys, especially if you have congestive heart failure. Your doctor should check your urine for changes during the first few months of treatment. Dosage adjustment is required if you have reduced kidney function.

ACE inhibitors can affect **white-blood-cell count**, possibly increasing your susceptibility to infection. Blood counts should be monitored periodically.

Possible Side Effects

▼ Most common: headache, dizziness, fatigue, nausea, diarrhea, and chronic cough. The cough is more common in women and usually goes away a few days after the medication is stopped.

▼ Less common: chest pain, low blood pressure, vomiting, upset stomach, breathing difficulties, rash, and muscle weakness.

▼ Rare: sweating, flushing, itching, impotence, reduced sex drive, muscle cramps, muscle and joint aches, arthritis, fainting, anemia, blurred vision, fever, blood vessel irritation, angina, heart attack, stroke, heart palpitations, dizziness when rising from a sitting or lying position, rapid heartbeat, abnormal heart rhythm, swelling in the arms or legs, sleep disturbances, sleepiness, confusion, depression, not feeling well, nervousness, tingling in the hands or feet, appetite loss, constipation, reduced urine flow, dry mouth, hepatitis, jaundice, urinary infection, pancreas inflammation, asthma, bronchitis, and sinus inflammation.

Drug Interactions

• The blood-pressure-lowering effect of lisinopril is additive with diuretic drugs and beta blockers. Any other drug that can reduce blood pressure should be used with caution if you are taking an ACE inhibitor.

• Lisinopril may increase your blood potassium levels, especially when taken with dyazide or other potassium-sparing diuretics.

• Lisinopril may increase the effects of lithium; this combination should be used with caution.

• Antacids may reduce the amount of lisinopril absorbed into the blood. Take these medications at least 2 hours apart.

• Capsaicin may trigger or aggravate lisinopril cough.

• Indomethacin may reduce the blood-pressure-lowering effect of lisinopril.

• Phenothiazine tranquilizers and antiemetics may increase the effects of lisinopril.

• The combination of allopurinol and lisinopril increases the chance of side effects.

• Lisinopril increases blood levels of digoxin, possibly increasing the chance of digoxin-related side effects.

Food Interactions

None known.

Usual Dose

5–40 mg a day. People with severe kidney disease should begin with 2.5 mg a day; dosage may then be increased up to 5–20 mg a day.

Overdosage

The principal effect of lisinopril overdose is a rapid drop in blood pressure, as evidenced by dizziness or fainting. Take the overdose victim to a hospital emergency room immediately. ALWAYS remember to bring the prescription bottle or container with you.

Special Information

Unexplained swelling of the face, lips, hands, and feet can also affect the larynx (throat) and tongue and interfere with breathing. If this happens, the victim should be taken to a hospital emergency room at once for treatment. Also, call your doctor if you develop a sore throat, mouth sores, abnormal heartbeat, chest pain, persistent rash, or loss of taste perception.

You may get dizzy if you rise quickly from a sitting or lying position.

Avoid strenuous exercise and/or very hot weather because heavy sweating or dehydration can cause a rapid drop in blood pressure.

Avoid over-the-counter diet pills, decongestants, and other stimulants that can raise blood pressure.

If you forget to take a dose of lisinopril, take it as soon as you remember. If it is within 8 hours of your next dose, skip the one you forgot and continue with your regular schedule. Do not take a double dose.

Special Populations

Pregnancy/Breast-feeding

ACE inhibitors have caused low blood pressure, kidney failure, slow formation of the skull, and death in fetuses when taken during the last 6 months of pregnancy. Women who are pregnant should not take lisinopril. Women who might become pregnant while taking lisinopril should use an effective contraceptive method and stop taking the medication if they do become pregnant.

It is not known if lisinopril passes into breast milk. However, nursing mothers who must take this drug should consider bottle-feeding: Infants, especially newborns, are more susceptible to the effects of this drug than are adults.

Seniors

Seniors may be more sensitive to the effects of lisinopril than younger adults because of age-related kidney impairment. Your lisinopril dosage must be individualized to your needs.

Generic Name

Lithium Carbonate

(LITH-ee-um CAR-buh-nate) G

Brand Names

Eskalith   Lithonate
Lithane   Lithotabs
Lithobid

The information in this profile also applies to the following drug:

Generic Ingredient: Lithium Citrate
Cibalith-S Ⓢ

Type of Drug

Antipsychotic and antimanic.

Prescribed for

Bipolar (manic-depressive) disorder, especially suppression of manic attacks or reduction in their number and intensity; also prescribed for cancer and AIDS, premenstrual tension, bulimia, postpartum depression, overactive thyroid, and alcoholism, especially in people who are also depressed. Lithium lotion has been used for genital herpes and dandruff.

General Information

Lithium carbonate and lithium citrate are the only effective antimanic drugs. They reduce the levels of manic episodes and may produce normal activity within the first 3 weeks of treatment. Typical manic symptoms include rapid speech, elation, hyperactive movements, little need for sleep, grandiose ideas, poor judgment, aggressiveness, and hostility.

Cautions and Warnings

This drug should not be given to anyone with **heart or kidney disease**, **dehydration**, **low blood sodium**, or to those taking **diuretic drugs**. If such people require lithium carbonate, they must be very carefully monitored by their doctors, and hospitalization may be needed until the lithium carbonate dose is stabilized.

A few people treated with both lithium carbonate and haloperidol or another antipsychotic have developed **encephalopathic syndrome** (symptoms include weakness, tiredness, fever, confusion, tremulousness, and uncontrollable muscle spasms). In addition, your doctor may find laboratory indicators of liver and/or kidney disease. Rarely, this combination of symptoms is followed by irreversible brain damage.

As many as 20% of people taking long-term lithium carbonate treatment develop **structural changes in their kidneys** and **reduced kidney function**.

Long-term use of this drug may also lead to **reduced thyroid activity, enlargement of the thyroid gland, and in-**

creased blood levels of thyroid-stimulating hormone. All of these conditions may be treated with thyroid hormone replacement therapy. **Overactive thyroid** has also occasionally occurred.

Frequent urination and thirst associated with lithium carbonate may be a sign of a condition known as diabetes insipidus, in which the kidney stops responding to a hormone called vasopressin, which causes the kidney to reabsorb water and make concentrated urine. Lithium carbonate may reverse the kidney's ability to perform this function, but things usually go back to normal when lithium carbonate treatment is stopped, dosage is reduced, or small doses of a thiazide diuretic are taken. Your lithium carbonate dosage may have to be temporarily reduced if you develop an infection or fever.

Some lithium carbonate products contain tartrazine dyes for product coloring purposes. Tartrazine can stimulate allergic responses in some people, including asthma. Ask your pharmacist or doctor for more information.

Possible Side Effects

Side effects of lithium carbonate are directly associated with the amount of drug in the bloodstream. Few side effects are seen if the blood level is less than 1.5 mEq/L, except in the occasional person who is sensitive to the drug. Mild to moderate side effects may occur at blood levels between 1.5 and 2.5 mEq/L. Moderate to severe reactions are seen when lithium carbonate blood levels range from 2 to 2.5 mEq/L.

▼ Most common: fine hand tremor, thirst, and excessive urination, especially when treatment is first started; mild nausea and discomfort during the first few days of treatment.

▼ Less common: diarrhea, vomiting, drowsiness, muscle weakness, poor coordination, giddiness, ringing or buzzing in the ears, and blurred vision.

▼ Rare: worsening symptoms in the muscles; nerves; central nervous system such as blackouts, seizures, dizziness, incontinence, slurred speech, and coma; heart and blood vessels; stomach and intestines such as diarrhea, nausea, and vomiting; kidney and urinary tract; skin; and thyroid gland. Lithium carbonate can also cause changes

---

Possible Side Effects *(continued)*

in tests used to monitor heart-brain function and can cause dry mouth and blurred vision.

Drug Interactions

• When lithium carbonate is combined with haloperidol, weakness, tiredness, fever, or confusion may result. In some people, these symptoms have been followed by permanent brain damage. Also, haloperidol may increase the effect of lithium carbonate.

• Combining lithium carbonate and chlorpromazine may reduce the effect of chlorpromazine and increase the lithium carbonate effect.

• The effect of lithium carbonate is counteracted by sodium bicarbonate, acetazolamide, urea, mannitol, and theophylline drugs, which increase the rate at which lithium carbonate is released from the body. Verapamil may reduce both blood levels of lithium carbonate and the chances of lithium carbonate toxicity.

• The effect of lithium carbonate may be increased by methyldopa, fluoxetine, carbamazepine, thiazide and loop diuretics, and nonsteroidal anti-inflammatory drugs (NSAIDs).

• Lithium carbonate may increase the effects of tricyclic antidepressant medications.

Food Interactions

It is essential to maintain a normal diet, including sodium (salt) and fluid intake, because lithium carbonate can cause a natural reduction in body-salt levels. Lithium carbonate should be taken immediately after meals or with food or milk.

Usual Dose

Dosage must be individualized to each person's needs. Most people will respond to 1800 mg a day at first. Once the person has responded to lithium carbonate, daily dosage is reduced to the lowest effective level, usually 300 mg 3–4 times a day.

Overdosage

Toxic blood levels of lithium carbonate are only slightly above the levels required for treatment. Blood levels should not exceed 2 mEq/L. Early signs of drug toxicity may be diarrhea, vomiting, nausea, tremors, drowsiness, and poor coordination. Later signs of toxicity include giddiness, weakness, blurred vision, ringing or buzzing in the ears, dizziness, fainting, confusion, muscle twitching, uncontrollable muscle movements, loss of bladder control, worsening of manic symptoms, overactive reflexes, and painful muscles or joints. If any of these symptoms occur, stop taking the medication and call your doctor immediately. ALWAYS bring the prescription bottle or container with you when you go to an emergency room.

Special Information

Lithium carbonate may cause drowsiness. Be cautious while driving or operating any hazardous machinery.

Lithium carbonate causes your body to lose sodium (salt). You must maintain a normal diet and salt intake and drink 8 to 12 full glasses of water a day while taking this drug. You may find that excessive sweating, which causes you to lose salt, or diarrhea makes you more sensitive to side effects.

Call your doctor if you develop diarrhea, vomiting, unsteady walking, tremors, drowsiness, or muscle weakness.

Your tolerance to a particular lithium carbonate dose may be reduced when your manic symptoms decline, causing a need for your doctor to modify your dose.

If you forget to take a dose of lithium carbonate, take it as soon as possible. However, if it is within 2 hours of your next dose, or 6 hours if you take the long-acting form, skip the missed dose and go back to your regular schedule. Do not take a double dose. Call your doctor if you miss more than 1 dose.

Special Populations

Pregnancy/Breast-feeding

Lithium carbonate can cause heart and thyroid birth defects, especially if taken during the first 3 months of pregnancy. It can also affect your newborn baby if the drug is present in your blood during delivery. These effects generally go away in a week or two, when the baby can eliminate the drug from his or her system. Talk with your doctor about the risks versus the benefits of taking this drug during your pregnancy.

Lithium carbonate passes readily into breast milk and can affect a nursing infant. Signs of these effects are weak muscle tone, low body temperature, bluish discoloration of the skin, and abnormal heart rhythm. You should bottle-feed your baby while taking this medication.

Seniors

Seniors are more sensitive than younger adults to the effects of lithium carbonate because their kidneys cannot clear it from their bodies as rapidly. It is potentially toxic to the central nervous system in older adults, even when lithium carbonate blood levels are in the desired range. Also, seniors taking lithium carbonate are more likely to develop an underactive thyroid.

Lo/Ovral

see **Contraceptives**, page 246

Lodine

see **Etodolac**, page 392

Type of Drug

Loop Diuretics

Brand Names

Generic Ingredient: Bumetanide Ⓖ
Bumex

Generic Ingredient: Ethacrynic Acid
Edecrin

Generic Ingredient: Furosemide Ⓖ
Lasix

Generic Ingredient: Torsemide
Demadex

Prescribed for

Congestive heart failure, cirrhosis of the liver, fluid accumulation in the lungs, kidney dysfunction, high blood pressure, and other conditions where it may be desirable to rid the body of excess fluid. Bumetanide can be used to treat people who urinate frequently at night. It does not work in prostatic hypertrophy.

General Information

Loop diuretics are strong drugs that work in a fashion similar to that of the less potent and more widely used thiazide diuretics. Not only do they affect the same part of the kidney as the thiazide diuretics, they also affect the portion of the kidney known as the "loop of Henle." This double action is what makes the loop diuretics such potent drugs. All 4 loop diuretics can be used for the same purposes, but their dosages are quite different.

Cautions and Warnings

Do not take these medications if you are **sensitive** or **allergic** to them. People allergic to sulfa drugs may also be allergic to furosemide, torsemide, or bumetanide.

Loop diuretics are potent drugs and can cause depletion of water and electrolytes. They should not be taken without constant medical supervision. You should not take these drugs if your urine production has been decreased abnormally by some type of **kidney disease**.

Excessive use of loop diuretics will result in **dehydration** or **reduction in blood volume**, and may cause circulatory collapse or other related problems, particularly in older adults.

Ringing or buzzing in the ears, hearing loss, deafness, fainting, and **fullness in the ears** can occur with these drugs. Hearing usually returns within 24 hours, but some loss may be permanent.

These drugs may worsen systemic **lupus erythematosus**. **Diarrhea** may occur with ethacrynic acid or furosemide solution because of the sorbitol content. On rare occasions, people taking bumetanide have developed **thrombocytopenia** (low blood-platelet count).

Because of the potent effect that these drugs have on **blood electrolytes** — potassium, sodium, carbon dioxide, and others — frequent laboratory evaluations of these electrolytes should be performed during the few months of therapy and periodically thereafter.

People taking a loop diuretic may develop **increased levels of total cholesterol, LDL cholesterol**, and **triglycerides**.

Possible Side Effects

▼ Common: Changes may develop in potassium and other electrolyte concentrations in your body. In the case of hypokalemia (low blood potassium), you may observe dryness of the mouth, excessive thirst, weakness, lethargy, drowsiness, restlessness, muscle pain or cramps, muscular tiredness, low blood pressure, decreased frequency of urination and decreased amount of urine produced, abnormal heart rate, and stomach upset, including nausea and vomiting. To compensate for this potassium loss, potassium supplements — tablets, liquids, or powders — and/or potassium-rich foods — bananas, citrus fruits, melons, and tomatoes — are recommended. Loop diuretics may change sugar metabolism in your body: If you have diabetes mellitus, you may develop high blood sugar or sugar in the urine. To treat this problem, the dosage of your antidiabetes drugs will have to be increased.

▼ Less common: abdominal discomfort, nausea, vomiting, diarrhea, rash, dizziness, light-headedness, headache, blurred vision, fatigue, weakness, jaundice (yellowing of the skin or whites of the eyes), acute gout attacks, dermatitis and other skin reactions, tingling in the extremities, dizziness upon rising quickly from a sitting or lying position, and anemia.

▼ Rare: a sweet taste in the mouth, a burning feeling in the stomach and/or mouth, excessive thirst, increased perspiration, and frequent urination.

Drug Interactions

• Loop diuretics increase the action of other blood-pressure-lowering drugs. This is beneficial and is frequently used to help lower blood pressure in patients with hypertension.

• The possibility of developing electrolyte imbalances in body fluids is increased if you take medications such as digitalis or adrenal corticosteroids while you are taking a loop diuretic. Be aware that the potassium loss caused by loop diuretics will significantly affect the toxicity of digitalis.

• Loop diuretics may increase the action of oral anticoagulants (blood-thinners); dosage adjustment may be needed if you are taking an anticoagulant.

• If you are taking an oral antidiabetes drug — except metformin — and begin taking a loop diuretic, the antidiabetes dosage may need to be altered.

• The action of theophylline may be altered by any loop diuretic. Your doctor should check your theophylline levels after you have started on a loop diuretic.

• If you are taking lithium carbonate, you should probably not take a diuretic, which greatly increases the risk of lithium toxicity by impairing the elimination of lithium from the blood.

• People taking chloral hydrate as a nighttime sedative may, in rare cases, experience hot flashes, high blood pressure, sweating, abnormal heart rhythm, weakness, and nausea when they also take a loop diuretic.

• Periodic hearing loss or ringing or buzzing in the ears may occur if a loop diuretic is taken with cisplatin (an anticancer drug) or an aminoglycoside antibiotic. Make sure your doctor knows you are taking a loop diuretic before giving you an injection of either of these.

• Clofibrate and thiazide diuretics increase the action of loop diuretics.

• Charcoal tablets, phenytoin, probenecid, aspirin and other salicylate drugs, and nonsteroidal anti-inflammatory drugs (NSAIDs) may decrease the effectiveness of loop diuretics.

• If you are taking a loop diuretic for high blood pressure or congestive heart failure, avoid over-the-counter cough, cold, and allergy products, which often contain stimulant drugs; check with your pharmacist before taking any over-the-counter drug if you're taking a loop diuretic.

Food Interactions

Loop diuretics rob your body of potassium. To counteract this effect, be sure to eat high-potassium foods, such as bananas, citrus fruits, melons, and tomatoes.

Furosemide should be taken on an empty stomach, at least 1 hour before or 2 hours after meals. The other loop diuretics, bumetanide, torsemide, and ethacrynic acid may be taken with food if they upset your stomach.

Usual Dose

Bumetanide
0.5–2 mg a day. It may also be taken every other day for 3 or 4 consecutive days followed by 1 or 2 days off the drug.

Ethacrynic Acid
Adult: 50–200 mg, taken every day or every other day.
Child: starting dose — 25 mg; increase slowly.

Furosemide
Adult: 20–80 mg a day, depending on your response. Doses of 600 mg or more a day have been prescribed.
Child: 0.9 mg per lb. of body weight in a single daily dose. If therapy is not successful, the dose may be increased in small steps, but not more than 2.7 mg per lb. a day.

Torsemide
Adult: 5–20 mg once a day. Doses up to 200 mg may be prescribed if necessary.
Child: not recommended.

Maintenance doses for all of the loop diuretics are adjusted to the minimum effective level to meet the individual's needs.

Overdosage

Symptoms include dehydration, reduced blood volume, passing of tremendous amounts of urine, weakness, dizziness, confusion, appetite loss, tiredness, vomiting, and cramps. Overdose victims should be taken to an emergency room for treatment. ALWAYS bring the prescription bottle or container with you.

Special Information

If, while taking a loop diuretic, the amount of urine you produce each day is dropping, or if you suffer from cramps, significant appetite loss, muscle weakness, tiredness, or nausea, contact your doctor immediately.

Loop diuretics are usually taken once a day after breakfast. If a second dose is needed, it should be taken no later than 2 p.m. to avoid nighttime urination.

To avoid the dizziness associated with these drugs, rise slowly and carefully from a sitting or lying position.

Loop diuretics can increase blood sugar. Diabetics may need their medication adjusted.

Loop diuretics can make some people very sensitive to the sun and to sunlamps. Avoid excess exposure, use sunscreens, and wear protective clothing.

If you forget to take a loop diuretic dose, take it as soon as you remember. If it is almost time for your next dose, skip the one you forgot and continue with your regular schedule. Do not take a double dose.

Special Populations

Pregnancy/Breast-feeding
Loop diuretics have been used to treat specific conditions in pregnancy, but they should be used only when absolutely necessary.

Loop diuretics may pass into breast milk. Bottle-feed your baby if you must take one of these drugs.

Seniors
Seniors are more sensitive to the effects of these drugs. Follow your doctor's directions and report any side effects at once.

Generic Name

Loperamide (loe-PER-uh-mide) [G]

Brand Name

Imodium

Type of Drug

Antidiarrheal.

Prescribed for

Acute and chronic diarrhea; also prescribed to reduce the amount of discharge in an ileostomy (surgical procedure in which a hole is made in the small intestine, usually through the abdominal wall).

General Information

Loperamide hydrochloride and other antidiarrheal agents should be used only for short periods; they will relieve diarrhea, but not its underlying causes. In some cases antidiarrheals should not be used at all; these drugs may harm people with certain bowel, stomach, or other diseases. Loperamide is not known to be addictive. It is available over-the-counter (OTC) under a variety of brand names. OTC loperamide products are used to treat acute diarrhea and traveler's diarrhea.

Cautions and Warnings

Do not use loperamide if you are **allergic or sensitive** to it, if you suffer from diarrhea associated with **colitis**, or if you have an **intestinal infection** of *Escherichia coli*, *Salmonella*, or *Shigella*. Loperamide should not be taken together with clindamycin.

If you have **ulcerative colitis** and start taking loperamide, stop the drug at once and call your doctor if you develop abdominal problems of any kind.

Possible Side Effects

The incidence of side effects from loperamide is low. Side effects are most likely to occur when loperamide is taken over longer periods to treat chronic diarrhea.

▼ Most common: stomach and abdominal pain, bloating or other discomfort, constipation, dry mouth, dizziness, tiredness, nausea and vomiting, and drug-sensitivity reactions, including rash.

Drug Interactions

• Loperamide depresses the central nervous system (CNS) and may make you tired and unable to concentrate; it may increase the effect of sleeping pills, tranquilizers, and alcohol. Avoid drinking alcoholic beverages while taking loperamide.

Food Interactions

Loperamide should be taken on an empty stomach.

Usual Dose

Acute Diarrhea

Adult and Child (age 12 and over): 4 mg to start, followed by 2 mg after each loose stool, up to 16 mg a day maximum. Improvement should be seen in 2 days.

Child (age 9–12): 2 mg 3 times a day to start, followed by 1 mg for every 22 lbs. of body weight after each loose stool, up to 6 mg a day maximum.

Child (age 6–8): 2 mg twice a day to start, followed by 1 mg for every 22 lbs. of body weight after each loose stool, up to 4 mg a day maximum.

Child (age 2–5): 1 mg 3 times a day to start, followed by 1 mg for every 22 lbs. of body weight after each loose stool, up to 3 mg a day maximum.

Chronic Diarrhea

Adult and child (age 12 and over): 4 mg to start, followed by 2 mg after each loose stool, until symptoms are controlled. Then dosage should be tailored to individual needs — usually 4–8 mg a day. Loperamide is usually effective within 10 days or not at all.

Overdosage

Symptoms of loperamide overdose are constipation, irritation of the stomach, and tiredness. Large doses usually cause vomiting. An overdose victim should be taken to the emergency room immediately. ALWAYS bring the prescription bottle or container with you.

Special Information

Loperamide may cause drowsiness and make it difficult to concentrate: Be careful while driving or operating any appliance or hazardous equipment.

Loperamide may cause dry mouth. Drink plenty of water or other clear fluids to prevent dehydration from the diarrhea. It is important to maintain a proper diet and to drink plenty of fluids to restore normal bowel function.

Call your doctor if diarrhea persists after a few days of loperamide treatment or if you develop abdominal discomfort or pain, fever, or other side effects.

If you forget to take a dose of loperamide, skip that dose and go back to your regular schedule. Do not take a double dose.

Special Populations

Pregnancy/Breast-feeding

Loperamide has not been found to cause birth defects; however, women who are or might be pregnant should not take this drug without their doctor's approval. When loperamide is considered crucial by your doctor, its benefits must be carefully weighed against its risks.

It is not known if loperamide passes into breast milk. Possible effects on your nursing infant must be considered if you breast-feed while taking loperamide.

Seniors

Seniors may be more sensitive to the constipating effects of loperamide.

Generic Name

Loratadine (lor-AH-tuh-dene)

Brand Name

Claritin

Type of Drug

Antihistamine.

Prescribed for

Stuffy and runny nose, itchy eyes, and scratchy throat caused by seasonal allergy and for other symptoms of allergy such as rash, itching, and hives; also prescribed for asthma triggered by an allergic reaction.

General Information

Antihistamines generally work by blocking the release of histamine (chemical released by body tissue during an allergic reaction) from the cell at the H_1 histamine receptor site, drying up secretions of the nose, throat, and eyes.

Loratadine causes less sedation than most antihistamines and appears to be just as effective. It has been widely used by those who find the drowsiness and tiredness caused by other antihistamines unacceptable.

Cautions and Warnings

Do not take loratadine if you are **allergic** to it.

People with liver disease should receive reduced doses of loratadine because they are unable to clear the drug rapidly from their bodies.

Possible Side Effects

▼ Most common: headache, dry mouth, drowsiness, and fatigue.

▼ Less common: sweating, tearing, impotence, thirst, flushing, blurred vision, conjunctivitis (pinkeye), earache, eye pain, ringing or buzzing in the ears, weight gain, back pain, leg cramps, chest pain, fever, chills, not feeling well, weakness, worsening of allergic symptoms, respiratory

---

Possible Side Effects *(continued)*

infection, breathing difficulties, blood-pressure changes, dizziness, fainting, heart palpitations, rapid heartbeat, hyperactivity, tingling in the hands or feet, eye-muscle spasms, migraine, tremors, nausea, vomiting, gas, abdominal distress, stomach irritation or upset, constipation, diarrhea, changes in sense of taste, changes in appetite, toothache, joint or muscle aches or pains, anxiety, depression, agitation, sleeplessness, memory lapse, loss of concentration, paranoia, confusion, nervousness, loss of sex drive, breast pain, vaginal irritation, menstrual changes, dry nose, stuffy nose, runny nose, nosebleeds, sore throat, coughing, sneezing, vomiting blood, bronchitis, bronchial spasm, laryngitis, itching, rash, dry hair or skin, unusual sensitivity to the sun, black-and-blue marks, altered urination, and urine discoloration.

▼ Rare: swelling in the legs, ankles, or feet; yellowing of the skin or whites of the eyes; hepatitis; hair loss; seizures; breast enlargement; and erythema multiforme (skin reaction).

Drug Interactions

• Unlike most antihistamines, loratadine is not known to interact with alcohol or other nervous-system depressants to produce drowsiness or loss of coordination.

• Loratadine, like other nonsedating antihistamines, may interact with ketoconazole, erythromycin, cimetidine, ranitidine, or theophylline. Conclusive evidence for these interactions has not yet been established due to the small number of people taking these drug combinations. If you are taking any of these drugs with loratadine, be sure to report any problems to your doctor.

Food Interactions

Loratadine should be taken on an empty stomach 1 hour before or 2 hours after eating; it may be taken with food or milk if it upsets your stomach.

Usual Dose

Adult and Child (over age 12): 10 mg once a day. People with liver disease should take 10 mg every other day.

Overdosage

Loratadine overdose is likely to cause drowsiness, headache, and rapid heartbeat. Severe side effects may also occur. Overdose victims should be given ipecac syrup — available at any pharmacy — to make them vomit and be taken to a hospital emergency room for treatment. Call your local poison control center or hospital emergency room for instructions. ALWAYS bring the prescription bottle or container with you.

Special Information

Dizziness or fainting may be the first sign of a serious side effect. Call your doctor at once if this happens to you.

Report sore throat; unusual bleeding, bruising, tiredness, or weakness; or any other unusual side effect to your doctor.

If you forget to take a dose of loratadine, take it as soon as you remember. If it is almost time for your next dose, skip the one you forgot and continue with your regular schedule. Do not take a double dose.

Special Populations

Pregnancy/Breast-feeding

Antihistamines have not been proven to cause birth defects in humans. Animal studies of loratadine have not revealed any adverse effect on the fetus. Do not take any antihistamine without your doctor's knowledge if you are or might be pregnant — especially during the last 3 months of pregnancy, because newborns may have severe reactions to antihistamines.

Loratadine passes into breast milk and may affect a nursing infant. Nursing mothers who must take loratadine should bottle-feed their infants.

Seniors

Seniors are unlikely to experience nervous-system effects with loratadine as opposed to the older, more sedating antihistamines. However, seniors, especially those with liver disease, are more likely to experience side effects than are younger adults. Report any unusual side effects to your doctor.

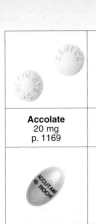		
Accolate 20 mg p. 1169	**Accupril** 10 mg p. 951	**Accutane** 20 mg p. 538

Accutane 40 mg p. 538	**Achromycin V** 250 mg p. 1064	**Adalat CC** 30 mg p. 781
Adalat CC 60 mg p. 781	**Adalat CC** 90 mg p. 781	**Aldactazide** 25/25 mg p. 357

Aldomet 250 mg p. 680	**Aldomet** 500 mg p. 680

Allegra 60 mg p. 178	**Altace** 2.5 mg p. 951	**Altace** 5 mg p. 951	**Alupent** 10 mg p. 665

A

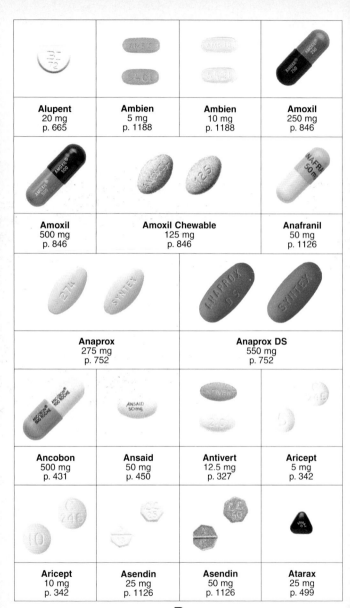

Alupent 20 mg p. 665	**Ambien** 5 mg p. 1188	**Ambien** 10 mg p. 1188	**Amoxil** 250 mg p. 846
Amoxil 500 mg p. 846	**Amoxil Chewable** 125 mg p. 846		**Anafranil** 50 mg p. 1126
Anaprox 275 mg p. 752		**Anaprox DS** 550 mg p. 752	
Ancobon 500 mg p. 431	**Ansaid** 50 mg p. 450	**Antivert** 12.5 mg p. 327	**Aricept** 5 mg p. 342
Aricept 10 mg p. 342	**Asendin** 25 mg p. 1126	**Asendin** 50 mg p. 1126	**Atarax** 25 mg p. 499

B

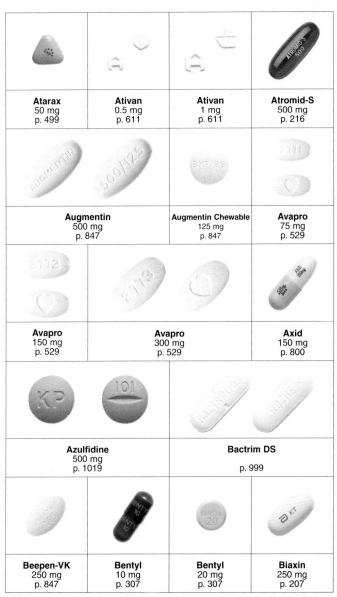

Atarax 50 mg p. 499	**Ativan** 0.5 mg p. 611	**Ativan** 1 mg p. 611	**Atromid-S** 500 mg p. 216

Augmentin 500 mg p. 847	**Augmentin Chewable** 125 mg p. 847	**Avapro** 75 mg p. 529

Avapro 150 mg p. 529	**Avapro** 300 mg p. 529	**Axid** 150 mg p. 800

Azulfidine 500 mg p. 1019	**Bactrim DS** p. 999

Beepen-VK 250 mg p. 847	**Bentyl** 10 mg p. 307	**Bentyl** 20 mg p. 307	**Biaxin** 250 mg p. 207

C

Biaxin 500 mg p. 207	**Blocadren** 10 mg p. 1093	**Blocadren** 20 mg p. 1093	**Brethine** 2.5 mg p. 1054
Brethine 5 mg p. 1054	**Bricanyl** 2.5 mg p. 1054	**Bricanyl** 5 mg p. 1054	**Bumex** 1 mg p. 600
BuSpar 5 mg p. 139	**Calan** 40 mg p. 1153	**Calan SR** 240 mg p. 1153	
Capoten 12.5 mg p. 149	**Capoten** 25 mg p. 149	**Capoten** 50 mg p. 149	**Capoten** 100 mg p. 149
Capozide 25/15 mg p. 149	**Capozide** 25/25 mg p. 149	**Cardizem** 30 mg p. 324	**Cardizem** 60 mg p. 324

D

Cardizem CD 180 mg p. 324	**Cardizem CD** 240 mg p. 324	**Cardizem CD** 300 mg p. 324	**Cardizem SR** 60 mg p. 324
Cardizem SR 90 mg p. 324	**Cardizem SR** 120 mg p. 324	**Cardura** 2 mg p. 350	**Cartrol** 2.5 mg p. 160
Cartrol 5 mg p. 160	**Catapres** 0.1 mg p. 224	**Catapres** 0.2 mg p. 224	**Ceclor** 500 mg p. 169
Ceftin 125 mg p. 169	**Ceftin** 500 mg p. 169		**Cefzil** 500 mg p. 169
CellCept 250 mg p. 744	**Cipro** 250 mg p. 433	**Cipro** 500 mg p. 433	**Cipro** 750 mg p. 433

E

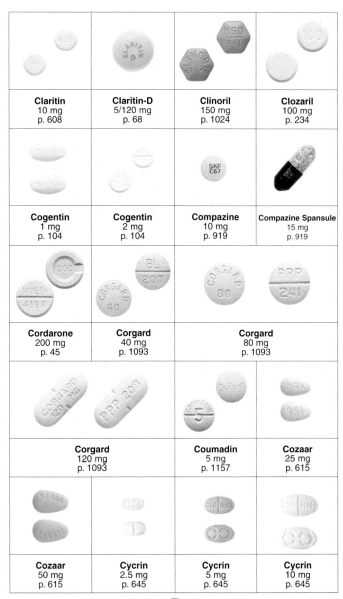

Claritin 10 mg p. 608	**Claritin-D** 5/120 mg p. 68	**Clinoril** 150 mg p. 1024	**Clozaril** 100 mg p. 234
Cogentin 1 mg p. 104	**Cogentin** 2 mg p. 104	**Compazine** 10 mg p. 919	**Compazine Spansule** 15 mg p. 919
Cordarone 200 mg p. 45	**Corgard** 40 mg p. 1093	**Corgard** 80 mg p. 1093	
Corgard 120 mg p. 1093		**Coumadin** 5 mg p. 1157	**Cozaar** 25 mg p. 615
Cozaar 50 mg p. 615	**Cycrin** 2.5 mg p. 645	**Cycrin** 5 mg p. 645	**Cycrin** 10 mg p. 645

F

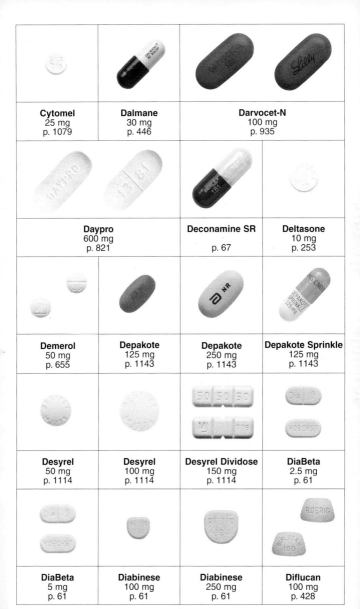

Cytomel 25 mg p. 1079	**Dalmane** 30 mg p. 446	**Darvocet-N** 100 mg p. 935	
Daypro 600 mg p. 821		**Deconamine SR** p. 67	**Deltasone** 10 mg p. 253
Demerol 50 mg p. 655	**Depakote** 125 mg p. 1143	**Depakote** 250 mg p. 1143	**Depakote Sprinkle** 125 mg p. 1143
Desyrel 50 mg p. 1114	**Desyrel** 100 mg p. 1114	**Desyrel Dividose** 150 mg p. 1114	**DiaBeta** 2.5 mg p. 61
DiaBeta 5 mg p. 61	**Diabinese** 100 mg p. 61	**Diabinese** 250 mg p. 61	**Diflucan** 100 mg p. 428

G

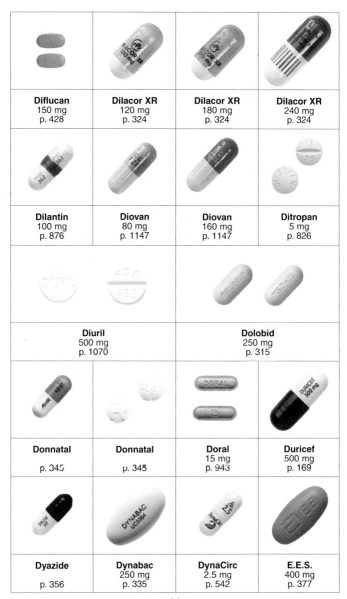

Diflucan 150 mg p. 428	**Dilacor XR** 120 mg p. 324	**Dilacor XR** 180 mg p. 324	**Dilacor XR** 240 mg p. 324
Dilantin 100 mg p. 876	**Diovan** 80 mg p. 1147	**Diovan** 160 mg p. 1147	**Ditropan** 5 mg p. 826
Diuril 500 mg p. 1070		**Dolobid** 250 mg p. 315	
Donnatal p. 345	**Donnatal** p. 345	**Doral** 15 mg p. 943	**Duricef** 500 mg p. 169
Dyazide p. 356	**Dynabac** 250 mg p. 335	**DynaCirc** 2.5 mg p. 542	**E.E.S.** 400 mg p. 377

H

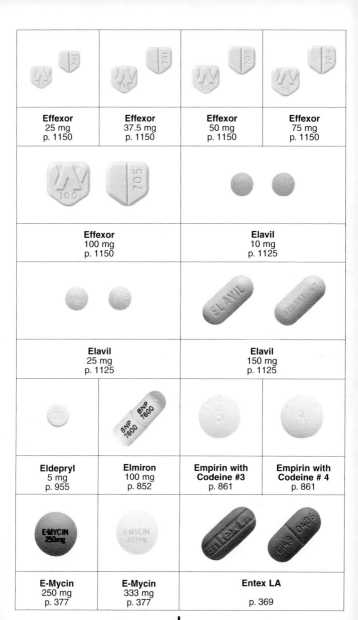

Effexor 25 mg p. 1150	**Effexor** 37.5 mg p. 1150	**Effexor** 50 mg p. 1150	**Effexor** 75 mg p. 1150

Effexor 100 mg p. 1150	**Elavil** 10 mg p. 1125

Elavil 25 mg p. 1125	**Elavil** 150 mg p. 1125

Eldepryl 5 mg p. 955	**Elmiron** 100 mg p. 852	**Empirin with Codeine #3** p. 861	**Empirin with Codeine # 4** p. 861

E-Mycin 250 mg p. 377	**E-Mycin** 333 mg p. 377	**Entex LA** p. 369

I

Equagesic p. 372	**EryPed Chewable** 200 mg p. 377
Ery-Tab 250 mg p. 377	**Ery-Tab** 333 mg p. 377	**Erythrocin Stearate** 250 mg p. 377

Erythrocin Stearate 500 mg p. 377	**Erythromycin Base Filmtab** 250 mg p. 377

Esidrix 50 mg p. 1070	**Eskalith** 300 mg p. 595	**Eskalith CR** 450 mg p. 595	**Estrace** 1 mg p. 386

Ethmozine 200 mg p. 732	**Ethmozine** 250 mg p. 732

J

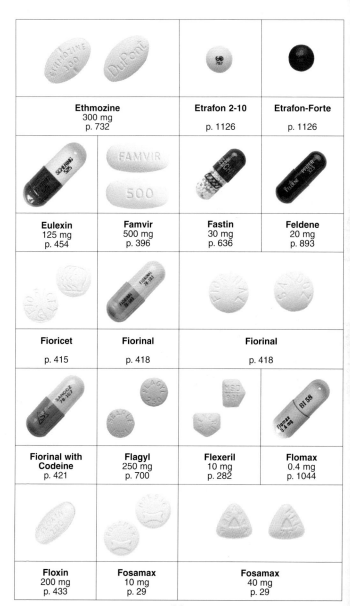

Ethmozine 300 mg p. 732	**Etrafon 2-10** p. 1126	**Etrafon-Forte** p. 1126
Eulexin 125 mg p. 454	**Famvir** 500 mg p. 396	**Fastin** 30 mg p. 636	**Feldene** 20 mg p. 893
Fioricet p. 415	**Fiorinal** p. 418	**Fiorinal** p. 418
Fiorinal with Codeine p. 421	**Flagyl** 250 mg p. 700	**Flexeril** 10 mg p. 282	**Flomax** 0.4 mg p. 1044
Floxin 200 mg p. 433	**Fosamax** 10 mg p. 29	**Fosamax** 40 mg p. 29

K

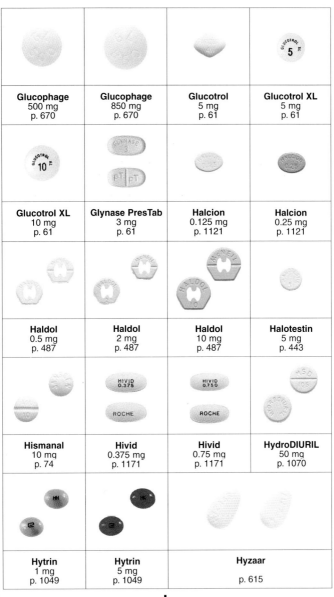

Glucophage 500 mg p. 670	**Glucophage** 850 mg p. 670	**Glucotrol** 5 mg p. 61	**Glucotrol XL** 5 mg p. 61
Glucotrol XL 10 mg p. 61	**Glynase PresTab** 3 mg p. 61	**Halcion** 0.125 mg p. 1121	**Halcion** 0.25 mg p. 1121
Haldol 0.5 mg p. 487	**Haldol** 2 mg p. 487	**Haldol** 10 mg p. 487	**Halotestin** 5 mg p. 443
Hismanal 10 mg p. 74	**Hivid** 0.375 mg p. 1171	**Hivid** 0.75 mg p. 1171	**HydroDIURIL** 50 mg p. 1070
Hytrin 1 mg p. 1049	**Hytrin** 5 mg p. 1049	**Hyzaar** p. 615	

L

Imdur 60 mg p. 534	**Imdur** 120 mg p. 534	**Imitrex** 25 mg p. 1028	**Imitrex** 50 mg p. 1028
Inderal 40 mg p. 938	**Inderal** 80 mg p. 938	**Inderal LA** 60 mg p. 938	**Inderal LA** 120 mg p. 938
Inderide 40/25 mg p. 938	**Inderide** 80/25 mg p. 938		**Inderide LA** 80/50 mg p. 938
Inderide LA 120/50 mg p. 938	**Indocin** 50 mg p. 512	**Indocin SR** 75 mg p. 512	**Ionamin** 30 mg p. 636
Isoptin 40 mg p. 1153	**Isoptin** 120 mg p. 1153		**Isoptin SR** 120 mg p. 1153

M

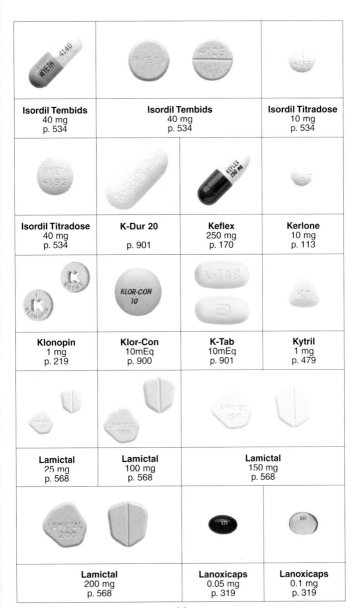

Isordil Tembids 40 mg p. 534	**Isordil Tembids** 40 mg p. 534	**Isordil Titradose** 10 mg p. 534
Isordil Titradose 40 mg p. 534	**K-Dur 20** p. 901	**Keflex** 250 mg p. 170	**Kerlone** 10 mg p. 113
Klonopin 1 mg p. 219	**Klor-Con** 10mEq p. 900	**K-Tab** 10mEq p. 901	**Kytril** 1 mg 479
Lamictal 25 mg p. 568	**Lamictal** 100 mg p. 568	**Lamictal** 150 mg p. 568	
Lamictal 200 mg p. 568	**Lanoxicaps** 0.05 mg p. 319	**Lanoxicaps** 0.1 mg p. 319

N

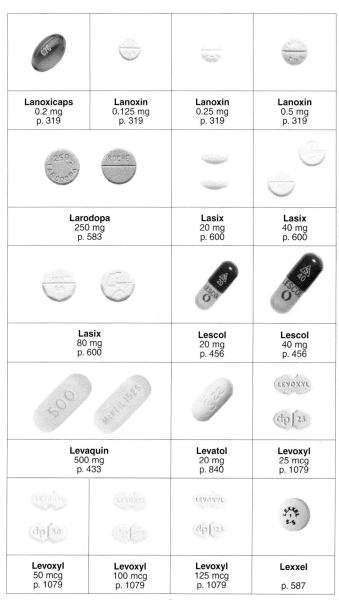

Lanoxicaps 0.2 mg p. 319	**Lanoxin** 0.125 mg p. 319	**Lanoxin** 0.25 mg p. 319	**Lanoxin** 0.5 mg p. 319
Larodopa 250 mg p. 583		**Lasix** 20 mg p. 600	**Lasix** 40 mg p. 600
Lasix 80 mg p. 600		**Lescol** 20 mg p. 456	**Lescol** 40 mg p. 456
Levaquin 500 mg p. 433		**Levatol** 20 mg p. 840	**Levoxyl** 25 mcg p. 1079
Levoxyl 50 mcg p. 1079	**Levoxyl** 100 mcg p. 1079	**Levoxyl** 125 mcg p. 1079	**Lexxel** p. 587

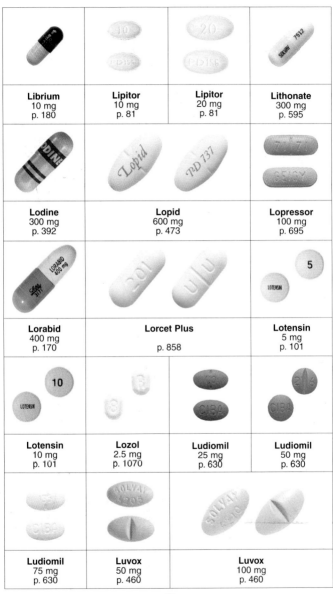

Librium 10 mg p. 180	**Lipitor** 10 mg p. 81	**Lipitor** 20 mg p. 81	**Lithonate** 300 mg p. 595
Lodine 300 mg p. 392	**Lopid** 600 mg p. 473		**Lopressor** 100 mg p. 695
Lorabid 400 mg p. 170	**Lorcet Plus** p. 858		**Lotensin** 5 mg p. 101
Lotensin 10 mg p. 101	**Lozol** 2.5 mg p. 1070	**Ludiomil** 25 mg p. 630	**Ludiomil** 50 mg p. 630
Ludiomil 75 mg p. 630	**Luvox** 50 mg p. 460	**Luvox** 100 mg p. 460	

P

Macrobid p. 792	**Macrodantin** 50 mg p. 792	**Maxaquin** 400 mg p. 433	**Maxzide** p. 356
Maxzide-25MG p. 356	**Mazanor** 1 mg p. 636	**Megace** 40 mg p. 653	**Mellaril** 25 mg p. 189
Mellaril 200 mg p. 189		**Mevacor** 20 mg p. 623	**Mevacor** 40 mg p. 623
Micro-K Extencaps 10 mEq p. 901	**Micronase** 1.25 mg p. 61	**Minipress** 1 mg p. 912	**Minipress** 2 mg p. 912
Minizide 1 p. 912	**Minizide 2** p. 912	**Minocin** 50 mg p. 1064	**Minocin** 100 mg p. 1064

Q

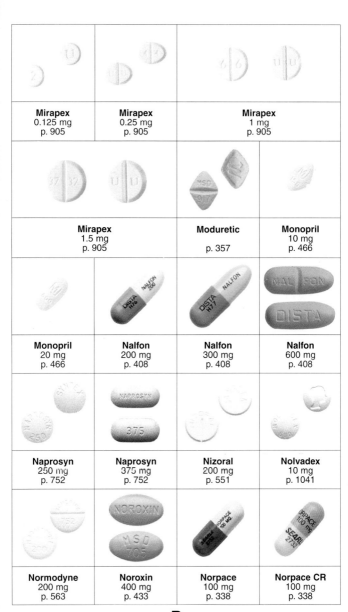

Mirapex 0.125 mg p. 905	**Mirapex** 0.25 mg p. 905	**Mirapex** 1 mg p. 905

Mirapex 1.5 mg p. 905	**Moduretic** p. 357	**Monopril** 10 mg p. 466

Monopril 20 mg p. 466	**Nalfon** 200 mg p. 408	**Nalfon** 300 mg p. 408	**Nalfon** 600 mg p. 408

Naprosyn 250 mg p. 752	**Naprosyn** 375 mg p. 752	**Nizoral** 200 mg p. 551	**Nolvadex** 10 mg p. 1041

Normodyne 200 mg p. 563	**Noroxin** 400 mg p. 433	**Norpace** 100 mg p. 338	**Norpace CR** 100 mg p. 338

R

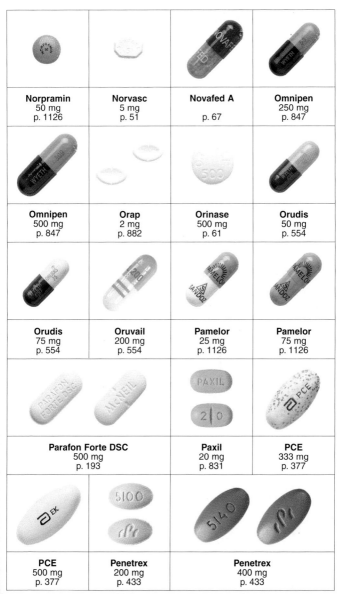

Norpramin 50 mg p. 1126	**Norvasc** 5 mg p. 51	**Novafed A** p. 67	**Omnipen** 250 mg p. 847
Omnipen 500 mg p. 847	**Orap** 2 mg p. 882	**Orinase** 500 mg p. 61	**Orudis** 50 mg p. 554
Orudis 75 mg p. 554	**Oruvail** 200 mg p. 554	**Pamelor** 25 mg p. 1126	**Pamelor** 75 mg p. 1126
Parafon Forte DSC 500 mg p. 193		**Paxil** 20 mg p. 831	**PCE** 333 mg p. 377
PCE 500 mg p. 377	**Penetrex** 200 mg p. 433	**Penetrex** 400 mg p. 433	

S

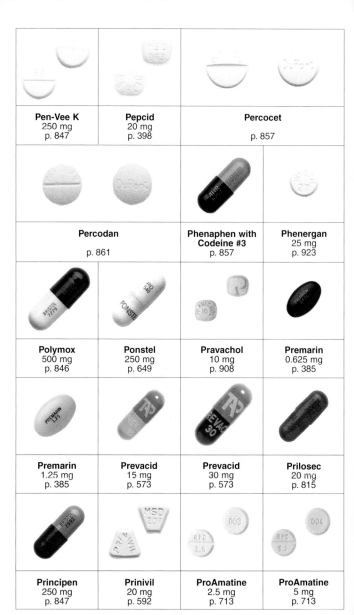

Pen-Vee K 250 mg p. 847	**Pepcid** 20 mg p. 398	**Percocet** p. 857

Percodan p. 861	**Phenaphen with Codeine #3** p. 857	**Phenergan** 25 mg p. 923

Polymox 500 mg p. 846	**Ponstel** 250 mg p. 649	**Pravachol** 10 mg p. 908	**Premarin** 0.625 mg p. 385

Premarin 1.25 mg p. 385	**Prevacid** 15 mg p. 573	**Prevacid** 30 mg p. 573	**Prilosec** 20 mg p. 815

Principen 250 mg p. 847	**Prinivil** 20 mg p. 592	**ProAmatine** 2.5 mg p. 713	**ProAmatine** 5 mg p. 713

T

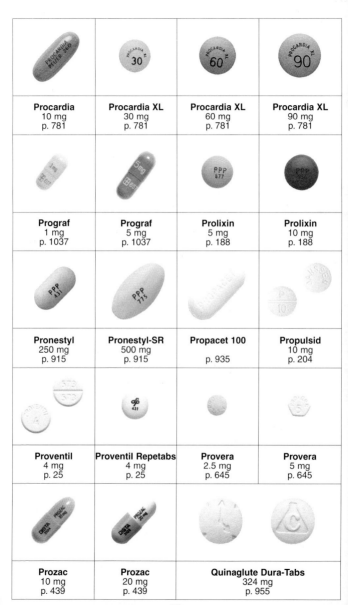

Procardia 10 mg p. 781	**Procardia XL** 30 mg p. 781	**Procardia XL** 60 mg p. 781	**Procardia XL** 90 mg p. 781
Prograf 1 mg p. 1037	**Prograf** 5 mg p. 1037	**Prolixin** 5 mg p. 188	**Prolixin** 10 mg p. 188
Pronestyl 250 mg p. 915	**Pronestyl-SR** 500 mg p. 915	**Propacet 100** p. 935	**Propulsid** 10 mg p. 204
Proventil 4 mg p. 25	**Proventil Repetabs** 4 mg p. 25	**Provera** 2.5 mg p. 645	**Provera** 5 mg p. 645
Prozac 10 mg p. 439	**Prozac** 20 mg p. 439	**Quinaglute Dura-Tabs** 324 mg p. 955	

U

Quinidex Extentabs 300 mg p. 955	**Reglan** 5 mg p. 691	**Reglan** 10 mg p. 691	**Relafen** 500 mg p. 748
	Remeron 30 mg p. 722	**Restoril** 30 mg p. 1121	**Retrovir** 100 mg p. 1176
	Rezulin 300 mg p. 1133		**Rezulin** 400 mg p. 1133
Rimactane 300 mg p. 968	**Risperdal** 1 mg p. 977	**Risperdal** 2 mg p. 977	**Risperdal** 3 mg p. 977
Risperdal 4 mg p. 977	**Ritalin** 10 mg p. 684	**Ritalin-SR** 20 mg p. 684	**Rythmol** 150 mg p. 928

V

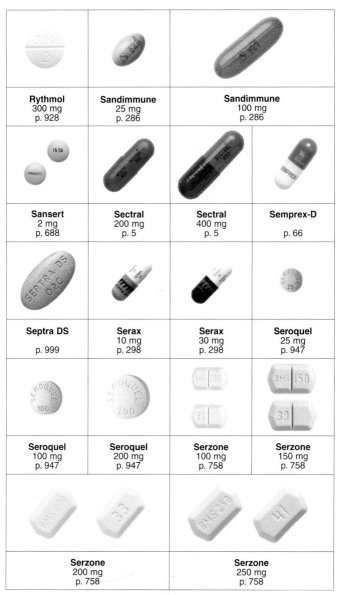

Rythmol 300 mg p. 928	**Sandimmune** 25 mg p. 286	**Sandimmune** 100 mg p. 286
Sansert 2 mg p. 688	**Sectral** 200 mg p. 5	**Sectral** 400 mg p. 5	**Semprex-D** p. 66
Septra DS p. 999	**Serax** 10 mg p. 298	**Serax** 30 mg p. 298	**Seroquel** 25 mg p. 947
Seroquel 100 mg p. 947	**Seroquel** 200 mg p. 947	**Serzone** 100 mg p. 758	**Serzone** 150 mg p. 758
Serzone 200 mg p. 758		**Serzone** 250 mg p. 758

W

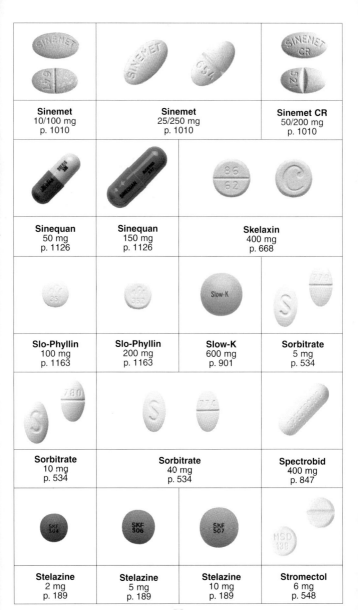

Sinemet 10/100 mg p. 1010	**Sinemet** 25/250 mg p. 1010	**Sinemet CR** 50/200 mg p. 1010
Sinequan 50 mg p. 1126	**Sinequan** 150 mg p. 1126	**Skelaxin** 400 mg p. 668

Slo-Phyllin 100 mg p. 1163	**Slo-Phyllin** 200 mg p. 1163	**Slow-K** 600 mg p. 901	**Sorbitrate** 5 mg p. 534
Sorbitrate 10 mg p. 534	**Sorbitrate** 40 mg p. 534		**Spectrobid** 400 mg p. 847
Stelazine 2 mg p. 189	**Stelazine** 5 mg p. 189	**Stelazine** 10 mg p. 189	**Stromectol** 6 mg p. 548

X

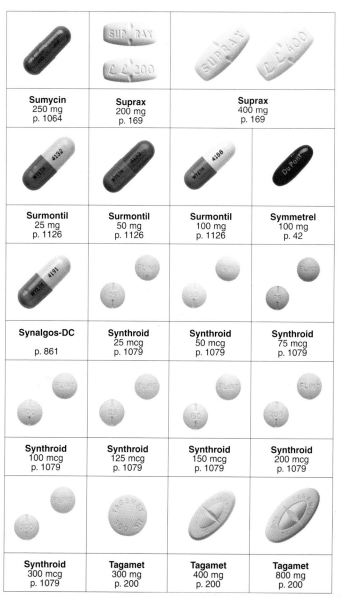

Sumycin 250 mg p. 1064	**Suprax** 200 mg p. 169	**Suprax** 400 mg p. 169
Surmontil 25 mg p. 1126	**Surmontil** 50 mg p. 1126	**Surmontil** 100 mg p. 1126	**Symmetrel** 100 mg p. 42
Synalgos-DC p. 861	**Synthroid** 25 mcg p. 1079	**Synthroid** 50 mcg p. 1079	**Synthroid** 75 mcg p. 1079
Synthroid 100 mcg p. 1079	**Synthroid** 125 mcg p. 1079	**Synthroid** 150 mcg p. 1079	**Synthroid** 200 mcg p. 1079
Synthroid 300 mcg p. 1079	**Tagamet** 300 mg p. 200	**Tagamet** 400 mg p. 200	**Tagamet** 800 mg p. 200

Y

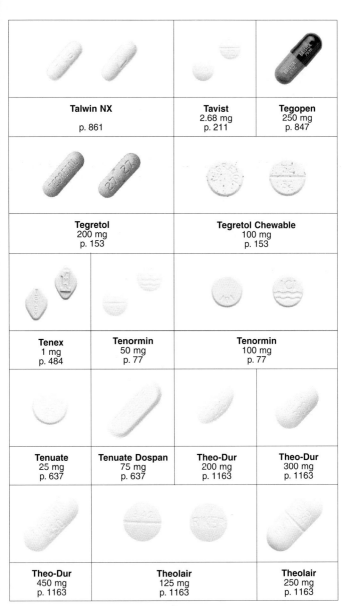

Talwin NX p. 861	**Tavist** 2.68 mg p. 211	**Tegopen** 250 mg p. 847
Tegretol 200 mg p. 153	**Tegretol Chewable** 100 mg p. 153	
Tenex 1 mg p. 484	**Tenormin** 50 mg p. 77	**Tenormin** 100 mg p. 77
Tenuate 25 mg p. 637	**Tenuate Dospan** 75 mg p. 637	**Theo-Dur** 200 mg p. 1163 / **Theo-Dur** 300 mg p. 1163
Theo-Dur 450 mg p. 1163	**Theolair** 125 mg p. 1163	**Theolair** 250 mg p. 1163

Z

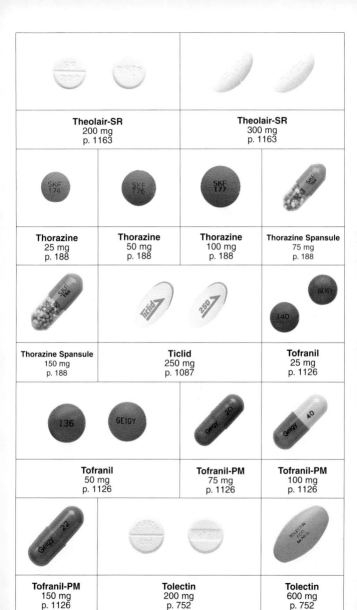

Theolair-SR
200 mg
p. 1163

Theolair-SR
300 mg
p. 1163

Thorazine
25 mg
p. 188

Thorazine
50 mg
p. 188

Thorazine
100 mg
p. 188

Thorazine Spansule
75 mg
p. 188

Thorazine Spansule
150 mg
p. 188

Ticlid
250 mg
p. 1087

Tofranil
25 mg
p. 1126

Tofranil
50 mg
p. 1126

Tofranil-PM
75 mg
p. 1126

Tofranil-PM
100 mg
p. 1126

Tofranil-PM
150 mg
p. 1126

Tolectin
200 mg
p. 752

Tolectin
600 mg
p. 752

AA

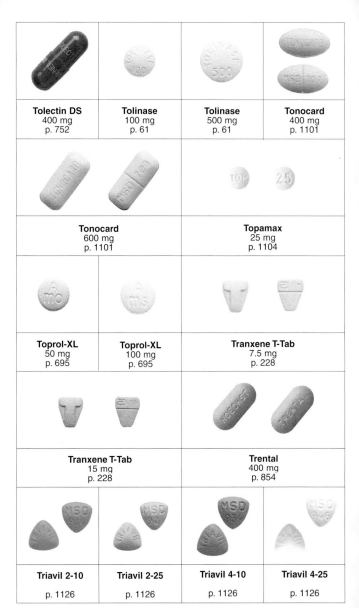

Tolectin DS 400 mg p. 752	**Tolinase** 100 mg p. 61	**Tolinase** 500 mg p. 61	**Tonocard** 400 mg p. 1101
Tonocard 600 mg p. 1101		**Topamax** 25 mg p. 1104	
Toprol-XL 50 mg p. 695	**Toprol-XL** 100 mg p. 695	**Tranxene T-Tab** 7.5 mg p. 228	
Tranxene T-Tab 15 mg p. 228		**Trental** 400 mg p. 854	
Triavil 2-10 p. 1126	**Triavil 2-25** p. 1126	**Triavil 4-10** p. 1126	**Triavil 4-25** p. 1126

BB

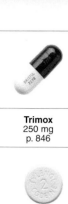		
Trimox 250 mg p. 846	**Trimox** 500 mg p. 846	**Tritec** 400 mg p. 965

Tylenol with Codeine #2	**Tylenol with Codeine #3**
p. 857	p. 857

Tylox p. 857	**Ultram** 50 mg p. 1107	**Valium** 5 mg p. 298

Valium 10 mg p. 298	**Vaseretic** 10/25 mg p. 365	**Vasotec** 5 mg p. 365	**Vasotec** 10 mg p. 365

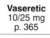		
Vasotec 20 mg p. 365	**Veetids** 250 mg p. 847	**Veetids** 500 mg p. 847

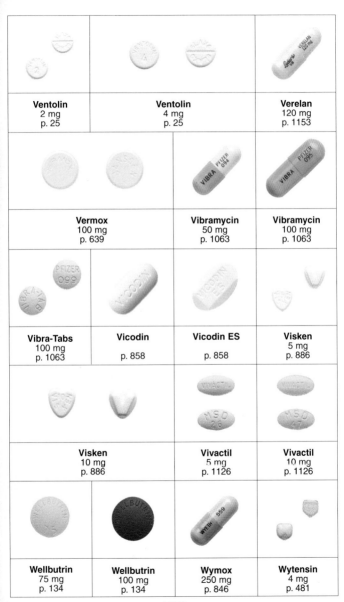

Ventolin 2 mg p. 25	**Ventolin** 4 mg p. 25	**Verelan** 120 mg p. 1153
Vermox 100 mg p. 639	**Vibramycin** 50 mg p. 1063	**Vibramycin** 100 mg p. 1063
Vibra-Tabs 100 mg p. 1063	**Vicodin** p. 858	**Vicodin ES** p. 858	**Visken** 5 mg p. 886
Visken 10 mg p. 886	**Vivactil** 5 mg p. 1126	**Vivactil** 10 mg p. 1126
Wellbutrin 75 mg p. 134	**Wellbutrin** 100 mg p. 134	**Wymox** 250 mg p. 846	**Wytensin** 4 mg p. 481

DD

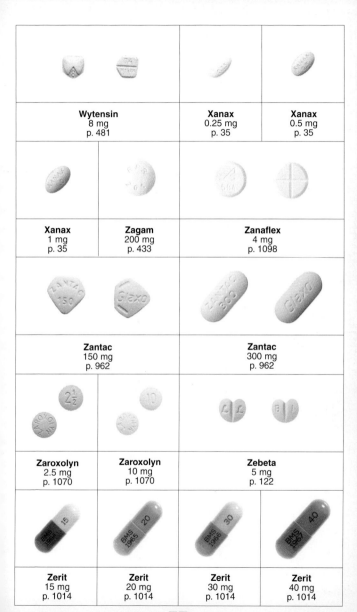

Wytensin 8 mg p. 481	**Xanax** 0.25 mg p. 35	**Xanax** 0.5 mg p. 35

Xanax 1 mg p. 35	**Zagam** 200 mg p. 433	**Zanaflex** 4 mg p. 1098

Zantac 150 mg p. 962	**Zantac** 300 mg p. 962

Zaroxolyn 2.5 mg p. 1070	**Zaroxolyn** 10 mg p. 1070	**Zebeta** 5 mg p. 122

Zerit 15 mg p. 1014	**Zerit** 20 mg p. 1014	**Zerit** 30 mg p. 1014	**Zerit** 40 mg p. 1014

EE

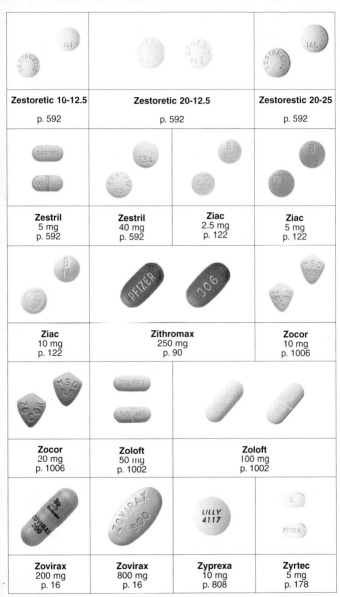

Zestoretic 10-12.5 p. 592	**Zestoretic 20-12.5** p. 592	**Zestorestic 20-25** p. 592

Zestril 5 mg p. 592	**Zestril** 40 mg p. 592	**Ziac** 2.5 mg p. 122	**Ziac** 5 mg p. 122

Ziac 10 mg p. 122	**Zithromax** 250 mg p. 90	**Zocor** 10 mg p. 1006

Zocor 20 mg p. 1006	**Zoloft** 50 mg p. 1002	**Zoloft** 100 mg p. 1002

Zovirax 200 mg p. 16	**Zovirax** 800 mg p. 16	**Zyprexa** 10 mg p. 808	**Zyrtec** 5 mg p. 178

FF

Generic Name

Lorazepam (lor-AZ-uh-pam) [G]

Brand Name

Ativan

Type of Drug

Benzodiazepine tranquilizer.

Prescribed for

Anxiety, tension, fatigue, and agitation; also prescribed for irritable bowel syndrome, panic attacks, and chronic sleeplessness.

General Information

Lorazepam is a member of a group of drugs known as benzodiazepines. All have some activity as antianxiety agents, anticonvulsants, or sedatives. Some are more suited to a specific role because of differences in their chemical makeup that give them greater activity in a certain area; others have particular characteristics that make them more desirable for certain functions. Often, individual drugs are limited by the applications for which their research has been sponsored.

Benzodiazepines work by a direct effect on the brain. They can relax you and make you more tranquil or sleepier, or they can slow nervous-system transmissions in such a way as to act as an anticonvulsant: The exact effect varies according to drug and dosage. Many doctors prefer the benzodiazepines to other drugs that can be used to similar effect because they tend to be safer, have fewer side effects, and are usually as effective, if not more so.

Cautions and Warnings

Do not take lorazepam if you know you are **sensitive** or **allergic** to it or another member of the group, including clonazepam.

Lorazepam can aggravate narrow-angle glaucoma, but you may take it if you have open-angle glaucoma. Check with your doctor.

Other conditions in which lorazepam should be avoided are severe **depression**, severe **lung disease, sleep apnea** (inter-

mittent cessation of breathing during sleep), **liver disease,**
drunkenness, and **kidney disease.** In each of these conditions,
the depressive effects of lorazepam may be enhanced and/or
could be detrimental to your overall condition.

Lorazepam should not be taken by **psychotic patients**
because it is not effective for them and can trigger unusual
excitement, stimulation, and rage.

Lorazepam is not intended to be used for more than 3 to 4
months at a time. Your doctor should reassess your condition
before continuing your prescription beyond that period.

Lorazepam may be **addictive,** and you can experience drug
withdrawal symptoms if you suddenly stop taking it after as
little as 4 to 6 weeks of treatment. Withdrawal symptoms are
more likely when short-acting drugs such as lorazepam are
taken for long periods. Withdrawal generally begins with
increased feelings of anxiety; it continues with tingling in the
extremities, sensitivity to bright light or to the sun, long
periods of sleep or sleeplessness, a metallic taste, flu-like
illness, fatigue, difficulty concentrating, restlessness, appetite
loss, nausea, irritability, headache, dizziness, sweating, muscle
tension or cramps, tremors, and feeling uncomfortable or ill
at ease. Other major withdrawal symptoms include confusion, abnormal perception of movement, depersonalization,
paranoid delusions, hallucinations, psychotic reactions, muscle
twitching, seizures, and memory loss.

Possible Side Effects

Weakness and confusion may occur, especially in seniors
and in those who are sickly. If these effects persist,
contact your doctor.

▼ Most common: mild drowsiness during the first few
days of therapy.

▼ Less common: depression, lethargy, disorientation,
headache, inactivity, slurred speech, stupor, dizziness,
tremors, constipation, dry mouth, nausea, inability to
control urination, sexual difficulties, irregular menstrual
cycle, changes in heart rhythm, low blood pressure, fluid
retention, blurred or double vision, itching, rash, hiccups,
nervousness, inability to fall asleep, and occasional liver
dysfunction. If you experience any of these symptoms,
stop taking the drug and contact your doctor immediately.

Possible Side Effects *(continued)*

▼ Rare: constipation, diarrhea, dry mouth, coated tongue, sore gums, vomiting, appetite changes, difficulty swallowing, increased salivation, upset stomach, incontinence, changes in sex drive, urinary difficulties, changes in heart rate, palpitations, swelling, stuffy nose, difficulty hearing, hair loss, hairiness, sweating, fever, tingling in the hands or feet, breast pain, muscle disturbances, breathing difficulties, changes in blood components, and joint pain.

Drug Interactions

• Lorazepam is a central-nervous-system depressant. Avoid taking it with alcohol, other tranquilizers, narcotics, barbiturates, monoamine oxidase inhibitors (MAOIs), antihistamines, and antidepressants. Taking lorazepam with these drugs may result in excessive depression, tiredness, sleepiness, difficulty breathing, or similar symptoms.

• Smoking may reduce the effectiveness of lorazepam by increasing the rate at which it is broken down by the body.

• The effects of lorazepam may be prolonged when it is taken together with cimetidine, oral contraceptives, disulfiram, fluoxetine, isoniazid, ketoconazole, metoprolol, probenecid, propoxyphene, propranolol, rifampin, or valproic acid. Theophylline may reduce lorazepam's sedative effects.

• If you take antacids, separate them from your lorazepam dose by at least 1 hour to prevent them from interfering with the absorption of lorazepam into the bloodstream.

• Lorazepam may increase blood levels of digoxin and the chances for digoxin toxicity. The effect of levodopa may be decreased if it is taken together with lorazepam. Combining lorazepam with phenytoin may increase phenytoin blood concentrations and the chances of phenytoin toxicity.

Food Interactions

Lorazepam is best taken on an empty stomach but may be taken with food if it upsets your stomach.

Usual Dose

Adult: 2–10 mg a day, individualized for maximum benefit. Symptoms and response to treatment may call for a dose outside this range. Most people require 2–6 mg a day. For sleep, 2–4 mg may be taken at bedtime.

Senior: A smaller dose is usually needed to control anxiety and tension.

Child: not recommended.

Overdosage

Symptoms of overdose are confusion, sleepiness, poor coordination, lack of response to pain such as a pinprick, loss of reflexes, shallow breathing, low blood pressure, and coma. The victim should be taken to a hospital emergency room for treatment. ALWAYS bring the prescription bottle or container with you.

Special Information

Lorazepam can cause tiredness, drowsiness, inability to concentrate, or similar symptoms. Be careful if you are driving, operating machinery, or performing other activities that require concentration.

People taking lorazepam for more than 3 or 4 months at a time may develop drug withdrawal reactions if the medication is stopped suddenly (see "Cautions and Warnings").

If you forget a dose of lorazepam, take it as soon as you remember. If it is almost time for your next dose, skip the dose you forgot and return to your regular schedule. Do not take a double dose.

Special Populations

Pregnancy/Breast-feeding

Lorazepam may cause birth defects if taken during the first 3 months of pregnancy; avoid taking it while pregnant.

Lorazepam passes into breast milk. Because infants break down the drug more slowly than do adults, they may accumulate enough lorazepam in their systems to produce undesirable effects. Bottle-feed your baby while taking this drug.

Seniors

Seniors, especially those with liver or kidney disease, are more sensitive to the effects of lorazepam and generally require smaller doses to achieve the same effect. Follow your doctor's directions and report any side effects at once.

Generic Name

Losartan (loe-SAR-tan)

Brand Name

Cozaar

Combination Products

Generic Ingredients: Losartan Potassium +
Hydrochlorothiazide
Hyzaar

Type of Drug

Angiotensin II antagonist.

Prescribed for

Hypertension (high blood pressure).

General Information

Losartan potassium was the first of a new class of drugs for high blood pressure called angiotensin II receptor antagonists. Losartan works by interfering with the special sites in blood vessels and other tissues where angiotensin II, a potent hormone which normally works as part of the body's system for maintaining blood pressure, exerts its effect. Losartan is different from angiotensin-converting enzyme (ACE) inhibitors that interrupt the body's production of angiotensin II.

After you take losartan, most of it is transformed in the liver to another, longer lasting compound that is responsible for most of the drug's effect, which lasts 1 day.

If additional blood-pressure lowering is required, your doctor may add a thiazide-type diuretic to your medication regimen.

Losartan is also being studied for heart failure.

Cautions and Warnings

Do not take losartan if you are **sensitive or allergic** to it.

People with serious **liver disease or cirrhosis** should receive a reduced dosage of losartan.

Some people may develop kidney function changes while taking losartan; this effect may be similar to that seen in some people who take ACE inhibitors.

Possible Side Effects

In studies of losartan, the risk of experiencing side effects was similar in people taking losartan and those taking a placebo (sugar pill).

▼ Most common: diarrhea, upset stomach, muscle cramps, muscle aches, back and leg pain, dizziness, sleeplessness, stuffy nose, cough, respiratory infection, and sinusitis and other sinus disorders.

▼ Less common: weakness, tiredness, swelling, abdominal pain, chest pain, nausea, headache, and sore throat.

▼ Rare: drug allergy or hypersensitivity and peeling skin. Other side effects may occur in virtually any body system.

Drug Interactions

• Losartan may interfere with the breakdown of other drugs in the liver. Studies of losartan and hydrochlorothiazide, digoxin, warfarin, phenobarbital, and cimetidine have shown no important interactions.

• Combining losartan with another blood-pressure-lowering drug such as hydrochlorothiazide reduces blood pressure more efficiently than either drug taken alone. People who are already taking a diuretic and start taking losartan may experience rapid blood-pressure lowering at first and should start with a lower losartan dosage.

Food Interactions

Food slows the absorption of losartan into the blood but will not affect your overall response to the drug. You may take it without regard to food or meals.

Usual Dose

Adult: 25–50 mg once a day to start, increasing gradually up to 100 mg in 1 or 2 doses a day.

Child: Losartan has not been studied in children under age 18 and should not be given to young children.

Overdosage

Animal studies indicate that losartan may be lethal in massive overdose. Little is known about human overdose. The most likely effects of losartan overdose are very low blood pressure and rapid heartbeat. Overdose victims should be taken to a hospital emergency room for evaluation and treatment. ALWAYS bring the prescription bottle or container with you.

Special Information

Studies show that losartan is much less effective in African Americans than in people of other ethnic backgrounds.

Women tend to absorb twice as much losartan as men, but the amount of active drug in the blood is about the same; no dosage adjustments are needed.

Avoid strenuous exercise and/or very hot weather because heavy sweating or dehydration may cause a rapid blood-pressure drop.

Avoid over-the-counter diet pills, decongestants, and stimulants that may raise blood pressure.

If you take losartan once a day and forget to take a dose, take it as soon as you remember. If it is within 8 hours of your next dose, skip the one you forgot and continue with your regular schedule. If you take losartan twice a day and forget to take a dose, take it as soon as you remember. If it is within 4 hours of your next dose, take one dose as soon as you remember and another in 5 or 6 hours, then continue with your regular schedule. Never take a double dose.

Special Populations

Pregnancy/Breast-feeding

Losartan should not be taken during the last 6 months of pregnancy because it may directly affect the fetus, possibly causing fetal injury or death. You should take another hypertension drug if you are or might be pregnant.

Animal studies show that losartan passes into breast milk, but it is not known if this occurs in humans. Nursing mothers who must take losartan should bottle-feed their infants.

Seniors

Seniors may take losartan without special precaution.

Lotensin

*see **Benazepril**, page 101*

Brand Name

Lotrel

Generic Ingredients

Amlodipine + Benazepril Hydrochloride

Type of Drug

Antihypertensive.

Prescribed for

Hypertension (high blood pressure).

General Information

Lotrel combines a calcium channel blocker — amlodipine — and an angiotensin-converting enzyme (ACE) inhibitor — benazepril. Both these drugs are often prescribed individually for hypertension. Lotrel is not intended as a first treatment for hypertension. You should take Lotrel only after you have tried an ACE inhibitor or calcium channel blocker alone and your doctor feels you need an additional drug to control your blood pressure. (See the "Amlodipine" and "Benazepril" profiles for more information.)

Cautions and Warnings

Do not take Lotrel if you are **sensitive or allergic** to any of its ingredients. People taking any ACE inhibitor may experience severe drug reactions, including swelling of the face, throat, lips, tongue, hands, and feet. In studies, this reaction occurs in about 5 of every 1000 people taking benazepril.

In rare instances, people taking a calcium channel blocker who have severe **heart disease** have developed increased angina pain and/or a heart attack.

In people with **heart failure**, ACE inhibitors may cause very low blood pressure, rare kidney failure, and death. Although ACE inhibitors are currently considered the most beneficial treatment for heart failure, people with heart failure who start Lotrel must be under a doctor's care.

Another ACE inhibitor has caused depression of bone marrow and reduced white-blood-cell counts, especially in people with **kidney failure**. Fever and chills can be a sign of this problem. Lotrel should be used with caution by people with kidney failure.

In rare instances, people taking ACE inhibitors have developed **liver failure**.

All ACE inhibitors may cause a persistent **cough**.

Possible Side Effects

Lotrel side effects are generally considered mild and temporary.

▼ Most common: cough, headache, dizziness, and swelling.

▼ Less common: allergic reactions, weakness, fatigue, dry mouth, nausea, abdominal pain, constipation, diarrhea, upset stomach, throat irritation, low blood-potassium levels, back pain, muscle cramps and pain, sleeplessness, nervousness, anxiety, tremors, reduced sex drive, sore throat, flushing, hot flashes, rash, impotence, and frequent urination.

▼ Rare: inflammation of the pancreas, hemolytic anemia, chest pain, abnormal heart rhythms, gout, neuritis, and ringing or buzzing in the ears.

Drug Interactions

• Combining a diuretic with Lotrel will lower blood pressure, possibly excessively.

• Combining a potassium-sparing diuretic such as spironolactone, amiloride, or triamterene with benazepril increases the risk of high blood potassium. High blood-potassium levels may lead to abnormal heart rhythms.

• Combining lithium with an ACE inhibitor such as benazepril may increase blood-lithium levels and lead to lithium side effects.

Food Interactions

Food does not affect individual tablets of amlodipine and benazepril, but the effects of food on Lotrel have not been studied. Until more information is available, take Lotrel on an empty stomach, or 1 hour before or 2 hours after meals.

Usual Dose

Adult: Daily doses range from 2.5 mg of amlodipine and 10 mg of benazepril, to 5 mg of amlodipine and 20 mg of benazepril. Dosage depends on your need for each of the 2 ingredients. Small or frail individuals and people with liver failure should follow dosage recommendations for seniors.

Senior: Start with 2.5 mg of amlodipine and 10 mg of benazepril a day and increase gradually. You may need to take amlodipine and benazepril in separate pills until your daily needs are established.

Overdosage

A few cases of overdose from amlodipine and benazepril taken separately have occurred. One person who took 70 mg of amlodipine and an unknown amount of a benzodiazepine tranquilizer died. No Lotrel overdoses have been reported. Call your local poison control center for more information. Overdose victims should be taken to a hospital emergency room for treatment. ALWAYS bring the prescription bottle or container with you.

Special Information

Be sure to continue taking your medication and follow all instructions, including diet restriction and other treatments. Hypertension is a condition with few recognizable symptoms; it may seem to you that you are taking a drug for no good reason. Ask your doctor or pharmacist if you have any questions.

Call your doctor if you develop swelling in the hands, feet, face, or throat; if you have sudden breathing difficulties; if you develop a sore throat, mouth sores, abnormal heartbeat, increased heart pain, persistent rash, constipation, nausea, weakness, dizziness, loss of the sense of taste; or any other particularly bothersome or persistent side effect.

You may get dizzy if you rise to your feet quickly from a sitting or lying position.

Avoid strenuous exercise and/or very hot weather because heavy sweating or dehydration may lead to a rapid drop in blood pressure.

Avoid over-the-counter stimulants that can raise blood pressure, including diet pills and decongestants.

It is important to maintain good dental hygiene while taking Lotrel and to use extra care when using your toothbrush or dental floss because of the chance that the drug may make you more susceptible to oral infections.

If you forget to take a dose of Lotrel, take it as soon as you remember. If it is within 8 hours of your next dose, skip the one you forgot and continue with your regular schedule. Do not take a double dose.

Special Populations

Pregnancy/Breast-feeding

Lotrel should not be taken by pregnant women, because ACE inhibitors may cause fetal damage or death. If you are taking Lotrel and become pregnant, see your doctor at once about changing drugs.

Small amounts of both active ingredients in Lotrel pass into breast milk. Nursing mothers who must take this product should bottle-feed their babies.

Seniors

Seniors may take this product without special restrictions; they should begin with the lowest strength of Lotrel available — 2.5 mg of amlodipine and 10 mg of benazepril.

Brand Name

Lotrisone

Generic Ingredients

Betamethasone Dipropionate + Clotrimazole

Type of Drug

Steroid-antifungal combination.

Prescribed for

Severe fungal infection or rash.

General Information

Lotrisone is one of a number of products that combine a steroid and an antifungal and are available by prescription. The steroid in Lotrisone is betamethasone dipropionate; the antifungal is clotrimazole. The other combination products have different generic ingredients but can be used for the same purposes. Lotrisone is used to relieve the symptoms of itching, rash, or skin inflammation associated with a severe fungal infection. It may treat the underlying cause of the skin problem by killing the fungus and relieving the associated inflammation.

Creams that contain only clotrimazole and only betamethasone — as betamethasone dipropriornate or in a slightly different form called betamethasone valerate — may be more effective than a combination product for certain skin conditions; use Lotrisone only upon your doctor's recommendation.

Improvement usually occurs within the first week of treatment. If you do not see results after 4 weeks, your doctor may need to prescribe a different medication.

Cautions and Warnings

Do not use Lotrisone if you are **sensitive** or **allergic** to either of its active ingredients.

Do not apply Lotrisone near or in your eyes. Avoid using this product on the ear if the eardrum is perforated, unless specifically directed to do so by your doctor.

Check with your doctor before using the contents of an old tube of Lotrisone for a new skin problem.

Possible Side Effects

▼ Most common: itching, stinging, burning, peeling skin, and swelling.

Drug Interactions

None known.

Usual Dose

Gently rub a thin film onto affected area(s) and surrounding skin.

Overdosage

Swallowing Lotrisone may cause nausea and vomiting. Call your local poison control center for more information.

Special Information

Apply a thin film of Lotrisone to the affected area(s). Washing or soaking the skin before applying the medication may increase the amount that penetrates into your skin.

Lotrisone should not be applied to the face, underarms, groin, genitals or genital areas, abdomen, or between the toes for more than a few days. Excessive use on these areas may result in stretch marks.

Do not wear tight clothing after applying Lotrisone, especially when applied to the genitals or genital areas.

Stop using the medication and call your doctor if Lotrisone causes itching, burning, or skin irritation.

If you forget to apply a dose of Lotrisone, apply it as soon as you remember. If it is almost time for your next application, skip the dose you forgot and continue with your regular schedule.

Special Populations

Pregnancy/Breast-feeding
Women in the first 3 months of pregnancy should not use this product when it is to be applied over large areas of skin, because Lotrisone can adversely affect fetal development.

Nursing mothers should not apply Lotrisone to the nipple or breast.

Seniors
Seniors may use Lotrisone without special restriction.

Generic Name

Lovastatin (loe-vuh-STAT-in)

Brand Name
Mevacor

Type of Drug
Cholesterol-lowering agent.

Prescribed for
High blood-cholesterol and LDL-cholesterol levels, in conjunction with a low-cholesterol diet program; also prescribed to slow the progression of atherosclerosis (hardening of the arteries), reduce the risk of death in people with heart disease, and treat inherited blood-lipid problems or lipid problems associated with diabetes or kidney disease.

General Information
Lovastatin is one of several cholesterol-lowering drugs that work by inhibiting an enzyme called HMG-CoA reductase. They interfere with the natural process for manufacturing cholesterol in your body, altering that process in order to

produce a harmless by-product. Studies have closely related high blood-fat levels — total cholesterol, LDL cholesterol, and triglycerides — to heart and blood-vessel disease. Drugs that reduce levels of any of these blood fats and increase HDL cholesterol — "good" cholesterol — have been assumed for several years to reduce the risk of death and heart attack. Recently, medication in this class has been proven to slow the formation of blood-vessel plaque — associated with atherosclerosis — and reduce the risk of heart attack and death related to heart disease.

Lovastatin reduces total triglyceride, cholesterol, and LDL-cholesterol counts while increasing HDL cholesterol. A very small amount of the drug actually reaches the body's circulation. Most is broken down and eliminated by the liver; 10% to 20% of the drug is released from the body through the kidneys. A significant blood-fat-lowering response is seen after 1 to 2 weeks of treatment. Blood-fat levels are lowest within 4 to 6 weeks after you start lovastatin and remain low as long as you continue to take the drug. The effect is known to persist for 4 to 6 weeks after you stop taking it.

Lovastatin generally does not benefit anyone under age 30, so it is not usually recommended for children. It may, under special circumstances, be prescribed for teenagers in the same dose as adults.

Cautions and Warnings

Do not take lovastatin if you are **allergic** to it or to any other HMG-CoA reductase inhibitor.

People with a history of **liver disease** and **those who drink large amounts of alcohol** should avoid lovastatin because it may aggravate or cause liver disease. Your doctor should take a blood sample to test your liver function every month or so during the first year of treatment to be sure that the drug is not adversely affecting you.

Lovastatin causes **muscle aches and/or muscle weakness** in a small number of people, which may be a sign of a more serious condition.

At doses between 50 and more than 100 times the maximum human dose, lovastatin has caused central-nervous-system lesions, liver tumors, and male infertility in lab animals. The importance of this information for people is not known.

Possible Side Effects

Most people who take lovastatin tolerate it quite well.

▼ Most common: headache.

▼ Common: nausea, vomiting, diarrhea, stomach cramps or pain, stomach gas, itching, and rash.

▼ Less common: constipation; heartburn; upset stomach; muscle aches, cramps, or pain; dizziness; eye irritation; and blurred vision.

▼ Rare: changes in sense of taste; dry mouth; acid regurgitation; leg, shoulder, or local pain; joint pain; sleeplessness; tingling in the hands or feet; chest pain; and hair loss. Other effects may occur in virtually any part of the body. Report anything unusual to your doctor.

Drug Interactions

• The cholesterol-lowering effects of lovastatin and colestipol or cholestyramine are additive when the drugs are taken together. Take lovastatin 1 hour before or 4 hours after either of these drugs.

• Lovastatin may increase the effects of warfarin or digoxin. If you take either of these drugs with lovastatin you should be periodically checked by your doctor.

• The combination of cyclosporine, erythromycin, gemfibrozil, or niacin with lovastatin may cause severe muscle aches or degeneration or other muscle problems. These combinations should be avoided.

• Propranolol can interfere with the action of lovastatin, reducing its effectiveness.

• The effect of lovastatin can be reduced by taking it with isradipine.

• Itraconazole can increase HMG-CoA reductase inhibitor levels by 20 times. Avoid this combination by temporarily stopping lovastatin if you take itraconazole.

Food Interactions

Take lovastatin with food to maximize the amount of drug absorbed. Continue your low-cholesterol diet while taking it.

Usual Dose

20–80 mg a day, usually with your evening meal. Your daily dosage of lovastatin should be adjusted monthly, based on

your doctor's assessment of how well the drug is working to
reduce your blood cholesterol.

Overdosage

A person suspected of having taken an overdose of lovastatin
should be taken to a hospital emergency room for evaluation
and treatment. The effects of lovastatin overdose are not well
understood, since only a few cases have occurred and all
victims recovered; the largest single lovastatin overdose was
6000 mg.

Special Information

Call your doctor if you develop blurred vision or muscle
aches, pain, tenderness, or weakness, especially if you are
also feverish or feel sick.

Lovastatin is always prescribed in combination with a
low-fat diet. Be sure to follow your doctor's dietary instructions, since both diet and medication are necessary to treat
your condition.

Lovastatin may cause unusual sensitivity to the sun. Use
sunscreen and wear protective clothing while in the sun until
you determine if you are affected.

Do not take more cholesterol-lowering medication than
your doctor has prescribed or stop taking the medication
without your doctor's knowledge.

If you forget to take a dose of lovastatin, take it as soon as
you remember. If it is almost time for your next dose, skip the
one you forgot and continue with your regular schedule. Do
not take a double dose.

Special Populations

Pregnancy/Breast-feeding

Women who are or might be pregnant should not take
lovastatin. Studies show that daily doses of lovastatin cause
malformation of the fetal skeleton in animals. Also, cholesterol is essential to the health and development of a fetus;
anything that interferes with that process will damage the
developing brain and nervous system.

Because hardening of the arteries is a long-term process,
you should be able to stop this medication during pregnancy
without developing atherosclerosis. If you become pregnant
while taking lovastatin, stop the drug immediately and call
your doctor.

Lovastatin may pass into breast milk. Women taking it should bottle-feed their infants to avoid interfering with their baby's development.

Seniors

Seniors may take lovastatin without special precaution. Be sure to report any side effects to your doctor.

Macrobid

see **Nitrofurantoin**, page 792

Generic Name

Malathion (MAL-uh-thye-on)

Brand Name

Ovide

Type of Drug

Scabicide.

Prescribed for

Head lice.

General Information

Originally used as an agricultural insecticide, malathion has been found to be effective against common lice and the eggs they leave behind in the scalp. Malathion works by interfering with the normal breakdown of acetylcholine, a common carrier of nervous-system impulses. The excess acetylcholine produced by malathion makes it toxic to the lice and eggs.

After it has been applied to the hair, malathion binds slowly with the hair shaft, providing some protection against future infestations. This binding process, and the protection it carries, takes about 6 hours to develop and reaches its maximum effect in about 12 hours.

Cautions and Warnings

Malathion is an extremely **toxic substance if swallowed** (see

"Overdosage" for more information). People with proven malathion **sensitivity** should not use this product. Normally, about 89% of the malathion applied to the skin is absorbed into the bloodstream, but larger quantities may be absorbed if the lotion is applied to broken skin or open sores. In rare situations, there may be a toxic reaction if too much malathion is absorbed through your skin into the blood.

Malathion lotion is **flammable**. Do not expose the lotion or hair that is still wet with the lotion to an open flame or an electric dryer because of the possibility of fire. Allow hair to dry naturally after application.

Malathion can severely **damage your eyes**. If some of it gets into your eyes, flush them with water immediately.

People with any of the following conditions should be cautious when using malathion because it can precipitate an attack or worsen your condition: **asthma**, very **slow heartbeat**, **low blood pressure**, **stomach spasms** or **ulcer**, recent **heart attack**, or **Parkinson's disease**.

Malathion can worsen the following conditions: severe **anemia**, **dehydration**, **insecticide exposure effects**, **liver disease** or **cirrhosis**, **malnutrition**, **myasthenia** or other neuromuscular diseases, and **seizure disorders**.

People with recent **brain surgery** should be concerned about using this product because it can initiate toxic nervous-system effects, including seizures.

Possible Side Effects

▼ Common: scalp irritation. Malathion is extremely toxic if it is swallowed or gets into your eyes (see "Overdosage" for more information).

▼ Rare: Convulsions and other drug effects can occur if enough drug is absorbed into the blood through the scalp (see "Overdosage" for more information).

Drug Interactions

• No drug interactions have been reported. However, unusually large amounts of malathion could interact with aminoglycosides (injectable antibiotics) to cause breathing problems, with local anesthetics to interfere with their breakdown and cause systemic side effects, and with some eyedrops used to treat glaucoma — physostigmine, echothiophate, demecarium, and isoflurophate — to cause side effects. Consult your doctor or pharmacist for more information.

Usual Dose

Adult and Child (age 2 and over): Apply to the hair and scalp and repeat after 7–9 days, if necessary.

Overdosage

If swallowed or absorbed through your skin, malathion can cause serious problems. Symptoms of malathion toxicity include abdominal cramps; anxiety; restlessness; clumsiness or unsteadiness; confusion; depression; diarrhea; dizziness; drowsiness; increased sweating; watery eyes or mouth; loss of bowel or bladder control; muscle twitching in the eyelids, face, or neck; pinpointed pupils; difficulty breathing; seizures; slow heartbeat; trembling; and weakness.

Malathion overdose is potentially deadly. People who swallow this product may not experience toxic effects for up to 12 hours. However, victims should be made to vomit with ipecac syrup — available at any pharmacy — to remove any remaining drug from the stomach. Anyone who swallows malathion MUST be taken to a hospital emergency room for treatment. ALWAYS bring the prescription bottle or container with you.

If any malathion gets into your eyes, IMMEDIATELY flush them with water to remove the insecticide and to avoid damage to your vision, then go to a hospital.

Special Information

Follow your prescription exactly, and do not use this product without your doctor's approval.

Sprinkle the lotion onto dry hair and rub in until the hair and scalp are wet. Pay special attention to the back of your head and neck. Avoid contact with the eyes. Immediately after applying the lotion, wash your hands to remove any remaining malathion from your skin. Allow the treated hair to dry naturally; do not cover it or use an electric dryer or other heat source. Do not shampoo the hair and scalp for 8 to 12 hours to allow the medicine to work. After 8 to 12 hours have passed, wash your hair with a plain shampoo. Remove the dead lice and eggs from the scalp with a fine-toothed comb.

Pregnant women should not handle this medication or apply it to others.

Other household members also may have lice and require malathion treatments. Call your doctor for information.

After head lice have been found, be sure to practice good hygiene to prevent spreading the lice and possible reinfestation of the treated scalp. Wash all clothing, bedding, towels, and washcloths in very hot water or dry-clean them to kill any lice or eggs. Hairbrushes or combs used by people with head lice infestation must be washed in very hot, soapy water to remove any remaining lice or eggs. Do not share brushes and combs because they may spread the lice. Thoroughly clean the entire living area, including furniture and clothing, with a vacuum cleaner to remove any remaining lice or eggs.

Be careful to avoid exposure to other insecticides while being treated with malathion.

Special Populations

Pregnancy/Breast-feeding
Malathion may be absorbed into the fetal bloodstream and can affect the fetus. Women who are or might be pregnant should not use it or apply it to others.

It is not known if malathion passes into breast milk. There is a risk that some of the insecticide may be absorbed into the bloodstream and possibly passed on to the nursing infant. Nursing mothers should bottle-feed their babies if using this drug.

Seniors
Seniors may use this product without special restriction.

Generic Name

Maprotiline (muh-PROE-tih-lene) G

Brand Name

Ludiomil

Type of Drug

Antidepressant.

Prescribed for

Depression and panic disorder.

General Information

Maprotiline hydrochloride blocks the movement of certain stimulant chemicals in and out of nerve endings and has a sedative effect. It also has anticholinergic activity and counteracts the effects of the neurohormone acetylcholine. Recent antidepressant theory says that antidepressant drugs work by changing the sensitivity and function of nerve endings, which over time leads to long-term changes in the nerve-ending activity. Thus, although maprotiline and other antidepressants immediately block neurohormones, it takes 2 to 4 weeks for their clinical effects to come into play. If your symptoms are unchanged after 6 to 8 weeks of treatment with an antidepressant, contact your doctor. Maprotiline elevates mood, increases physical activity and mental alertness, and improves appetite and sleep patterns in a depressed person. Maprotiline is also a mild sedative and is useful in treating mild forms of depression associated with anxiety. Maprotiline is broken down in the liver.

Cautions and Warnings

Do not take maprotiline if you are **allergic** or sensitive to it.

Do not take maprotiline if you are **recovering from a heart attack**. Take maprotiline with caution if you have a history of **epilepsy** or other convulsive disorders, **urinary difficulties, glaucoma, heart disease, liver disease**, or **hyperthyroidism**. Antidepressants may aggravate the condition of people who are **schizophrenic** or **paranoid** and may cause people with **bipolar (manic-depressive) disorder** to switch phase. These reactions are also possible when changing or stopping antidepressants. **Suicide** is always a possibility in severely depressed people, who should only be allowed to have minimal quantities of medication in their possession at any one time.

Because maprotiline lowers the seizure threshold, seizures may occur at usual doses as well as with overdoses.

Possible Side Effects

▼ Most common: sedation and anticholinergic effects, including blurred vision, disorientation, confusion, hallucination, muscle spasms or tremors, seizures, convulsions, dry mouth, constipation, urinary difficulties, worsened glaucoma, and sensitivity to bright light or sunlight.

Possible Side Effects *(continued)*

▼ Less common: blood-pressure changes, abnormal heart rate, heart attack, anxiety, restlessness, excitement, numbness or tingling in the extremities, poor coordination, rash, itching, fluid retention, fever, allergy (symptoms include breathing difficulties, skin rash, itching), changes in blood composition, nausea, vomiting, appetite loss, upset stomach, diarrhea, breast enlargement in both males and females, changes in sex drive, and blood-sugar changes.

▼ Rare: agitation, insomnia, nightmares, feelings of panic, a peculiar taste in the mouth, stomach cramps, black discoloration of the tongue, yellowing of the skin or whites of the eyes, changes in liver function, weight changes, excessive perspiration, flushing, frequent urination, drowsiness, dizziness, weakness, headache, hair loss, and not feeling well.

Drug Interactions

• Combining maprotiline with a monoamine oxidase inhibitor (MAOI) antidepressant may cause high fever and convulsions; this combination is potentially fatal. Do not take an MAOI until at least 2 weeks after maprotiline has been stopped. People who take both maprotiline and an MAOI require close medical observation.

• Maprotiline interacts with guanethidine and clonidine used to treat high blood pressure. Tell your doctor if you are taking any drug for high blood pressure.

• Maprotiline increases the effects of alcohol, barbiturates, tranquilizers, and other sedative drugs. In addition, barbiturates may decrease the effectiveness of maprotiline. Taking maprotiline and thyroid medication together will enhance the effects of both drugs and possibly cause abnormal heart rhythms.

• The combination of maprotiline and reserpine may cause overstimulation.

• Oral contraceptives may reduce the effect of maprotiline, as may smoking. Charcoal tablets may prevent maprotiline's absorption into the bloodstream. Estrogens may increase or decrease the effect of maprotiline.

• Drugs such as bicarbonate of soda, acetazolamide, quinidine, and procainamide increase the effect of maprotiline. Cimetidine, methylphenidate, and phenothiazine drugs, such as thorazine and compazine, block the liver metabolism of maprotiline and cause it to stay in the body longer, which may cause severe side effects.

Food Interactions

You may take maprotiline with food if it upsets your stomach.

Usual Dose

Adult: 75–225 mg a day. Hospitalized patients may need up to 300 mg a day. Dosage must be tailored to your needs.

Senior: Lower doses are recommended for people over age 60, usually 50–75 mg a day.

Overdosage

Symptoms of maprotiline overdose include confusion, inability to concentrate, hallucinations, drowsiness, lowered body temperature, abnormal heart rate, heart failure, enlarged pupils, seizures, convulsions, very low blood pressure, stupor, and coma. Agitation, stiffening of muscles, vomiting, and high fever may also develop. The victim should be taken to a hospital emergency room immediately. ALWAYS bring the prescription bottle or container with you.

Special Information

Avoid alcohol and other depressants while taking maprotiline. Do not stop taking this drug unless your doctor has specifically told you to do so: Abruptly stopping maprotiline may cause nausea, headache, and feelings of ill health.

Maprotiline may cause drowsiness, dizziness, and blurred vision. Be careful when driving or operating hazardous machinery. Avoid prolonged exposure to the sun or sun lamps.

Call your doctor at once if you develop seizures, difficult or rapid breathing, fever, sweating, blood pressure changes, muscle stiffness, loss of bladder control, or unusual tiredness or weakness.

Dry mouth may lead to an increase in cavities, gum bleeding, and gum disease. People taking maprotiline should pay special attention to dental hygiene.

If you forget a dose of maprotiline, skip it and go back to your regular schedule. Do not take a double dose.

Special Populations

Pregnancy/Breast-feeding

Maprotiline crosses into fetal circulation; birth defects have been reported. Avoid taking this drug while pregnant.

Maprotiline passes into breast milk in concentrations equal to those in the mother's blood. Nursing mothers taking maprotiline should consider bottle-feeding.

Seniors

Seniors may be especially sensitive to the side effects of maprotiline, especially constipation and heart-related effects such as abnormal rhythms. Seniors usually require a lower dose than younger adults to achieve the same result. Follow your doctor's directions and report any unusual effects at once.

Generic Name

Masoprocol (MAY-soe-proe-col)

Brand Name

Actinex

Type of Drug

Antiproliferative (growth slower).

Prescribed for

Premalignant skin lesions usually associated with excessive exposure to the sun.

General Information

Masoprocol has an antiproliferative effect on cell cultures, but how this drug works on the skin is not known. It is prescribed to treat lesions where the horny layer of the skin grows at a much faster rate than the other skin layers. This condition, known as actinic keratosis, is thought to be a precursor to the development of skin cancer.

Cautions and Warnings

Do not cover masoprocol cream with clear plastic wrap or another dressing that obstructs the skin.

Masoprocol contains sulfites as preservatives. If you are allergic to sulfites, exposure to masoprocol may cause hives, itching, wheezing, or severe allergic reaction.

Possible Side Effects

Skin reactions to masoprocol are common, but they usually resolve within 2 weeks of starting the drug.

▼ Most common: skin redness and irritation, itching, dryness, flaking, swelling, burning, and soreness.

▼ Less common: bleeding, crusting, eye irritation, oozing, rash, stinging, tightness, and tingling.

▼ Rare: blistering, eczema, cuts or abrasions in the skin, cracking of the skin, a leathery feeling, wrinkling, and skin roughness.

Drug Interactions

• Do not use other skin products or cosmetics when using masoprocol.

Usual Dose

Adult: Wash and dry the areas to which masoprocol cream is to be applied. Gently massage the cream into the affected areas until it is evenly distributed. Masoprocol should be used morning and night for 28 days.

Overdosage

Animals receiving high doses of masoprocol developed liver and stomach problems. Anyone who swallows masoprocol should be made to vomit with ipecac syrup — available at any pharmacy — as soon as possible in order to remove existing material from the stomach. Call your local poison control center for more information and instructions. ALWAYS bring the prescription bottle or container with you if you go to a hospital emergency room for treatment.

Special Information

Masoprocol frequently causes allergic contact dermatitis (skin reaction). If this happens to you, stop using the cream and call your doctor.

If you apply masoprocol directly with your fingers, you must thoroughly wash your hands after each application. Consider using disposable gloves to apply the cream.

You should be careful not to get masoprocol cream into your eyes. If it does get into your eyes, it must be washed out immediately with water.

You should avoid the sun if you are using this product. The lesions being treated are caused by excessive sun exposure and can only be worsened by continuing sun exposure.

Masoprocol cream may stain your skin, clothing, sheets, or furniture.

If you forget to apply a dose of masoprocol, do so as soon as you remember. If it almost time for your next dose, skip the one you forgot and continue with your regular schedule.

Special Populations

Pregnancy/Breast-feeding
There is no reliable information about the effect of this drug on pregnant women. It should be used during pregnancy only when absolutely necessary.

It is not known if masoprocol passes into breast milk. Nursing mothers should use this medication with caution.

Seniors
Seniors may use this medication without special restriction.

Generic Name

Mazindol (MAY-zin-dol)

Brand Names

Mazanor   Sanorex

The information in this profile also applies to the following drugs:

Generic Ingredient: Phentermine Hydrochloride
Adipex-P   Obe-Nix
Fastin   Obephen
Ionamin

Generic Ingredient: Phendimetrazine
Anorex   Obalan
Bontril PDM   Wehless

Generic Ingredient: Sustained-Release Phendimetrazine
Bontril Slow Release   Prelu-2
Dyrexan-OD   Wehless Timecelles
Melfiat-105

Generic Ingredient: Diethylpropion

Tenuate						Tepanil
Tenuate Dospan					Tepanil Ten-Tab

Type of Drug

Non-amphetamine appetite suppressant.

Prescribed for

Short-term appetite suppression in the treatment of obesity; also prescribed for Duchenne's muscular dystrophy.

General Information

Although this drug is not an amphetamine, it has many amphetamine-like effects. It suppresses appetite by working on specific areas in the brain, although studies have shown that appetite suppressants are more effective when combined with behavior therapy than when they are taken without such supportive therapy. Each dose of mazindol works for 8 to 15 hours. Mazindol should only be used for 2 to 3 months.

Cautions and Warnings

Do not take mazindol if you have **heart disease, high blood pressure, thyroid disease,** or **glaucoma**, or if you are **sensitive** or **allergic** to it or any other appetite suppressant. Do not use mazindol if you are prone to **emotional agitation** or **substance abuse**, since appetite suppressants can be easily abused.

Possible Side Effects

▼ Common: a false sense of well-being, nervousness, euphoria (feeling high), overstimulation, restlessness, and trouble sleeping.

▼ Less common: palpitations, high blood pressure, drowsiness or sedation, weakness, dizziness, tremors, headache, dry mouth, nausea, vomiting, diarrhea or other intestinal disturbances, rash, itching, changes in sex drive, hair loss, muscle pains, difficulty urinating, sweating, chills, blurred vision, and fever.

Drug Interactions

• Combining other stimulants — including decongestants,

some asthma drugs, and over-the-counter cold remedies — with mazindol may result in excessive stimulation.

• Taking this medication within 2 weeks of taking any monoamine oxidase inhibitor (MAOI) may result in very high blood pressure.

• Appetite suppressants may reduce the effects of some drugs used to treat high blood pressure.

• One case of lithium toxicity occurred in a person taking lithium in combination with mazindol.

Food Interactions

Do not crush or chew this product. Mazindol may be taken on a full stomach to reduce stomach upset caused by the drug.

Usual Dose

1 mg 3 times a day, 1 hour before meals; or 2 mg once a day, before lunch.

Overdosage

Symptoms of overdose are restlessness, tremors, shallow breathing, confusion, hallucinations, and fever. Fatigue and depression may follow these symptoms. Additional symptoms are changes in blood pressure, cold and clammy skin, nausea, vomiting, diarrhea, and stomach cramps. Take the victim to a hospital emergency room immediately, and ALWAYS bring the prescription bottle or container with you.

Special Information

Do not take any appetite suppressant as part of a weight-control program for more than 12 weeks, and take it only under a doctor's supervision. This drug will not reduce body weight by itself. You must limit or modify your diet and follow your exercise regimen, if applicable.

Appetite suppressants often cause dry mouth, which increases the chances of dental cavities and gum disease. Pay special attention to oral hygiene if you are taking this medicine. Dry mouth usually can be relieved with sugarless candy, gum, or ice chips.

If you forget to take a dose of mazindol, skip the dose you forgot and continue with your regular schedule. Do not take a double dose.

Special Populations

Pregnancy/Breast-feeding

Studies have shown that large doses of mazindol may damage the fetus. All appetite suppressants, including mazindol, should be avoided by women who are or might be pregnant. In cases where your doctor considers this drug crucial, its potential benefits must be weighed against its risks.

It is not known if mazindol passes into breast milk. Nursing mothers should not take any appetite suppressant.

Seniors

Seniors should not take this drug unless supervised by a doctor. It can aggravate diabetes or high blood pressure, conditions common in older adults.

Generic Name

Mebendazole (meh-BEN-duh-zole)

Brand Name

Vermox

Type of Drug

Anthelmintic.

Prescribed for

Whipworm, pinworm, roundworm, hookworm, and mixed-worm infections.

General Information

Mebendazole blocks the mechanism by which susceptible worms get sugar, effectively starving the organism. This is a slow process; it may take 3 days or more for the worm to be eliminated from the body. Most of the drug passes out of the body unchanged in the feces.

Cautions and Warnings

Do not take mebendazole if you are **sensitive** or **allergic** to it.

Possible Side Effects

Side effects are infrequent and passing; most common are pain and diarrhea in cases of massive infection. Fever has also occurred.

Drug Interactions

• Carbamazepine and phenytoin-type drugs may reduce blood levels of mebendazole, possibly interfering with its effect.

Food Interactions

Chew or crush the mebendazole tablet and mix it with food, especially fatty food, to increase the amount of drug absorbed.

Usual Dose

1 tablet in the morning and at night for 3 consecutive days, although one type of worm infection may be treated with a single tablet.

Overdosage

Stomach cramps and pain may develop several hours after an overdose. Overdose victims should be given ipecac syrup — available in any pharmacy — to induce vomiting. Call your local poison control center for more information.

Special Information

The same dosage is prescribed to everyone who takes mebendazole, regardless of age.

Each dose of mebendazole should be chewed or crushed and taken with food.

In the case of pinworm infection, all family members must take a 3-day course of mebendazole, even if only one member was infected; a second treatment is usually required in 2 or 3 weeks. Wash — do not shake — all bedclothes after treatment to prevent reinfection.

In the case of hookworm or whipworm, take an iron supplement every day during treatment with mebendazole. If you are anemic you may have to take iron treatment for up to 6 months after treatment is completed.

Call your doctor if you do not begin to get better in a few days. If the infection is not cured in 3 weeks, you may need another course of treatment.

It is essential that you follow the dosage schedule prescribed by your doctor. If you forget a dose take it as soon as you remember. If it is almost time for your next dose, skip the dose you forgot and continue with your regular schedule. Do not take a double dose.

Special Populations

Pregnancy/Breast-feeding

Mebendazole is toxic to animal fetuses and causes birth defects in animals. It is not recommended for use by pregnant women and should be used only if absolutely necessary.

It is not known if mebendazole passes into breast milk. Nursing mothers should take this drug with caution.

Seniors

Seniors may use this medication without special precaution.

Generic Name

Meclofenamate (mec-loe-FEN-uh-mate)

Brand Name

Meclomen

Type of Drug

Nonsteroidal anti-inflammatory drug (NSAID).

Prescribed for

Rheumatoid arthritis, osteoarthritis, mild to moderate pain, sunburn, migraine headache, menstrual headache, and discomfort associated with excessive menstrual bleeding.

General Information

Meclofenamate is one of 16 NSAIDs, which are used to relieve pain and inflammation. We do not know exactly how NSAIDs work, but part of their action may be due to their ability to inhibit the body's production of a hormone called prostaglandin as well as the action of other body chemicals, including cyclooxygenase, lipoxygenase, leukotrienes, and lysosomal enzymes. NSAIDs are generally absorbed into the bloodstream quickly. Pain relief comes within 1 hour after taking the first dose of meclofenamate, but its anti-inflammatory effect generally takes several days to become apparent and may take 2 to 3 weeks to reach maximum effect. Meclofenamate is broken down in the liver and eliminated through the kidneys.

Cautions and Warnings

People who are **allergic** to meclofenamate or any other

NSAID and those with a history of **asthma** attacks brought on by an NSAID, iodides, or aspirin should not take meclofenamate.

Meclofenamate can cause **gastrointestinal (GI) bleeding, ulcers,** and **stomach perforation**. This can occur at any time, with or without warning, in people who take meclofenamate regularly. People with a history of **active GI bleeding** should be cautious about taking any NSAID. People who develop bleeding or ulcers and continue NSAID treatment should be aware of the possibility of developing more serious drug toxicity.

Meclofenamate can affect **platelets and blood clotting** at high doses, and should be avoided by people with clotting problems and by those taking warfarin.

People with **heart problems** who use meclofenamate may experience swelling in their arms, legs, or feet.

Meclofenamate can cause severe toxic effects to the **kidney**. Report any unusual side effects to your doctor, who may need to periodically test your kidney function.

Meclofenamate can make you unusually photosensitive (sensitive to the effects of the sun).

Possible Side Effects

▼ Most common: diarrhea, nausea, vomiting, constipation, stomach gas, stomach upset or irritation, and appetite loss — especially during the first few days of treatment.

▼ Less common: stomach ulcers, GI bleeding, hepatitis, gallbladder attacks, painful urination, poor kidney function, kidney inflammation, blood and protein in the urine, dizziness, fainting, nervousness, depression, hallucinations, confusion, disorientation, tingling in the hands or feet, light-headedness, itching, increased sweating, dry nose and mouth, heart palpitations, chest pain, difficulty breathing, and muscle cramps.

▼ Rare: severe allergic reactions including closing of the throat, fever and chills, changes in liver function, jaundice (yellowing of the skin or whites of the eyes), and kidney failure. People who experience such effects must be promptly treated in a hospital emergency room or doctor's office. NSAIDs have caused severe skin reac-

> **Possible Side Effects** *(continued)*
>
> tions; if this happens to you, see your doctor immediately.

Drug Interactions

• Meclofenamate can increase the effects of oral anticoagulant (blood-thinning) drugs such as warfarin. You may take this combination, but your doctor might have to reduce your anticoagulant dose.

• Taking meclofenamate with cyclosporine may increase the toxic kidney effects of both drugs. Methotrexate toxicity may be increased in people also taking meclofenamate.

• Meclofenamate may reduce the blood-pressure-lowering effect of beta blockers and loop diuretics.

• Meclofenamate may increase phenytoin blood levels, leading to increased side effects. Lithium blood levels may be increased in people taking meclofenamate.

• Meclofenamate blood levels may be affected by cimetidine.

• Probenecid may interfere with the elimination of meclofenamate from the body, increasing the risk of meclofenamate side effects.

• Aspirin and other salicylates may decrease the amount of meclofenamate in your blood. These drugs should never be combined with meclofenamate.

Food Interactions

Take meclofenamate with food or a magnesium/aluminum antacid if it upsets your stomach.

Usual Dose

Adult and Child (age 14 and over): 200–400 mg a day.
Child (under age 14): not recommended.

Overdosage

People have died from NSAID overdoses. The most common signs of overdose are drowsiness, nausea, vomiting, diarrhea, abdominal pain, rapid breathing, rapid heartbeat, increased sweating, ringing or buzzing in the ears, confusion, disorientation, stupor, and coma. Take the victim to a hospital emergency room at once. ALWAYS bring the prescription bottle or container with you.

Special Information

Take each dose with a full glass of water and then do not lie down for 15 to 30 minutes afterward. Meclofenamate can make you drowsy and/or tired: Be careful when driving or operating hazardous equipment. Do not take any over-the-counter products containing acetaminophen or aspirin while taking meclofenamate. Avoid alcoholic beverages.

Contact your doctor if you develop skin rash or itching, visual disturbances, weight gain, breathing difficulties, fluid retention, hallucinations, black or tarry stools, persistent headache, or any unusual or intolerable side effect.

If you forget to take a dose of meclofenamate, take it as soon as you remember. If you take meclofenamate once a day and it is within 8 hours of your next dose, skip the dose you forgot and continue with your regular schedule. If you take several doses a day and it is within 4 hours of your next dose, skip the one you forgot and continue with your regular schedule. Never take a double dose.

Special Populations

Pregnancy/Breast-feeding

NSAIDs may cross into fetal blood circulation. They have not been found to cause birth defects, but animal studies indicate that they may affect the fetal heart during the second half of pregnancy. Pregnant women should not take meclofenamate without their doctor's approval, particularly during the last 3 months of pregnancy. When the drug is considered crucial by your doctor, its potential benefits must be carefully weighed against its risks.

NSAIDs may pass into breast milk but have caused no problems in breast-fed infants, except for seizures in a baby whose mother was taking the NSAID indomethacin. Other NSAIDs have caused problems in animal studies. There is a possibility that a nursing mother taking meclofenamate could affect her baby's heart or cardiovascular system. If you must take meclofenamate, bottle-feed your baby.

Seniors

Seniors may be more susceptible to meclofenamate side effects, especially ulcers.

Generic Name

Medroxyprogesterone Acetate

(med-rok-see-proe-JES-ter-one) [G]

Brand Names

Amen   Cycrin
Curretab   Provera

The information in this profile also applies to the following drugs:

Generic Ingredient: Norethindrone Acetate
Aygestin

Generic Ingredient: Progesterone
Crinone

Type of Drug

Progestin.

Prescribed for

Irregular menstrual bleeding, endometrial or kidney cancer, and menopause — in conjunction with estrogen replacement therapy (ERT); also prescribed to stimulate breathing in people who suffer from sleep apnea and for other conditions in which breathing rate is abnormally slow or stops completely for short periods of time. Norethindrone acetate may be used for endometriosis. Progesterone has been used to treat premenstrual syndrome (PMS), prevent spontaneous abortion in early stages of pregnancy, prevent premature labor in later stages of pregnancy, and support embryo implantation and help maintain pregnancy in some Assisted Reproductive Technology procedures.

General Information

Progesterone is the principal hormone involved in the process of pregnancy. It works through other hormone systems on almost every phase of the preparation of the womb for acceptance of the fertilized egg and the maintenance of conditions needed for the growth and development of the fetus.

The decision to take medroxyprogesterone acetate on a regular basis should be made carefully by you and your doctor because of the possibility of developing problems related to medroxyprogesterone acetate. Your need for medroxyprogesterone acetate treatment should be evaluated at least every 6 months.

Other progestins have been prescribed for additional medical uses, including acquired immunodeficiency syndrome (AIDS) Wasting Syndrome.

Cautions and Warnings

Do not take this drug if you are **sensitive** or **allergic** to it or to any of the progestins, have a history of **blood clotting** or similar disorders, or if you have had **convulsions**, **liver disease**, known or suspected **breast cancer**, undiagnosed **vaginal bleeding**, or a **miscarriage**. Medroxyprogesterone and other progestins should not be used regularly to avoid weight loss.

Though megestrol, a progestin, has been widely used for endometrial and breast cancer, its use in **HIV infected women** has been limited; all such women experienced breakthrough bleeding during drug trials.

Like medroxyprogesterone acetate, progestins have been used to **prevent spontaneous abortion**. Such treatment can harm a fetus if given during the first 4 months of pregnancy. This drug may delay a spontaneous abortion by relaxing the uterus. However, most abortions are caused by a defective egg, a circumstance that the drug cannot affect.

Medroxyprogesterone acetate use should be carefully considered if you have had **asthma**, **cardiac insufficiency**, **epilepsy**, **migraine headaches**, **kidney problems**, **diabetes**, **ectopic pregnancy**, **high blood-fat levels**, or **depression**.

Possible Side Effects

There is a strong relationship between the use of progestin drugs and the development of blood clots in the veins, lungs, or brain.

Medroxyprogesterone Acetate and Norethindrone Acetate

▼ Most common: breakthrough bleeding, spotting, changes in or loss of menstrual flow, water retention,

Possible Side Effects (continued)

increase or decrease in body weight, breast tenderness, jaundice, acne, skin rash with or without itching, and depression.

▼ Common: changes in libido or sex drive, changes in appetite and mood, headache, nervousness, dizziness, tiredness, backache, loss of scalp hair, growth of hair in unusual quantities or places, itching, symptoms similar to urinary infections, and unusual rashes.

▼ Rare: allergy, fatigue, fever, flu-like symptoms, bloating, asthma, back or leg pain, sinus inflammation, respiratory infection, upset stomach, stomach gas or noise, emotional instability, sleeplessness, acne, itching, painful urination, urinary infections.

Progesterone Gel
Side effects are less common if you use this drug once a day.

▼ Most common: pelvic or abdominal pain or cramps, tiredness, headache, nervousness, depression, reduced sex drive, constipation, nausea, breast enlargement, and nighttime urination.

▼ Common: bloating, dizziness, diarrhea, vomiting, painful intercourse, joint pain, itching, and vaginal infection or discharge.

Drug Interactions

• Rifampin may increase the rate at which medroxyprogesterone acetate is broken down in the liver, decreasing its effectiveness. Aminoglutethimide may increase the rate at which medroxyprogesterone is broken down in the liver, possibly reducing its effectiveness.

• Diabetics may experience a decrease in glucose tolerance, worsening their condition.

Food Interactions

You may take this drug with food it it upsets your stomach.

Usual Dose

Medroxyprogesterone Acetate: 5–10 mg a day for 5–10 days, beginning on what is assumed to be the sixteenth to twenty-first day of the menstrual cycle.

Norethindrone Acetate: For endometriosis: starting dosage —
5 mg a day for 14 days. Increase gradually up to 15 mg a day.
Treatment may be continued for 6–9 months. For abnormal
periodic bleeding or no period: 2.5–10 mg a day for 5–10
days during the second half of the menstrual cycle.

Progesterone Gel: Apply a single-use disposable unit once or
twice a day.

Overdosage

Medroxyprogesterone acetate overdose may result in severe
side effects. In many cases, small overdoses will result in no
unusual symptoms. Call your local poison control center or
hospital emergency room for more information.

Special Information

Stop taking this drug immediately and call your doctor at
the first sign of sudden, partial, or complete loss of vision;
double vision; sudden falling; calf pain, swelling, and redness; numbness in an arm or leg; leg cramp; water retention;
unusual vaginal bleeding; migraine or a sudden and severe
headache; depression; or if you think you have become
pregnant.

Medroxyprogesterone acetate may make you unusually
sensitive to the sun or bright light. Avoid the sun whenever
possible, and use extra sunscreen and protective clothing if
you must be outdoors.

Medroxyprogesterone acetate may mask the symptoms of
menopause.

If you forget to take a dose of medroxyprogesterone acetate, take it as soon as you remember. If it is almost time for
your next dose, skip the one you forgot and continue with
your regular schedule. Do not take a double dose.

Special Populations

Pregnancy/Breast-feeding

Medroxyprogesterone acetate and norethindrone may cause
birth defects or interfere with fetal development; it can double
the rate of certain birth defects if used during the first 4
months of pregnancy. It is not considered safe for use during
pregnancy, except under very specific circumstances. Progesterone gel is used to support the embryo implantation and
help maintain pregnancies in some Assisted Reproductive
Technology procedures.

Medroxyprogesterone acetate passes into breast milk. This drug may increase the volume of milk and length of time you make milk if given after birth. The effect of the drug on a nursing infant is not known.

Seniors

Seniors with severe liver disease are more sensitive to the effects of this drug. Follow your doctor's directions and report any side effects at once.

Generic Name

Mefenamic Acid (MEF-eh-NAM-ik AH-sid)

Brand Name

Ponstel

Type of Drug

Nonsteroidal anti-inflammatory drug (NSAID).

Prescribed for

Short-term treatment of sunburn, migraine attacks, menstrual pain, menstrual headache, and premenstrual syndrome (PMS).

General Information

Mefenamic acid is one of 16 NSAIDs, which are used to relieve pain and inflammation. We do not know exactly how NSAIDs work, but part of their action may be due to their ability to inhibit the body's production of a hormone called prostaglandin as well as the action of other body chemicals, including cyclooxygenase, lipoxygenase, leukotrienes, and lysosomal enzymes. NSAIDs are generally absorbed into the bloodstream quickly. Pain relief comes within 1 hour after taking the first dose of mefenamic acid, but its anti-inflammatory effect generally takes several days to 2 weeks to become apparent and may take a month or more to reach maximum effect. Mefenamic acid is broken down in the liver and eliminated through the kidneys. It should only be used for less than 1 week.

Cautions and Warnings

People who are **allergic** to mefenamic acid or any other

NSAID and those with a history of **asthma** attacks brought on by an NSAID, iodides, or aspirin should not take mefenamic acid.

Mefenamic acid can cause **gastrointestinal (GI) bleeding, ulcers,** and **stomach perforation**. This can occur at any time, with or without warning, in people who take mefenamic acid regularly. People with a history of **active GI bleeding** should be cautious about taking any NSAID. People who develop bleeding or ulcers and continue NSAID treatment should be aware of the possibility of developing more serious drug toxicity.

Mefenamic acid can affect **platelets and blood clotting** at high doses, and should be avoided by people with clotting problems and by those taking warfarin.

People with **heart problems** who use mefenamic acid may experience swelling in their arms, legs, or feet.

Mefenamic acid can cause severe toxic effects to the **kidney**. Report any unusual side effects to your doctor, who may need to periodically test your kidney function.

Mefenamic acid can make you unusually photosensitive (sensitive to the effect of the sun).

Possible Side Effects

▼ Most common: diarrhea, nausea, vomiting, constipation, stomach gas, stomach upset or irritation, and appetite loss — especially during the first few days of treatment.

▼ Less common: stomach ulcers, GI bleeding, hepatitis, gallbladder attacks, painful urination, poor kidney function, kidney inflammation, blood and protein in the urine, dizziness, fainting, nervousness, depression, hallucinations, confusion, disorientation, tingling in the hands or feet, light-headedness, itching, increased sweating, dry nose and mouth, heart palpitations, chest pain, breathing difficulties, and muscle cramps.

▼ Rare: severe allergic reactions including closing of the throat, fever and chills, changes in liver function, jaundice (yellowing of the skin or whites of the eyes), and kidney failure. People who experience such effects must be promptly treated in a hospital emergency room or doctor's office. NSAIDs have caused severe skin reac-

Possible Side Effects *(continued)*

tions; if this happens to you, see your doctor immediately.

Drug Interactions

• Mefenamic acid can increase the effects of oral anticoagulant (blood-thinning) drugs such as warfarin. You may take this combination, but your doctor might have to reduce your anticoagulant dose.

• Taking mefenamic acid with cyclosporine may increase the toxic kidney effects of both drugs. Methotrexate toxicity may be increased in people also taking mefenamic acid.

• Mefenamic acid may reduce the blood-pressure-lowering effect of beta blockers and loop diuretics.

• Mefenamic acid may increase phenytoin blood levels, leading to increased side effects. Lithium blood levels may be increased in people taking mefenamic acid.

• Mefenamic acid blood levels may be affected by cimetidine.

• Probenecid may interfere with the elimination of this drug from the body, increasing the risk for mefenamic acid toxic reactions.

• Aspirin and other salicylates may decrease the amount of mefenamic acid in your blood. These drugs should never be combined with mefenamic acid.

Food Interactions

Take mefenamic acid with food or a magnesium/aluminum antacid if it upsets your stomach.

Usual Dose

Adult and Child (age 14 and over): 500 mg to start, then 250 mg every 6 hours.

Child (under age 14): not recommended.

Overdosage

People have died from NSAID overdoses. The most common signs of overdose are drowsiness, nausea, vomiting, diarrhea, abdominal pain, rapid breathing, rapid heartbeat, increased sweating, ringing or buzzing in the ears, confusion, disorientation, stupor, and coma. Take the victim to a hospital emergency room at once. ALWAYS bring the prescription bottle or container with you.

Special Information

Take each dose with a full glass of water and do not lie down for 15 to 30 minutes afterward. Mefenamic acid can make you drowsy and/or tired: Be careful when driving or operating hazardous equipment. Do not take any over-the-counter products containing acetaminophen or aspirin while taking mefenamic acid. Avoid alcoholic beverages.

Contact your doctor if you develop skin rash or itching, visual disturbances, weight gain, breathing difficulties, fluid retention, hallucinations, black or tarry stools, persistent headache, or any unusual or intolerable side effect.

If you forget to take a dose of mefenamic acid, take it as soon as you remember. If you take mefenamic acid once a day and it is within 8 hours of your next dose, skip the dose you forgot and continue with your regular schedule. If you take several doses a day and it is within 4 hours of your next dose, skip the one you forgot and continue with your regular schedule. Never take a double dose.

Special Populations

Pregnancy/Breast-feeding

NSAIDs may cross into fetal blood circulation. They have not been found to cause birth defects, but animal studies indicate that they may affect the fetal heart during the second half of pregnancy. Pregnant women should not take mefenamic acid without their doctor's approval, particularly during the last 3 months of pregnancy. When the drug is considered crucial by your doctor, its potential benefits must be carefully weighed against its risks.

NSAIDs may pass into breast milk but have caused no problems in breast-fed infants, except for seizures in a baby whose mother was taking the NSAID indomethacin. There is a possibility that a nursing mother taking mefenamic acid could affect her baby's heart or cardiovascular system. If you must take mefenamic acid, bottle-feed your baby.

Seniors

Seniors may be more susceptible to mefenamic acid side effects, especially ulcer disease.

Generic Name

Megestrol (meh-JES-trol) G

Brand Name

Megace

Type of Drug

Progestin.

Prescribed for

Cancer of the breast or endometrium; also prescribed for decreased appetite and weight loss associated with acquired immunodeficiency syndrome (AIDS).

General Information

Megestrol acetate has been used successfully in the treatment of the cancers mentioned above. This medication acts as a hormonal counterbalance in areas of the body rich in estrogen such as the breast and the endometrium. Other progestins, including norethindrone, may be used to treat cancer of the endometrium or uterus or to correct hormone imbalance.

Megestrol's role in treating the appetite loss, weight loss, and poor physical condition experienced by people with AIDS is not fully understood. We do know that megestrol stimulates appetite and adds muscle and lean body mass whereas many other dietary supplements add fat.

Cautions and Warnings

Megestrol should be used only for its 2 specific indications, and users of this drug should be closely and regularly monitored by their doctors. Megestrol use should be carefully considered if you have a history of **blood clots or similar disorders, convulsions, liver disease, undiagnosed vaginal bleeding, asthma, cardiac insufficiency, epilepsy, migraine, kidney problems, diabetes, ectopic pregnancy, high blood-fat levels**, or **depression**.

If you experience a partial or complete loss of vision,

double vision, migraine headache, or a sudden fall, stop taking the medication and call your doctor immediately.

Possible Side Effects

▼ Common: weight gain due to increased appetite, not fluid retention. When megestrol is used for weight gain in AIDS, the most common side effect is impotence.

▼ Less common: back or stomach pain, headache, nausea, and vomiting. If you develop any of these symptoms, call your doctor immediately.

▼ Rare: diarrhea, stomach gas, rash, swelling in the legs or feet, and weakness.

Drug Interactions

• Megestrol may interfere with the effects of bromocriptine; do not combine these drugs.

• Rifampin may reduce the effectiveness of megestrol by increasing the rate at which it is broken down by the liver.

Food Interactions

Megestrol is best taken on an empty stomach but may be taken with food if it upsets your stomach.

Usual Dose

Breast or Endometrial Cancer: 40–320 mg a day.

AIDS-related Weight Loss: 800 mg 4 times a day

Overdosage

Megestrol overdose may result in severe side effects. In many cases, small overdoses will not result in unusual symptoms. Call your local poison control control center or hospital emergency room for more information.

Special Information

Continuous treatment for 2 months is usually required to determine if megestrol is effective for your condition.

Call your doctor if you develop back or abdominal pain, headache, nausea, vomiting, breast tenderness, or other persistent, severe, or bothersome side effects.

Women of childbearing age taking megestrol should use an effective contraceptive because this drug causes birth defects.

People with AIDS who take megestrol for weight gain should continue taking it until they reach their desired weight and then stop taking the drug until needed again.

If you forget to take a dose of megestrol, take it as soon as you remember. If it is almost time for your next dose, skip the dose you forgot and continue with your regular schedule. Do not take a double dose.

Special Populations

Pregnancy/Breast-feeding

Megestrol is known to cause birth defects and interferes with fetal development. This drug should not be used during the first 4 months of pregnancy. Call your doctor at once if you are taking this medication and become pregnant.

Megestrol passes into breast milk but has caused no problems among breast-fed infants. However, you must consider possible effects on the nursing infant.

Seniors

Seniors with severe liver disease are more sensitive to the effects of megestrol. Follow your doctor's directions and report any side effects at once.

Generic Name

Meperidine (muh-PER-ih-dine) G

Brand Name

Demerol

Type of Drug

Narcotic analgesic (pain reliever).

Prescribed for

Moderate to severe pain.

General Information

Meperidine hydrochloride is a potent narcotic analgesic and cough suppressant. It is also used before surgery to reduce anxiety and help bring the patient into early stages of anesthesia. Meperidine is probably the most widely used narcotic in American hospitals. Its effects compare favorably with those of morphine sulfate, the standard for narcotic analgesics.

It is useful for mild to moderate pain; 25 to 50 mg of meperidine are approximately equal in pain-relieving effect to 2 325-mg aspirin tablets. Meperidine may be less active than aspirin for pain associated with inflammation because aspirin reduces inflammation whereas meperidine does not. Meperidine suppresses the cough reflex but does not cure the underlying cause of the cough. In certain instances, it may be inappropriate to overly suppress a cough because cough suppression reduces your ability to naturally eliminate excess mucus produced as a result of respiratory disease.

Cautions and Warnings

Do not take meperidine if you are **allergic or sensitive** to it. Use this drug with extreme caution if you suffer from **asthma or other breathing problems**. Chronic (long-term) use of meperidine may cause **drug dependence or addiction**. Narcotic side effects are severe in the presence of a **head injury, brain tumor, or other head problem**; use meperidine with extreme caution if any of these apply to you. Narcotics may also hide the symptoms of head injury.

Possible Side Effects

▼ Most common: light-headedness, dizziness, sleepiness, nausea, vomiting, appetite loss, and increased sweating. These side effects usually will disappear if you lie down. More serious side effects of meperidine are shallow breathing or breathing difficulties.

▼ Less common: euphoria (feeling high), weakness, headache, agitation, uncoordinated muscle movement, minor hallucinations, disorientation, visual disturbances, dry mouth, constipation, flushing of the face, rapid heartbeat, palpitations, faintness, urinary difficulties or hesitancy, reduced sex drive or potency, itching, rash, anemia, lowered blood sugar, and yellowing of the skin or whites of the eyes. Narcotic analgesics may aggravate convulsions in those who have had them in the past.

Drug Interactions

• Because of its depressant effect and potential effect on breathing, meperidine should be taken with extreme care in combination with alcohol, sleeping medication, tranquilizers, or other depressant drugs.

• People taking cimetidine and a narcotic analgesic may experience confusion, disorientation, nervous-system depression, seizure, or breathing difficulties.

• When this drug is combined with a monamine oxidase inhibitor (MAOI) antidepressant, unusual and possibly fatal reactions may occur. Do not take meperidine within 2 weeks of your last dose of an MAOI. Symptoms that have occurred include breathing difficulties; blood-pressure changes; bluish discoloration of the lips, fingernails, or skin; and coma.

Food Interactions

Meperidine may be taken with food to reduce upset stomach.

Usual Dose

Adult: 50–150 mg every 3–4 hours as needed.
Child: 0.5–0.8 mg per lb. every 3–4 hours as needed, up to the adult dosage.

Overdosage

Symptoms of overdose include slow breathing, extreme tiredness progressing to stupor and then coma, pinpointed pupils, no response to pain stimulation, cold or clammy skin, slow heartbeat, low blood pressure, convulsions, and cardiac arrest. The victim should be taken to a hospital emergency room immediately. ALWAYS bring the prescription bottle or container with you.

Special Information

If you are taking meperidine, be extremely careful while driving or operating complicated or hazardous machinery. Avoid alcoholic beverages.

Call your doctor if this drug makes you very nauseous or constipated, if you experience breathing difficulties, or if any prominent or persistent side effect occurs.

Consider asking your doctor to lower your meperidine dosage if you experience light-headedness, dizziness, sleepiness, nausea, vomiting, appetite loss, or increased sweating.

If you forget to take a dose of meperidine, take it as soon as you remember. If it is almost time for your next dose, skip the one you forgot and continue with your regular schedule. Do not take a double dose.

Special Populations

Pregnancy/Breast-feeding

Animal studies show that narcotics may cause problems in the fetus. Women who are or might be pregnant while using this drug should talk to their doctors about the risks of taking it versus the benefits it may provide.

Meperidine passes into breast milk, but no problems in nursing infants have been seen. Nursing mothers who must take this drug should bottle-feed their infants.

Large amounts of any narcotic, including meperidine, taken on a long-term basis during pregnancy or breast-feeding may cause the baby to become dependent on the narcotic. Narcotics may also cause breathing difficulties in the infant during delivery.

Seniors

Seniors are more likely to be sensitive to meperidine's side effects and should take the smallest effective dosage.

Generic Name

Meprobamate (muh-PROE-buh-mate) G

Brand Names

Equanil	Miltown
Meprospan	Neuramate

Type of Drug

Antianxiety agent.

Prescribed for

Short-term anxiety and tension of less than 4 months' duration.

General Information

Meprobamate works by directly affecting several areas of the brain. It can relax you, relieve anxiety, and act as a muscle relaxant, anticonvulsant, or sleeping pill. This drug should be used only for short-term relief of anxiety and tension.

Cautions and Warnings

Do not take meprobamate if you are **allergic** to it or to a related drug such as carbromal, carisoprodol, felbamate, or mebutamate. Meprobamate may cause seizures in epileptic patients.

Long-term meprobamate users have developed severe physical and psychological **drug dependence.** It can produce chronic intoxication after prolonged use or if used in greater than recommended doses: Symptoms include slurred speech, dizziness, general sleepiness, and depression. Suddenly stopping meprobamate after prolonged and excessive use may result in drug withdrawal symptoms, including severe anxiety, vomiting, appetite loss, sleeplessness, tremors, muscle twitching, severe sleepiness, confusion, hallucinations, and convulsions. Withdrawal symptoms usually begin 12 to 48 hours after meprobamate has been stopped and may last 1 to 4 days. When stopping treatment with meprobamate, the drug should be reduced gradually over 1 or 2 weeks.

People with **kidney or liver disease** need to take lower doses of meprobamate because these conditions will cause the drug to accumulate in your body.

Possible Side Effects

▼ Most common: drowsiness, sleepiness, dizziness, slurred speech, poor muscle coordination, headache, weakness, tingling in the arms and legs, and euphoria (feeling high).

▼ Less common: nausea, vomiting, diarrhea, abnormal heart rhythm, excitement or overstimulation, low blood pressure, itching, rash, and changes in various blood components.

▼ Rare: allergic reactions, including high fever, chills, bronchospasm (closing of the throat), and reduced urinary function.

Drug Interactions

• Combining meprobamate with nervous-system depressants, including alcohol, other tranquilizers, narcotics, barbiturates, sleeping pills, or antihistamines, can cause excess tranquilization, depression, sleepiness, or fatigue.

Food Interactions

Take this drug with food if it upsets your stomach.

Usual Dose

Adult and Child (age 13 and over): 1200–1600 mg a day in divided doses; maximum daily dose, 2400 mg.
Child (age 6–12): 100–200 mg 2–3 times a day.
Child (under age 6): not recommended.

Overdosage

In attempted suicide or accidental overdose, symptoms are extreme drowsiness, lethargy, stupor, and coma, with possible shock and respiratory collapse, when breathing stops. Some people have died after taking only 30 tablets, while others have survived after taking 100. If alcohol or another depressant has also been taken, a much smaller dose of meprobamate can be fatal. After a large overdose, the victim will go to sleep very quickly, and blood pressure, pulse, and breathing levels will drop rapidly. The overdose victim must immediately be taken to a hospital emergency room, where his or her stomach will be pumped and respiratory assistance and other supportive therapy given. ALWAYS bring the prescription bottle or container with you.

Special Information

Take this drug according to your doctor's direction. Do not change your dose without your doctor's approval.

This drug causes drowsiness and poor concentration. Be careful when driving or performing complex activities. Avoid alcohol and other nervous-system depressants because they increase these effects.

Call your doctor if you develop fever, sore throat, rash, mouth sores, nosebleeds, unexplained black-and-blue marks, or easy bruising or bleeding, or if you become pregnant.

If you forget to take a dose of meprobamate and you remember within about 1 hour of your regular time, take it right away. If you do not remember until later, skip the dose you forgot and go back to your regular schedule. Do not take a double dose.

Special Populations

Pregnancy/Breast-feeding

Meprobamate has been shown to increase the risk of birth defects, particularly during the first 3 months of pregnancy. Inform your doctor immediately if you are or might be pregnant. There are few good reasons for pregnant women to take meprobamate.

Meprobamate passes into breast milk in concentrations 2 to 4 times greater than are found in the blood. It may cause tiredness in nursing infants. Nursing mothers who must take this drug should bottle-feed their babies.

Seniors

Seniors are more sensitive to the sedative and other effects of this drug, and should take the lowest dose possible. Report any side effects at once.

Generic Name

Mesalamine (meh-SAL-uh-mene)

Brand Names

Asacol   Rowasa
Pentasa

Type of Drug

Bowel anti-inflammatory.

Prescribed for

Oral Products: ulcerative colitis.

Rectal Products: distal ulcerative colitis, proctitis, and proctosigmoiditis.

General Information

Mesalamine is the breakdown product of sulfasalazine and olsalazine, two widely used treatments for ulcerative colitis and other inflammatory conditions. Mesalamine is the active agent in these drugs in treating symptoms of bowel inflammation. No one knows exactly how mesalamine, a chemical cousin of aspirin, produces its effect, but it is thought to have a local effect on the bowel. Mesalamine tablets are coated with an acrylic resin to delay drug release from the tablet until it reaches the colon. Little of the drug is absorbed into the blood; 70% to 90% stays in the colon.

Cautions and Warnings

Mesalamine may actually worsen **colitis** or cause **cramping**, sudden **abdominal pain, bloody diarrhea, fever, headache**, or **rash**. Call your doctor immediately and stop taking this drug at once if any of these symptoms develop.

People who are **allergic** to mesalamine or aspirin should not use this drug. Although people who are sensitive or allergic to sulfasalazine have generally been able to tolerate mesalamine because so little of the drug is absorbed into the bloodstream, they should be cautious.

Some people taking mesalamine have developed **kidney problems**. People with a current or past history of kidney disease should be cautious about using this drug. All people taking mesalamine should have kidney function tests before starting this drug and while they are taking it.

Possible Side Effects

Mesalamine is generally well tolerated. Mesalamine tablets have the most side effects, suppositories the least.

Tablets
▼ Most common: abdominal pain, cramps, or discomfort; stomach rumbling; and generalized pain.
▼ Common: constipation, diarrhea, upset stomach, vomiting, muscle weakness, dizziness, fever, runny nose, rashes, skin spots, achy joints, back pain, and stiff muscles.
▼ Less common: worsening of colitis, flatulence or gas, chills, sweating, feeling unwell, tiredness, acne, itching, arthritis, muscle aches, chest pain, pinkeye, painful menstruation, swelling, and flu symptoms.
▼ Rare: sleeplessness, hair loss, and urinary burning or infection. Other rare side effects can affect almost any body system.

Capsules
▼ Less common: abdominal pain, cramps, or discomfort; diarrhea; nausea; headache; rash; and skin spots.
▼ Rare: worsening of colitis, constipation, stomach gas, vomiting, dizziness, fever, sleeplessness, sweating, feeling unwell, tiredness, itching, acne, achy joints, leg or joint pain, muscle aches, pinkeye, swelling, and hair loss. Other rare side effects can affect almost any body system.

Suppositories
▼ Common: headache.

Possible Side Effects *(continued)*

▼ Less common: abdominal pain, cramps, or discomfort; diarrhea; worsening of colitis; flatulence or gas; nausea; rectal pain, soreness, or burning; muscle weakness; dizziness; fever; sore throat; cold symptoms; acne; rash; skin spots; and swelling.

Rectal Suspension
▼ Common: abdominal pain, cramps, or discomfort; flatulence or gas; nausea; headache; and flu-like symptoms.

▼ Less common: bloating; diarrhea; hemmorhoids; pain on enema insertion; rectal pain, soreness, or burning; dizziness; fever; feeling unwell; tiredness; cold symptoms; sore throat; itching; rash; skin spots; back pain; leg pain; and joint pain.

▼ Rare: constipation, muscle weakness, sleeplessness, swelling, hair loss, and urinary burning or infection.

Drug Interactions

None known.

Food Interactions

Take this drug with food if it upsets your stomach.

Usual Dose

Capsules: 1000 mg 4 times a day for up to 8 weeks.

Tablets: 800 mg 3 times a day for 6 weeks.

Rectal Suspension: 1 bottle of suspension taken as an enema at bedtime every night for 3–6 weeks. The enema liquid should be retained for about 8 hours.

Suppositories: 1 suppository 2 times a day for 3–6 weeks. Retain the suppository for 1–3 hours for maximum benefit.

Overdosage

Symptoms are likely to be similar to those of an aspirin overdose: ringing or buzzing in the ears, fainting or dizziness, headache, confusion, drowsiness, sweating, rapid breathing, vomiting, and diarrhea. Overdose victims should be made to vomit with ipecac syrup—available at any pharmacy—to remove the medication from the stomach; they should then be taken to a hospital emergency room for treatment. In one case of accidental overdose in a 3-year-old boy who took 2000 mg, treatment with ipecac syrup and charcoal — to absorb any remaining medicine — resulted in no serious consequences. Call your local poison control center before giving the ipecac syrup. ALWAYS take the prescription bottle or container with you when you go for treatment.

Special Information

Mesalamine tablets must be swallowed whole. The outer coating is designed to protect the mesalamine until it reaches the colon. Call your doctor if you pass whole tablets.

When using suppositories, remove the foil wrapper and insert into the rectum, pointed end first, with as little handling as possible to prevent it from accidentally melting.

When using the rectal suspension, shake the bottle well and remove the protective sheath from the applicator tip. Lie on your left side with your lower leg extended and the upper leg flexed to maintain balance. Gently insert the applicator tip in the rectum pointing toward your navel. Steadily squeeze the bottle to discharge most of the contents into your colon.

Call your doctor if you develop chest pains, breathing difficulties, urinary difficulties, worsening of your colitis, or any other side effect that is bothersome or persistent.

If you forget a dose of mesalamine, take it as soon as you remember. If you take mesalamine tablets and it is within 4 hours of your next dose, skip the dose you forgot and continue with your regular schedule. If you take mesalamine suppositories or rectal solution and you do not remember until it is almost time for the next dose, skip the one you forgot and continue with your regular schedule. Never take a double dose.

Special Populations

Pregnancy/Breast-feeding

Mesalamine passes into the circulation of the fetus. Pregnant women should consult their doctors before using mesalamine.

Small amounts of mesalamine pass into breast milk, although the importance of this is not known. Nursing mothers taking mesalamine should exercise caution.

Seniors

Seniors may use this drug without special restriction. Be sure to report any unusual side effects to your doctor.

Generic Name

Metaproterenol (met-uh-proe-TER-uh-nol) [G]

Brand Names

Alupent Inhalation Aerosol	Metaprel Inhalation Aerosol
Alupent Solution	Metaprel Solution
Alupent Syrup	Metaprel Syrup
Alupent Tablets	Metaprel Tablets

Type of Drug

Bronchodilator.

Prescribed for

Asthma and bronchospasm.

General Information

Metaproterenol sulfate can be taken both by mouth as a tablet or syrup and by inhalation. This drug may be used with other drugs to produce relief from asthma symptoms. Oral metaproterenol begins working 15 to 30 minutes after a dose; its effects may last for up to 4 hours. Metaproterenol inhalation begins working in 5 to 30 minutes and lasts for 2 to 6 hours.

Cautions and Warnings

This drug should be used with caution by people with a history of **angina pectoris, heart disease, high blood pressure, stroke, seizures, diabetes, thyroid disease, prostate disease,** or **glaucoma.** Excessive use of metaproterenol could lead to worsening of your condition.

Using excessive amounts of metaproterenol can lead to increased breathing difficulties rather than relief. In the most extreme cases, people have had heart attacks after using excessive amounts of inhalant.

Possible Side Effects

▼ Common: heart palpitations, rapid heartbeat, tremors, convulsions, shakiness, nervous tension, dizziness, fainting, headache, heartburn, upset stomach, nausea

Possible Side Effects *(continued)*

and vomiting, cough, dry or sore and irritated throat, muscle cramps, and urinary difficulties.

▼ Less common: high blood pressure, abnormal heart rhythms, and angina. Metaproterenol inhalation is less likely to cause these effects than some of the older drugs. It can also cause diarrhea, unusual tastes or smells, dry mouth, drowsiness, hoarseness, stuffy nose, worsening of asthma, backache, fatigue, and rash.

Drug Interactions

• The effect of this drug may be increased by antidepressant drugs, some antihistamines, levothyroxine, and monoamine oxidase inhibitors (MAOIs).

• The chances of cardiac toxicity may be increased in people combining metaproterenol and theophylline.

• Metaproterenol is antagonized by beta-blocking drugs such as propranolol.

• Metaproterenol may antagonize the effects of blood-pressure-lowering drugs, especially reserpine, methyldopa, and guanethidine.

Food Interactions

If the tablets upset your stomach, they may be taken with food.

Usual Dose

Tablets or Syrup
   Adult and Child (age 10 and over or 60 lbs.): 60–80 mg a day.
   Child (age 6–9 or under 60 lbs.): 30–40 mg a day.
   Child (under age 6): 0.6–1.2 mg per lb. of body weight a day. Children this age should be treated only with metaproterenol syrup.

Inhalation
   Adult and Child (age 12 and over): 2–3 puffs every 3–4 hours.
   Child (under age 12): not recommended.

Each canister contains about 300 inhalations. Do not use more than 12 puffs a day.

Overdosage

Symptoms of metaproterenol overdose are palpitations, abnormal heart rhythm, rapid or slow heartbeat, chest pain, high blood pressure, fever, chills, cold sweat, blanching of the skin, nausea, vomiting, sleeplessness, delirium, tremor, pinpoint pupils, convulsions, coma, and collapse. The victim should see a doctor or be taken to a hospital emergency room. ALWAYS bring the prescription bottle or container with you.

Special Information

Be sure to follow your doctor's instructions for using metaproterenol. Using more than the amount prescribed can lead to drug tolerance and actually worsen your symptoms. If your condition worsens rather than improves after taking metaproterenol, stop taking it and call your doctor.

Metaproterenol inhalation should be breathed in during the second half of your inward breath, since this allows it to reach more deeply into your lungs.

Call your doctor immediately if you develop chest pain, palpitations, rapid heartbeat, muscle tremors, dizziness, headache, facial flushing, or urinary difficulty, or if you still have trouble breathing after using this medication.

If you miss a dose of metaproterenol, take it as soon as possible. Take the rest of that day's dose at regularly spaced time intervals. Go back to your regular schedule the next day.

Special Populations

Pregnancy/Breast-feeding
This drug should be used by women who are pregnant only when absolutely necessary. The potential hazard to the fetus is not known at this time. However, metaproterenol has caused birth defects when given in large amounts to pregnant animals.

It is not known if metaproterenol passes into breast milk. Nursing mothers who are taking this drug must watch for side effects in their infants. You may want to consider bottle-feeding.

Seniors
Seniors are more sensitive to the effects of this drug. Closely follow your doctor's directions and report any side effects at once.

Generic Name

Metaxalone (meh-TAX-uh-lone)

Brand Name

Skelaxin

Type of Drug

Skeletal muscle relaxant.

Prescribed for

Muscle spasms.

General Information

Metaxalone is prescribed as a part of a coordinated program of rest, physical therapy, and other measures for the relief of acute, painful spasm conditions. Metaxalone does not directly relax skeletal muscles; exactly how it works is unknown.

Cautions and Warnings

Metaxalone should be taken with caution if you have had a **reaction** to it in the past, if you have a tendency toward **anemia**, or if you have **poor kidney or liver function**.

Possible Side Effects

▼ Most common: nausea, vomiting, upset stomach, stomach cramps, drowsiness, dizziness, headache, nervousness, and irritability.

▼ Less common: rapid or pounding heartbeat, fainting, convulsions, hallucinations, depression, clumsiness or unsteadiness, constipation, diarrhea, heartburn, hiccups, black or tarry bowel movements, vomiting of material that resembles coffee grounds, agranulocytosis (symptoms include fever with or without chills, sore throat, and sores or white spots on the lips or mouth), uncontrolled eye movement, stuffy nose, stinging or burning eyes, bloodshot eyes, weakness, unusual tiredness, chest tightness, swollen glands, unusual bleeding or bruising, and breathing difficulties.

Possible Side Effects *(continued)*

▼ Rare: liver inflammation, yellowing of the skin or whites of the eyes, and drug-sensitivity reactions (symptoms include rash, hives, itching, changes in facial color, fast or irregular breathing, troubled breathing, and wheezing).

Drug Interactions

• Tranquilizers, alcohol, and other nervous system depressants may increase the depressant effects of metaxalone.

Food Interactions

Metaxalone may be taken with food or meals if it upsets your stomach.

Usual Dose

Adult and Child (age 13 and over): 800 mg 3 or 4 times a day.
Child (under age 13): not recommended.

Overdosage

Symptoms of metaxalone overdose are likely to be severe side effects but may include some less common reactions as well. Overdose victims should be taken to a hospital emergency room for treatment. ALWAYS bring the prescription bottle or container.

Special Information

Long-term metaxalone treatment may cause liver toxicity or damage. If you are using this medicine for an extended period, your doctor should check your liver function about every 1 to 2 months.

Metaxalone may cause tiredness, dizziness, and lightheadedness. Be careful when driving or performing tasks that require concentration and coordination.

Call your doctor if you develop breathing difficulties, unusual tiredness or weakness, fever, chills, cough or hoarseness, lower back or side pain, painful urination, yellowing of the skin or whites of the eyes, rash, hives, itching, redness, or any other bothersome or persistent symptom.

If you miss a dose of metaxalone, take it as soon as you

remember. If it is almost time for your next dose, take 1 dose as soon as you remember, another in 3 or 4 hours, and then go back to your regular schedule. Do not take a double dose.

Special Populations

Pregnancy/Breast-feeding

There are no cases of metaxalone-related birth defects. As with all drugs, pregnant women should not use metaxalone unless its benefits have been carefully weighed against its risks.

It is not known if metaxalone passes into breast milk. Nursing mothers should use this drug with caution.

Seniors

No serious problems have been reported in older adults taking metaxalone. However, the fact that seniors are likely to have some loss of kidney and/or liver function should be taken into account when determining dosage.

Generic Name

Metformin (met-FOR-min)

Brand Name

Glucophage

Type of Drug

Biguanide antihyperglycemic.

Prescribed for

Diabetes mellitus.

General Information

Metformin is chemically different from all other antidiabetes drugs, which belong to the sulfonylurea group. Generally, people are not given metformin until they have tried one of the sulfonylureas without a satisfactory response. If neither drug works alone, it is possible that a combination of metformin and a sulfonylurea may be effective in controlling your diabetes, since the two drugs work by different methods. Metformin can moderately lower blood fats, while sulfonylureas tend to raise blood fat levels; however, the combination of metformin with a sulfonylurea still lowers blood-fat levels.

Cautions and Warnings

Do not take metformin if you have had an **allergic** reaction to it or if you have **heart failure**. Metformin should not be taken by people with **kidney disease** because the drug is cleared by the kidneys. If you are having surgery or an x-ray that requires the injection of an iodine-based contrast material, you should temporarily stop taking metformin because the combination could result in acute kidney problems.

Metformin is related to an older antidiabetes drug that was moderately popular but was removed from the market because of the possibility of a very rare but serious complication known as **lactic acidosis**. When lactic acidosis does develop, it is fatal approximately half of the time. Lactic acidosis may also occur in association with a number of conditions, including diabetes mellitus. The risk of lactic acidosis increases with age, heart failure, and worsening kidney function. Regular monitoring of kidney function minimizes the chances of developing lactic acidosis, as does the use of the minimum effective dose of metformin. Metformin should not be taken by people with acidosis, including those with diabetic ketoacidosis. Diabetic ketoacidosis should be treated with insulin.

People with **liver disease** should not take metformin because of the increased chance of lactic acidosis.

People taking oral antidiabetes drugs are generally more likely to develop **heart disease**, compared with people taking insulin or those treated by diet alone.

Possible Side Effects

People who have been stabilized on metformin should not consider gastrointestinal (GI) symptoms to be related to the drug unless other causes or lactic acidosis have been excluded.

▼ Most common: diarrhea, nausea, vomiting, abdominal bloating, stomach gas, and appetite loss. These symptoms tend to occur when you first start taking metformin but are generally transient and resolve on their own. Occasionally, temporary dose reduction may be useful.

▼ Rare: Metformin can cause about 3 in every 100 people to develop an unpleasant or metallic taste in the

Possible Side Effects *(continued)*

mouth. This usually resolves on its own. About 9 of every 100 people taking metformin alone develop low blood levels of vitamin B_{12}, without any associated symptoms. This also occurs in 6 of every 100 people on combined metformin-sulfonylurea therapy. Blood folic acid levels do not decrease significantly when vitamin B_{12} is affected. Blood levels of vitamin B_{12} should be periodically checked, or you may take a B_{12} supplement.

Drug Interactions

• Metformin may reduce the effect of glyburide, a sulfonylurea, but this interaction is highly variable from one person to another.

• Alcohol increases the chance of developing lactic acidosis while taking metformin.

• Metformin may interfere with amiloride, digoxin, morphine, procainamide, quinine, quinidine, ranitidine, triamterene, trimethoprim, and vancomycin. Careful monitoring is necessary to avoid any possible problems.

• Cimetidine and furosemide can cause a large increase in metformin blood levels and possible side effects. Furosemide levels are reduced by metformin.

• Nifedipine increases metformin absorption into the bloodstream, blood levels of metformin, and the amount of metformin that is cleared through the kidneys.

Food Interactions

Metformin may be taken with food to reduce upset stomach.

Usual Dose

Adult: 500 mg twice daily, increased gradually to a maximum daily dose of 2550 mg. Starting dosage can be 850 mg in the morning.

Senior: Older adults should start with regular doses but generally are not given the maximum daily dose of 2550 mg a day.

Child: not recommended.

Overdosage

Contrary to what you might expect, low blood sugar is not

common with metformin overdose—it did not even occur in the case of someone swallowing up to 85 g of metformin—although lactic acidosis has occurred in cases of metformin overdose. Overdose victims should be taken to the hospital for treatment at once. ALWAYS bring the prescription bottle or container with you.

Special Information

Diet and exercise are the mainstays of diabetes treatment. Be sure to follow your doctor's directions in these areas even though you are also taking medication.

Avoid excessive alcohol intake since alcohol increases the chance of developing lactic acidosis while you are taking metformin.

Lactic acidosis is a medical emergency that must be treated in a hospital. Metformin treatment must be stopped immediately if you develop lactic acidosis. This disease is often subtle, and is accompanied only by nonspecific symptoms such as feeling unwell, muscle aches, breathing difficulties, tiredness, and nonspecific upset stomach. Low body temperature, low blood pressure, and slow heartbeat can develop with more severe acidosis. Call your doctor at once if you develop these symptoms while taking metformin.

Stomach and intestine metformin side effects may be reduced by gradually increasing your metformin dose and by taking metformin with meals.

Metformin should be temporarily stopped if you have severe diarrhea and/or vomiting because dehydration and reduced kidney function may develop. However, do not stop taking your medication without first consulting your doctor.

If you forget a dose of metformin, take it as soon as you remember. If it is almost time for your next dose, skip the dose you forgot and continue with your regular schedule. Do not take a double dose.

Special Populations

Pregnancy/Breast-feeding

Diabetic women who are or might be pregnant should be taking insulin injections during their pregnancy. The safety of metformin during pregnancy is not known.

Metformin passes into breast milk. Nursing mothers who must take metformin should consider bottle-feeding their babies.

Seniors

Seniors retain more metformin than do younger adults because of the normal decline in kidney function that accompanies aging; they need less medication to effectively lower their blood sugar levels.

Generic Name

Methenamine Mandelate

(meth-EN-uh-meen MAN-deh-late) G

Brand Name

Mandelamine

The information in this profile also applies to the following drug:

Generic Ingredient: Methenamine Hippurate
Hiprex   Urex

Type of Drug

Urinary anti-infective.

Prescribed for

Chronic urinary-tract infections.

General Information

The methenamine anti-infectives work by turning into formaldehyde and ammonia when the urine is acidic. The formaldehyde kills bacteria in the urinary tract. These drugs do not break down in the blood. You may need to make your urine more acidic by taking 4 to 12 g a day of ascorbic acid (vitamin C) or ammonium chloride.

Cautions and Warnings

People who are **allergic** to any form of methenamine, and those with **kidney disease, severe dehydration,** or severe **liver disease** should not use this drug. Methenamine anti-infectives should not be taken with a sulfa drug because sulfa drugs form an insoluble substance in the kidneys when mixed with formaldehyde.

Large doses — 8 g or more a day — of methenamine can

cause bladder irritation, painful and frequent urination, and protein and blood in the urine.

People with **gout** who take methenamine may experience some kidney pain due to formation of urate crystals in the kidney.

Possible Side Effects

Methenamine side effects are relatively rare.

▼ Most common: nausea, vomiting, stomach cramps, diarrhea, appetite loss, and stomach irritation. Large doses over long periods may cause bladder irritation, painful or frequent urination, and protein or blood in the urine. This drug may also cause elevation in liver enzymes.

▼ Less common: headache, breathing difficulties, swelling, lung irritation, and rash.

▼ Rare: itching and rash.

Drug Interactions

• Do not take methenamine with sulfa drugs (see "Cautions and Warnings").

• Sodium bicarbonate and acetazolamide will decrease the effect of methenamine by making the urine less acidic.

Food Interactions

Take methenamine with food to minimize stomach upset. Methenamine's action is decreased by foods that reduce urine acidity, including dairy products. Avoid large amounts of these foods.

Usual Dose

Adult and Child (age 12 and over): 1 g 2–4 times a day.
Child (age 6–11): 0.5–1 g 2–4 times a day.
Child (under age 6): not recommended.

Overdosage

Upset stomach and exaggerated side effects are indicators of methenamine overdose. Call a poison control center or emergency room for more information. ALWAYS bring the prescription bottle or container with you if you go to the hospital for treatment.

Special Information

Make sure you take all the medication your doctor has prescribed. Stopping too soon can lead to a relapse of your infection.

Take each dose with at least 8 oz. of water.

Call your doctor if you develop pain on urinating, a skin rash, or a severe upset stomach while taking this drug.

If you miss a dose of methenamine, take it as soon as possible. Take the rest of that day's doses at regularly spaced time intervals. Go back to your regular schedule the next day.

Special Populations

Pregnancy/Breast-feeding

Methenamine crosses into the fetal circulation but has not been found to cause birth defects. It has been used during the last 3 months of pregnancy—when many drugs are considered especially dangerous to the fetus—though its safety has never been proven. When the drug is considered crucial by your doctor, its potential benefits must be carefully weighed against its risks.

This drug passes into breast milk in concentrations similar to those found in blood, but has caused no problems among breast-fed infants. Nursing mothers taking methenamine should exercise caution.

Seniors

Seniors without severe kidney or liver disease may take this medication without special restriction. Follow your doctor's directions and report any side effects at once.

Generic Name

Methotrexate (meth-oe-TREK-sate) Ⓖ

Brand Name

Rheumatrex

Type of Drug

Antimetabolite, antiarthritic, and anti-inflammatory.

Prescribed for

Cancer chemotherapy, psoriasis, psoriatic arthritis, adult and juvenile rheumatoid arthritis, mycosis fungoides, Reiter's disease, and severe asthma.

General Information

Methotrexate sodium was one of the first drugs found to be effective against certain cancers in the late 1940s. More recent research with smaller doses of this drug has resulted in its acceptance as a treatment for other conditions that respond to immune-system suppressants. Methotrexate dosages differ dramatically for each drug use, but you should be aware that methotrexate may be extremely toxic even in the relatively low doses prescribed for rheumatoid arthritis. This drug should be considered "last-resort" therapy for all non-cancer patients, to be used only in severe cases that have not responded to other treatments. Methotrexate should be prescribed only by doctors who are familiar with the drug and its potential for producing toxic effects.

Cautions and Warnings

Methotrexate can trigger a unique and dangerous form of **lung disease** at any time during your course of therapy. This reaction can occur at doses as low as 7.5 mg per week — the antiarthritis dose. Symptoms of this condition are cough, respiratory infection, difficulty breathing, abnormal chest x-ray, and low blood-oxygen levels. Report any change in your breathing or lung status to your doctor.

Methotrexate can cause severe **liver damage**; this usually occurs only after taking it over a long period. Changes in liver enzymes — measured by a blood test — are common.

Methotrexate should be used with caution, and the dosage should be reduced for people with **kidney disease**.

Methotrexate can cause severe lowering of **red- and white-blood-cell** and **blood-platelet counts**.

Your doctor should periodically test your kidney and liver function and your blood components.

Methotrexate can cause severe **diarrhea, stomach irritation**, and **mouth or gum sores**. Death can result from **intestinal perforation** caused by methotrexate.

Aspirin, nonsteroidal anti-inflammatory drugs (NSAIDs), and low-dose corticosteroid treatment may be continued while you are taking methotrexate for rheumatoid arthritis, although an increase in drug toxicity is possible. Previous studies of methotrexate in rheumatoid arthritis were usually done in people already taking an NSAID.

Methotrexate has been studied as an abortion drug in combination with misoprostol, see "Misoprostol."

Possible Side Effects

▼ Most common: liver irritation, loss of kidney function, reduced blood platelet count, nausea, vomiting, diarrhea, stomach upset and irritation, itching, rash, hair loss, dizziness, and increased susceptibility to infection.

▼ Less common: reduced red-blood-cell count, unusual sensitivity to the sun, acne, headache, drowsiness, blurred vision, respiratory infection and breathing problems, appetite loss, muscle aches, chest pain, coughing, painful urination, eye discomfort, nosebleeds, fever, infections, blood in the urine, sweating, ringing or buzzing in the ears, defective sperm production, reduced sperm count, menstrual dysfunction, vaginal discharge, convulsions, and slight paralysis.

Drug Interactions

• Fatal reactions have developed in 4 people taking methotrexate with certain NSAIDs—3 with ketoprofen, 1 with naproxen. Do not take another anti-inflammatory or antiarthritic drug—even over-the-counter drugs such as ibuprofen or naproxen—with methotrexate unless specifically directed to do so by your doctor.

• Combining phenylbutazone and methotrexate increases the risk of severe white-blood-cell count reductions, but may be medically necessary. In these cases, your doctor will watch especially closely for signs of drug toxicity (see "Cautions and Warnings").

• Aspirin and other salicylates, certain other anticancer drugs, etretinate, procarbazine, probenecid, and sulfa drugs can increase the therapeutic and toxic effects of methotrexate.

• Folic acid counteracts the effects of methotrexate.

• Methotrexate may lower phenytoin blood levels, possibly reducing phenytoin's effectiveness.

Food Interactions

Food interferes with methotrexate absorption into the bloodstream. The drug is best taken on an empty stomach, at least

1 hour before or 2 hours after meals, but may be taken with food if it upsets your stomach.

Usual Dose

Methotrexate dosage varies with the condition being treated. Some cancers can be treated with 10–30 mg a day, while others are treated with hundreds or thousands of mg given by intravenous injection in the hospital.

Rheumatoid Arthritis: starting dosage — 7.5 mg a week by mouth, either as a single dose or in 3 separate doses of 2.5 mg taken every 12 hours. Weekly dosage may be increased gradually up to 20 mg. Doses above 20 mg a week are more likely to cause severe side effects.

Psoriasis: 2.5–6.5 mg a day by mouth, not to exceed 30 mg a week. In severe cases, dosage may be increased to 50 mg a week.

Overdosage

Methotrexate overdose can be serious and life-threatening. Victims should be taken to a hospital emergency room immediately. A specific antidote to the effects of methotrexate, calcium leucovorin, is available in every hospital. ALWAYS bring the prescription bottle or container with you if you go to the emergency room for treatment.

Special Information

If you vomit after taking a dose of methotrexate, do not take a replacement dose unless instructed to do so by your doctor.

Women taking this drug must use effective birth control.

To avoid possible birth defects, men should not attempt to father a child during treatment or for 3 months after treatment has been completed.

Call your doctor immediately if you develop diarrhea, fever or chills, skin reddening, mouth or lip sores, stomach pain, unusual bleeding or bruising, blurred vision, seizures, cough, or breathing difficulties. The following symptoms are less severe but should still be reported to your doctor: back pain, darkened urine, dizziness, drowsiness, headache, unusual tiredness or sickness, and yellowing of the skin or whites of the eyes.

If you forget a dose of methotrexate, skip the dose you forgot and continue with your regular schedule. Call your doctor at once. Do not take a double dose.

Special Populations

Pregnancy/Breast-feeding

Methotrexate can cause spontaneous abortion, stillbirth, and severe birth defects. Do not attempt to become pregnant during methotrexate treatment or for at least 1 menstrual cycle after the treatment is completed. Use effective birth control while taking this drug.

Men should not attempt to father a child during treatment or for 3 months after treatment has been completed to avoid possible birth defects. Methotrexate reduces sperm counts and may affect sperm structure.

Nursing mothers who must take methotrexate should bottle-feed their babies.

Seniors

Seniors may be more susceptible to side effects because of age-related impairment of kidney and liver function. Seniors may require smaller doses to obtain the same results.

Generic Name

Methyldopa (meth-ul-DOPE-uh) Ⓖ

Brand Name

Aldomet

Type of Drug

Antihypertensive.

Prescribed for

Hypertension (high blood pressure).

General Information

How methyldopa works is not well understood. Methyldopa's effect probably has to do with the fact that the drug is converted in the body to a form of norepinephrine that stimulates receptors in the central nervous system, which then leads to lower blood pressure. The drug may also interfere with the actions of norepinephrine, renin, and dopamine — all hormones with central roles in maintaining normal blood pressure. Methyldopa causes a reduction in the amounts of the neurohormones serotonin, dopamine, norepinephrine, and epinephrine in the body, which may play a part in reducing blood pressure. It takes about 2 days for methyldopa to reach its maximal antihypertensive (blood-pressure-lowering) effect.

Methyldopa is usually prescribed with one or more other antihypertensive drugs or a diuretic. Methyldopa does not cure hypertension but helps to control it.

Cautions and Warnings

Do not take methyldopa if you have ever developed a **reaction** to it. You should not take methyldopa if you have **hepatitis** or active **cirrhosis of the liver**. People taking this drug may develop a fever with changes in liver function within the first 3 weeks of treatment. Some people develop jaundice (symptoms include yellowing of the skin or whites of the eyes) during the first 2 or 3 months of treatment. Your doctor should periodically check your liver function during the first 3 months of methyldopa treatment, or if you develop an unexplained fever.

Methyldopa should be used with caution in people with severe **kidney disease**, who may need reduced dosages to avoid prolonged and severe lowering of blood pressure.

Possible Side Effects

Most people have little trouble with methyldopa, but it can cause temporary sedation in the first few weeks of treatment or when the dose is increased. Passing headache and weakness are other possible early side effects.

▼ Less common: dizziness; light-headedness; tingling in the extremities; muscle spasms or weakness; decreased mental acuity; psychological disturbances including nightmares, mild psychosis, and depression; changes in heart rate; increase of pain associated with angina pectoris; water retention, resulting in weight gain; dizziness when rising suddenly from a sitting or lying position; nausea;

Possible Side Effects *(continued)*

vomiting; constipation; diarrhea; mild dryness of the mouth; sore and/or black tongue; stuffy nose; male breast enlargement and/or pain; lactation in females; impotence or decreased sex drive in males; mild arthritis symptoms; and skin reactions.

▼ Rare: Methyldopa may affect white blood cells or blood platelets. It may also cause involuntary jerky movements, twitching, restlessness, and slow, continuous, wormlike movements of the fingers, toes, hands, or other body parts.

Drug Interactions

• Methyldopa increases the effect of other blood-pressure-lowering drugs. This is a desirable interaction for people with hypertension. Ironically, the combination of methyldopa with either propranolol or nadolol—two beta blockers often prescribed for hypertension—has sometimes, although rarely, caused an increase in blood pressure.

• Avoid over-the-counter (OTC) cough, cold, and allergy products containing stimulant drugs that may aggravate your hypertension. Ask your pharmacist which OTC products are safe for you.

• Methyldopa may increase the blood-sugar-lowering effect of tolbutamide or other sulfonylurea-types of oral antidiabetic drugs.

• If methyldopa is combined with phenoxybenzamine, urinary incontinence (inability to control the bladder) may result.

• The effect of methyldopa may be reduced by barbiturates and by tricyclic antidepressants.

• The combination of methyldopa and lithium may cause symptoms of lithium overdose—upset stomach, frequent urination, muscle weakness, tiredness, and tremors—even though blood levels of lithium have not changed.

• Methyldopa in combination with haloperidol may produce irritability, aggressiveness, assaultive behavior, or other psychiatric symptoms.

• When methyldopa and levodopa are combined, the effects of both drugs may be increased.

• People taking methyldopa and a monoamine oxidase inhibitor (MAOI) antidepressant may experience excessive stimulation.

• Combining methyldopa with stimulants or a phenothiazine-type drug may lead to a serious increase in blood pressure.

Food Interactions

Methyldopa is best taken on an empty stomach, but you may take it with food if it upsets your stomach.

Usual Dose

Adult: starting dose — 250 mg tablet 2–3 times per a day for the first 2 days. Dosage may then be increased until lower blood pressure is achieved. Maintenance dose — 500–3000 mg a day in 2–4 divided doses, depending on individual need.

Senior: Lower doses may be needed.

Child: 5 mg per lb. of body weight a day in 2–4 divided doses, depending on individual need. Do not exceed 30 mg per lb. of body weight a day, or 3000 mg a day.

Overdosage

Symptoms of methyldopa overdose are sedation, very low blood pressure, weakness, dizziness, light-headedness, fainting, slow heartbeat, constipation, abdominal gas or bulging, nausea, vomiting, and coma. Overdose victims should be made to vomit if they are still conscious by using ipecac syrup — available at any pharmacy — and then taken to a hospital emergency room for treatment. If some time has passed since the overdose was taken, just take the victim directly to an emergency room. ALWAYS bring the prescription bottle or container with you.

Special Information

Take methyldopa exactly as prescribed to maintain maximum control of your hypertension. Do not stop taking this drug unless you are told to do so by your doctor.

A mild sedative effect is to be expected from methyldopa and will resolve within several days.

Your urine may darken if left exposed to air. This is normal and should not be a cause for alarm.

Call your doctor if you develop fever, prolonged general tiredness, or unusual dizziness. If you develop involuntary muscle movements, fever, or jaundice, stop taking the drug and contact your doctor immediately. If these reactions are due to methyldopa, your temperature and/or liver abnormalities will begin to normalize as soon as you stop taking it.

If you forget to take a dose of methyldopa, take it as soon as you remember. If it is almost time for your next dose, skip the one you forgot and continue with your regular schedule. Do not take a double dose.

Special Populations

Pregnancy/Breast-feeding
Methyldopa crosses into the fetal circulation, but it has not been found to cause birth defects. Women who are or might be pregnant should not take this drug without their doctor's approval. When the drug is considered crucial by your doctor, its potential benefits must be carefully weighed against its risks.

Only small amounts of methyldopa pass into breast milk. Women taking methyldopa may nurse their babies.

Seniors
Seniors are more sensitive to the sedating and blood-pressure-lowering effects of methyldopa and may experience dizziness or fainting. Older adults should receive lower doses to account for this sensitivity. Follow your doctor's directions, and report any side effects at once.

Generic Name

Methylphenidate (meth-ul-FEN-ih-date) G

Brand Names

Ritalin   Ritalin-SR

Type of Drug

Mild central-nervous-system stimulant.

Prescribed for

Attention-deficit hyperactivity disorder (ADHD) in children; also prescribed for psychological, educational, or social disorders; narcolepsy and mild depression of the elderly. Methylphenidate is also used to treat cancer, to help stroke victims recover, and, with variable success, in treating hiccups after anesthesia.

General Information

Methylphenidate hydrochloride is primarily used for the treatment of ADHD in children. It should be used only after a complete evaluation of the child and should depend on the frequency and severity of symptoms and their appropriateness for the age of the child, not solely on the presence of one or more behavioral characteristics. Common symptoms of ADHD are short attention span, easy distractibility, emotional instability, impulsiveness, and moderate to severe hyperactivity. Children who suffer from ADHD will find it difficult to learn. Many professionals feel that methylphenidate offers only a temporary solution because it does not permanently change behavior patterns. It must be used with other special psychological measures. Stimulants like methylphenidate are not for children whose symptoms are related to environmental factors or to primary psychiatric conditions, including psychosis. Methylphenidate should not be used to treat a primary stress reaction.

Cautions and Warnings

Chronic or abusive use of methylphenidate can lead to **drug dependence or addiction**. This drug can also cause severe psychotic episodes.

Take methylphenidate with caution if you have **glaucoma** or other **visual problems**, **high blood pressure**, a **seizure disorder**, if you are extremely **tense** or **agitated**, or if you are **allergic** to this drug.

Possible Side Effects

Adult

▼ Most common: nervousness and inability to sleep, which your doctor generally controls by reducing or eliminating the afternoon or evening dose.

▼ Rare: skin rash, itching, fever, symptoms similar to arthritis, appetite loss, nausea, dizziness, abnormal heart rhythm, headache, drowsiness, changes in blood pressure or pulse, chest pain, stomach pain, psychotic reac-

---

Possible Side Effects *(continued)*

---

tions, effects on components of the blood, and loss of some scalp hair.

Child

▼ Most common: appetite loss; stomach pains; weight loss, especially during prolonged therapy; sleeping difficulties; and abnormal heart rhythm.

Drug Interactions

• Methylphenidate will reduce the effectiveness of guanethidine, a drug used to treat high blood pressure.

• Interaction with monoamine oxidase inhibitors (MAOIs) may vastly increase the effect of methylphenidate, causing problems.

• Mixing methylphenidate with a tricyclic antidepressant may lead to increased amounts of the antidepressant in your blood, increasing the risk of side effects.

• If you take methylphenidate regularly, avoid alcoholic beverages: This combination will enhance drowsiness.

Food Interactions

This medication is best taken 30 to 45 minutes before meals.

Usual Dose

Dosages should be tailored to individual needs; those listed here are only guidelines. SR-tablets are designed to last for 8 hours and may be used in place of more frequent doses during the same period of time. These tablets must be swallowed whole, never crushed or chewed.

Adult: Average doses range from 20–30 mg a day but can be prescribed in doses as high as 60 mg a day. The drug is taken in divided doses, 2–3 times a day.

Child (age 6 and over): starting dose—5 mg before breakfast and lunch. Increase in increments of 5–10 mg each week as required, not to exceed 60 mg a day.

Overdosage

An overdose of methylphenidate results in stimulation of the nervous system. Symptoms include vomiting, agitation, uncontrollable twitching of the muscles, convulsions followed by coma, euphoria (feeling high), confusion, hallucinations, delirium, sweating, flushing (redness of the face, hands, and extremities), headache, high fever, abnormal heart rate, high blood pressure, and dryness of the mouth and nose. The victim should be taken to a hospital emergency room immediately. ALWAYS bring the prescription bottle or container with you.

Special Information

Methylphenidate is a stimulant that can mask the signs of temporary drowsiness or fatigue: Be careful while driving or operating hazardous machinery. Take your last daily dose no later than 6 p.m. to avoid sleeping difficulties.

Call your doctor if you develop any unusual, persistent, or bothersome side effects. Do not increase your dose of this drug if the medicine seems to be losing its effect without first talking to your doctor.

If you miss a dose of methylphenidate, take it as soon as possible. Take the rest of that day's doses at regularly spaced time intervals. Go back to your regular schedule the next day.

Special Populations

Pregnancy/Breast-feeding

Methylphenidate crosses into fetal circulation but has not been found to cause birth defects. Women who are or might be pregnant should not take this drug without their doctor's approval. When the drug is considered crucial by your doctor, its potential benefits must be carefully weighed against its risks.

The amount of drug that passes into breast milk is not known, but it has caused no problems among breast-fed infants. You must consider the potential effect on the nursing infant if breast-feeding while taking this medication.

Seniors

Seniors may take this medication without special restriction. Follow your doctor's directions and report any side effects at once.

Generic Name

Methysergide (meth-ih-SER-jide)

Brand Name

Sansert

Type of Drug

Migraine preventive.

Prescribed for

Preventing or reducing the intensity of severe migraine.

General Information

Methysergide maleate is prescribed to prevent or reduce the number and intensity of migraine attacks in people who regularly suffer at least 1 migraine per week or whose headaches are severe.

Methysergide is derived from ergot, a natural plant fungus. The way that methysergide produces its effects is not known, but it does block the effects of serotonin, a hormone that is active in many portions of the brain and central nervous system and in blood vessels that carry blood to the brain. Serotonin inhibition may be the key to the action of this drug.

Methysergide must be taken for 1 to 2 days before you feel the effect of the drug. Its effects will persist for 1 to 2 days after you stop taking it.

Cautions and Warnings

This drug should be used only by people whose headaches are **severe and uncontrollable** and who are under close **medical supervision**.

People who are **sensitive** or **allergic** to methysergide or any other ergot-derived medicine should not take this drug. Those with **vascular (blood vessel) disease**, **severe hardening of the arteries**, very **high blood pressure**, **angina** or other signs of **coronary artery disease**, **disease of the heart valves**, **phlebitis**, **pulmonary disease**, **connective tissue disease** such as lupus, **liver or kidney disease**, or **serious infections** and those who are **severely ill** should be cautious about taking this medication.

People taking methysergide for long periods of time may

develop **thickening of tissues surrounding the lung**, making it more difficult to breathe; **thickening of the heart valves**, which may interfere with heart function; and **fibrous tissues in the abdomen**. To prevent these effects, you should take a "drug holiday," or drug-free period, of 3 to 4 weeks every 6 months before resuming methysergide therapy.

Methysergide tablets contain **tartrazine dye**, which should be avoided by asthmatics, people with aspirin allergy, and those who are allergic to tartrazine. Ask your pharmacist about obtaining tartrazine-free methysergide.

Possible Side Effects

Side effects are experienced by 30% to 50% of people taking methysergide.

▼ Most common: nausea, vomiting, constipation, diarrhea, heartburn, and abdominal pain usually develop early in drug treatment; they can be avoided by gradually increasing the dosage and by taking the drug with food.

▼ Less common: sleeplessness, drowsiness, mild euphoria (feeling high), light-headedness, dizziness, weakness, feelings of disassociation or hallucinations, flushing, raised red spots appearing on the skin, temporary hair loss, swelling, alterations in some blood components, muscle and joint aches, and weight gain.

▼ Rare: lung fibrosis—experienced as chest or abdominal pain or cold, numb, painful hands or feet with possible tingling and loss of pulse in the arms or legs; visual changes; clumsiness; rash; and depression.

Drug Interactions

• Alcohol, tranquilizers, and other nervous-system depressants will increase the depressant effects of this drug. Also, alcohol worsens migraine.

• Beta blockers and methysergide may cause reduced blood flow to hands and feet, leading to cold hands or feet and, possibly, gangrene.

Food Interactions

Take this drug with food or milk to avoid stomach upset.

Usual Dose

4–8 mg daily, taken with food.

Overdosage

Overdose symptoms include cold and pale hands or feet, severe dizziness, excitement, and convulsions. Overdose victims should be taken to a hospital emergency room for treatment. ALWAYS bring the prescription bottle or container with you.

Special Information

Do not take methysergide for more than 6 months at a time without a 3- to 4-week drug-free period. Do not stop taking it without your doctor's knowledge and approval. Withdrawal headaches can occur if the drug is stopped suddenly. It should be gradually stopped over 2 to 3 weeks.

If methysergide does not produce an improvement within the first 3 weeks of use, it is unlikely that the drug will be effective for you. Other treatments may be needed.

Heavy smokers experience blood-vessel constriction while taking methysergide, leading to cold hands or feet, chest and abdominal pain, itching, numbness, and tingling of the toes, fingers, or face. Call your doctor if any of these symptoms develop, especially if you do not smoke. Call your doctor if you develop visual changes, clumsiness, stimulation, swelling, changes in heart rate, fever, chills, cough, hoarseness, lower back or side pain, urinary difficulties, depression, skin rash, redness or darkening of the face, red spots on the skin, leg cramps, appetite loss, breathing difficulties, or swelling of the hands, legs, ankles, or feet. Call your doctor if any infection develops; infections can increase your sensitivity to the effects of methysergide.

People taking methysergide must be careful when driving or engaging in other activities that require concentration and coordination because this drug can cause tiredness, dizziness, or light-headedness.

Exposure to extremely cold weather may worsen feelings of coldness, tingling, or pain caused by methysergide. Protect yourself from cold winter weather.

If you take methysergide 2 times a day and forget a dose, take it as soon as you remember. If it is almost time for your next dose, take one dose as soon as you remember and another in 5 or 6 hours, then go back to your regular schedule. Do not take a double dose.

If you take methysergide 3 times a day and forget a dose,

take it as soon as you remember. If it is almost time for your next dose, take one dose as soon as you remember and another in 3 or 4 hours, then go back to your regular schedule. Do not take a double dose.

Special Populations

Pregnancy/Breast-feeding
Methysergide must not be taken by pregnant women because the drug can cause miscarriage.

Methysergide passes into breast milk and may cause the nursing baby to develop vomiting, diarrhea, or seizures. Nursing mothers who must take methysergide should bottle-feed their infants.

Seniors
Seniors taking this drug may develop hypothermia (low body temperature) and other complications. Seniors are likely to need less methysergide than younger adults because of age-related impairment of kidney function.

Generic Name

Metoclopramide (met-oe-KLOE-pruh-mide) Ⓖ

Brand Names

Clopra   Octamide
Maxolon   Reglan*

*Some products in this brand-name group are alcohol or sugar free. Consult your pharmacist.

Type of Drug

Antiemetic and gastrointestinal (GI) stimulant.

Prescribed for

Nausea and vomiting related to cancer chemotherapy, surgery, pregnancy, labor, and other causes; also prescribed for the nausea, vomiting, heartburn, fullness after meals, and appetite loss of diabetic gastroparesis (stomach paralysis associated with diabetes) and for gastroesophageal reflux disease (GERD), stomach ulcer, anorexia nervosa, and bleeding from blood vessels in the esophagus—often associated with severe liver disease. It also facilitates diagnostic x-ray procedures and improves the absorption of anti-migraine medication and narcotic pain relievers. Nursing mothers are occasionally given metoclopramide to increase milk production.

General Information

Metoclopramide stimulates movement of the upper GI tract but does not stimulate excess stomach acids or other secretions. Its effect against nausea and vomiting may be caused by the drug's direct effect on dopamine receptors in the brain. It also affects the secretion of a variety of hormones in the body and may improve drug absorption into the bloodstream by slowing the movement of the stomach and intestines, keeping the drug in an area where it may be absorbed for a longer period of time.

Cautions and Warnings

People with **high blood pressure, Parkinson's disease, asthma, liver or kidney failure,** or **seizure disorders** should use metoclopramide with caution. Do not take this drug if you are **allergic** to it. Metoclopramide should not be used if you have a **bleeding ulcer** or if the presence of **other conditions makes stimulation of the GI tract dangerous**.

Mild to severe depression has occurred in people taking metoclopramide. People with a history of depression should use this product only if its potential benefits outweigh its risks.

Uncontrollable motions similar to those that develop in Parkinson's disease have developed as a side effect of this drug. These generally occur within 6 months after starting metoclopramide and generally subside within 2 to 3 months.

This drug may cause extrapyramidal side effects similar to those caused by phenothiazine drugs. Do not take the 2 classes of drugs together. Extrapyramidal effects occur in 0.2% of the people taking the drug; effects include restlessness and involuntary movements of the arms and legs, face, tongue, lips, or other parts of the body.

Women taking this drug develop chronic elevations of a hormone called prolactin. About 33% of breast tumors are prolactin-dependent, a factor that should be taken into account when this drug is prescribed.

Possible Side Effects

Mild side effects that usually go away when the drug is stopped occur in 20% to 30% of people who take metoclopramide. Side effects are more common as the dosage increases or if you take the drug for long periods of time.

▼ Most common: restlessness, drowsiness, fatigue, sleeplessness, dizziness, anxiety, loss of muscle control, headache, muscle spasm, confusion, severe depression, convulsions, and hallucinations.

▼ Less common: rash, diarrhea, blood-pressure changes, abnormal heart rhythms, slow heartbeat, oozing from the nipples, tender nipples, loss of regular menstrual periods, breast swelling and tenderness, impotence, reduced white-blood-cell counts, frequent urination, loss of urinary control, visual disturbances, or worsening of bronchial spasm.

▼ Rare: People taking this drug may develop a group of possibly fatal symptoms collectively called neuroleptic malignant syndrome. These symptoms include very high fever, semi-consciousness, rigid muscles, flushing of the face and upper body, and liver toxicity after high doses.

Drug Interactions

• The effects of metoclopramide on the stomach are antagonized by narcotics and anticholinergic drugs.

• Metoclopramide may increase the effects of alcoholic beverages and cyclosporine by increasing the amount absorbed by the bloodstream.

• Metoclopramide may increase the sedative effects of nervous-system depressants including tranquilizers and sleeping pills.

• Metoclopramide and levodopa have opposite effects on the same nervous-system receptors and will antagonize each other.

• Metoclopramide may reduce the effects of digitalis drugs and cimetidine.

• Combining metoclopramide with a monoamine oxidase inhibitor (MAOI) antidepressant may cause very high blood pressure.

Food Interactions

Take this drug 30 minutes before meals and at bedtime.

Usual Dose

Adult and Child (age 15 and over): 5–15 mg before meals and at bedtime. Single doses of 10–20 mg are used before x-ray diagnostic procedures.

Senior: starting dosage — 5 mg.

Child (age 6–14): ¼–½ the adult dosage.

Child (under age 6): 0.05 mg per lb. of body weight per dose.

Overdosage

Symptoms of overdose include drowsiness, disorientation, restlessness, or uncontrollable muscle movement; these usually disappear within 24 hours after the drug has been stopped. Anticholinergic drugs will antagonize these symptoms.

Special Information

Call your doctor if you develop chills, fever, sore throat, dizziness, severe or persistent headache, feeling unwell, rapid or irregular heartbeat, difficulty speaking or swallowing, loss of balance, stiffness of the arms or legs, a shuffling walk, a mask-like face, lip-smacking or puckering, puffing of the cheeks, rapid, worm-like tongue movement, uncontrollable chewing movement, uncontrolled arm and leg movement, or any other persistent or intolerable side effect.

Metoclopramide may cause dizziness, confusion, and drowsiness. Take care while driving or operating hazardous equipment. Avoid alcohol and be cautious about taking tranquilizers or sleeping pills while you are on this drug.

If you forget to take a dose of metoclopramide, take it as soon as you remember. If it is almost time for your next dose, skip the forgotten dose and continue with your regular schedule. Do not take a double dose.

Special Populations

Pregnancy/Breast-feeding

Metoclopramide crosses into the fetal circulation but has not been found to cause birth defects. When this drug is considered crucial by your doctor, its potential benefits must be carefully weighed against its risks.

Nursing mothers may occasionally be given metoclopramide to increase milk production. This drug passes into breast milk but there appears to be no risk for the infant whose nursing mother is taking 45 mg or less a day. Always consider possible effects on the nursing infant if breast-feeding while taking this medication.

Seniors

Seniors, especially women, are more sensitive to the side effects of this drug (see "Cautions and Warnings"). Follow your doctor's directions and report any side effects at once.

Generic Name

Metoprolol (meh-TOPE-roe-lol) [G]

Brand Names

Lopressor   Toprol XL

Type of Drug

Beta-adrenergic blocking agent.

Prescribed for

High blood pressure, angina pectoris, abnormal heart rhythms, prevention of second heart attack, migraine headache, tremors, aggressive behavior, side effects of antipsychotic drugs, improving cognitive performance, congestive heart failure, and bleeding from the esophagus.

General Information

Metoprolol is one of 15 beta-adrenergic-blocking drugs, or beta blockers, that interfere with the action of a specific part of the nervous system. Beta receptors are found all over the body and affect many body functions. This accounts for the usefulness of beta blockers against a wide variety of conditions. The oldest of these drugs, propranolol, affects the entire beta-adrenergic range of the nervous system. Newer, more refined beta blockers affect only a portion of that system, making them more useful in the treatment of cardiovascular disorders and less useful for other purposes. Other of the newer beta blockers act as mild stimulants to the heart or have particular characteristics that make them more adapted for specific purposes or certain people. One of these, carvedilol, was approved for heart failure in 1997.

Metoprolol has been studied in heart failure for many years; some doctors use small doses of metoprolol to help heart failure patients. Compared with other beta blockers, metoprolol has less of an effect on pulse and bronchial muscles — which affect asthma — and less of a rebound effect when discontinued; it also causes less tiredness, depression, and intolerance to exercise. Metoprolol is available in a sustained-release formulation, taken only once a day, that maintains a steady blood level of the drug for a full 24 hours.

Cautions and Warnings

You should be cautious about taking metoprolol if you have **asthma**, a **very slow heart rate**, or **heart block (disruption of the electrical impulses that control heart rate)** because the drug may aggravate these conditions.

People with **angina** who take metoprolol for high blood pressure risk aggravating their angina if they suddenly stop taking the drug. These people should have their drug dosage reduced gradually over 1 to 2 weeks.

Metoprolol should be used with caution if you have **liver or kidney disease** because your ability to eliminate the drug from your body may be impaired.

Metoprolol reduces the amount of blood pumped by the heart with each beat. This reduction in blood flow may aggravate the condition of people with **poor circulation** or **circulatory disease**.

If you are undergoing major surgery, your doctor may want you to stop taking metoprolol at least 2 days before to permit the heart to respond more acutely to stresses that can occur during the procedure. This practice is still controversial and may not hold true for all surgeries.

Possible Side Effects

Metoprolol side effects are relatively uncommon and usually mild; normally they develop early in the course of treatment and are rarely a reason to stop taking meto-prolol.

▼ Most common: impotence.

▼ Less common: unusual tiredness or weakness, slow heartbeat, heart failure (symptoms include swelling of the legs, ankles, or feet), dizziness, breathing difficulties,

---

Possible Side Effects *(continued)*

bronchospasm, depression, confusion, anxiety, nervousness, sleeplessness, disorientation, short-term memory loss, emotional instability, cold hands and feet, constipation, diarrhea, nausea, vomiting, upset stomach, increased sweating, urinary difficulties, cramps, blurred vision, skin rash, hair loss, stuffy nose, facial swelling, aggravation of lupus erythematosus (chronic condition affecting the body's connective tissue), itching, chest pain, back or joint pain, colitis, drug allergy (symptoms include fever and sore throat), and liver toxicity.

Drug Interactions

• Metoprolol may interact with surgical anesthetics to increase the risk of heart problems during surgery. Some anesthesiologists recommend having gradually stopped the drug 2 days before surgery.

• Metoprolol may interfere with the normal signs of low blood sugar and with the action of oral antidiabetes medications.

• Metoprolol increases the blood-pressure-lowering effects of other blood-pressure-reducing agents, including clonidine, guanabenz, and reserpine; and calcium-channel blockers, such as nifedipine.

• Aspirin-containing drugs, indomethacin, sulfinpyrazone, and estrogen drugs may interfere with the blood-pressure-lowering effect of metoprolol.

• Cocaine may reduce the effectiveness of all beta blockers.

• Metoprolol may worsen the problem of cold hands and feet associated with taking ergot alkaloids, used to treat migraine headache. Gangrene is a possibility in people taking both an ergot and metoprolol.

• The effect of benzodiazepine antianxiety drugs may be increased by metoprolol.

• Metoprolol will counteract thyroid hormone replacements.

• Calcium channel blockers, flecainide, hydralazine, oral contraceptives, propafenone, haloperidol, phenothiazine tranquilizers—molindone and others—quinolone antibacterials, and quinidine may increase the amount of metoprolol in the bloodstream and lead to increased metoprolol effects.

• Metoprolol should not be taken within 2 weeks of taking a monoamine oxidase inhibitor (MAOI) antidepressant.

• Cimetidine increases the amount of metoprolol absorbed into the bloodstream from oral tablets.

• Metoprolol may interfere with the effectiveness of some asthma medications, including theophylline and aminophylline, and especially ephedrine and isoproterenol.

• Combining metoprolol with phenytoin or digitalis drugs may result in excessive slowing of the heart, possibly causing heart block.

• If you stop smoking while taking metoprolol, your dose may have to be reduced because your liver will break down the drug more slowly afterward.

Food Interactions

Sustained-release metoprolol — Toprol XL — may be taken with food if it upsets your stomach. Because food increases the amount of short-acting metoprolol — Lopressor — absorbed into the blood, take the short-acting form without food.

Usual Dose

100–450 mg a day; dosage must be tailored to your specific needs.

Overdosage

Symptoms of overdose include changes in heartbeat — unusually slow, unusually fast, or irregular — severe dizziness or fainting, breathing difficulties, bluish-colored fingernails or palms, and seizures. The victim should be taken to a hospital emergency room. ALWAYS bring the prescription bottle or container with you.

Special Information

Metoprolol should be taken continuously. When ending metoprolol treatments, dosage should be lowered gradually over a period of about 2 weeks. Do not stop taking this drug unless directed to do so by your doctor: Abrupt withdrawal may cause chest pain, breathing difficulties, increased sweating, and unusually fast or irregular heartbeat.

Call your doctor at once if you develop back or joint pain, breathing difficulties, cold hands or feet, depression, skin rash, or changes in heartbeat. This drug may produce an undesirable lowering of blood pressure, leading to dizziness or fainting; call your doctor if this happens to you. Call your doctor if you experience persistent or bothersome nausea or vomiting, upset stomach, diarrhea, constipation, impotence, headache, itching, anxiety, nightmares or vivid dreams, trouble sleeping, stuffy nose, frequent urination, unusual tiredness, or weakness.

Metoprolol can cause drowsiness, light-headedness, dizziness, or blurred vision. Be careful when driving or performing complex tasks.

It is best to take your metoprolol at the same time each day. If you forget a dose, take it as soon as you remember. If you take metoprolol once a day and it is within 8 hours of your next dose, skip the dose you forgot and continue with your regular schedule. If you take it twice a day and it is within 4 hours of your next dose, skip the one you forgot and continue with your regular schedule. Never take a double dose.

Special Populations

Pregnancy/Breast-feeding

Infants born to women who took a beta blocker while pregnant had lower birth weights, low blood pressure, and reduced heart rates. Metoprolol should be avoided by women who are or might be pregnant. When the drug is considered crucial by your doctor, its potential benefits must be carefully weighed against its risks.

Small amounts of metoprolol pass into breast milk, but problems are rare. Still, nursing mothers taking metoprolol should bottle-feed their babies.

Seniors

Seniors may absorb and retain more metoprolol and may require less of the drug to achieve results. Your doctor should adjust your dosage to meet your individual needs. Seniors taking metoprolol may be more likely to suffer from cold hands and feet, reduced body temperature, chest pain, general feelings of ill health, sudden breathing difficulties, increased sweating, or changes in heartbeat.

Generic Name

Metronidazole (met-roe-NYE-duh-zole) Ⓖ

Brand Names

Flagyl   MetroGel
Metizol   Protostat
MetroCream

Type of Drug

Amoebicide and antibiotic.

Prescribed for

Acute amoebic dysentery and infections of the vagina, bone,
brain, nervous system, urinary tract, abdomen, and skin.
Metronidazole may also be prescribed for pneumonia, inflammatory bowel disease, colitis caused by other antibiotics,
periodontal (gum) infection, and some complications of severe liver disease. Metronidazole gel may be applied to the
skin to treat acne. It can also be used for severe decubitus
(skin) ulcers and inflammation of the skin around the mouth.
Metronidazole given by intravenous injection may be used
before, during, and after bowel surgery to prevent infectious
complications.

General Information

Metronidazole is effective against infections caused by a
variety of fungi and some bacteria. Metronidazole kills these
microorganisms by disrupting the DNA of the organism after
it enters body cells. Metronidazole may be prescribed for
symptomless diseases when the doctor feels that an underlying infection may be involved. For example, asymptomatic
women may be treated with this drug when vaginal examination shows evidence of *Trichomonas*. Because vaginal
trichomonal infection is a venereal disease, asymptomatic
sexual partners of female patients should also be treated if
the organism has been found in the woman's genital tract.
This is needed to prevent reinfection of the partner. The
decision to treat an asymptomatic male partner without
evidence of infection must be made by a doctor.

Cautions and Warnings

You should not use this drug if you have a history of **blood**

disease or if you know that you are **sensitive** or **allergic** to metronidazole.

People taking this medication have experienced **seizures** and **numbness or tingling in the hands or feet**. This effect is rare with low doses but may be more common in people taking larger doses for long periods, such as in Crohn's disease. If this happens to you, stop taking the drug and call your doctor at once. Metronidazole should be taken with caution if you have active **nervous system disease,** including **epilepsy,** or if you have **severe liver problems**.

Possible Side Effects

▼ Most common: gastrointestinal (GI) symptoms, including nausea sometimes accompanied by headache, dizziness, appetite loss, vomiting, diarrhea, upset stomach, abdominal cramping, and constipation. A sharp, unpleasant metallic taste is also associated with the use of this drug.

▼ Less common: numbness or tingling in the extremities, joint pain, confusion, irritability, depression, difficulty sleeping, and weakness. Itching and a sense of pelvic pressure also have been reported.

▼ Rare: clumsiness or poor coordination, fever, increased urination, seizure, incontinence, and reduced sex drive.

Drug Interactions

• Avoid alcoholic beverages: Interaction with metronidazole may cause abdominal cramps, nausea, vomiting, headaches, and flushing. Modification of the taste of alcoholic beverages has also been reported. Metronidazole should not be used if you are taking disulfiram (drug used to maintain alcohol abstinence) because the combination may cause confusion and psychotic reactions.

• People taking oral anticoagulant (blood-thinning) drugs such as warfarin will have to have their anticoagulant dosage reduced because metronidazole increases the effect of anticoagulants.

• Metronidazole increases lithium blood levels, effects, and side effects.

• Cimetidine may interfere with the liver's ability to break down metronidazole, causing increased blood levels of metronidazole. Metronidazole dosage may have to be reduced if you are also taking cimetidine.

• Phenobarbital and other barbiturates may increase the rate at which metronidazole is broken down, compromising its effectiveness.

• Drugs that cause nervous system toxicity — such as mexiletine, ethambutol, isoniazid, lindane, lincomycin, lithium, pemoline, quinacrine, and long-term high-dose pyridoxine (vitamin B_6) — should not be taken with metronidazole because nervous-system side effects may be increased.

• Metronidazole may increase blood levels of phenytoin by interfering with its breakdown in the liver. This could increase the risk of phenytoin side effects. Your doctor may need to adjust your phenytoin dosage.

Food Interactions

This drug is best taken with food to avoid stomach upset.

Usual Dose

Adult: amoebic dysentery — 500–750 mg 3 times a day for 5–10 days. Trichomonal infection — 250 mg 3 times a day for 7 days; or 2 g in 1 dose.

Senior: Reduced adult dosages may be necessary.

Child: amoebic dysentery — 16–23 mg per lb. of body weight daily, divided in 3 equal doses for 10 days.

Overdosage

Single doses as large as 15,000 mg have been taken in suicide attempts and accidental doses. Overdose symptoms include nausea, vomiting, clumsiness, unsteadiness, seizures, and pain or tingling in the hands or feet. Call your local poison control center for more information. ALWAYS bring the prescription bottle or container with you if you go for treatment.

Special Information

Call your doctor if you become dizzy or light-headed while taking this drug, or if you develop numbness, tingling, pain, or weakness in your hands or feet. Seizures are also possible with high doses of metronidazole. Rare side effects that demand your doctor's attention include clumsiness or unsteadiness; mood changes; unusual vaginal irritation, discharge, or dryness; rash, hives, or itching; and severe pain of the back or abdomen accompanied by vomiting, appetite loss, or nausea. Call your doctor if any other side effects become particularly bothersome or persistent.

Metronidazole may cause darkening of your urine; this is probably not important, but inform your doctor if it happens.

Follow your doctor's dosage instructions faithfully and do not stop until the full course of metronidazole has been completed.

Metronidazole may cause dry mouth, which usually can be relieved with ice, hard candy, or gum. Call your doctor or dentist if dry mouth persists for more than 2 weeks.

If you forget to take a dose of metronidazole, take it as soon as you remember. If it is almost time for your next dose, skip the dose you forgot and continue with your regular schedule. Do not take a double dose.

Special Populations

Pregnancy/Breast-feeding

Metronidazole passes into fetal blood circulation soon after it is taken. This drug should not be taken during the first 3 months of pregnancy and should be used with caution during the last 6 months.

About the same amount of metronidazole passes into breast milk as is present in the mother's blood. Breast-feeding while taking this drug may cause side effects in infants. If you must take metronidazole, bottle-feed your baby. After you have finished metronidazole treatment, express any milk produced while you were taking the drug and discard it along with any pumped breast milk you might have saved. Nursing can be resumed 1 or 2 days after stopping metronidazole.

Seniors

Seniors, particularly those with advanced liver disease, are more sensitive to the effects of this drug and may require lower dosages. Follow your doctor's directions and report any side effects at once.

Mevacor

*see **Lovastatin**, page 623*

Generic Name

Mexiletine (mek-SIL-eh-tene)

Brand Name

Mexitil

Type of Drug

Antiarrhythmic.

Prescribed for

Abnormal heart rhythms. Mexiletine may be helpful in treating the pain, tingling, and loss of the sense of touch that may come with severe diabetes.

General Information

Mexiletine works on the heart in the same way as lidocaine, a commonly used injectable antiarrhythmic drug. It slows the speed at which nerve impulses are carried through the heart's ventricles, helping the heart to maintain a stable rhythm by making heart muscle cells less easily excited. Mexiletine affects different areas of the heart than many other oral antiarrhythmic drugs. It is usually prescribed for people with life-threatening arrhythmias as a follow-up to intravenous lidocaine, and should be prescribed only after other drugs have been tried. When mexiletine is replacing other drug treatments, it may be taken 6 to 12 hours after the last dose of quinidine or disopyramide, 3 to 6 hours after the last dose of procainamide, or 12 hours after the last dose of tocainide.

Cautions and Warnings

Because this drug is broken down by the liver and can cause some liver problems, people with **severe liver disease** must be cautious while taking it. Special considerations also must be made if you have a history of **heart block, heart failure, heart attack, low blood pressure,** or **seizure disorders** and intend to take mexiletine.

   Like other antiarrhythmic drugs, mexiletine may occasionally worsen heart-rhythm problems. It has not actually been proven to help people live longer.

Possible Side Effects

▼ Most common: nausea, vomiting, diarrhea, constipation, tremors, dizziness, light-headedness, nervousness, and poor coordination. These can be reversed if drug dose is reduced, if it is taken with food or antacids, or if the drug is stopped.

▼ Less common: heart palpitations, chest pain, angina, change in appetite, abdominal pain or cramps, stomach ulcers and bleeding, difficulty swallowing, dry mouth, changes in sense of taste, changes in the saliva and mucous membranes of the mouth, tingling or numbness in the hands or feet, weakness, fatigue, ringing or buzzing in the ears, depression, speech difficulties, rash, breathing difficulties, and swelling.

▼ Rare: abnormal heart rhythms, memory loss, hallucinations and other psychological problems, fainting, low blood pressure, slow heartbeat, hot flashes, high blood pressure, shock, joint pain, fever, increased sweating, hair loss, impotence, decreased sex drive, not feeling well, difficulty urinating, hiccups, and dry skin.

Drug Interactions

• Mexiletine's effects are reduced by aluminum-magnesium antacids, atropine, ammonium chloride, and vitamin C. Phenytoin, rifampin, phenobarbital, narcotics, and other drugs that stimulate the liver to break down drugs more rapidly also reduce this drug's effect.

• Smoking stimulates drug breakdown by the liver, reducing mexiletine's effectiveness.

• Bicarbonates and acetazolamide decrease the clearance of mexiletine through the kidney, thus increasing its effects.

• Cimetidine may raise or lower blood levels of mexiletine.

• Other drugs for abnormal heart rhythms may produce an additive effect on the heart, although sometimes drug combinations are the only way to control an abnormal rhythm.

• Mexiletine may increase blood levels of theophylline. Your theophylline dose may have to be lowered if you take this combination.

• Mexiletine may reduce the effects of caffeine on your body.

Food Interactions

Take mexiletine with food if it upsets your stomach.

Usual Dose

600–1200 mg a day in 2 or 3 doses.

Overdosage

Mexiletine overdose can be fatal. The first overdose symptoms are generally dizziness, drowsiness, nausea, low blood pressure, slow pulse, seizures, and tingling in the hands or feet. Coma or respiratory failure can occur after a massive overdose. Overdose victims should be taken to a hospital emergency room immediately. ALWAYS bring the prescription bottle or container with you.

Special Information

Call your doctor if you develop chest pain, a fast or irregular heartbeat, breathing difficulties, seizures, tiredness, yellow skin or eyes, sore throat, fever or chills, unexplained bruising or bleeding, or if any side effect becomes intolerable.

Avoid diets that can change the acidity of your urine. A high-acid diet—such as one containing large quantities of citrus fruits—will increase the rate at which mexiletine is removed from your body; a low-acid diet will cause the drug to be retained in your body. Your doctor or pharmacist can give you more information.

If you miss a dose of mexiletine, take it as soon as you can. If it is more than 4 hours past your regular dose time, skip the dose you forgot and continue with your regular schedule. Do not take a double dose.

Special Populations

Pregnancy/Breast-feeding

Mexiletine passes into the fetal blood circulation. It is not known to cause human birth defects, but animal experiments have shown some negative effects. When the drug is considered crucial by your doctor, its potential benefits must be carefully weighed against its risks.

This drug passes into breast milk in amounts as high or higher than those in the mother's blood. Nursing mothers who must take mexiletine should bottle-feed their babies.

Seniors

Seniors with severe liver disease are more sensitive to the

effects of this drug; others may take it without special restriction. Follow your doctor's directions and report any side effects at once.

Generic Name

Mibefradil (mih-BEF-ruh-dil)

Brand Name

Posicor

Type of Drug

Calcium channel blocker.

Prescribed for

Hypertension (high blood pressure) and chronic angina pain.

General Information

Calcium flows into muscle cells through two known channels. They are the T-type (low-voltage) channel and the L-type (high voltage) channel. Mibefradil dihydrochloride is the first calcium channel blocker to interfere with the flow of calcium into muscle cells through both channels. Other calcium channel blockers block only the L-type channel. The movement of calcium into and out of muscle cells is an essential factor in muscle contraction, especially in the heart and smooth muscle of the blood vessels. Calcium channel blockers interfere with the contraction of these muscles, which in turn dilates (widens) blood vessels, leading to a reduction in blood pressure. The amount of oxygen used by the heart is also reduced. The ability of mibefradil to block calcium flow more completely than other calcium channel blockers may mean it is more effective, although this has not yet been definitely proven.

The blood-pressure-lowering effect of mibefradil is dosage-related. That is, a larger dosage lowers blood pressure more than a smaller dosage. In addition, people with higher blood pressures initially can expect a better response to mibefradil than people with lower blood pressures before treatment. The blood-pressure-lowering effect of mibefradil is the same in people of all races and is not affected by diabetes, body weight, or heart disease.

The way that mibefradil helps people with chronic angina is not exactly known; however, angina pains develop when arteries are narrowed and there is not enough oxygen-carrying blood flowing to heart muscle cells. Mibefradil allows the heart to use less oxygen and to work at a slower, easier rate during exercise. Anything that helps the heart to receive more blood and use less oxygen will help angina pains. Like other calcium channel blockers, mibefradil affects the flow of nerve impulses through the heart, producing a slight slowing of the heartbeat.

Approximately 70% of each mibefradil tablet is absorbed into the bloodstream. Mibefradil is broken down in the liver.

Cautions and Warnings

People who are **sensitive** or **allergic** to mibefradil should not take this drug.

People with **heart block** (disruption of the electrical impulses that control heart rate) or **sick sinus syndrome** who do not have a pacemaker should not take mibefradil; neither should people who are taking **simvastatin, lovastatin, terfenadine, astemizole,** or **cisipride** (see "Drug Interactions").

People with severe **liver disease** may have more difficulty breaking down mibefradil and their blood pressure and heart rate should be closely monitored.

Mibefradil may change the appearance of an **electrocardiogram** (EKG). This can be confusing to doctors not familiar with the effect; some EKGs have been misread. It is especially important to be aware of mibefradil's potential to change EKG readings because the effects of some other heart medications are checked by an EKG test. In these cases, other, non-EKG tests should be used to assess drug effectiveness.

Mibefradil should be taken with caution if you have a **slow heart rate**—less than 55 beats a minute; **heart failure;** or a **heart ventricle problem.**

Possible Side Effects

Most mibefradil side effects are mild or moderate, tend to increase with the dosage, and go away on their own without having to stop the drug.

▼ Most common: headache.

▼ Less common: leg swelling, runny nose, abdominal pain, light-headedness, and upset stomach.

Possible Side Effects *(continued)*

▼ Rare: sweating, dizziness or fainting when rising quickly from a sitting or lying position, weakness, trauma, slow heart rate, heart failure, chest pain, low blood pressure, tingling in the hands or feet, diarrhea, intestinal gas, stomach irritation, rectal bleeding, ringing or buzzing in the ears, ear infection, local swelling, arthritis, back pain, muscle cramps, arm or leg pain, sprains or strains, depression, sleeplessness, impotence, bronchitis, coughing, breathing difficulties, stuffy nose, sore throat, sinus irritation, rash, urinary infection, and pinkeye.

Drug Interactions

• The blood-pressure-lowering effect of mibefradil is increased by diuretics, beta blockers, and angiotensin-converting enzyme (ACE) inhibitor drugs.

• Mibefradil interferes with the breakdown of many drugs in the liver, including terfenadine, astemizole, and cisapride. Excess quantities of these drugs in the bloodstream have been associated with severe cardiac side effects; they should not be combined with mibefradil.

• Mibefradil may slow the rate at which the body breaks down the cholesterol-lowering drugs lovastatin and simvastatin. People combining these drugs with mibefradil have developed severe drug-induced muscle damage, which may lead to kidney or heart damage. The severity of this interaction may be intensified if cyclosporine or tacrolimus — used to prevent organ transplant rejection — is also being taken. Do not mix these drugs. This interaction is not expected with fluvastatin or pravastatin because their breakdown is not affected by mibefradil. Information on the interaction between mibefradil and atorvastatin or cerivistatin is not conclusive, but these drugs should not be combined with mibefradil until more is known.

• Mibefradil drastically reduces the rate at which tricyclic antidepressants are broken down in the body. Reduction of antidepressant dosages is necessary when these drugs are combined with mibefradil.

• The dosage of benzodiazepine-type antianxiety drugs, beta blockers, other calcium channel blockers, cyclosporine, flecainide, mexiletine, propafenone, and quinidine may have to be adjusted if these drugs are combined with mibefradil.

• The risk of muscle aches and destruction while taking a statin-type cholesterol lowering drug may be increased if you are also taking mibefradil. Be sure to report any problems to your doctor.

Food Interactions

None known.

Usual Dose

Adult: 50–100 mg once a day.
Child: not recommended.

Overdosage

There has been no experience with mibefradil overdose. Overdose symptoms are likely to include low blood pressure, slow heartbeat, dizziness, and fainting. Victims should be taken to a hospital emergency room for treatment. ALWAYS bring the prescription bottle or container with you.

Special Information

Call your doctor if you become light-headed, dizzy, or faint while taking mibefradil.

Do not crush or chew mibefradil tablets.

If you forget a dose of mibefradil, take it as soon as you remember. If it is almost time for your next dose, skip the dose you forgot and continue with your regular schedule. Do not take a double dose.

Special Populations

Pregnancy/Breast-feeding

Pregnant animals treated with very high doses of mibefradil have given birth to babies with heart problems. There is no information about the effect of mibefradil in humans; tell your doctor if you are pregnant. This drug should be taken during pregnancy only if its possible benefits outweigh its risks. All calcium channel blockers should be avoided during labor and delivery.

Large amounts of mibefradil are found in the milk of lab animals. If the same is true in humans, a nursing infant would receive a significant dose of the drug. Nursing mothers who must take mibefradil should bottle-feed their babies.

Seniors

Seniors with a slow heart rate — less than 55 beats a minute — should not combine mibefradil and a beta blocker because of the risk of excessive slowing of the heart.

Generic Name

Miconazole (mye-KON-uh-zole) Ⓖ

Brand Name

Monistat

The information in this profile also applies to the following drug:

Generic Ingredient: Tioconazole
Vagistat-1

Type of Drug

Antifungal.

Prescribed for

Fungal infections of the vagina, skin, and blood.

General Information

Miconazole nitrate is used to treat a wide variety of fungal infections. Monistat-Derm Cream is applied directly to the skin to treat common fungal infections of the skin, including ringworm, athlete's foot, and jock itch. Monistat 3 is used to treat vaginal infections. Hospitalized patients may receive this drug by intravenous injection to ward off serious fungal infections. When used for vaginal or topical infections, it is effective against several nonfungal organisms, as well as fungal-type infections.

Cautions and Warnings

Do not use miconazole if you are **allergic** to it. Proper diagnosis is essential for effective treatment. Do not use this product without first consulting your doctor.

Possible Side Effects

Intravenous Injection
   ▼ Common: vein irritation, itching, rash, nausea, vomiting, fever, drowsiness, diarrhea, loss of appetite, and flushing.

Vaginal Administration
   ▼ Common: itching, burning, and irritation.
   ▼ Less common: pelvic cramps, hives, rash, and headache.

Topical Application
   ▼ Less common: skin irritation or burning.

Drug and Food Interactions

None known.

Usual Dose

Vaginal Suppositories and Cream: 1 applicatorful or suppository into the vagina at bedtime for 3–7 days.

Topical Cream, Lotions, and Powder: Apply to affected areas 2 times a day for up to 1 month.

Overdosage

If accidentally swallowed, little of the drug passes into the bloodstream. Upset stomach may develop. Call your local poison control center or hospital emergency room for more information.

Special Information

When using the vaginal cream, insert the whole applicator of cream high into the vagina and be sure to complete the full course of treatment prescribed for you. Call your doctor if you develop burning or itching.

   If you forget to take a dose of miconazole, take it as soon as you remember. If it is almost time for your next dose, skip the dose you forgot and continue with your regular schedule. Do not take a double dose.

Special Populations

Pregnancy/Breast-feeding

Pregnant women should avoid using the vaginal cream

during the first 3 months of pregnancy, and use it during the next 6 months only if it is absolutely necessary. Your doctor may want you to avoid using a vaginal applicator during pregnancy; instead, insert miconazole vaginal suppositories by hand.

Miconazole has not been shown to cause problems in breast-fed infants.

Seniors

Seniors may take this medication without special restriction. Follow your doctor's directions and report any side effects at once.

Generic Name

Midodrine (MYE-doe-drene)

Brand Name

ProAmatine

Type of Drug

Alpha stimulant.

Prescribed for

Dizziness or fainting, when rising from a sitting or standing position, that cannot be controlled with other medications. Midodrine is also used for poor urinary control.

General Information

Midodrine is recommended only if other medical treatments for dizziness or fainting have failed and symptoms are interfering with your daily routine. After you take midodrine tablets, the drug is converted to its active form in the body. Once converted, it stimulates nerve endings in small veins and arteries, "tightening" them slightly to raise blood pressure. This helps control dizziness and fainting caused by poor blood flow to the brain. Your systolic blood pressure (usually, the higher of the two readings) goes up by 15 to 30 points 1 hour after taking 10 mg of midodrine. The effect lasts about 2 to 3 hours.

Cautions and Warnings

Do not take this drug if you **retain urine** or have **severe heart**

disease, active kidney disease, diabetes, pheochromocytoma (adrenal gland tumor), a severely **overactive thyroid gland, visual problems,** or excessive and persistent **high blood pressure when lying down**, because it can worsen these problems.

High blood pressure—especially when you are lying down—can be the most serious side effect of midodrine. This problem may be prevented by not completely reclining, or raising the head of your bed, when you sleep.

The active form of midodrine is eliminated from your body through the kidneys. People with kidney disease will have more medicine in the blood and can expect higher blood pressure; they should take a lower dose of midodrine.

People with **liver disease** should be cautious about using midodrine because it may be partially broken down in the liver.

Your doctor should check your kidney and liver function periodically while you are taking midodrine.

Your heart rate may slow slightly after you start taking midodrine.

Possible Side Effects

▼ Most common: tingling in the hands or feet, pain, itching, goosebumps, painful urination, high blood pressure when lying down, and chills.

▼ Less common: rash, headache, feeling a fullness or pressure in your head, facial flushing, confusion, abnormal thinking, dry mouth, nervousness, anxiety, and rash.

▼ Rare: visual problems; dizziness; skin that is sensitive to touch, temperature, or pain; sleeplessness; tiredness; canker sores; dry skin; urinary difficulties; weakness; backache; nausea; upset stomach; stomach gas; heartburn; and leg cramps.

Drug Interactions

• Midodrine increases the effects of digoxin or digitoxin and similar drugs, psychoactive medications, beta blockers, and other stimulants. Be very cautious when combining these drugs with midodrine.

• People who take both midodrine and fludrocortisone must have their fludrocortisone dose reduced or lower their salt intake before starting midodrine. Fludrocortisone also worsens glaucoma and raises pressure inside the eye.

• Alpha blockers like prazosin, terazosin, and doxazosin can block the effects of midodrine.

Food Interactions

None known.

Usual Dose

Dizziness or Fainting
   Adult: 10 mg 3 times a day. People with kidney failure should start with 2.5 mg.
   Child: not recommended.

Urinary Incontinence
   Adult: 2.5–5 mg 2–3 times a day.
   Child: not recommended.

Overdosage

Symptoms can include high blood pressure, goosebumps, feeling cold, and difficulty urinating. There are two reported instances of midodrine overdose; both people survived. Overdose victims should be taken to a hospital emergency room. ALWAYS bring the prescription bottle or container with you.

Special Information

Midodrine should be taken during the day while you are awake and active. Your doctor may suggest that you take the medication about every 4 hours: when you get up, around noon, and in the late afternoon—no later than 6 p.m. The drug may also be taken every 3 hours to control symptoms.

   Do not take midodrine after dinner or less than 4 hours before you go to bed.

   Continue taking midodrine only if it works for you. If you forget a dose of midodrine, take it as soon as you remember. If it is almost time for your next dose, skip the dose you forgot and continue with your regular schedule. Call your doctor if you forget to take 2 or more doses in a row.

Special Populations

Pregnancy/Breast-feeding
Midodrine should be taken by pregnant women only if the possible benefits outweigh the risks. Discuss this with your doctor before taking midodrine.

   It is not known if midodrine passes into breast milk.

Nursing mothers who must take it should watch their babies for drug side effects.

Seniors
Seniors may take midodrine without special precautions.

Generic Name

Miglitol (mig-LIH-tol)

___

Brand Name

Glyset

Type of Drug

Antidiabetic.

Prescribed for

Non-insulin-dependent diabetes, together with a diabetic diet program; also prescribed with another antidiabetic drug if the effect of that drug alone is not enough to adequately control blood sugar levels.

General Information

Miglitol works differently from other antidiabetes drugs taken by mouth. The sulfonylurea-type antidiabetics stimulate the pancreas to release more insulin into the blood stream to help metabolize, or break down, the excess sugar in the blood that is the major sign of diabetes. Metformin helps body cells utilize insulin to metabolize blood sugar more efficiently. Miglitol, however, delays the digestion of carbohydrates (sugars) by acting in the small cells that line the small intestine, where sugar is absorbed. This results in less sugar being absorbed into the blood and, therefore, a lower blood-sugar level. Miglitol also has some effect against the enzyme lactase, but usually does not cause lactose intolerance.

Hypoglycemia (very low blood sugar) is unlikely with miglitol because of the way the drug works in diabetes. Miglitol may increase the risk of hypoglycemia if taken with a sulfonylurea-type antidiabetes drug.

People taking miglitol should have their blood sugar checked periodically to see how well the drug is working. Home glucose monitors are available to allow you to do this for yourself. Blood sugar may go up if you have an infection, stress, fever, a trauma, or surgery. Insulin injections may be needed temporarily.

Cautions and Warnings

Do not take miglitol if you are **sensitive** or **allergic** to it. Miglitol should be used with caution if you have **diabetic ketoacidosis, inflammatory bowel disease, ulcers in the colon, partial obstruction of your intestine,** or **absorption** or **digestion diseases.**

People with kidney disease build up higher levels of miglitol in the blood, but this does not affect the drug's action because it acts locally in cells lining the small intestine. Those with severe **kidney disease** should not take this drug because of excess buildup in the blood.

Possible Side Effects

Most side effects of miglitol go away with continued use of the drug.
  ▼ Most common: gas, diarrhea, and abdominal pain.
  ▼ Common: skin rash and low blood iron.

Drug Interactions

• Miglitol interferes with the absorption of several drugs into the blood, including propranolol and ranitidine. Your doctor may need to adjust your dose of these drugs.

• Digestive enzymes, charcoal, and kaolin — an ingredient in Kaopectate — reduce the effects of miglitol.

Food Interactions

Miglitol must be taken with the first bite of each main meal.

Usual Dose

Adult: 25–100 mg with breakfast, lunch, and dinner.
Child: not recommended.

Overdosage

Unlike other antidiabetic medicines, a miglitol overdose does not cause hypoglycemia. Overdose symptoms are likely to be stomach gas, diarrhea, and pain. Call your local poison control center or hospital emergency room for more information.

Special Information

Take your dose with the first bite of each meal. The drug has
to be present in your intestine to prevent the absorption of
sugar into your blood.

If you forget to take a dose of miglitol with your meal, skip
the forgotten dose, since it cannot work unless there is food
in your stomach. Continue with your regular dose at the
beginning of your next meal.

Special Populations

Pregnancy/Breast-feeding

Little is known about the effects of this drug during pregnancy. Miglitol should be used only by pregnant women who
have discussed its possible risks and benefits with their
doctors. Diabetes that develops during pregnancy is usually
treated with insulin injections.

Small amounts of miglitol pass into breast milk. Nursing
mothers who must take this medication should bottle-feed
their babies.

Seniors

Seniors may take this drug with no special precautions.

Generic Name

Minoxidil (mih-NOX-ih-dil) [G]

Brand Names

Loniten   Rogaine

Type of Drug

Antihypertensive; and hair-growth stimulant.

Prescribed for

Hypertension (high blood pressure), male-pattern baldness,
and alopecia areata.

General Information

Minoxidil reduces blood pressure by dilating peripheral blood
vessels, allowing more blood to flow through the arms and
legs. This increased blood flow reduces the resistance levels

MINOXIDIL

in central blood vessels — for example in the heart, lungs, and kidneys — and therefore reduces blood pressure. Minoxidil's effect on blood pressure is seen 30 minutes after a dose is taken and lasts up to 3 days. Patients usually take this drug once or twice a day. Minoxidil reaches maximum drug effect as soon as 3 days after the drug is started, if the dose is large enough — 40 mg a day. Minoxidil is prescribed for severe hypertension that has not responded to other drugs.

Minoxidil stimulates hair growth in men and women with hereditary hair loss. It is also used to treat alopecia areata, a condition in which patches of hair fall out all over the body. No one knows exactly how minoxidil produces this effect and it does not work for everyone. The ideal candidate for minoxidil's hair-restoring effect is a man who has just started to lose his hair. Women may be helped by minoxidil lotion, too. The drug does not help unless hair in the balding area is at least ½ in. long, and it takes 4 to 6 months of applications before any effect can be expected. The application regimen must be followed carefully; stopping the drug will nullify any benefit that has been gained and new hair that has grown in will fall out. Some men who used minoxidil lotion continuously for a year found that their hair loss continued, but at a slower rate.

Cautions and Warnings

The oral form of minoxidil may cause severe **adverse effects on the heart**, including angina pain and fluid around the heart, which affects cardiac function. Oral minoxidil should be taken only by people who do not respond to other antihypertensive (blood-pressure-lowering) treatments. It is usually prescribed with a beta-blocking antihypertensive drug — such as propranolol, metoprolol, nadolol — to prevent rapid heartbeat, and a diuretic to prevent fluid accumulation. Hospitalization may be recommended for some patients when they start minoxidil to avoid too rapid a drop in blood pressure.

This drug should not be used by people with **pheochromocytoma** (adrenal gland tumor).

This drug has not been carefully studied in people who have suffered a **heart attack** within a month of beginning minoxidil treatment; cardiac side effects may be particularly serious in people with a history of heart disease. People who use minoxidil for hair growth must have a healthy scalp and no heart disease.

Possible Side Effects

Tablets

Water and sodium retention may develop, which can worsen heart failure. Some patients taking minoxidil may develop fluid in the sacs surrounding the heart, which is usually treated with a diuretic.

▼ Most common: 80% of people experience thickening, elongation, and darkening of body hair within 3 to 6 weeks, first noticed on the temples, between the eyebrows, on the forehead, or on the upper cheek. Later it may extends to the back, arms, legs, and scalp. This effect stops when the drug is stopped, and symptoms usually disappear in 1 to 6 months. Heart rhythm changes can be detected with electrocardiogram in 60% of people, but they are usually not associated with any symptoms. Some laboratory tests, such as blood, liver, kidney tests, may be affected by minoxidil.

▼ Less common: bronchitis or other respiratory infections, sinus inflammation, rash, eczema, fungal infection, itching, redness, dry skin or scalp, flaking, worsening of hair loss, triggering hair loss where none was present, diarrhea, nausea, vomiting, headache, dizziness, lightheadedness, fainting, back pain, broken bones, tendinitis, aches and pains, swelling of the arms or legs, chest pain, blood-pressure changes, heart palpitations, pulse-rate changes, allergic reactions (symptoms include breathing difficulties, rash, and itching), hives, runny nose, facial swelling, conjunctivitis (pinkeye), ear infection, visual disturbances, weight gain, urinary infection, inflammation of the prostate or urethra, vaginal discharge, pain during sex, anxiety, depression, fatigue, menstrual changes, nonspecific breast symptoms, and pain, inflammation, or redness of the testes, vagina, or vulva.

Lotion

People using 2% minoxidil lotion may experience irritation or itching. The amount of minoxidil absorbed into the bloodstream is too small to affect blood pressure or cause serious side effects.

Drug Interactions

• Minoxidil may interact with guanethidine to produce

severe dizziness when rising from a sitting or lying position. These drugs should not be taken together.

• Do not take over-the-counter (OTC) products that contain stimulants. If you are unsure about which OTC products to avoid, ask your doctor or pharmacist.

Food Interactions

None known.

Usual Dose

Tablets

Adult and Child (age 12 and over): 5 mg a day to start; may be increased to 40 mg a day. Do not exceed 100 mg a day. Dosage must be tailored to individual needs. Follow your doctor's directions exactly.

Child (under age 12): 0.1 mg per lb. of body weight a day to start; may be increased to 0.5 mg per lb. of body weight a day. Do not exceed 50 mg a day. Dosage must be tailored to the child's specific needs.

Minoxidil is usually taken with a diuretic — such as 100 mg a day of hydrochlorothiazide, 50–100 mg a day of chlorthalidone, or 80 mg a day of furosemide — and a beta blocker — such as 80–160 mg a day of propranolol, or the equivalent dose of another beta blocker. People who cannot take beta blockers may take 500–1500 mg a day of methyldopa, or 0.2–0.4 mg a day of clonidine.

Lotion

Apply to scalp twice a day.

Overdosage

Symptoms of minoxidil overdose may include dizziness, fainting, and rapid heartbeat. Contact your local poison control center or hospital emergency room for instructions. ALWAYS bring the prescription bottle or container with you if you must go for treatment.

Special Information

Oral minoxidil is usually prescribed with 2 other drugs — a beta blocker and a diuretic; do not discontinue any of these drugs unless told to do so by your doctor. Take all medication exactly as prescribed.

The effect of this drug on body hair (see "Possible Side

Effects") is more of a nuisance than a risk and is not a reason to stop taking it.

Call your doctor if you experience an increase in your pulse of 20 or more beats per minute; weight gain of more than 5 lbs; unusual swelling of your arms, legs, face, or stomach; chest pain; breathing difficulties; dizziness; or fainting spells.

If you forget to take a dose of minoxidil, take it as soon as you remember. If it is almost time for your next regularly scheduled dose, skip the dose you forgot and continue with your regular schedule. Do not take a double dose.

Special Populations

Pregnancy/Breast-feeding

Minoxidil crosses into the circulation of the fetus but has not been found to cause human birth defects. Women who are or might be pregnant should not take minoxidil. When the drug is considered crucial by your doctor, its potential benefits must be carefully weighed against its risks.

This drug passes into breast milk and should not be used while nursing. Nursing mothers who must take minoxidil should bottle-feed their babies.

Seniors

Minoxidil clears the body through the kidneys. Seniors may be more sensitive to the blood-pressure-lowering effects of the drug because of a normal loss of kidney capacity due to age or other factors. Follow your doctor's directions, and report any side effects at once.

Generic Name

Mirtazapine (mur-TAZ-uh-pene)

Brand Name

Remeron

Type of Drug

Antidepressant.

Prescribed for

Depression.

General Information

The exact way that mirtazapine works is not known. It blocks the movement of certain stimulant chemicals in and out of nerve endings and has a sedative effect. Mirtazapine also moderately counteracts the effects of the neurohormone acetylcholine. Recent theory says that antidepressant drugs work by changing the sensitivity and function of nerve endings, which over time leads to long-term changes in nerve-ending activity. Thus, although mirtazapine and other antidepressants immediately block neurohormones, it takes 2 to 4 weeks for their clinical effects to come into play. If your symptoms are unchanged after 6 to 8 weeks of treatment with an antidepressant, contact your doctor. Mirtazapine elevates mood, increases physical activity and mental alertness, and improves appetite and sleep patterns in a depressed person. Mirtazapine is also a mild sedative and is useful in treating mild forms of depression associated with anxiety. Mirtazapine is broken down in the liver. The drug clears the system slower in women than in men.

Cautions and Warnings

Do not take mirtazapine if you are **allergic** or **sensitive** to it.

Mirtazapine should be taken with care if you are **recovering from a heart attack**.

Take this drug with caution if you have a history of **epilepsy** or other convulsive disorders, **urinary difficulties, glaucoma, heart disease, liver disease**, or **hyperthyroidism**. Antidepressants may aggravate the condition of people who are **schizophrenic** or **paranoid,** and may cause people with **bipolar (manic depressive) disorder** to switch phase. These reactions are also possible when changing or stopping antidepressants. **Suicide** is always a possibility in severely depressed people, who should only be allowed to have minimal quantities of medication in their possession at any one time.

Seizures are rare and can be minimized by starting with a low mirtazapine dose and staying with the lowest effective dose. Dosage should be increased gradually and only after at least 2 weeks on the starting dose.

People taking mirtazapine may develop very **low white-blood-cell counts,** leading to infections, fever, and related problems. Call your doctor at once if you develop a sore throat, fever, infection, or mouth sores while taking this drug.

Mirtazapine should be taken with care if you have **severe kidney or liver disease**.

Possible Side Effects

▼ Most common: tiredness, dizziness, dry mouth, constipation, increased appetite, weight gain, large increases in blood cholesterol and/or triglyceride levels, weakness, and flu symptoms.

▼ Less common: back pain, nausea, vomiting, muscle ache, abnormal dreaming or thinking, anxiety, agitation, confusion, tremors, itching, rash, breathing difficulties, and frequent urination.

▼ Rare: blood-pressure changes, weakness, hair loss, uncontrollable muscle spasms or movements, hallucinations, manic reactions, and liver function changes. Other infrequent or rare side effects of mirtazapine may affect virtually any system of the body.

Drug Interactions

• Combining mirtazapine with a monoamine oxidase inhibitor (MAOI) antidepressant may cause high fevers and convulsions. This combination is potentially fatal. Do not take an MAOI until at least 2 weeks after mirtazapine has been stopped. People who take both mirtazapine and an MAOI require close medical observation.

• Mirtazapine increases the effects of alcohol, tranquilizers, and other sedative drugs.

Food Interactions

You may take mirtazapine with food if it upsets your stomach.

Usual Dose

Adult: 15 mg at bedtime. Dosage must be tailored to your needs.

Overdosage

There is little experience with mirtazapine overdose. Reported symptoms have been limited to disorientation, drowsiness, memory loss, and rapid heartbeat. The victim should be taken to a hospital emergency room immediately. ALWAYS bring the prescription bottle or container with you.

Special Information

Do not stop taking this drug unless your doctor has specifically told you to do so: Abruptly stopping mirtazapine may cause nausea, headache, and feelings of ill health.

Mirtazapine may cause drowsiness and dizziness. Be careful when driving or operating hazardous machinery. Avoid alcohol and other depressant drugs while taking this medication. Avoid prolonged exposure to the sun or sun lamps.

Be careful when taking over-the-counter (OTC) medications because mirtazapine may interact with sedative ingredients in OTC products.

Call your doctor at once if you develop chills, difficult or rapid breathing, fever, sweating, blood pressure changes, muscle stiffness, loss of bladder control, or unusual tiredness or weakness.

If you forget a dose of mirtazapine, skip it and go back to your regular schedule. Do not take a double dose.

Special Populations

Pregnancy/Breast-feeding

Mirtazapine crosses into the fetal blood circulation and birth defects have been reported. Pregnant women should take mirtazapine only if it is absolutely necessary.

It is not known if mirtazapine passes into breast milk. Nursing mothers taking mirtazapine should watch their babies for possible side effects.

Seniors

Seniors should take mirtazapine with caution because they are more sensitive to its side effects. Seniors usually require a lower dose than younger adults to achieve the same result. This difference is more striking among men than women. Follow your doctor's directions and report any unusual side effects at once.

Generic Name

Misoprostol (mye-soe-PROS-tol)

Brand Name

Cytotec

Type of Drug

Antiulcer.

Prescribed for

Stomach ulcer associated with nonsteroidal anti-inflammatory drugs (NSAIDs), duodenal (intestinal) ulcer, and, in combination with other drugs, prevention of kidney rejection after transplant.

General Information

Like cimetidine and other of the antiulcer drugs, misoprostol suppresses stomach acid. It has a demonstrated ability to protect the stomach lining from damage, although the exact way misoprostol works is not known. Misoprostol may increase production of stomach lining and the thickness of the protective gel layer lining the stomach. It may also increase blood flow in and subsequent healing of the stomach lining, and increase production of bicarbonate, a natural antacid found in the stomach.

Misoprostol is intended to prevent severe stomach irritation and stomach ulcers in people taking an NSAID. It is helpful for seniors and others with a history of ulcer or stomach disease who have been otherwise unable to tolerate NSAID treatment for arthritis. Misoprostol is also used to treat duodenal ulcers, although it will not prevent them. It is likely to be an effective ulcer treatment for people who have not responded to cimetidine, ranitidine, famotidine, or nizatidine, or who are unable to take one of these drugs because of side effects or adverse drug interactions.

Misoprostol is known to cause the pregnant uterus to contract and has been studied as a vaginal abortion drug. It works in the same way and is as effective as the controversial French abortion drug RU-486. Oral misoprostol plus one dose of methotrexate is as effective an abortifacient as vaginal misoprostol.

Cautions and Warnings

Misoprostol may make both men and women **less fertile**. People who are **allergic** to misoprostol or any prostaglandin agent should not take this drug.

People with **kidney disease** routinely have misoprostol blood levels that are about twice as high as those with normal kidney function. This is not a problem for most people, but dosage may have to be reduced if side effects become intolerable.

People with **epilepsy** or **blood-vessel disease** in the heart or brain should be cautious about taking misoprostol.

Possible Side Effects

▼ Most common: diarrhea and abdominal pain. Most cases of diarrhea are mild and last no more than 2 to 3 days.

▼ Less common: headache, nausea, vomiting, and stomach upset or gas.

▼ Rare: spotting, cramps, excessive menstrual bleeding, painful menstruation or other menstrual disorders, and vaginal bleeding.

Drug Interactions

• Because misoprostol reduces stomach acid, it may interfere with the absorption of drugs that can depend upon the presence of stomach acid for absorption, such as diazepam and theophylline.

• Antacids reduce the amount of misoprostol absorbed into the bloodstream, but this usually does not interfere with misoprostol's effectiveness. Magnesium-containing antacids may worsen misoprostol-induced diarrhea.

Food Interactions

Food interferes with the passage of misoprostol into the bloodstream; it should be taken with or after meals, and at bedtime to minimize the drug's gastrointestinal (GI) side effects.

Usual Dose

Adult: 200 mcg 4 times a day.

Overdosage

The toxic dose of misoprostol in humans is not known; up to 1600 mcg a day have been taken with only minor discomfort. Overdose symptoms are sedation; tremors; convulsions; breathing difficulties; stomach pain; diarrhea; fever; changes in heart rate, either very fast or very slow; and low blood pressure. Overdose victims should be taken to a hospital emergency room for treatment. ALWAYS bring the prescription bottle or container with you.

Special Information

Do not stop taking misoprostol without your doctor's knowledge, and keep your follow-up appointments. Do not take this drug for more than 4 weeks without your doctor's permission. Never share your misoprostol prescription with anyone, particularly a woman of childbearing age.

Call your doctor if side effects, especially diarrhea or abdominal or stomach pain, become severe or intolerable. Women who experience misoprostol-related menstrual problems and postmenopausal women who experience vaginal bleeding should discuss these side effects with their doctors.

If you forget to take a dose of misoprostol, take it as soon as you remember. If it is almost time for your next dose, skip the dose you forgot and continue with your regular schedule. Do not take a double dose.

Special Populations

Pregnancy/Breast-feeding

Misoprostol makes the pregnant uterus contract and will cause a spontaneous miscarriage. Within 2 weeks of starting misoprostol treatment, you must have had a negative result of a BLOOD test for pregnancy—an over-the-counter urine test is not sufficient. Afterward, start taking misoprostol on day 2 or 3 of your period and use effective contraception for the entire time you are taking the drug. PREGNANT WOMEN SHOULD NOT TAKE THIS DRUG. Women of childbearing age should take misoprostol only if they absolutely must take an NSAID and already have, or are at a high risk of developing, stomach ulcers.

Misoprostol is not likely to pass into breast milk because it is broken down rapidly in the body. However, this drug may cause major diarrhea in breast-fed infants and should be avoided by nursing mothers. If you must take misoprostol, you should bottle-feed your baby.

Seniors

Seniors absorb more misoprostol than younger adults, although generally without suffering increased side effects. Dosage should be reduced if intolerable side effects develop.

Generic Name

Moexipril (moe-EX-uh-pril)

Brand Name

Univasc

Type of Drug

Angiotensin converting enzyme (ACE) inhibitor.

Prescribed for

Hypertension (high blood pressure).

General Information

Moexipril hydrochloride belongs to the class of drugs known as angiotensin-converting enzyme (ACE) inhibitors. The ACE inhibitors work by preventing the conversion of a hormone called angiotensin I to another hormone called angiotensin II, a potent blood-vessel constrictor. Preventing this conversion relaxes blood vessels, thus reducing blood pressure and relieving the symptoms of heart failure by making it easier for a failing heart to pump blood through the body. Moexipril also affects production of other hormones and enzymes that participate in the regulation of blood vessel dilation; this action probably increases the drug's effectiveness. Moexipril begins working about 1 hour after you take it and continues to work for 24 hours.

Some people who start taking an ACE inhibitor after they are already on a diuretic (agent that increases urination) experience a rapid drop in blood pressure after their first doses or when the dosage is increased. To prevent this from happening, you may be told to stop taking the diuretic 2 or 3 days before starting the ACE inhibitor, or to increase your salt intake during that time. The diuretic may then be restarted gradually. Heart failure patients generally will have been on digoxin and a diuretic before beginning their ACE inhibitor.

Cautions and Warnings

Do not take moexipril if you have had an **allergic reaction** to it in the past.

Moexipril occasionally causes very **low blood pressure**.

Moexipril may cause a **decline in kidney function**, especially if you have congestive heart failure. It is advisable for your doctor to check your urine for changes during the first few months of treatment. Dosage adjustment of moexipril may be necessary.

Moexipril can occasionally affect **white-blood-cell count**, possibly increasing your susceptibility to infection. Blood counts should be monitored periodically.

Possible Side Effects

▼ Most common: dizziness, tiredness, headache, nausea, low blood pressure, chest pain, and chronic cough. The cough usually goes away a few days after you stop taking the medicine.

▼ Less common: chest pain, angina, dizziness when rising from a sitting or lying position, fainting, abdominal pain, nausea, vomiting, diarrhea, bronchitis, urinary tract infection, breathing difficulties, weakness, and skin rash.

▼ Rare: itching, fever, heart attack, stroke, abnormal heart rhythm, heart palpitations, difficulty sleeping, tingling in the hands or feet, appetite loss, abnormal tastes, upset stomach, hepatitis and jaundice, pancreatitis, blood in the stool, swollen tongue, hair loss, rash, unusual sensitivity to the sun, flushing, anxiety, sleeplessness, nervousness, reduced sex drive, muscle cramps or weakness, impotence, arthritis, muscle aches, asthma, respiratory infection, sinus irritation, confusion, depression, not feeling well, sweating, kidney problems, anemia, blurred vision, and swelling of the arms, legs, lips, face, and throat.

Drug Interactions

• The blood-pressure-lowering effect of moexipril is increased by taking diuretic drugs and beta blockers. Any other drug that causes a rapid drop in blood pressure should be used with caution if you are taking an ACE inhibitor.

• Moexipril may increase potassium levels in your blood, especially when taken with dyazide or other potassium-sparing diuretics.

• Moexipril may increase the effects of lithium; this combination should be used with caution.

• Antacids may reduce the amount of moexipril absorbed into the blood. Separate doses of these medications by at least 2 hours.

• Capsaicin may trigger or aggravate the cough associated with moexipril therapy.

• Indomethacin may reduce the blood-pressure-lowering effects of moexipril.

• Phenothiazine tranquilizers and antiemetics may increase the effects of moexipril.

• The combination of allopurinol and moexipril increases the chance of side effects.

• Moexipril increases the levels of digoxin in the blood, possibly increasing the chance of digoxin-related side effects.

Food Interactions

Moexipril should be taken 1 hour before or 2 hours after meals.

Usual Dose

7.5–30 mg once a day. Some people may divide their total daily dosage into 2 doses. People with poor kidney function should take half the usual dose.

Overdosage

The principal effect of moexipril overdose is a rapid drop in blood pressure, as evidenced by dizziness or fainting. Take the overdose victim to a hospital emergency room immediately. ALWAYS bring the prescription bottle or container with you.

Special Information

Call your doctor if you develop swelling of the face or throat, if you have sudden difficulty in breathing or if you develop swelling of the face or throat, a sore throat, mouth sores, abnormal heartbeat, chest pain, persistent rash, or loss of taste perception.

Moexipril can cause unexplained swelling of the face, lips, hands, and feet. This swelling can also affect the larynx (throat) and tongue and interfere with breathing. If this happens, the victim should be taken to a hospital emergency room at once for treatment.

You may get dizzy if you rise to your feet quickly from a sitting or lying position.

Avoid strenuous exercise and/or very hot weather because heavy sweating or dehydration can cause a rapid blood pressure drop.

Avoid over-the-counter diet pills, decongestants, and other stimulants that can raise blood pressure.

If you take moexipril once a day and forget to take a dose, take it as soon as you remember. If it is within 8 hours of your next dose, skip the one you forgot and continue with your regular schedule. If you take moexipril twice a day and forget a dose, take it as soon as you remember. If it is within 4 hours of your next dose, take one dose as soon as you remember and another in 5 or 6 hours, then go back to your regular schedule. Never take a double dose.

Special Populations

Pregnancy/Breast-feeding

ACE inhibitors have caused low blood pressure, kidney failure, slow formation of the skull, and death in fetuses when taken during the last 6 months of pregnancy. Women who are pregnant should not take moexipril. Women who may become pregnant while taking moexipril should use an effective contraceptive method and stop taking the medication if they do become pregnant.

Relatively small amounts of moexipril pass into breast milk, and the effect on a nursing infant is likely to be minimal. However, nursing mothers who must take this drug should consider bottle-feeding: Infants, especially newborns, are more susceptible than adults to the drug's effects.

Seniors

Seniors may be more sensitive to the effects of moexipril than younger adults because of the possibility of kidney impairment. Your dosage must be individualized to your needs.

Monopril

see *Fosinopril, page 466*

Generic Name

Moricizine (mor-IH-sih-zene)

Brand Name

Ethmozine

Type of Drug

Antiarrhythmic.

Prescribed for

Life-threatening cardiac arrhythmias.

General Information

Moricizine treatment should always be started in a hospital because of the close cardiac monitoring required during the first phase of drug treatment. It should not be prescribed for minor arrhythmias or those that do not cause symptoms of their own. Moricizine works by stabilizing heart tissues and making them less sensitive to excessive stimulation. Moricizine starts working 2 hours after it is taken and lasts for 10 to 24 hours. People with heart failure are usually able to tolerate this drug but should be closely monitored for any sign that the condition is worsening.

Cautions and Warnings

Ironically, moricizine can cause abnormal rhythms of its own or worsen existing rhythm problems. This calls for close monitoring by your doctor. It is often impossible to distinguish between a **drug-induced arrhythmia** and one that occurs naturally, except when the problem occurs soon after drug treatment has been started and the patient is on continuous heart monitoring. Arrhythmias can be serious and life-threatening.

Do not take this drug if you are **allergic** to it. People with **heart block** should avoid moricizine.

Moricizine should be used with caution in patients with a form of heart disease called **"sick sinus syndrome,"** in which the part of the heart that initiates heart contractions is not working properly.

Moricizine causes **changes in electrocardiograms** and may change the actual conduction of electrical impulses throughout the heart.

People with **pacemakers** who start taking moricizine may need their pacemakers reset because of changes in the sensitivity of heart tissue to electrical impulses.

Because moricizine is partially broken down by the liver and passes out of the body through the kidneys, these organs are essential to the efficient removal of the drug from the body. People with **kidney or liver disease** should receive lower-than-usual doses of the drug and be monitored more closely for unwanted drug effects.

Some people taking moricizine may develop **fevers** or other drug sensitivity reactions. If fever develops, it should subside within 2 days after the drug is stopped.

As is the case with other antiarrhythmic drugs, people taking moricizine have not been proven to live longer than those who do not take it.

Possible Side Effects

▼ Most common: dizziness, nausea, vomiting, headache, pain, breathing difficulties, fatigue, and drug-induced abnormal heart rhythms—this is the most dangerous.

▼ Common: heart palpitations, chest pain, heart failure, heart attack, cardiac death, changes in blood pressure, fainting, very slow heart rate, blood clots in the lungs, stroke, muscle weakness, nervousness, tingling in the hands or feet, sleep difficulties, tremors, anxiety, depression, euphoria (feeling high), confusion, agitation, seizure, coma, difficulty walking, hallucinations, blurred or double vision, speech difficulties, memory loss, coordination difficulties, and ringing or buzzing in the ears.

▼ Less common: urinary difficulty, loss of urinary control, kidney pain, loss of sex drive, male impotence, hyperventilation, asthma, sore throat, cough, sinus irritation, abdominal pain, upset stomach, diarrhea, loss of appetite, a bitter taste, stomach gas and cramps, difficulty swallowing, sweating, dry mouth, muscle pain, drug fever, low body temperature, intolerance to heat or cold, eye pain, rash, itching, dry skin, swelling of the lips or tongue, and swelling around the eyes.

▼ Rare: hepatitis or jaundice (symptoms include yellowing of the skin or whites of the eyes).

Drug Interactions

• Cimetidine, propranolol, and digoxin may increase the amount of moricizine in the blood, increasing the possibility of drug side effects.

• Moricizine may drastically decrease the amount of theophylline in the blood by increasing the rate at which theophylline is cleared from the body. Dosage adjustment may be required.

Food Interactions

Taking moricizine 30 minutes after eating delays the absorption of the drug into the blood, but does not affect the total amount of drug absorbed. You may take moricizine with food if it upsets your stomach.

Usual Dose

Adult: 600–900 mg a day.

Senior: A lower starting dose is recommended; the dose should gradually be increased until the maximum effect is achieved. People with kidney or liver disease—same as dosage for seniors.

Overdosage

Symptoms are vomiting, lethargy, fainting, coma, low blood pressure, abnormal heart rhythms, worsening of heart failure, heart attack, and breathing difficulties. Death has occurred after doses of 2250 mg (17 250-mg tablets) and 10,000 mg (33 300-mg tablets). Victims should be taken to an emergency room immediately. ALWAYS bring the prescription bottle or container with you.

Special Information

People switching to moricizine from another antiarrhythmic should not take their first dose of moricizine until several hours after their last dose of the old drug. This is necessary to allow most of the latter to clear from the body. The waiting period varies from 3 to 12 hours, depending on which antiarrhythmic is being discontinued.

Some side effects may be related to the size of an individual dose. Therefore, it is usually better to divide the total daily dose into 3 separate doses, rather than 1 or 2 doses.

Call your doctor if you develop cardiac problems; dizziness; anxiety; fever; swelling of the tongue, the lips, or the area around the eyes; visual or urinary difficulties; yellowing of the skin or whites of the eyes; severe nausea; diarrhea; vomiting; or other persistent or intolerable side effects.

If you take moricizine twice a day and forget a dose, take it as soon as you remember. If it is almost time for your next dose, take one dose as soon as you remember and another in 5 or 6 hours, then go back to your regular schedule. If you take moricizine 3 times a day and forget a dose, take it as soon as you remember. If it is almost time for your next dose, take one dose as soon as you remember and another in 3 or 4 hours, then go back to your regular schedule. Never take a double dose.

Special Populations

Pregnancy/Breast-feeding
In animal studies, doses of moricizine almost 7 times larger than the maximum human dose affected the size and weight of offspring or development of the fetus. However, there is no information on the effect of moricizine in pregnant women. When this drug is considered crucial by your doctor, its potential benefits should carefully be weighed against its risks.

Moricizine passes into breast milk. Nursing mothers who must take this drug should bottle-feed their babies.

Seniors
Seniors generally experience the same side effects as younger adults, although studies of the drug showed that stopping drug treatment because of newly discovered arrhythmias was more common among older adults.

Seniors are also more likely to have a kidney and/or liver problem. Those conditions call for starting moricizine at a lower dose and increasing the dosage more cautiously.

Brand Name

Motofen

Generic Ingredients
Difenoxin + Atropine Sulfate

Type of Drug
Antidiarrheal.

Prescribed for
Acute and chronic diarrhea that does not respond to other treatments.

General Information
Difenoxin is an antidiarrheal agent related to meperidine. Meperidine is a narcotic analgesic (pain reliever) and an

ingredient in Demerol. Difenoxin works by slowing the rate at which intestinal-wall muscles contract. It is a chemical by-product of diphenoxylate, another popular antidiarrheal. Atropine sulfate is added to prevent drug overdose and product abuse because difenoxin can be addicting. Atropine causes undesirable effects at small doses, thus deterring users from taking larger Motofen doses.

Motofen and other antidiarrheals should be used only for short periods; they relieve diarrhea, but do nothing for the underlying cause. Some people should not use this drug even if diarrhea is present: People with some types of stomach, bowel, or other conditions may be harmed by antidiarrheal drugs. Do not use Motofen without your doctor's advice.

Cautions and Warnings

Do not take Motofen if you are **allergic** to any of its ingredients, including atropine, or to Lomotil. Avoid Motofen if you have advanced **liver disease**, if you have **jaundice** (yellowing of the skin or whites of the eyes), or if your diarrhea was caused by taking **clindamycin** or another antibiotic.

Possible Side Effects

▼ Most common: nausea, vomiting, dry mouth, dizziness, light-headedness, drowsiness, and headache.

▼ Less common: constipation, upset stomach, confusion, and tiredness or sleeplessness.

▼ Rare: burning eyes, blurred vision, dry skin, rapid heartbeat, elevated temperature, and urinary difficulties.

Drug Interactions

• Motofen may increase the effects of alcohol, tranquilizers, pain relievers, and other nervous-system depressants. Avoid these combinations if possible.

• Monoamine oxidase inhibitor (MAOI) antidepressants may, in theory, produce a high-blood-pressure crisis in combination with Motofen. Do not use Motofen if you are taking an MAOI unless you are under a doctor's care.

Food Interactions

None known.

Usual Dose

Adult and Child (age 12 and over): 2 tablets to start, then 1 after each loose stool or every 3 to 4 hours, as needed; up to 8 tablets in any day. Treatment for more than 2 consecutive days is usually not needed.

Child (under age 12): not recommended.

Overdosage

Overdose symptoms include the following: dry skin, mouth, and nose; flushing; fever; and rapid heartbeat. These symptoms may be followed by loss of natural reflexes, pinpointed pupils, droopy eyelids, breathing difficulty, and lethargy or coma. Take the victim to a hospital emergency room immediately. ALWAYS bring the prescription bottle or container with you.

Special Information

Be careful when driving or performing complex tasks because Motofen can make you tired, dizzy, or light-headed. Alcohol, tranquilizers, or other nervous-system depressants will increase the depressant effects of this drug.

Your doctor may prescribe fluid and salt mixtures to replace the body fluids you lose while taking Motofen.

Call your doctor if you develop heart palpitations or if your symptoms do not clear up in 2 days. You may need a different dose or a different drug for your problem.

If you forget to take a dose of Motofen, take it as soon as you remember. If it is almost time for your next dose, skip the one you forgot and continue with your regular schedule. Do not take a double dose.

Special Populations

Pregnancy/Breast-feeding
Animal studies with very large doses of Motofen showed no evidence of birth defects, but showed some increase in stillbirths. Pregnant women should not use Motofen unless its potential benefits have been carefully weighed against its risks.

Nursing mothers taking Motofen should bottle-feed their babies.

Seniors
No special problems have been reported in seniors. However, those with severe kidney and/or liver disease need lower doses of Motofen.

Generic Name

Mupirocin (mue-PYE-roe-sin)

Brand Name

Bactroban

Type of Drug

Topical antibiotic.

Prescribed for

Impetigo (streptococcal skin infections), eczema, inflammation of the hair follicles, and minor bacterial skin infections. Mupirocin nasal is used to prevent resistant *Staphylococcus aureus* infections from spreading during outbreaks of the infection.

General Information

Mupirocin is a unique, non-penicillin product that works against the common microorganisms that cause impetigo in children. It is used to supplement other treatments for impetigo, although many doctors prefer to prescribe oral medication for the condition. Mupirocin works by interfering with bacteria's ability to make the proteins it needs for survival. Large amounts of mupirocin kill bacteria and smaller amounts stop the bacteria from growing. It may be effective against antibiotic-resistant bacteria.

Cautions and Warnings

Do not use a mupirocin product if you are **allergic** to any of its components. Mupirocin ointment is **not for use in the eye**.

Mupirocin nasal should **not be used to prevent Staphylococcus aureus infections**, but only to treat people who are already infected with the organism.

Large quantities of mupirocin ointment should **not be applied to an open wound** because polyethylene glycol—used as a base in mupirocin ointment—may be absorbed through the wound and damage the kidneys.

Possible Side Effects

Ointment

▼ Less common: burning, itching, rash, stinging or pain where the ointment is applied, nausea, skin redness, dry skin, tenderness, swelling, and increased oozing from impetigo lesions.

Nasal Ointment

▼ Most common: headache and runny nose.

▼ Less common: respiratory congestion, sore throat, changes in sense of taste, burning/stinging, cough, and itching.

▼ Rare: eyelid inflammation, diarrhea, dry mouth, ear pain, nosebleeds, nausea, and rash.

Drug and Food Interactions

• Do not use mupirocin nasal at the same time as any other prescription or over-the-counter nasal drug product.

• Taking antibiotics while using a mupirocin product can lead to the development of resistant bacteria.

Usual Dose

Ointment: Apply a small amount to the affected area 3 times a day. Cover with gauze if desired.

Nasal Ointment: Put half the ointment from a single use tube in each nostril morning and evening for 5 days. After the ointment is applied, squeeze your nostrils closed and allow them to open again. Repeat this continuously for about 1 minute.

Overdosage

There are few reports of mupirocin overdose or accidental ingestion. Call your local poison control center or hospital emergency room for more information.

Special Information

Call your doctor if this medication does not work within 3 to 5 days or if any of the following symptoms develop: dry skin or redness, rash, itching, stinging, pain, or other possible drug reactions.

If you forget to apply a dose of mupirocin, do so as soon as you remember. If it is almost time for your next dose, skip the one you forgot and continue with your regular schedule. Do not apply a double dose.

Special Populations

Pregnancy/Breast-feeding

Animal studies have revealed no fetal damage. Still, pregnant women should use this drug only if absolutely necessary.

It is not known if mupirocin passes into breast milk. Nursing mothers who must take this drug should bottle-feed their babies.

Seniors

Seniors may use mupirocin without special restriction.

Generic Name

Muromonab-CD3 (muh-ROE-moe-nab)

Brand Name

Orthoclone OKT3

Type of Drug

Immunosuppressant.

Prescribed for

Kidney, heart, and liver transplantation.

General Information

Muromonab-CD3, a product of biotechnology processes, is an important alternative to cyclosporine in preventing organ transplant rejection. Muromonab-CD3 acts against human T-cells, which normally protect the body from foreign bodies. By acting against T-cells, this drug suppresses the immune system and prevents organ rejection. The drug starts working minutes after it is first given and continues working for as long as it is used. T-cells rapidly return to normal within 1 week after the medication is stopped.

Cautions and Warnings

This drug should not be used by people with untreated **heart failure**, **fluid overload**, or a history of **seizures**.

Muromonab-CD3 is made in cells from mouse tissue and causes the **development of anti-mouse antibodies** in humans. People who have received other drugs made in this way may already have high levels of this kind of antibody in their blood and, if they do, should not be treated with muromonab-CD3. Your doctor will test for antibody levels.

People who receive this drug usually develop **cytokine release syndrome** (CRS) from 30 minutes to 2 days after the first dose is given. CRS symptoms range from mild, flu-like symptoms such as fever, chills, joint aches, weakness, and headaches, to a less common, life-threatening shock-like reaction that involves the heart and nervous system. Some of the more severe symptoms of CRS are shortness of breath; high fever—up to 107°F; wheezing; rapid heartbeat; chest pains; respiratory collapse or failure; heart attack; severe drug reactions; seizures; confusion; hallucinations; stiff neck; brain swelling; and headache. People who are at risk for more severe forms of CRS include those with a recent heart attack or uncontrolled angina pectoris, heart failure, fluid in the lungs, serious lung disease, and a history of seizure or shock. CRS may be prevented or minimized by giving methylprednisolone 1 to 4 hours before the first dose of muromonab-CD3.

People receiving this drug or other immunosuppressants are more likely to develop infection. Preventive antibiotic therapy is sometimes used to reduce the risk of infection.

Possible Side Effects

More than 90% of people receiving muromonab-CD3 experience some form of CRS, though it is usually mild (see "Cautions and Warnings").

▼ Rare: increased infection risk, rash, itching, increased sweating, flushing, diarrhea, nausea, vomiting, abdominal gas and pain, reductions in various blood-cell counts, blood-clotting abnormalities, liver inflammation, muscle and joint stiffness and pain, arthritis, blindness, blurred or double vision, hearing loss, middle-ear infection, ringing or buzzing in the ears, dizziness, fainting, conjunctivitis (pink-eye), stuffy nose or ears, sensitivity to bright light, and kidney damage.

Drug Interactions

- Other immunosuppressants—corticosteroids, cyclosporine, and azathioprine—and indomethacin increase the effect of muromonab-CD3, increasing the risk of CRS.

Food Interactions

Muromonab-CD3 may be taken without regard to food.

Usual Dose

Adult and Child (age 12 and over): 5 mg intravenously a day for 10–14 days.

Child (under age 12): 0.1 mg intravenously for every 2.2 lbs. of body weight a day for 10–14 days.

Overdosage

Call your poison control center for information.

Special Information

Call your doctor at the first sign of rash, itching, rapid heartbeat, difficulty swallowing, breathing difficulties, unusual swelling, allergic reaction, or if you experience any other serious or bothersome side effects. It is essential to maintain close contact with your doctor while taking muromonab-CD3.

Mild reactions due to CRS may be treated by taking acetaminophen or antihistamines. Your body temperature should be no higher than 100°F when each dose is given.

Avoid exposure to bacterial infection and immunizations while you are taking this drug. If an infection develops, your doctor will have to stop muromonab-CD3 treatments and treat the infection.

It is important to maintain good dental hygiene while taking muromonab-CD3 and to use extra care when using your toothbrush or dental floss because of the risk that the drug will make you more susceptible to oral infection. See your dentist regularly while taking this drug.

This drug may cause confusion or interfere with your alertness, dexterity, or coordination. Take care if you are driving or doing anything that requires close concentration.

It is essential to complete the full course of treatment. This medication should not be stopped unless an infection or other severe side effect develops. If you miss a dose, take it as soon as you remember and call your doctor.

Special Populations

Pregnancy/Breast-feeding

Muromonab-CD3 may cross into the fetal circulation but its

effect is not known. Women who are or might be pregnant should consider the risks of muromonab-CD3.

It is not known if muromonab-CD3 passes into breast milk. Nursing mothers who must take this drug should bottle-feed their infants.

Seniors

Seniors may use this drug without special restriction.

Generic Name

Mycophenolate (mye-coe-FEN-oe-late)

Brand Name

CellCept

Type of Drug

Immunosuppressant.

Prescribed for

Kidney transplantation.

General Information

Mycophenolate mofetil is used with corticosteroids and cyclosporine to prevent the rejection of transplanted kidneys. In animals, mycophenolate extends the survival of kidney, heart, liver, intestine, limb, small bowel, pancreas cell, and bone marrow transplants. The drug is rapidly absorbed into the bloodstream where it is metabolized into MPA, the active form of mycophenolate. MPA inhibits the ability of T and B lymphocytes, key elements of the immune system, to respond in their usual way. MPA also suppresses antibody formation and may act directly on inflammation sites and organ rejection sites to prevent the tissue rejection process from proceeding. People with moderate to severe loss of kidney function may have to have their daily dosage adjusted.

Cautions and Warnings

As with other immunosuppressants, people taking mycophenolate are at increased risk of developing a **lymphoma or other malignancy**. The risk increases with the degree of immune suppression and the length of time that the drug is taken.

Two of every 100 people receiving mycophenolate develop severe **reductions in the number of certain white-blood-cells**. Call your doctor if you develop symptoms of viral infection or other unusual symptoms.

Bleeding in the stomach or intestines occurs in about 3 of every 100 people who take this drug, though many of these people are also taking other drugs that may affect the gastrointestinal (GI) tract. People with **stomach or intestinal disease** should take this drug with caution.

People with **kidney disease** should receive lower dosages of mycophenolate. People who experience post-transplant reduction in liver function may develop **kidney damage**.

Mild to moderate hypertension (high blood pressure) is a common side effect of mycophenolate and may be a sign of kidney damage. People taking this drug should measure their blood pressure regularly.

Possible Side Effects

▼ Most common: general pain, abdominal pain, fever, headache, infection, blood infection, weakness, chest pain, back pain, hypertension, anemia, reduced white-blood-cell and platelet counts, urinary infection, blood in the urine, swelling of the arms or legs, diarrhea, constipation, nausea, vomiting, upset stomach, oral fungus infection, respiratory infection, cough, breathing difficulties, and tremors.

▼ Common: kidney damage, urinary tract problems, high blood cholesterol, low blood-phosphate levels, fluid retention, changes in blood-potassium levels, high blood sugar, sore throat, pneumonia, bronchitis, acne, rash, sleeplessness, and dizziness.

▼ Less common: painful urination, impotence, frequent urination, pyelonephritis, urinary disorder, angina pain, heart palpitations, low blood pressure, dizziness when rising from a sitting or lying position, cardiovascular disorders, appetite loss, stomach gas, stomach irritation or bleeding, gum irritation or enlargement, liver irritation, mouth ulcer, asthma, lung disorder, stuffy or runny nose, sinus irritation, hair loss, itching, sweating, skin ulcer, anxiety, depression, stiff muscles, tingling in

---

Possible Side Effects *(continued)*

the hands or feet, joint or muscle pain, leg cramps, double vision, cataracts, conjunctivitis (pinkeye), chills and fever, abdominal enlargement, facial swelling, cysts, flu-like symptoms, bleeding, hernia, feeling sick, pelvic pain, and black-and-blue marks.

▼ Rare: lymphoma, skin cancer—not melanomas—and other malignancies, herpes, chickenpox or shingles, fungus infection, and pneumocystis and other opportunistic infections that usually only develop in people with suppressed immune systems.

Drug Interactions

• When mycophenolate is taken with acyclovir (an antiviral drug), the amount of both drugs in the blood rises.

• Use of cholestyramine and aluminum/magnesium antacids decreases the amount of mycophenolate absorbed by the blood and should be separated from mycophenolate use by at least 1 hour.

• Azathioprine, another immune-system suppressant, should not be taken with mycophenolate because of the risk of excess immune-system suppression.

• Taking probenecid with mycophenolate may double or triple the amount of the immunosuppressant in the blood. Aspirin also increases the amount of mycophenolate in the blood.

• Mycophenolate may moderately reduce the amount of phenytoin or theophylline in the blood.

Food Interactions

Mycophenolate should be taken 1 hour before or 2 hours after meals.

Usual Dose

Adult: 2–3 g a day divided into 2 doses.
Child: not recommended.

Overdosage

The largest dosage given to one person is 4 or 5 g a day. This dosage is associated with an increased risk of side effects—especially those that affect the stomach and intestines—and blood abnormalities. Any person who takes an overdose of mycophenolate must be taken to a hospital emergency room for treatment. ALWAYS bring the prescription bottle or container with you.

Special Information

It is extremely important for you to take this drug exactly as prescribed. If you forget a dose of mycophenolate, take it as soon as you remember. If it is almost time for your next dose, skip the forgotten dose and continue with your regular schedule. Do not take a double dose. Call your doctor if you forget 2 or more doses in a row.

Because this drug has been proven to cause birth defects in animals, take extra caution when handling the capsules. Do not open or crush the capsules. Avoid inhaling the powder or allowing it to touch your skin or the membranes inside your mouth or nose. If such contact does occur, wash thoroughly with soap and water. If the powder gets into your eyes, rinse them thoroughly with plain water.

People taking mycophenolate require regular testing to monitor their progress.

Call your doctor at the first sign of fever; sore throat; tiredness; weakness; nervousness; unusual bleeding or bruising; tender or swollen gums; convulsions; irregular heartbeat; confusion; numbness or tingling of your hands, feet, or lips; breathing difficulties; severe stomach pain with nausea; or blood in the urine. Other side effects are less serious but should be brought to your doctor's attention, particularly if they are unusually bothersome or persistent.

It is important to maintain good dental hygiene while taking mycophenolate and to use extra care when using your toothbrush or dental floss because of the risk that the drug will make you more susceptible to dental infection. Mycophenolate suppresses the normal body systems that fight infection. See your dentist regularly while taking this medication.

This drug should be continued for as long as prescribed by your doctor. Do not stop taking it because of side effects or other problems unless directed to do so by your doctor.

Special Populations

Pregnancy/Breast-feeding

Animal studies show that mycophenolate may be highly toxic to the fetus. Women of childbearing age should have a negative pregnancy test at least 1 week before treatment is started. They should either use 2 effective contraceptive methods before treatment is started and continuing until 6 weeks after mycophenolate is discontinued or they should practice abstinence during this period. Should you accidentally become pregnant during mycophenolate treatment, discuss with your doctor the advisability of continuing the pregnancy. When this drug is considered crucial by your doctor, its potential benefits must be carefully weighed against its risks.

Nursing mothers who must take mycophenolate should bottle-feed their infants.

Seniors

Seniors may take mycophenolate but their dosage may have to be reduced to accommodate normal loss of kidney function.

Generic Name

Nabumetone (nah-BUE-meh-tone)

Brand Name

Relafen

Type of Drug

Nonsteroidal anti-inflammatory drug (NSAID).

Prescribed for

Rheumatoid arthritis and osteoarthritis.

General Information

Nabumetone is one of 16 NSAIDs, which are used to relieve pain and inflammation. We do not know exactly how NSAIDs work, but part of their action may be due to their ability to inhibit the body's production of a hormone called prostaglandin as well as the action of other body chemicals, including cyclooxygenase, lipoxygenase, leukotrienes, and lysosomal enzymes. NSAIDs are absorbed into the blood quickly. Pain relief generally comes within 1 hour after taking the first dose of nabumetone, but its anti-inflammatory effect takes several days to 2 weeks to become apparent and may take a month or more to reach maximum effect. Nabumetone is broken down in the liver, where it must be converted to its active form before it can have an effect.

Cautions and Warnings

People who are **allergic** to nabumetone or any other NSAID and those with a history of **asthma** attacks brought on by an NSAID, iodides, or aspirin should not take nabumetone.

Nabumetone can cause **gastrointestinal (GI) bleeding, ulcers,** and **stomach perforation**. This can occur at any time, with or without warning, in people who take nabumetone regularly. People with a history of **active GI bleeding** should be cautious about taking any NSAID. People who develop bleeding or ulcers and continue NSAID treatment should be aware of the possibility of developing more serious side effects.

Nabumetone can affect platelets and **blood clotting** at high doses, and should be avoided by people with clotting problems and by those taking warfarin.

People with **heart problems** who use nabumetone may experience swelling in their arms, legs, or feet.

Nabumetone can cause severe toxic effects to the **kidney**. Report any unusual side effects to your doctor, who may need to periodically test your kidney function.

Nabumetone can make you unusually sensitive to the effects of the sun.

Possible Side Effects

▼ Most common: diarrhea, nausea, vomiting, constipation, stomach gas, stomach upset or irritation, and appetite loss, especially during the first few days of treatment.

▼ Less common: stomach ulcers, GI bleeding, hepatitis, gallbladder attacks, painful urination, poor kidney function, kidney inflammation, blood and protein in the urine, dizziness, fainting, nervousness, depression, hallucinations, confusion, disorientation, tingling in the hands or feet, light-headedness, itching, increased sweating, dry nose and mouth, heart palpitations, chest pain, breathing difficulties, and muscle cramps.

▼ Rare: severe allergic reactions including closing of the throat, fever and chills, changes in liver function,

Possible Side Effects *(continued)*

jaundice (yellowing of the skin or whites of the eyes), and kidney failure. People who experience such effects must be promptly treated in a hospital emergency room or doctor's office.

NSAIDs have caused severe skin reactions; if this happens to you, see your doctor immediately.

Drug Interactions

• Nabumetone can increase the effects of oral anticoagulant (blood-thinning) drugs such as warfarin. You may take this combination, but your doctor might have to reduce your anticoagulant dose.

• Combining nabumetone with cyclosporine may increase the toxic kidney effects of both drugs. Methotrexate toxicity may be increased in people also taking nabumetone.

• Nabumetone may reduce the blood-pressure-lowering effect of beta blockers and loop diuretics.

• Nabumetone may increase phenytoin blood levels, leading to increased side effects. Lithium blood levels may be increased in people taking nabumetone.

• Nabumetone blood levels may be affected by cimetidine.

• Probenecid may interfere with the elimination of nabumetone from the body, increasing the chances for nabumetone side effects.

• Aspirin and other salicylates may decrease the amount of nabumetone in your blood. These drugs should never be combined with nabumetone.

Food Interactions

Take nabumetone with food or a magnesium-aluminum antacid if it upsets your stomach.

Usual Dose

1000–2000 mg a day, taken in 1 or 2 doses.

Overdosage

People have died from NSAID overdoses. The most common signs of overdose are drowsiness, nausea, vomiting, diarrhea, abdominal pain, rapid breathing, rapid heartbeat, increased sweating, ringing or buzzing in the ears, confusion, disorientation, stupor, and coma. Take the victim to a hospital emergency room at once. ALWAYS bring the prescription bottle or container with you.

Special Information

Take each dose with a full glass of water and do not lie down for 15–30 minutes afterward.

Nabumetone can make you drowsy and/or tired: Be careful when driving or operating hazardous equipment. Do not take any over-the-counter products containing acetaminophen or aspirin while taking nambumetone. Avoid alcoholic beverages.

Contact your doctor if you develop skin rash or itching, visual disturbances, weight gain, breathing difficulties, fluid retention, hallucinations, black or tarry stools, persistent headache, or any unusual or intolerable side effect.

If you forgot to take a dose of nabumetone, take it as soon as you remember. If you take nabumetone once a day and it is within 8 hours of your next dose, skip the dose you forgot and continue with your regular schedule. If you take several doses a day and it is within 4 hours of your next dose, skip the one you forgot and continue with your regular schedule. Never take a double dose.

Special Populations

Pregancy/Breast-feeding

NSAIDs may cross into the fetal blood circulation. They have not been found to cause birth defects, but animal studies indicate that they may affect a fetal heart during the second half of pregnancy. Pregnant women should not take nabumetone without their doctor's approval, particularly during the last 3 months of pregnancy. When the drug is considered crucial by your doctor, its potential benefits must be carefully weighed against its risks.

NSAIDs may pass into breast milk but have caused no problems in breast-fed infants, except for seizures in a baby whose mother was taking the NSAID indomethacin. Other NSAIDs have caused problems in animal studies. There is a possibility that a nursing mother taking nabumetone could affect her baby's heart or cardiovascular system. If you must take nabumetone, bottle-feed your baby.

Seniors

Seniors may be more susceptible to nabumetone side effects, especially ulcer disease.

Generic Name

Naproxen/Naproxen Sodium

(nah-PROX-en) Ⓖ

Brand Names

Aleve	EC-Naprosyn	Napron X
Anaprox	Naprelan	Naprosyn

The information in this profile also applies to the following drugs:

Generic Ingredient: Tolmetin Sodium
Tolectin   Tolectin DS

Type of Drug

Nonsteroidal anti-inflammatory drug (NSAID).

Prescribed for

Rheumatoid arthritis, osteoarthritis, ankylosing spondylitis, mild to moderate pain, tendinitis, bursitis, gout, fever, sunburn, migraine prevention, menstrual pain, and menstrual headache. Only naproxen is prescribed for juvenile rheumatoid arthritis, only naproxen sodium for migraine attacks and premenstrual syndrome (PMS).

General Information

Naproxen is one of 16 NSAIDs, which are used to relieve pain and inflammation. We do not know exactly how NSAIDs work, but part of their action may be due to their ability to inhibit the body's production of a hormone called prostaglandin as well as the action of other body chemicals, including cyclooxygenase, lipoxygenase, leukotrienes, and lysosomal enzymes. Pain relief comes within 1 hour after taking the first dose of naproxen and lasts for about 7 hours, but its anti-inflammatory effect takes several days to 2 weeks to become apparent and may take a month to reach maximum effect.

Cautions and Warnings

People who are **allergic** to naproxen or any other NSAID and those with a history of **asthma** attacks brought on by an NSAID, iodides, or aspirin should not take naproxen.

Naproxen can cause **gastrointestinal (GI) bleeding, ulcers,** and **stomach perforation.** This can occur at any time, with or without warning, in people who take naproxen regularly. People with a history of **active GI bleeding** should be cautious about taking any NSAID. People who develop bleeding or ulcers and continue NSAID treatment should be aware of the possibility of developing more serious side effects.

Naproxen can affect platelets and **blood clotting** at high doses, and should be avoided by people with clotting problems and by those taking warfarin.

People with **heart problems** who use naproxen may experience swelling in their arms, legs, or feet.

Naproxen dosage should be reduced in people with severe **liver disease**.

Naproxen can cause severe toxic effects to the **kidney**. Report any unusual side effects to your doctor, who may need to periodically test your kidney function.

Naproxen can make you unusually sensitive to the effects of the sun.

Possible Side Effects

▼ Most common: diarrhea, nausea, vomiting, constipation, stomach gas, stomach upset or irritation, and appetite loss, especially during the first few days of treatment.

▼ Less common: stomach ulcers, GI bleeding, hepatitis, gallbladder attacks, painful urination, poor kidney function, kidney inflammation, blood and protein in the urine, dizziness, fainting, nervousness, depression, hallucinations, confusion, disorientation, tingling in the hands or feet, light-headedness, itching, increased sweating, dry nose and mouth, heart palpitations, chest pain, difficulty breathing, and muscle cramps.

▼ Rare: severe allergic reactions including closing of the throat, fever and chills, changes in liver function, jaundice (yellowing of the skin or whites of the eyes), and kidney failure. People who experience such effects must be promptly treated in a hospital emergency room or doctor's office. NSAIDs have caused severe skin reactions; if this happens to you, see your doctor immediately.

Drug Interactions

• Naproxen can increase the effects of oral anticoagulant (blood-thinning) drugs such as warfarin. You may take this combination, but your doctor might have to change your anticoagulant dose.

• The combination of naproxen and a thiazide diuretic affects the amount of diuretic in your blood. Naproxen may reduce the effect of the diuretic.

• Taking naproxen with cyclosporine may increase the toxic kidney effects of both drugs. Methotrexate toxicity may be increased in people also taking naproxen.

• Naproxen may reduce the blood-pressure-lowering effect of beta blockers—except atenolol—and loop diuretics.

• Naproxen may increase phenytoin blood levels, leading to increased side effects. Lithium blood levels may be increased in people taking naproxen.

• Naproxen blood levels may be affected by cimetidine.

• Probenecid may interfere with the body's elimination of naproxen, increasing the risk of naproxen side effects.

• Aspirin and other salicylates may decrease the amount of naproxen in your blood. These drugs should never be combined with naproxen.

Food Interactions

Take naproxen with a full glass of water. Take it with food or a magnesium-aluminum antacid if it upsets your stomach.

Usual Dose

Naproxen
    Adult: starting dose—250–375 mg a.m. and p.m.; up to 1250 mg a day if needed. For mild to moderate pain take 250–275 mg every 6–8 hours.
    Child (age 2 and over): 4.5 mg per lb. of body weight divided into 2 doses a day.
    Child (under age 2): not recommended.

Overdosage

People have died from NSAID overdoses. The most common signs of overdose are drowsiness, nausea, vomiting, diarrhea, abdominal pain, rapid breathing, rapid heartbeat, increased sweating, ringing or buzzing in the ears, confusion, disorientation, stupor, and coma. Take the victim to a hospital emergency room at once. ALWAYS bring the prescription bottle or container with you.

Special Information

Take each dose with a full glass of water and do not lie down for 15 to 30 minutes afterward.

Naproxen can make you drowsy and/or tired: Be careful when driving or operating hazardous equipment. Do not take any over-the-counter products containing acetaminophen or aspirin while taking naproxen. Avoid alcoholic beverages.

Contact your doctor if you develop skin rash or itching, visual disturbances, weight gain, breathing difficulties, fluid retention, hallucinations, black or tarry stools, persistent headache, or any unusual or intolerable side effect.

If you forget a dose of naproxen, take it as soon as you remember. If you take naproxen once a day and it is within 8 hours of your next dose, skip the dose you forgot and continue with your regular schedule. If you take several doses a day and it is within 4 hours of your next dose, skip the one you forgot and continue with your regular schedule. Never take a double dose.

Special Populations

Pregnancy/Breast-feeding

NSAIDs may cross into fetal blood circulation. They have not been found to cause birth defects, but may affect fetal heart development during the second half of pregnancy. Pregnant women should not take naproxen without their doctor's approval, particularly during the last 3 months of pregnancy. When the drug is considered crucial by your doctor, its potential benefits must be carefully weighed against its risks.

NSAIDs may pass into breast milk but have caused no problems in breast-fed infants, except for seizures in a baby whose mother was taking the NSAID indomethacin. Other NSAIDs have caused problems in animal studies. There is a possibility that a nursing mother taking naproxen could affect her baby's heart or cardiovascular system. If you must take naproxen, talk to your doctor about bottle-feeding your baby.

Seniors

Seniors may be more susceptible to naproxen side effects, especially ulcer disease.

Generic Name

Nedocromil (neh-DOK-ruh-mil)

Brand Name

Tilade

Type of Drug

Antiasthmatic.

Prescribed for

Mild to moderate bronchial asthma.

General Information

Nedocromil sodium is an anti-inflammatory agent that is inhaled in order to prevent bronchial asthma by minimizing the body's usual response to asthma-triggering inhaled substances. The drug does not have specific effects of its own that would treat or prevent asthma; it works only by limiting the body's response. Very little of this drug is absorbed into the blood after it has been inhaled into your lungs. Clinical studies have shown that nedocromil improves asthma symptoms and lung function when used with an inhaled bronchodilator as needed.

Cautions and Warnings

Nedocromil should never be used to treat an **acute asthma attack**. It can be used only to prevent or reduce the number of asthma attacks and their intensity.

Do not use this product if you are **allergic** to nedocromil or to any of the ingredients in the aerosol.

People taking **corticosteroids**, either inhaled or oral, may still need them after starting on nedocromil; however, the daily corticosteroid dose will likely be reduced.

Cough or **bronchial spasm** may occasionally occur after the inhalation of a nedocromil dose. If this happens, stop taking the drug and talk to your doctor about using a different medication.

Possible Side Effects

This drug is generally very well tolerated.

▼ Most common: coughing, sore throat, runny nose, upper respiratory infection, bronchospasm, nausea, headache, chest pain, and unpleasant taste.

▼ Less common: increased sputum production, distressed breathing, bronchitis, vomiting, upset stomach, diarrhea, abdominal pain, dry mouth, dizziness, hearing disturbances, fatigue, and viral infections.

Possible Side Effects *(continued)*

▼ Rare: rash, arthritis, tremors, a feeling of warmth, and liver inflammation.

Drug Interactions

None known.

Food Interactions

Make sure you have nothing in your mouth when you inhale nedocromil.

Usual Dose

Adult and Child (age 12 and over): 2 puffs 3–4 times a day. Each puff provides 1.75 mg of nedocromil.

Overdosage

There is little potential for serious effects from an overdose of this drug. Call your local poison control center or hospital emergency room for more information.

Special Information

Nedocromil is taken to prevent or minimize severe asthma attacks. It is imperative that you take this medication on a regular basis to maintain its protection. Follow the directions in the instructional leaflet that comes with the aerosol. Store the drug at room temperature.

Call your doctor if you develop wheezing, coughing, or an allergic drug reaction. Other side effects should be reported if they are severe or bothersome. Report any symptoms that do not improve or that worsen while you are taking this drug.

Nedocromil's effectiveness depends on taking it regularly. If you forget a dose of nedocromil, take it as soon as you remember and space the remaining doses equally throughout the rest of the day. Do not take a double dose. Call your doctor if symptoms of your condition return because you have skipped too many doses.

Special Populations

Pregnancy/Breast-feeding

There are no reports of birth defects with nedocromil. However, pregnant women should not use nedocromil unless its advantages have been carefully weighed against possible dangers.

It is not known if nedocromil passes into breast milk. No drug-related problems have been known to occur, but nursing mothers who use nedocromil should be cautious.

Seniors

No special problems have been reported.

Generic Name

Nefazodone (neh-FAZ-oe-don)

Brand Name

Serzone

Type of Drug

Antidepressant.

Prescribed for

Depression.

General Information

Nefazodone is a unique compound whose chemical structure is unrelated to other antidepressant drugs. Nefazodone interferes with the ability of nerve endings in the brain to take up serotonin and norepinephrine, two key neurohormones. Nefazodone is rapidly absorbed, but about 80% of each dose is quickly broken down during its first pass through the liver. Severe liver disease may increase the amount of nefazodone in the body by 25%. Very little of the drug is released through the kidneys.

Cautions and Warnings

The possibility of **suicide** must always be considered in severely depressed people. Persons taking this drug who are at high risk for suicide should be carefully watched at all times until their condition has significantly improved.

People with a history of **seizure disorders** may experience seizures while taking nefazodone.

Recent **heart attack** patients should use this drug with caution because it can substantially reduce heart rate.

Possible Side Effects

▼ Most common: weakness, dry mouth, nausea, constipation, blurred or abnormal vision, tiredness, dizziness, light-headedness, and confusion.

▼ Common: upset stomach, increased appetite, cough, memory loss, tingling in the hands or feet, flushing or feelings of warmth, poor muscle coordination, and dizziness when rising from a lying or sitting position.

▼ Less common: low blood pressure, fever, chills, flu-like symptoms, joint pain, stiff neck, itching, rash, diarrhea, nausea, vomiting, thirst, sore throat, changes in sense of taste, ringing or buzzing in the ear, unusual dreams, poor coordination, tremors, muscle stiffness, reduced sex drive, urinary difficulties including infection, vaginitis, and breast pain.

▼ Rare: drug allergy, feeling unwell, swelling, sensitivity to the sun, pelvic pain, hernia, bad breath, high blood pressure, dizziness, angina pain, periodontal abcess, gum disease, abnormal liver tests, tongue swelling, difficulty swallowing, stomach bleeding, liver inflammation, arthritis, eye pain, impotence, and breast enlargement.

Drug Interactions

• People taking nefazodone within 2 weeks after having taken a monoamine oxidase inhibitor (MAOI) antidepressant may experience severe reactions including high fever, muscle rigidity or spasm, mental changes, and fluctuations in pulse, temperature, and breathing rate. People stopping nefazodone should wait at least 1 week before starting an MAOI.

• Nefazodone increases blood levels of astemizole and terfenadine, two nonsedating antihistamines, which may lead to cardiac side effects associated with those drugs. Nefazodone may increase blood levels of alprazolam and triazolam, two benzodiazepine anti-anxiety drugs. Lorazepam, another benzodiazepine drug, was not affected by nefazodone. Do not combine these drugs with nefazodone.

• Blood levels of digoxin may be substantially increased by nefazodone. People taking these drugs together should have their digoxin blood levels checked periodically.

• The clearance of haloperidol, an antipsychotic drug, may be drastically reduced by nefazodone; the implications of this are not clear.

• Combining nefazodone with propranolol may cause substantial reductions in propranolol blood levels and substantial increases in nefazodone blood levels. Do not take these 2 drugs together.

• Drinking alcohol while taking nefazodone may make you very tired; avoid this combination.

Food Interactions

Food delays the absorption of nefazodone and may reduce nefazodone blood levels by 20%. Take this drug on an empty stomach, at least 1 hour before or 2 hours after meals.

Usual Dose

Adult: 100 mg twice a day to start. Dosage may be increased by 100 mg a week to a maximum daily dose of approximately 600 mg.

Senior: Start at half the regular adult dose and increase as needed up to 600 milligrams a day.

Child (under age 18): not recommended.

Overdosage

Symptoms of nefazodone overdose include nausea, vomiting, and sleepiness. There are no reports of death due to nefazodone overdose. Nevertheless, overdose victims should be taken to a hospital emergency room for treatment. ALWAYS bring the prescription bottle or container with you.

Special Information

Several weeks of treatment may be needed to see the effects of nefazodone. Continue taking the medication during this period even though you may see no changes. Be sure to continue taking it once changes have taken place.

Call your doctor at once if you develop hives, rash, or other allergic side effects while taking nefazodone.

Nefazodone may make you drowsy. Be careful when driving, performing complex tasks, or operating equipment. Avoid alcoholic beverages.

Check with your pharmacist or doctor before you take any over-the-counter medication because of the possibility of drug interactions with nefazodone.

Special Populations

Pregnancy/Breast-feeding

Animal studies with large doses of this drug have indicated

the possibility of decreased fertility and increased risk to the fetus, but no human data are available. Pregnant women or women who may become pregnant should take nefazodone only if it is absolutely necessary.

It is not known if nefazodone or its by-products pass into breast milk. Women who must take this drug while breast-feeding should watch their infants for possible side effects.

Seniors

Seniors, especially women, have difficulty breaking nefazodone down and should start treatment at half the usual dose. Dosage may be gradually increased as needed, up to the maximum recommended dosage.

Generic Name

Nelfinavir (nel-FIN-uh-vere)

Brand Name

Viracept

Type of Drug

Protease inhibitor.

Prescribed for

Human immunodeficiency virus (HIV) infection.

General Information

Part of the triple-drug cocktail responsible for the most important gains in the fight against acquired immuno-deficiency syndrome (AIDS), nelfinavir belongs to a group of anti-HIV drugs called protease inhibitors. Triple-drug cocktails are considered responsible for the first overall reduction in the AIDS death rate, recorded in 1996. When the HIV virus attacks a cell, it must be converted into viral DNA. Older drugs known as reverse transcriptase inhibitors interfered with this step but are inferior to protease inhibitors. Protease inhibitors work at the end of the process of HIV reproduction, at the point when proteins are "cut" into strands of exactly the right size to duplicate HIV; these proteins are cut by protease enzymes. Protease inhibitors prevent the mature HIV virus from being formed by interfering with this cutting process. Proteins that are cut to the wrong length or remain uncut are inactive. Protease inhibitors are not a cure for HIV infection or AIDS.

Protease inhibitors are always taken with 1 or 2 nucleoside antiviral drugs such as AZT, ddI, ddC, or 3TC. Protease inhibitors revolutionized HIV treatment because, when taken in combination with other drugs, they reduce the amount of HIV virus in the bloodstream to levels that are often undetectable by current methods such as CD_4 cell counts of immune system cells and viral load (amount of virus in the blood) measurements. Multiple-drug therapy has changed the current view of HIV disease from a fatal disease to a manageable chronic (long-term) illness.

People taking a protease inhibitor may still develop infection or other conditions normally associated with HIV disease. Because of this, it is very important for you to remain under the care of a doctor or other health care provider. The long-term effects of nelfinavir are not known. You may be able to transmit the HIV virus to others even if you are on triple-drug therapy.

Cautions and Warnings

Do not take nelfinavir if you are **allergic** to it. People with **liver disease** or **cirrhosis** break down nelfinavir more slowly than do those with normal liver function.

Nelfinavir may raise **blood sugar**, worsen **diabetes**, or bring out latent diabetes. Diabetics who take nelfinavir may have to have the dosage of their antidiabetes medication adjusted for this effect.

Possible Side Effects

▼ Most common: diarrhea.

▼ Common: liver inflammation.

▼ Less common: nausea, abdominal pain, stomach gas, weakness, and rash.

▼ Rare: Other side effects may occur in almost any body part or system. These include back pain, fever, allergic reaction, headache, feeling unwell, appetite loss, upset stomach, stomach bleeding, mouth sores, vomiting, pancreas inflammation, anemia, low blood platelets,

---

Possible Side Effects *(continued)*

arthritis, muscle cramp or pain, muscle ache, weakness, anxiety, depression, dizziness, emotional instability, stimulation, sleeplessness, migraine, tingling in the hands or feet, seizure, suicidal thoughts, sleepiness, breathing difficulties, sore throat, runny nose, sinus irritation, itching, sweating, kidney stones, sexual problems, and eye disorders.

Drug Interactions

• Anticonvulsant medication such as carbamazepine, phenytoin, or phenobarbital may reduce the amount of nelfinavir in the blood.

• Combining nelfinavir with indinavir or saquinavir, other protease inhibitors, results in large increases in the amounts of both drugs in the blood. Other drugs that increase the amount of nelfinavir in the blood are ketoconazole and ritonavir.

• Combining rifabutin with nelfinavir lowers the amount of nelfinavir in the blood and raises the amount of rifabutin. Rifabutin dosage should be cut in half when this combination is used.

• Combining rifampin and nelfinavir significantly reduces the amount of nelfinavir in the blood. Do not combine these drugs.

• Nelfinavir interferes with the liver's ability to break down terfenadine and astemizole. Combining nelfinavir with these drugs may lead to severe side effects; avoid these combinations.

• Nelfinavir reduces the amount of oral contraceptive hormones in your bloodstream. Oral contraceptives may not be reliable if you are taking nelfinavir. A condom or other contraceptive method should be used.

• Combining nelfinavir, lamivudine, and zidovudine (an AIDS drug—also known as AZT) results in a reduced amount of AZT in the blood. If you are taking this combination, your AZT dosage may have to be increased.

Food Interactions

Take nelfinavir with food.

Usual Dose

Adult and Child (age 14 and over): 250 mg every 8 hours around the clock.

Child (age 2–13): 9–13 mg per lb. of body weight.

Overdosage

Consequences of nelfinavir overdose other than severe side effects are not known. Take overdose victims to a hospital emergency room for treatment. ALWAYS bring the prescription bottle or container with you.

Special Information

It is imperative for you to take your HIV medication exactly as prescribed. Missing or skipping doses of nelfinavir increases your risk of becoming resistant to the drug and losing the benefits of nelfinavir therapy.

Nelfinavir does not cure AIDS. It will not prevent you from transmitting the HIV virus to another person; you must still practice safe sex.

Diarrhea associated with nelfinavir may be controlled by using loperamide, an over-the-counter remedy.

Do not depend on oral contraceptives while taking nelfinavir. Use another contraceptive method.

Report anything unusual to your doctor.

If you forget a dose of nelfinavir, take it as soon as you remember. If it is almost time for your next dose, skip the dose you forgot and continue with your regular schedule. Do not take a double dose.

Special Populations

Pregnancy/Breast-feeding

If you are or might be pregnant while taking nelfinavir, consult your doctor. There is little information about how nelfinavir affects pregnant women or the fetus.

Nursing mothers who must take nelfinavir should bottle-feed their babies. In any case, nursing mothers should bottle-feed their babies to avoid transmitting the virus through their milk.

Seniors

Seniors may take nelfinavir without special restriction.

Brand Name

Neosporin Ophthalmic

Generic Ingredients

Gramicidin + Neomycin Sulfate + Polymyxin B Sulfate Ⓖ

Other Brand Names
AK-Spore

Type of Drug

Ophthalmic-antibiotic combination.

Prescribed for

Superficial eye infection.

General Information

Neosporin Ophthalmic is a combination of antibiotics that is effective against the most common types of eye infection. It is most useful when the infecting organism is one known to be sensitive to any of the 3 antibiotics contained in Neosporin Ophthalmic. It may also be useful when the infecting organism is not known because of the drug's broad range of coverage.

Prolonged use of any antibiotic product in the eye should be avoided because of the risk of developing sensitivity to the antibiotic. Frequent or prolonged use of antibiotics in the eye may result in the growth of other organism such as fungi. If the infection does not clear up within a few days, call your doctor.

Neosporin or its generic equivalent is also available as an eye ointment with a minor formula change—bacitracin is substituted for gramicidin. Both the eyedrops and eye ointment are used for the same kinds of eye infection.

Cautions and Warnings

Do not use Neosporin Ophthalmic if you are **allergic or sensitive** to it or any of its ingredients.

Possible Side Effects

▼ Less common: occasional eye irritation, itching, or burning.

Drug Interactions

None known.

Usual Dose

1-2 drops in the affected eye 2-4 times a day or more frequently if the infection is severe.

Overdosage

The amount of medication contained in each bottle of Neosporin Ophthalmic is too small to cause serious problems. Call your doctor, hospital emergency room, or local poison control center for more information.

Special Information

To administer eyedrops, lie down or tilt your head back. Hold the dropper above your eye, gently squeeze your lower lid to form a small pouch, and release the drop or drops of medication inside your lower lid while looking up. Release the lower lid, keeping your eye open. Do not blink for 40 seconds. Press gently on the bridge of your nose at the inside corner of your eye for 1 minute to help circulate the drug in your eye. To avoid infection, do not touch the dropper tip to your finger, eyelid, or any other surface. Wait at least 5 minutes before using another eyedrop or eye ointment.

Call your doctor if the itching or burning does not go away after a few minutes, or if redness, irritation, swelling, visual disturbance, loss of vision, or eye pain persists.

In general, you should not wear contact lenses if you have an eye infection but your doctor may determine that the use of lenses is acceptable in your situation.

If you forget to take a dose of Neosporin Ophthalmic, take it as soon as you remember. If it is almost time for your next dose, skip the forgotten dose and continue with your regular schedule. Do not take a double dose.

Special Populations

Pregnancy/Breast-feeding

This drug has been found to be safe for use during pregnancy and breast-feeding. Remember to check with your doctor before taking any drug if you are pregnant.

Seniors

Seniors may take this drug without special restriction.

Generic Name

Nevirapine (nev-EYE-ruh-pene)

Brand Name

Viramune

Type of Drug

Antiviral.

Prescribed for

Human immunodeficiency virus (HIV), specifically HIV-1 infection in adults whose condition has deteriorated on other anti-HIV treatments.

General Information

Nevirapine is a non-nucleoside reverse transcriptase inhibitor (NNRTI). Nevirapine inhibits the reverse transcriptase (RT) enzyme, necessary for reproduction of HIV in body cells, by binding directly to it. The duration of any benefit from taking this drug may be limited because HIV can become resistant to nevirapine. In one study of nevirapine plus zidovudine (AZT), resistance began to develop in some people as soon as 2 weeks after treatment began. For this reason, nevirapine is generally prescribed as part of an anti-HIV "cocktail" of 2 or 3 antivirals.

HIV that is resistant to one NNRTI—including nevirapine—may also be resistant to other NNRTIs. Cross resistance is unlikely between nevirapine and the protease inhibitor antivirals. Information on cross resistance between NNRTIs and nucleoside-type antivirals is limited.

Nevirapine is readily absorbed into the blood after it is swallowed. It is broken down in the liver by the same enzyme systems that break down other drugs, although the effect of liver or kidney disease in nevirapine treatment is not known. One small study of nevirapine in people of different races showed no differences in blood levels; other possible effects of ethnicity on nevirapine have not been studied.

Cautions and Warnings

People who are **allergic or sensitive** to nevirapine should avoid it.

Severe and potentially fatal **skin reactions** may develop in people taking this drug, including Stevens-Johnson syndrome (symptoms include fever, skin blisters, mouth sores, eye irritation, swelling, muscle or joint aches, and not feeling well). Call your doctor at once if any of these symptoms or any other skin reactions develop. Most rashes occur within the first 6 weeks of nevirapine treatment.

If adding nevirapine to your anti-HIV treatment does not help or your condition continues to worsen, further changes in your treatment program may be needed.

Possible Side Effects

▼ Most common: rash, fever, nausea, headache, and changes in liver function tests.

▼ Less common: abdominal pain, mouth or throat sores, tingling in the hands or feet, muscle aches, and liver inflammation.

▼ Rare: diarrhea, pain, and changes of sensation in the arms or legs.

Drug Interactions

• Rifampin and rifabutin may stimulate liver enzymes that break down nevirapine, reducing the amount of nevirapine in the blood. Neither of these drugs should be combined with nevirapine.

• The enzyme systems that break down protease inhibitors are stimulated by nevirapine. Combining nevirapine and a protease inhibitor may reduce the amount of protease inhibitor in the blood, reducing its effectiveness and increasing the chance of protease inhibitor resistance.

• Combining nevirapine with an oral contraceptive may reduce the effectiveness of the contraceptive by lowering the amount of hormone in the blood.

Food Interactions

None known.

Usual Dose

Adult: Starting dose—200 mg a day for 2 weeks. Maintenance dose—200 mg twice a day in combination with a nucleoside-type antiviral, such as didanosine and AZT.

Child: not recommended.

Overdosage

The effects of nevirapine overdose are not well known. One person who took a nevirapine overdose did not experience any problems. Call your local emergency room or poison control center for more information. ALWAYS bring the prescription bottle or container with you if you take an overdose victim to the emergency room.

Special Information

Call your doctor at once if you develop any rash or other skin side effect (see "Cautions and Warnings").

Nevirapine does not cure AIDS. It will not prevent you from transmitting HIV to another person; you must still practice safe sex.

Take nevirapine according to your doctor's direction; this is very important in preventing the development of drug-resistant HIV. If you do forget a dose of nevirapine, take it as soon as you remember. If it almost time for your next dose, skip the dose you forgot and continue with your regular schedule. If you do not take your nevirapine for a week, you will have to start the treatment program all over again, beginning with 200 mg a day for 2 weeks.

Special Populations

Pregnancy/Breast-feeding

Animal studies of the use of nevirapine during pregnancy showed no effects, but the drug's effect on pregnant women is not known. When this drug is considered crucial by your doctor, its potential benefits must be weighed against its risks.

Nevirapine passes into breast milk. In any case, mothers who are HIV positive should bottle-feed their babies to avoid transmitting the virus through their milk.

Seniors

Seniors may take nevirapine without special restriction.

Generic Name

Niacin (NYE-uh-sin) Ⓖ

Brand Names

Niacor   Nicolar

Type of Drug

Vitamin.

Prescribed for

Pellagra (niacin deficiency); also prescribed for high blood levels of cholesterol and triglycerides and to dilate (widen) blood vessels.

General Information

Niacin, also known as vitamin B_3 and nicotinic acid, is essential to normal body function through the part it plays in enzyme activity. It is effective in lowering blood fat levels and helps to dilate blood vessels, but we do not know exactly how it works. The effect of niacin on blood fats is seen as early as 1 week after treatment is started. Normally, individual requirements of niacin are easily supplied in a balanced diet.

Some experts have suggested using megadoses of niacin in the treatment of schizophrenia although there is no good evidence for this use.

Cautions and Warnings

Do not take niacin if you are **sensitive or allergic** to it or to any related drugs or if you have **liver disease, stomach ulcer, severely low blood pressure, gout,** or **hemorrhage (bleeding)**.

When you are taking niacin in therapeutic dosages, your doctor should periodically check your liver function and blood-sugar level. Diabetics may experience an **increase in blood sugar**.

Blood levels of uric acid may rise; people who are prone to gout may experience an attack.

Possible Side Effects

▼ Most common: flushing, which may occur within 2 hours of taking the first dose of niacin.

▼ Less common: decreased sugar tolerance in diabetics, activation of stomach ulcer, jaundice (symptoms include yellowing of the skin or whites of the eyes), upset stomach, oily or dry skin, aggravation of skin conditions such as acne, itching, high blood levels of uric acid, low

---

Possible Side Effects *(continued)*

blood pressure, headache, tingling feeling in the hands or feet, rash, abnormal heartbeats, and dizziness.

Drug Interactions

• Niacin may intensify the effect of blood-pressure-lowering drugs, causing postural hypotension (dizziness when rising quickly from a sitting or lying position).

• Niacin may interfere with the effect of sulfinpyrazone (a gout medication).

• Combining lovastatin taken together with niacin may lead to the destruction of skeletal-muscle cells. One case of this interaction has been reported.

Food Interactions

Take niacin with or after meals to reduce the risk of upset stomach.

Usual Dose

Vitamin Supplement: 25 mg a day.

Niacin Deficiency: not more than 100 mg a day.

Pellagra: not more than 500 mg a day.

High Blood-Fat Levels: Initial dose, 1–2 g 3 times a day to start; take with a glass of cold water to help you swallow. The dosage should be increased slowly to the maximum so you can watch for side effects.

Overdosage

Symptoms of overdose may include side effects (see "Possible Side Effects"). Take the victim to a hospital emergency room for treatment. ALWAYS bring the prescription bottle or container with you.

Special Information

Skin reactions may occur within 2 hours after taking the first niacin dose and may include flushing and warmth, especially in the face, ears, or neck; tingling; and itching. Headache may also occur. Call your doctor if these effects do not disappear as you continue taking niacin.

If you forget to take a dose of niacin, take it as soon as you remember. If it is almost time for your next dose, skip the missed dose and continue with your regular schedule. Do not take a double dose.

Special Populations

Pregnancy/Breast-feeding
When used in normal dosages, niacin may and should be taken by pregnant women as part of a prenatal vitamin formulation. But if it is used in high dosages—to help lower blood-fat levels—there may be problems.

Although this drug has not been shown to cause birth defects or problems in breast-fed infants, consult with your doctor about taking high dosages of niacin if you are nursing.

Seniors
Seniors may take this medication without special restriction. Follow your doctor's directions and report any side effects at once.

Generic Name

Nicardipine (nye-KAR-dih-pene)

Brand Name
Cardene

Type of Drug
Calcium channel blocker.

Prescribed for
Angina pectoris, high blood pressure, and congestive heart failure.

General Information
Nicardipine hydrochloride is one of many calcium channel blockers available in the U.S. These drugs block the passage of calcium, an essential factor in muscle contraction, into the heart and smooth muscles. Such blockage of calcium interferes with the contraction of these muscles, which in turn dilates (widens) the veins and vessels that supply blood to them. This action has several beneficial effects. Because

arteries are dilated, they are less likely to spasm. In addition, because blood vessels are dilated, both blood pressure and the amount of oxygen used by the heart muscle are reduced. Nicardipine is therefore useful in treating not only high blood pressure but also angina pectoris (brief attacks of chest pain), a condition related to poor oxygen supply to the heart muscle. Other calcium channel blockers are prescribed for abnormal heart rhythm, heart failure, cardiomyopathy (loss of blood-pumping ability due to damaged heart muscle), and diseases that involve blood-vessel spasm, such as migraine headache and Raynaud's syndrome.

Nicardipine affects the movement of calcium only into muscle cells; it has no effect on calcium in the blood.

Cautions and Warnings

Nicardipine can **slow your heart rate** and interfere with normal electrical conduction in heart muscle. For some people, this action can result in temporary heart stoppage, but such a reaction will not occur in people whose hearts are otherwise healthy.

You should not use nicardipine if you have had a **stroke** or bleeding in the brain or if you have advanced **hardening of the arteries**—particularly the aorta—because the drug can cause heart failure.

People who take nicardipine for congestive **heart failure** should be aware that the drug may aggravate the condition by reducing the effectiveness of the heart in pumping blood.

If you are also taking a **beta blocker**, its dosage should be reduced gradually rather than stopped abruptly when starting on nicardipine.

Nicardipine dosage should be adjusted in the presence of **kidney or liver disease**, since both can prolong the release of nicardipine from the body.

Nicardipine may cause **angina** when treatment is first started, when dosage is increased, or if the drug is rapidly withdrawn. This can be avoided by reducing dosage gradually.

Studies of calcium channel blockers—usually those taken several times a day, not those taken only once daily—have shown that people taking them are more likely to have a **heart attack** than are people taking beta blockers or other medication for the same purposes. Discuss this with your doctor to be sure you are receiving the best possible treatment.

Possible Side Effects

The side effects of calcium channel blockers are generally mild and rarely cause people to stop taking them.

▼ Most common: dizziness or light-headedness; fluid accumulation in the hands, legs, or feet; headache; weakness or fatigue; heart palpitations; angina; and facial flushing.

▼ Less common: low blood pressure; abnormal heart rhythms; fainting; increase or decrease in heart rate; heart failure; nausea; skin rash; nervousness; tingling in the hands or feet; hallucinations; temporary memory loss; difficulty sleeping; weakness; diarrhea; vomiting; constipation; upset stomach; itching; unusual sensitivity to the sun; painful or stiff joints; liver inflammation; increased urination, especially at night; infection; allergic reactions; sore throat; and hyperactivity.

Drug Interactions

• Combining nicardipine with a beta-blocking drug in order to treat high blood pressure is usually well tolerated, but may lead to heart failure in susceptible people.

• Blood levels of cyclosporine may be increased by nicardipine, increasing the chance for cyclosporine-related kidney damage.

• The effect of quinidine (an antiarrhythmic) may be altered by nicardipine.

• Cimetidine and ranitidine may increase the amount of nicardipine in the bloodstream.

• Combining nicardipine with fentanyl (a narcotic pain reliever) may cause very low blood pressure.

Food Interactions

Nicardipine is best taken on an empty stomach, at least 1 hour before or 2 hours after meals, but it may be taken with food or milk if it upsets your stomach.

Avoid high-fat meals while on this drug, since such a meal taken up to 3 hours after a dose of nicardipine can significantly reduce the amount of medication absorbed into the bloodstream. Do not drink grapefruit juice if you are taking nicardipine.

Usual Dose

Immediate-release: 20–40 mg 3 times a day. People with kidney disease should take 20 mg 3 times a day. People with liver disease should take 20 mg 2 times a day. Seniors should start with 20 mg 2–3 times a day and increase dosage gradually.

Sustained-release: 30–60 mg 2 times a day. People with kidney disease should take 30 mg 2 times a day.

Overdosage

The major symptoms of nicardipine overdose are very low blood pressure and reduced heart rate. Nicardipine can be removed from the victim's stomach by inducing vomiting with ipecac syrup—available at any pharmacy. This must be done within 30 minutes of the actual overdose, before the drug can be absorbed into the blood. Once symptoms develop or if more than 30 minutes have passed since the overdose, the victim must be taken to an emergency room. ALWAYS bring the prescription bottle or container with you.

Special Information

Call your doctor if you develop any of the following symptoms: worsening angina pain; swelling of the hands, legs, or feet; severe dizziness; constipation or nausea; or very low blood pressure.

Some people may experience a slight increase in blood pressure just before their next dose is due. You will be able to see this effect only if you use a home blood-pressure-monitoring device. If this happens, contact your doctor.

If you take nicardipine 3 times a day and forget a dose, take it as soon as you remember. If it is almost time for your next dose, take it and space the remaining doses evenly throughout the rest of the day. If you take nicardipine 2 times a day and forget a dose, take it as soon as you remember. If it is almost time for your next dose, skip the dose you forgot and continue with your regular schedule. Never take a double dose.

Special Populations

Pregnancy/Breast-feeding

In animal studies, large doses of nicardipine have been shown to harm the fetus. Nicardipine should be avoided by women who are or might be pregnant. When your doctor considers this drug crucial, its potential benefits must be carefully weighed against its risks.

Nicardipine passes into breast milk; nursing mothers should consider bottle-feeding their babies if they must take this drug.

Seniors

Seniors may be more sensitive to the side effects of nicardipine. Because of the possibility of reduced kidney and/or liver function in older adults, they should receive lower doses (see "Usual Dose").

Generic Name

Nicotine (NIK-uh-tene)

Brand Names

Habitrol	Nicotrol NS
Nicoderm CQ	ProStep
Nicorette	

Type of Drug

Smoking deterrent.

Prescribed for

Addiction to cigarettes in people who need another source of nicotine to help break the smoking habit. Nicotine gum has been prescribed with haloperidol for children with Tourette's syndrome.

General Information

Nicotine affects many brain functions: It improves memory, increases one's ability to perform a number of different tasks, reduces hunger, and increases tolerance to pain. Nicotine replacement products are prescribed for short-term treatment and make cigarette withdrawal much easier for many people.

Although these products are designed to fulfill a specific need in those trying to quit smoking, there are a great many other social and psychological needs filled by smoking. These must be dealt with through counseling or other psychological support in order for a program to be successful.

The major advantage of nicotine patches over chewing gum or nasal spray is their convenience and ease of use. Although a specific amount of nicotine is delivered through the skin directly into the blood, there are differences among the various patch products in terms of how much nicotine is absorbed. All of the products are labeled according to the amount of nicotine actually absorbed into the blood. Obese men absorb significantly less nicotine into their blood.

Each dose of the nasal spray contains 1 mg of nicotine, which is rapidly absorbed into the bloodstream. The spray should be used at least 8 times a day to ease symptoms of nicotine withdrawal.

You may be addicted to nicotine if you smoke more than 15 cigarettes a day; prefer unfiltered cigarettes or those with a high nicotine content; usually inhale the smoke; have your first cigarette within 30 minutes of getting up in the morning; find the first morning cigarette the hardest to give up; smoke most frequently in the morning hours; find it hard to obey "no smoking" rules; or smoke even when you are sick in bed.

Cautions and Warnings

Do not use nicotine if you are **sensitive or allergic** to it or to any component of nicotine replacement product.

Nicotine should be used only by smokers or others who are addicted to nicotine. It should not be used during the period immediately following a **heart attack** or if severe **abnormal heart rhythms** or **angina pains** are present.

People with severe **temporomandibular joint (TMJ) disease** should not chew nicotine gum.

People with other **heart conditions** must be evaluated by a cardiologist before starting treatment with nicotine. Liver disease or severe kidney disease may affect how the body breaks down or eliminates nicotine.

Nicotine should be used with caution by **diabetics** being treated with insulin and by people with an **overactive thyroid, kidney or liver disease, pheochromocytoma, hypertension (high blood pressure), stomach ulcer,** or **chronic dental problems** that might be worsened by nicotine chewing gum.

The nasal spray should not be used by people who suffer from **asthma, bronchospasm, allergic rhinitis,** or **sinusitis** or who have nasal polyps.

It is possible for nicotine addiction to be transferred from cigarettes to the nicotine replacement product or for the addiction to worsen while using the product.

Possible Side Effects

Chewing Gum

▼ Most common: injury to gums, jaw, or teeth; sore mouth or throat; stomach growling due to swallowing air while chewing.

▼ Common: nausea, vomiting, upset stomach, and hiccups.

▼ Less common: excessive salivation, dizziness, lightheadedness, irritability, headache, increased bowel movement, diarrhea, constipation, gas pain, dry mouth, hoarseness, flushing, sneezing, coughing, sleeplessness, swelling of the arms or legs, hypertension, heart palpitations, rapid and abnormal heartbeat, confusion, convulsions, depression, euphoria (feeling high), numbness, tingling in the hands or feet, ringing or buzzing in the ears, fainting, weakness, skin redness, itching, and rash.

Transdermal Patch

▼ Most common: tiredness and irritation at the patch site. Transdermal systems may be more irritating to people with eczema or other skin conditions.

▼ Common: weakness, back pain, body ache, diarrhea, upset stomach, headache, sleeplessness, dizziness, nervousness, unusual dreams, increased cough or sore throat, muscle and joint pain, changes in sense of taste, and painful menstruation.

▼ Less common: chest pain, allergic reaction (symptoms include hives, breathing difficulties, and peeling skin), dry mouth, abdominal pain, vomiting, tiredness, poor concentration, tingling in the hands or feet, sinus irritation or inflammation, increased sweating, and hypertension.

Nasal Spray

▼ Most common: nose, throat, and eye irritation.

Drug Interactions

• Heavy smokers who suddenly stop smoking may experience an increase in the effects of drugs whose breakdown is known to be stimulated by cigarettes. If you are taking any of the following medications, your dosage may have to be reduced to account for this effect: acetaminophen, theophyl-

line, imipramine, pentazocine, furosemide, oxazepam, propranolol, and propoxyphene hydrochloride.

• Smoking increases the rate at which your body breaks
down caffeine. Stopping nicotine may make you more sensitive to the effects of caffeine in coffee or tea.

• Any drug that affects the nervous system—either blockers or stimulants—may be affected by nicotine because of its
effect on levels of certain circulating hormones naturally
produced by the body. Your doctor should monitor for any
dosage adjustments that may be needed during nicotine
therapy.

• Smoking may reduce the effects of furosemide (a diuretic) on your body. Once you stop smoking, the drug's
effect may increase and your dosage may need adjustment.

• The absorption of glutethimide (a sleeping pill) may be
increased when you stop smoking. Also, more insulin may be
absorbed into the blood after each injection. Your doctor may
have to recheck your insulin dosage after you stop smoking.

• More propoxyphene (a pain reliever) may be absorbed by
the blood after you stop smoking, increasing the risk of side
effects.

Food Interactions

Caffeine containing food and drinks may interfere with the
absorption of nicotine from the chewing gum product.

Do not eat or drink anything while or immediately after you
chew nicotine gum.

Usual Dose

Chewing Gum: 1 piece of gum whenever you feel the urge
for a cigarette; do not chew more than 30 pieces of gum a day.
Gradually reduce the number of pieces you chew and the
time you chew each piece every 4–7 days. Substituting
sugarless gum for nicotine gum may help in the process of
gradual dosage reduction. Each piece contains 2–4 mg of
nicotine.

Transdermal Patch: Apply the nicotine patch to the skin as
soon as you remove it from the package. Nicotrol patches
should be placed when you get up in the morning and
removed at bedtime. Prescription nicotine patches should be
left on for 24 hours at a time. Use a different skin site when
you put on a new patch each day. The dosage of the patch will
be gradually reduced by your doctor to help wean you off
nicotine.

Nasal Spray: 1 or 2 sprays in each nostril up to five times an hour. Do not use more than 40 doses a day.

Overdosage

Nicotine overdosage may be deadly. Symptoms include excessive salivation, nausea, vomiting, diarrhea, abdominal pain, headache, cold sweats, dizziness, hearing and visual disturbances, weakness, and confusion. If untreated, these symptoms will be followed by fainting; very low blood pressure; a pulse that is weak, rapid, and irregular; convulsions; and death by paralysis of the muscles that control breathing. The lethal dose of nicotine is about 50 mg.

Nicotine stimulates the brain's vomiting center, making this reaction common but not automatic. Spontaneous vomiting may be sufficient to remove the poison from the victim's system. If this has not occurred, call your doctor or poison control center for instructions on how to make the victim vomit by giving ipecac syrup—available at any pharmacy. If the victim must be treated in a hospital emergency room, ALWAYS bring the nicotine package with you.

Special Information

Follow the instruction on the patient-information sheet included in each package. Chew each piece of gum slowly and intermittently for about 30 minutes to promote slow and even absorption of the nicotine through the tissues in your mouth. Too-rapid chewing releases the nicotine too quickly and may lead to side effects including nausea, hiccups, and throat irritation. Follow directions for gradually reducing your chewing time and substituting or reducing the number of pieces of nicotine gum you chew each day.

You will learn to control your daily dosage of nicotine chewing gum so that your smoking habit is broken and side effects are minimized. Do not chew more than 30 pieces of gum a day. The amount of gum chewed should be gradually reduced and stopped after 3 months of successful treatment.

When administering a dose of the nasal spray, tilt your head back slightly and do not sniff or inhale through your nose. A dose consists of one spray in each nostril. Administering less than 8 doses a day may not be effective. Do not exceed 40 doses a day.

Be careful to properly store and dispose of nicotine patches and nasal spray containers—used or unused—out of the reach of children or pets to avoid accidental poisoning. Do not store nicotine patches in an area that is warmer than 86°F, because the patches are heat sensitive. Slight discoloration is not a sign of loss of potency, but do not store a patch after you have removed it from its pouch. Nicotine patches should not be used for more than 3 months at a time. The nasal spray should not be used for longer than 6 months.

Special Populations

Pregnancy/Breast-feeding

Nicotine should not be used by women who are or might be pregnant; nicotine is known to cause fetal harm when taken during the last 3 months of pregnancy. Regardless of the source, nicotine interferes with the newborn baby's ability to breathe properly. Additionally, miscarriages have occurred in women using nicotine. Be sure to use effective contraceptive measures if there is a chance you will become pregnant while using a nicotine product.

Mothers should not breast-feed while using this product because nicotine passes into breast milk and may be harmful to a growing infant. Bottle-feed your baby if you must use a product containing nicotine.

Seniors

Seniors may be more sensitive to side effects of this drug including weakness, dizziness, and body aches. Follow your doctor's directions and report any side effects at once.

Generic Name

Nifedipine (nih-FED-ih-pene) Ⓖ

Brand Names

Adalat	Procardia
Adalat CC	Procardia XL

Type of Drug

Calcium channel blocker.

Prescribed for

Angina pectoris, Prinzmetal's angina, and high blood pressure; also prescribed for migraine headache prevention, asthma, heart failure, Raynaud's disease, disorders of the esophagus, gallbladder and kidney stone attacks, severe high blood pressure triggered by pregnancy, and premature labor.

General Information

Nifedipine is one of many calcium channel blockers available in the U.S. These drugs block the passage of calcium, an essential factor in muscle contractions, into the heart and smooth muscles. Such blockage of calcium interferes with the contraction of these muscles, which in turn dilates (widens) the veins and vessels that supply blood to them. This action has several beneficial effects. Because arteries are dilated, they are less likely to spasm. In addition, because blood vessels are dilated, both blood pressure and the amount of oxygen used by the heart muscle are reduced. Nifedipine is therefore useful in treating not only high blood pressure but also angina pectoris (brief attacks of chest pain), a condition related to poor oxygen supply to the heart muscle. Other calcium channel blockers are prescribed for abnormal heart rhythm, heart failure, cardiomyopathy (loss of blood-pumping ability due to damaged heart muscle), and diseases that involve blood-vessel spasm, such as migraine headache and Raynaud's syndrome.

Nifedipine affects the movement of calcium only into muscle cells; it has no effect on calcium in the blood.

Nifedipine capsules contain liquid medication. In cases in which the drug is needed in the blood immediately, the capsules may be punctured and their content squeezed under the tongue; the medication is rapidly absorbed into the blood when taken in this manner. Thus nifedipine capsules are particularly useful when extremely high blood pressure must be lowered as quickly as possible. Some researchers assert that biting the capsule and swallowing the contents is an even faster way of absorbing the drug.

Cautions and Warnings

Nifedipine may cause unwanted **low blood pressure** in some people who take it for reasons other than hypertension.

Patients taking a beta-blocking drug who begin taking nifedipine may develop an increase in incidences of **angina** pain. Angina may also intensify when nifedipine is first started, when it is increased, or if it is stopped abruptly.

Studies have shown that people taking calcium channel

blockers—usually those taken several times a day, not those that are taken only once daily—have a greater chance of having a **heart attack** than people taking beta blockers or other medications for the same purposes. Discuss this with your doctor to be sure you are receiving the best possible treatment.

Congestive **heart failure** has, on rare occasions, developed in people taking nifedipine. This happens because the drug can reduce the efficiency of an already compromised heart.

Do not take this drug if you have had an **allergic reaction** to it in the past.

Nifedipine may interfere with one of the mechanisms by which **blood clots** form, especially if you are also taking aspirin. Call your doctor if you develop unusual bruises, bleeding, or black-and-blue marks.

People with severe **liver disease** break down nifedipine much more slowly than people with mildly diseased or normal livers. **Kidney disease** can affect the release of nifedipine from your body. Your doctor should take these issues into account when determining your nifedipine dosage.

Possible Side Effects

Nifedipine side effects are generally mild and rarely cause people to stop taking the drug.

▼ Most common: swelling of the ankles, feet, and legs; dizziness or light-headedness; flushing; a feeling of warmth; and nausea.

▼ Less common: nervousness; headache; weakness, shakiness, or jitteriness; giddiness; muscle cramps, inflammation, and pain; nervousness; mood changes; heart palpitations; heart failure; heart attack; breathing difficulties; coughing; fluid in the lungs; wheezing; stuffy nose; fever and chills; and sore throat.

▼ Rare: low blood pressure; unusual heart rhythms; angina; fainting; shortness of breath; diarrhea; cramps; constipation; stomach gas; dry mouth; taste changes; frequent urination, especially at night; stiffness and inflammation of the joints; arthritis; psychotic reaction; anxiety; memory loss; paranoia; hallucinations; tingling in the hands or feet; tiredness; muscle weakness; liver inflammation; blurred vision; ringing or buzzing in the ears; difficulty sleeping; unusual dreams; respiratory in-

Possible Side Effects *(continued)*

fections; anemia, bleeding; bruising; nosebleeds; swollen
gums; weight gain; reduced white-blood-cell counts; difficulty maintaining balance; itching; rash; hair loss; painful breast inflammation; unusual sensitivity to the sun;
severe skin reactions; fever; sweating; chills; sexual difficulties; and increases in certain blood-sugar and enzyme
tests.

Drug Interactions

• Nifedipine may interact with beta-blocking drugs to cause
heart failure, very low blood pressure, or an increased incidence of angina pain. However, in many cases these drugs
have been taken together with no problem.

• Nifedipine may cause unexpected blood pressure reduction in patients who also take other drugs to control their high
blood pressure. Low blood pressure can also result from
taking nifedipine with fentanyl (a narcotic pain reliever).

• Cimetidine and ranitidine increase the amount of nifedipine in the blood and may account for a slight increase in
nifedipine's effect.

• The combination of quinidine (an antiarrhythmic) and
nifedipine must be used with caution because it can produce
low blood pressure, very slow heart rate, abnormal heart
rhythm, and swelling in the arms or legs.

• On rare occasions, nifedipine may increase the effects of
oral anticoagulant (blood-thinning) drugs.

• Nifedipine may intensify the effects of cyclosporine,
digoxin, and theophylline products, increasing the chances of
side effects from those drugs.

Food Interactions

Avoid drinking grapefruit juice if you are taking nifedipine.

Usual Dose

Immediate-release: 10–30 mg 3 times a day. Do not exceed
180 mg a day.

Sustained-release: 30–60 mg once a day.

Do not stop taking nifedipine abruptly. The dosage should
be reduced gradually.

Overdosage

Overdose of nifedipine can cause low blood pressure. If you think you have taken an overdose of nifedipine, call your doctor or go to a hospital emergency room. ALWAYS bring the prescription bottle or container with you.

Special Information

Call your doctor if you develop constipation, nausea, very low blood pressure, worsening angina, swelling in the hands or feet, breathing difficulties, increased heart pain, or dizziness or light-headedness, or if other side effects are particularly bothersome or persistent.

If you are taking nifedipine for high blood pressure, be sure to continue taking your medication and follow any instructions for diet restriction or other treatments. High blood pressure is a condition with few recognizable symptoms; it may seem to you that you are taking medication for no good reason. Call your doctor or pharmacist if you have any questions.

If you take Procardia XL, be sure not to break or crush the tablets. You may notice an empty tablet in your stool. This is not a cause for alarm, because the drug is normally released without actually destroying the tablet.

It is important to maintain good dental hygiene while taking nifedipine and to use extra care when using your toothbrush or dental floss: The drug may make you more susceptible to some infections.

If you forget a dose of nifedipine and you take it 3 or more times a day, take it as soon as you remember. If it is almost time for your next dose, take the dose you forgot and space the rest evenly throughout the remainder of the day. If you take nifedipine 2 times a day and forget to take a dose, take it as soon as you remember. If it is almost time for your next dose, skip the dose you forgot and continue with your regular schedule. Never a double dose.

Special Populations

Pregnancy/Breast-feeding

Nifedipine crosses into the fetal blood circulation. It has been used to treat severe high blood pressure associated with pregnancy without causing any unusual effect on the fetus. Nevertheless, women who are or might be pregnant should not take nifedipine without their doctor's approval. When the drug is considered crucial by your doctor, its potential benefits must be carefully weighed against its risks.

Small amounts of nifedipine may pass into breast milk, but the drug has caused no problems among breast-fed infants. You must consider the potential effect on the nursing infant if breast-feeding while taking this medication.

Seniors

Seniors are more sensitive to the effects of nifedipine and may develop low blood pressure because the drug takes longer to pass out of their bodies. Follow your doctor's directions and report any side effects at once.

Generic Name

Nimodipine (nih-MOE-dih-pene)

Brand Name

Nimotop

Type of Drug

Calcium channel blocker.

Prescribed for

Functional losses following a stroke and migraine and cluster headaches.

General Information

Nimodipine is one of many calcium channel blockers available in the U.S. Unlike the other members of this group, nimodipine has a negligible effect on the heart. It is unique because it is the only calcium channel blocker proven to improve neurological function after a stroke. Other calcium channel blockers are prescribed for abnormal heart rhythm, heart failure, cardiomyopathy (loss of blood-pumping ability due to damaged heart muscle), and diseases that involve blood-vessel spasm, such as migraine headache and Raynaud's syndrome.

Nimodipine readily dissolves in fatty tissues and reaches very high concentrations in the brain and spinal fluid. Because of this, it has a greater effect on blood vessels in the brain than on those in other parts of the body. Nimodipine relieves stroke symptoms but does not reduce spasms in brain blood vessels. A great deal of research still needs to be done to discover exactly how this drug works.

Cautions and Warnings

Nimodipine should not be taken if you are **sensitive** or **allergic** to it.

Liver disease, including cirrhosis, may slow the body's breakdown of nimodipine. Dosage reduction may be required.

Possible Side Effects

Side effects of calcium channel blockers are generally mild and rarely cause people to stop taking them.

▼ Most common: diarrhea, low blood pressure, and headache.

▼ Less common: swelling of the arms or legs, high blood pressure, heart failure, rapid heartbeat, changes in the electrocardiogram, depression, memory loss, psychosis, paranoid feelings, hallucinations, nausea, itching, acne, rash, anemia, bleeding or bruising, abnormal blood clotting, flushing, breathing difficulties, stomach bleeding, and muscle cramps.

▼ Rare: dizziness, heart attack, liver inflammation or jaundice, vomiting, and sexual difficulties.

Drug Interactions

• Calcium channel blockers may cause bleeding when taken alone or combined with aspirin.

• Combining nimodipine with a beta-blocking drug is usually tolerated well but may lead to heart failure in susceptible people.

• Calcium channel blockers, including nimodipine, may add to the effects of digoxin; this effect is not observed with any consistency, however, and only affects people with a large amount of digoxin already in their system.

Food Interactions

Nimodipine is best taken at least 1 hour before or 2 hours after meals, but may be taken with food or milk if it upsets your stomach. Avoid drinking grapefruit juice if you are taking this drug.

Usual Dose

Stroke: 60 mg 4 times a day, beginning within 96 hours after the stroke and continuing for 21 days.

Migraine Headache: 40 mg 3 times a day.

Overdosage

The major symptoms of nimodipine overdose are nausea, weakness, dizziness, drowsiness, confusion, and slurred speech. Blood pressure and heart rate may also be affected. Nimodipine can be removed from a victim's stomach by giving ipecac syrup—available at any pharmacy—to induce vomiting, but this should be done only under a doctor's supervision or direction. Once symptoms develop, the victim must be taken to a hospital emergency room for treatment. ALWAYS bring the prescription bottle or container with you.

Special Information

Call your doctor if you develop any of the following symptoms: swelling of the arms or legs, breathing difficulties, severe dizziness, constipation, or nausea.

Patients who are unable to swallow nimodipine capsules because of their condition may have the liquid withdrawn from the capsule with a syringe, mixed with other liquids, and given orally or through a feeding tube.

If you forget a dose of nimodipine, it should be taken as soon as you remember. If it is almost time for your next dose, skip the dose you forgot and continue with your regular schedule. Call your doctor if more than two consecutive doses are missed.

Special Populations

Pregnancy/Breast-feeding

Animal studies have shown that nimodipine may cause fetal malformation. Very high doses can cause poor growth, bone problems, and death in the fetus. Nimodipine should be avoided by women who are or might be pregnant. When your doctor considers this drug crucial, its potential benefits must be carefully weighed against its risks.

In animal studies, nimodipine has been shown to pass into breast milk. Nursing mothers who must take nimodipine should bottle-feed their babies.

Seniors

Seniors, especially those with severe liver disease, may be more sensitive to the side effects of nimodipine.

Generic Name

Nisoldipine (nih-SOL-dih-pene)

Brand Name

Sular

Type of Drug

Calcium channel blocker.

Prescribed for

Hypertension (high blood pressure).

General Information

Nisoldipine is one of many calcium channel blockers available in the U.S. These drugs block the passage of calcium, an essential factor in muscle contraction, into the heart and smooth muscles. Such blockage of calcium interferes with the contraction of these muscles, which in turn dilates (widens) the veins and vessels that supply blood to them. This action has several beneficial effects. Because arteries are dilated, they are less likely to spasm. In addition, because blood vessels are dilated, both blood pressure and the amount of oxygen used by the heart muscle are reduced. Nisoldipine is therefore useful in treating not only high blood pressure but also angina pectoris (brief attacks of chest pain), a condition related to poor oxygen supply to the heart muscle. Other calcium channel blockers are prescribed for abnormal heart rhythm, heart failure, cardiomyopathy (loss of blood-pumping ability due to damaged heart muscle), and diseases that involve blood-vessel spasm, such as migraine headache and Raynaud's syndrome.

Nisoldipine affects the movement of calcium only into muscle cells; it has no effect on calcium in the blood.

Cautions and Warnings

Do not take this drug if you have had an **allergic** reaction to it or to a chemically similar calcium channel blocker. Use nisoldipine with caution if you have **heart failure**, since calcium channel blockers may worsen the condition.

On rare occasions, nisoldipine may cause very **low blood pressure.** This may lead to stimulation of the heart and rapid heartbeat and can worsen angina in some people.

Nisoldipine may cause angina pain when treatment is first started, when dosage is increased or if the drug is rapidly withdrawn. This can be avoided by reducing dosage gradually.

Studies of calcium channel blockers—usually those taken several times a day and not those taken only once daily— show that people taking them are more likely to have a **heart attack** than are people taking beta blockers or other medication for the same purposes. Discuss this with your doctor to be sure you are receiving the best possible treatment.

Nisoldipine can slow heart rate, which may exacerbate **heart failure**.

People with severe **liver disease** break down nisoldipine much more slowly than people with less severe disease or normal livers. Blood levels can be 5 times as high in people with cirrhosis as in people with a normal liver. Your doctor will take this factor into account when determining your nisoldipine dosage.

Possible Side Effects

Nisoldipine side effects are generally mild.

▼ Most common: headache and swelling in the arms or legs.

▼ Common: sore throat, flushing, sinus irritation, and heart palpitations.

▼ Less common: chest pain, nausea, and rash.

▼ Rare side effects may affect almost any body system. Report any unusual symptom to your doctor.

Drug Interactions

• Nisoldipine may interact with beta-blocking drugs to cause heart failure, very low blood pressure, or an increased incidence of angina pain. However, in most cases these drugs can be taken together with no problem.

• When nisoldipine is combined with cimetidine, blood levels of nisoldipine increase substantially.

• Quinidine reduces the amount of nisoldipine in the blood

by about 25%, but maximum levels remain unaffected. The importance of this interaction is not known.

Food Interactions

Avoid fatty foods and any grapefruit product with your nisoldipine dose. Taking nisoldipine with these foods leads to high drug blood levels.

Usual Dose

Adult: starting dose—20 mg a day. Maintenance dose—40 or 60 mg, as needed.

Seniors and People with Liver Disease: starting dose—10 mg a day. Maintenance dose—40 or 60 mg, as needed and tolerated.

Child: not recommended.

Overdosage

There have been no cases of nisoldipine overdose. Overdose of chemically similar calcium channel blockers can cause very low blood pressure. Other possible effects include nausea, dizziness, weakness, drowsiness, confusion and slurred speech, reduced heart efficiency, and unusual heart rhythms. Victims of a nisoldipine overdose should be taken to a hospital emergency room. ALWAYS bring the prescription bottle or container with you.

Special Information

Do not crush, chew, or divide nisoldipine tablets. They must be swallowed whole.

Call your doctor if you develop swelling in the arms or legs, breathing difficulties, abnormal heartbeat, increased heart pain, dizziness, constipation, nausea, dizziness, light-headedness, or very low blood pressure.

If you forget to take a dose of nisoldipine, take it as soon as you remember. If it is almost time for your next regular dose, skip the forgotten dose and continue with your regular schedule. Do not take a double dose.

Special Populations

Pregnancy/Breast-feeding

Laboratory studies found nisoldipine to affect the development of animal fetuses at doses that were also toxic to the mother. It has not been found to cause human birth defects.

Women who are or might become pregnant should not take nisoldipine without their doctor's approval. When your doctor considers nisoldipine to be crucial, its potential benefits must be carefully weighed against its risks.

It is not known if nisoldipine passes into breast milk. Women who must take it should consider bottle-feeding their babies.

Seniors

Seniors may have 2 to 3 times as much nisoldipine in their blood as do younger adults. Lower starting doses of 10 mg should be used. Headache is less common in older adults than in younger people.

Generic Name

Nitrofurantoin (NYE-troe-few-RAN-toe-in)

Brand Names

Furadantin   Macrodantin
Macrobid

Type of Drug

Urinary anti-infective.

Prescribed for

Urinary tract infections, such as pyelonephritis, pyelitis, and cystitis.

General Information

Nitrofurantoin, like several other urinary anti-infectives, including nalidixic acid (NegGram), is helpful in treating urinary tract infections because large amounts of it pass into your urine. Nitrofurantoin works by interfering with the metabolism of carbohydrates, or sugars, in the infecting bacteria. It may also affect the formation of the bacterial cell wall. This drug is only used to treat urinary tract infections caused by organisms susceptible to nitrofurantoin. It should not be used to treat infections in other parts of the body.

Cautions and Warnings

Do not take nitrofurantoin if you have **kidney disease** or if you are **allergic** to this agent.

Rarely, **severe chest pain, breathing difficulties, cough, fever,** and **chills** may develop within a few hours to 3 weeks after taking nitrofurantoin. These symptoms usually go away within 1 to 2 days after you stop taking the drug. People who take nitrofurantoin for prolonged periods of time may develop cough, breathing difficulties, and feelings of ill health after 1 to 6 months or more of treatment. Respiratory failure and death have occurred in a few cases.

Nitrofurantoin may cause a rare reaction called **hemolytic anemia.** People with a deficiency of the enzyme G-6-PD are most susceptible to this reaction and should not take nitrofurantoin.

Rarely, nitrofurantoin causes **hepatitis,** which may lead to death. This appears to be a rare drug-sensitivity reaction and is most likely to develop if you are taking long-term nitrofurantoin treatment.

Possible Side Effects

Side effects are less prominent when Macrodantin, the large-crystal form of nitrofurantoin, is used rather than Furadantin, the regular-crystal form.

▼ Most common: loss of appetite, nausea, vomiting, stomach pain, and diarrhea. Some people develop hepatitis symptoms.

▼ Less common: fever, chills, cough, chest pain, breathing difficulties, and development of fluid in the lungs. If these reactions occur in the first week of therapy, they can generally be resolved by stopping the medication. If they develop after taking nitrofurantoin for a longer period, they are considered chronic and may be more serious.

▼ Rare: rash, itching, asthmatic attacks in patients with history of asthma, drug fever, symptoms similar to arthritis, jaundice (yellowing of the whites of the eyes or skin), effects on components of the blood, headache, dizziness, drowsiness, and temporary loss of hair.

This drug is known to cause changes in white and red blood cells. It should be used only under the strict supervision of your doctor.

Drug Interactions

• Nitrofurantoin may increase other drugs' toxic effects on

the liver and can increase the chances of hemolytic anemia
if you are taking another drug associated with that condition. These include oral antidiabetes drugs, methyldopa, primaquine, procainamide, quinidine, quinine, and sulfa drugs.

• Nitrofurantoin interferes with the effect of nalidixic acid.
Do not take these drugs together.

• Sulfinpyrazone or probenecid may interfere with the
passage of nitrofurantoin through the kidneys, increasing
blood levels of the drug. This reduces the drug's effectiveness
because nitrofurantoin depends on being present in the urine
in very large quantities. Some side effects may also be
increased by this interaction.

• Anticholinergic drugs, including propantheline, may increase the amount of nitrofurantoin absorbed into the bloodstream. This does not improve nitrofurantoin's antibacterial
effect but may increase the chance of side effects.

• Magnesium, found most commonly in antacids, delays
or decreases the amount of nitrofurantoin absorbed into the
blood.

• Drugs that cause nervous system toxicity, including metronidazole, mexiletine, ethambutol, isoniazid, lindane, lincomycin, lithium, pemoline, quinacrine, and long-term high-
dose pyridoxine (vitamin B_6), should not be taken with
nitrofurantoin because of the chance that nervous system
effects may be increased.

Food Interactions

Nitrofurantoin should be taken with food to help decrease
stomach upset, loss of appetite, nausea, or other gastrointestinal symptoms. Avoid eating citrus fruits or milk products
while taking nitrofurantoin. These foods can change the
acidity of your urine and affect the drug's action.

Usual Dose

Adult: 50–100 mg 4 times a day, with meals and at bedtime.
Child (over 1 month): 2–3 mg per lb. of body weight in 4
doses.
Child (under 1 month): not recommended.

Nitrofurantoin may be used in lower doses over a long
period by people with chronic urinary infections.

Overdosage

Overdose victims should be made to vomit with ipecac

syrup—available at any pharmacy—if they have not already done so. Call your local poison control center or hospital emergency room for more information. ALWAYS bring the prescription bottle or container with you if you go for treatment.

Special Information

Call your doctor if you develop chest pains or breathing difficulties, sore throat, pale skin, unusual tiredness or weakness, dizziness, drowsiness, headache, skin rash and itching, yellow skin, achy joints, fever and chills, or numbness, tingling, or burning of the face or mouth, or if other side effects are especially persistent or bothersome.

Continue to take this medicine for at least 3 days after you stop experiencing symptoms of urinary tract infection.

Nitrofurantoin may give your urine a brownish color: This is typical and not dangerous.

The liquid form of oral nitrofurantoin can stain your teeth if you do not swallow it rapidly.

If you miss a dose of nitrofurantoin, take it as soon as possible. If it is almost time for your next dose and you take it 3 or more times a day, space the missed dose and your next dose by 2 to 4 hours, or double your next dose and then continue with your regular schedule.

Special Populations

Pregnancy/Breast-feeding

Nitrofurantoin should be taken by pregnant women only if the benefits of taking the drug outweigh any possible risks. It should never be taken by pregnant women with G-6-PD deficiency and those who are near term, because it can interfere with the immature enzyme systems of the fetus and cause hemolytic anemia. Other urinary anti-infectives are preferred in these circumstances.

This drug passes into breast milk and may affect some nursing infants, especially those who are G-6-PD deficient. You may want to bottle-feed your baby while taking nitrofurantoin.

Seniors

Seniors with kidney disease may be more sensitive to nervous system and lung effects of this drug. Also, seniors are likely to have some reduction of kidney function and may therefore require a dosage reduction. Follow your doctor's directions and report any side effects at once.

Generic Name

Nitroglycerin (nye-troe-GLIH-ser-in) Ⓖ

Brand Names

Deponit	Nitrogard
Minitran	Nitroglyn
Nitro-Bid	Nitrol
Nitrocine	Nitrong
Nitrodisc	Nitrostat
Nitro-Dur	Transderm-Nitro

Type of Drug

Antianginal agent.

Prescribed for

Chest pain associated with angina pectoris; nitroglycerin injection is also used as a treatment after a heart attack, for heart failure, and for high blood pressure.

General Information

Nitroglycerin is available in several forms: sublingual tablets, which are taken under the tongue and allowed to dissolve; capsules, which are swallowed; transmucosal tablets, which are placed between the lip or cheek and gum and allowed to dissolve; oral sprays, which are sprayed directly onto or under the tongue; transdermal patches, which deliver nitroglycerin through the skin over a 24-hour period; and ointment, which is usually spread over the chest wall or another area of the body. Patients frequently use one or more forms of nitroglycerin to prevent and/or alleviate the attacks of chest pain associated with angina.

Cautions and Warnings

You should not take nitroglycerin if you are **allergic** to it or to another nitrate product, such as isosorbide.

Because nitroglycerin will increase the pressure of fluid inside your head, it should be taken with great caution if **head trauma** or **bleeding in the head** is present.

Other conditions in which the use of nitroglycerin may be inappropriate are severe **anemia, glaucoma,** severe **liver disease, overactive thyroid, cardiomyopathy** (loss of blood-pumping ability due to damaged heart muscle), **low blood pressure,** recent **heart attack,** severe **kidney problems,** and **overactive gastrointestinal tract.**

Possible Side Effects

Most common: flushing and headache, which may be severe or persistent.

▼ Less common: dizziness and weakness. Blurred vision may occur; if it does, stop taking the drug and call your doctor. Some people exhibit a marked sensitivity to the blood-pressure-lowering effect of nitroglycerin and may experience severe responses, including nausea, vomiting, weakness, restlessness, pallor (loss of facial color), increased perspiration, and collapse. Rash may also occur.

Drug Interactions

• Avoid over-the-counter drugs containing stimulants, such as cough, cold, and allergy remedies and appetite suppressants; they may aggravate your heart disease.

• Interaction with large amounts of alcoholic beverages may rapidly lower blood pressure, resulting in weakness, dizziness, and fainting.

• Aspirin and calcium channel blockers may lead to higher nitrate blood levels and increased side effects.

• Nitroglycerin may interfere with the effects of heparin, an injectable anticoagulant drug.

• Nitrates increase the amount of dihydroergotamine absorbed into the blood, which may raise blood pressure or inhibit the effects of nitroglycerin.

Food Interactions

Do not use any oral form of nitroglycerin with food or gum in your mouth. Nitroglycerin pills intended for swallowing are best taken on an empty stomach.

Usual Dose

Use only as much as is necessary to control chest pains.

Sublingual Tablets: Since this form acts within 10–15 seconds of being taken, the drug is taken only when necessary.

Transmucosal Tablets: The tablets are placed between the upper lip and gum or between the cheek and gum and allowed to dissolve over a 3- to 5-hour period. The rate at which the tablet releases the drug is increased by touching the tablet with your tongue or by drinking a hot liquid. Insert another tablet after the previous one is dissolved, so long as you are awake.

Sustained-release Capsules and Tablets: Generally, these are used to prevent chest pain associated with angina; the dose is 1 capsule or tablet every 8–12 hours.

Ointment: 1–2 in. squeezed from the tube onto a specially marked piece of paper—some people may require as much as 4–5 in. The ointment is spread on the skin every 3–4 hours as needed for control of chest pain. The medication is absorbed through the skin. The application sites should be rotated to prevent skin inflammation and rash.

Transdermal Patch: Patches are placed on the body in a hairless spot not associated with excess movement 1 a day, left on for 12–14 hours. Doses start at 0.2–0.4 mg per hour and go to 0.8 mg. Higher doses are preferable for once-daily patch applications.

Aerosol: 1–2 sprays (0.4–0.8 mg) under or on your tongue; repeat as needed to relieve an angina attack.

Overdosage

Nitroglycerin overdose can result in low blood pressure; very rapid heartbeat; flushing; increased perspiration followed by cold, bluish, and clammy skin; headache; heart palpitations; blurred vision and other visual disturbances; dizziness; nausea; vomiting; slow and difficult breathing; slow pulse; confusion; moderate fever; and paralysis. Overdose victims should be taken to a hospital emergency room immediately. ALWAYS bring the prescription bottle or container with you.

Special Information

Do not change brands of nitroglycerin without your doctor's and pharmacist's knowledge. A different product may require a different dosage to provide the same relief.

Sublingual nitroglycerin should be acquired from your pharmacist only in the original, unopened bottle; the tablets must not be transferred to another bottle or container because they may lose potency. Close the bottle tightly after each use or the drug may evaporate from the tablets.

Sublingual nitroglycerin should be taken while you are sitting down. This form of nitroglycerin frequently produces a burning sensation under the tongue. Some people may believe this indicates that the drug is potent and will produce the desired effect, but in fact the presence or absence of this sensation has no bearing on the tablet's strength. The only way to determine whether or not the tablets are working is to take them and see if they work. If 1 tablet does not relieve your symptoms in 5 minutes, take another. If the second one does not work, take a third. If the pain continues or worsens, call your doctor and/or go to an emergency room for treatment at once.

When applying nitroglycerin ointment, do not rub or massage it into the skin. Any excess ointment should be washed from the hands after application.

People who use transdermal patches for more than 12 hours a day for an extended period can build up a tolerance to the patch and may have to return to using other forms of nitroglycerin. Nitroglycerin patches contain a significant amount of medication even after they have been used. They can be a hazard to children and small pets—be certain to dispose of them properly.

Orthostatic hypotension may become a problem if you take nitroglycerin over a long period of time. More blood stays in the extremities and less becomes available to the brain, resulting in light-headedness or faintness if you stand up suddenly. Avoid prolonged standing and be careful to stand up slowly.

If you take nitroglycerin on a regular schedule and forget a dose, take it as soon as you remember. If you use immediate-release nitroglycerin tablets and it is within 2 hours of your next dose, skip the dose you forgot and continue with your regular schedule. If you take sustained-release nitroglycerin tablets or capsules and it is within 6 hours of your next dose, skip the dose you forgot and continue with your regular schedule.

Special Populations

Pregnancy/Breast-feeding

This drug crosses into the fetal circulation but has not been found to cause birth defects. Women who are or might be pregnant should not take nitroglycerin without their doctor's approval. When the drug is considered crucial by your doctor, its potential benefits must be carefully weighed against its risks.

This drug passes into breast milk, but has caused no problems among breast-fed infants. Nevertheless, you should consider the potential effects on the infant if you breast-feed while taking this medicine.

Seniors

Seniors may take nitroglycerin without special restriction. Be sure to follow your doctor's directions. Because saliva is necessary for the absorption of sublingual nitroglycerin, seniors with reduced saliva secretion may need to use another form of nitroglycerin or add a saliva substitute; this also applies to younger people with dry mouth.

Nitrostat

see **Nitroglycerin**, page 796

Generic Name

Nizatidine (nih-ZAY-tih-dene)

Brand Names

Axid   Axid-AR

Type of Drug

Histamine H_2 antagonist.

Prescribed for

Ulcers of the stomach and duodenum (upper intestine); also used to treat gastroesophageal reflux disease (GERD).

General Information

Like the other histamine H_2 antagonists, nizatidine works by turning off the system that produces stomach acid and other secretions. Nizatidine is effective in treating the symptoms of ulcer and preventing complications of the disease, although an ulcer that does not respond to another histamine H_2 antagonist will probably not respond to nizatidine because all these drugs work in exactly the same way. Histamine H_2 antagonists differ only in their potency. Cimetidine is the least potent; 1000 mg are roughly equal to 300 mg of either nizatidine or ranitidine, or 40 mg of famotidine. All these drugs have roughly equivalent success rates in treating ulcer disease and all carry comparable chances of side effects.

Cautions and Warnings

Do not take nizatidine if you have ever had an **allergic** reaction to it or to any histamine H_2 antagonist.

People with **kidney or liver disease** should take nizatidine with caution because ⅓ of each dose is broken down in the liver and the rest passes out of the body through the kidneys.

Possible Side Effects

Side effects are infrequent.

▼ Most common: tiredness and increased sweating.

▼ Rare: headache, dizziness, confusion, sleeplessness, mild diarrhea and constipation, abdominal discomfort, nausea, vomiting, liver inflammation and jaundice (symptoms include yellowing of the skin and whites of the eyes), reduced blood-platelet levels, rash, itching, abnormal heartbeat, heart attack, painful swelling of the breast, impotence, loss of sex drive, joint pain, fever, and high uric-acid blood levels unassociated with symptoms of gout.

Drug Interactions

• Antacids, anticholinergics, and metoclopramide may slightly reduce the amount of nizatidine absorbed into the blood, but no precaution is needed.

• Enteric-coated tablets should not be taken with nizatidine. The change in stomach acidity produced by nizatidine will cause the tablets to disintegrate prematurely in the stomach.

• Nizatidine may increase blood levels of aspirin in people taking very large doses of aspirin.

Food Interactions

You may take nizatidine without regard to food or meals.

Food may slightly increase the amount of drug absorbed, but without consequence.

Usual Dose

Adult: 300 mg at bedtime or 150 mg twice a day. Dosage is reduced in people with kidney disease.

Overdosage

There is little information on nizatidine overdosage. Overdose victims might be expected to show exaggerated side effect symptoms, but little else is known. Your local poison control center may advise giving the victim ipecac syrup— available at any pharmacy—to induce vomiting and remove any drug remaining in the stomach. Victims who have definite symptoms should be taken to a hospital emergency room. ALWAYS bring the prescription bottle or container with you.

Special Information

You must take nizatidine exactly as directed and follow your doctor's instructions regarding diet and other treatment to get the maximum benefit from the drug. Antacids may be taken together with nizatidine, if needed. Cigarette smoking is known to be associated with stomach ulcer and may reverse the effect of nizatidine on stomach acid.

Call your doctor at once if any unusual side effects develop. Especially important are unusual bleeding or bruising, unusual tiredness, diarrhea, dizziness, or rash. Black or tarry stools or vomiting material that resembles coffee grounds may indicate your ulcer is bleeding.

If you empty the nizatidine capsule and mix it with juice before taking it, you may keep it in the refrigerator. Do not store it for more than 2 days because the drug may lose potency.

If you forget to take a dose of nizatidine, take it as soon as you remember. If it is almost time for your next dose, skip the one you forgot and continue with your regular schedule. Do not take a double dose.

Special Populations

Pregnancy/Breast-feeding

Studies with laboratory animals reveal no damage to the fetus, but it is recommended that nizatidine be avoided by women who are or might be pregnant. When the drug is considered crucial by your doctor, nizatidine's potential benefits must be carefully weighed against its risks.

Very small amounts of nizatidine may pass into breast milk. No problems have been identified in breast-fed babies, but nursing mothers should consider the risk of side effects in their babies.

Seniors

Seniors respond well to nizatidine. They may need lower doses to achieve results, because the drug is eliminated through the kidneys and kidney function tends to decline with age. Seniors may be more susceptible to nizatidine side effects.

Brand Name

Norgesic Forte

Generic Ingredients

Aspirin + Caffeine + Orphenadrine Citrate

Other Brand Names

Norgesic

Type of Drug

Analgesic combination.

Prescribed for

Pain of muscle spasms, sprains, strains, or back pain.

General Information

The main ingredient in Norgesic Forte is orphenadrine citrate, a pain reliever. The aspirin in Norgesic Forte adds extra pain relief.

Norgesic Forte cannot treat the cause of muscle spasm; it can only temporarily relieve the pain. You must follow any additional advice from your doctor to help solve the underlying problem.

Cautions and Warnings

Do not take Norgesic Forte if you have **glaucoma, stomach**

**ulcer, heart disease, intestinal obstruction, difficulty in pass-
ing urine,** or known **sensitivity** or **allergy** to this drug or any of
its ingredients.

Orphenadrine can make you **light-headed** or dizzy. Be
careful doing anything that requires concentration or alertness.

Norgesic Forte should not be taken by children.

Possible Side Effects

▼ Most common: dryness of the mouth.

▼ Less common: rapid heartbeat, palpitations, difficulty
in urination, blurred vision, enlarged pupils, weakness,
nausea, vomiting, headache, dizziness, constipation,
drowsiness, skin rash or itching, runny or stuffy nose,
hallucinations, agitation, tremors, and stomach upset.
These side effects increase as dosage increases.

▼ Large doses or prolonged therapy with Norgesic
Forte may lead to aspirin poisoning, (symptoms include
ringing in the ears, fever, confusion, sweating, thirst,
dimness of vision, rapid breathing, increased pulse rate,
and diarrhea).

Drug Interactions

• The aspirin in Norgesic Forte may interact with anticoagulant (blood-thinning) drugs, increase the effect of
probenecid, and increase the blood-sugar-lowering effects of
antidiabetic drugs.

• Combining Norgesic Forte with propoxyphene (Darvon)
may cause confusion, anxiety, and tremors or shaking.

• Long-term users should avoid alcohol, which may worsen
stomach upset and bleeding.

Food Interactions

Take this medication with food or at least half a glass of water
to prevent stomach upset.

Usual Dose

½–1 tablet 3–4 times a day.

Overdosage

A single dose of 40 to 60 Norgesic Forte tablets is lethal to
adults, and large overdoses below this level can rapidly

become fatal. The victim must be taken to a hospital emergency room immediately. ALWAYS bring the prescription bottle or container with you.

Special Information

Norgesic Forte may make you drowsy. Be careful while driving or operating complex or hazardous equipment.

Call your doctor if you develop skin rash or itching, rapid heart rate, palpitations, confusion, or if side effects are persistent or bothersome.

Avoid alcoholic beverages, which can increase the stomach irritation and depressive effects caused by this drug.

If you forget to take a dose of Norgesic Forte and you remember within about 1 hour of your regular time, take the dose right away. If you do not remember until later, skip the missed dose and go back to your regular schedule. Do not take a double dose.

Special Populations

Pregnancy/Breast-feeding

Taking too much aspirin late in pregnancy can decrease a newborn's weight and cause other problems. When Norgesic Forte is considered essential by your doctor, its potential benefits must be carefully weighed against its risks.

The ingredients in Norgesic Forte may pass into breast milk. Nursing mothers who must take this product should watch their infants for drug-related side effects.

Seniors

Seniors may be more sensitive to the side effects of this medication and should take the lowest effective dose of Norgesic Forte. Seniors may experience some degree of mental confusion in reaction to this medication.

Norvasc

see *Amlodipine*, page 51

Generic Name

Nystatin (nye-STAH-tin) G

Brand Names

Mycostatin   Nilstat

Type of Drug

Antifungal.

Prescribed for

Fungal infections.

General Information

Nystatin is a versatile antifungal agent that is available in a number of different dosage forms. It can be prescribed in any situation where fungus infection is a possible complication either of a disease or of a treatment. Generally, nystatin will relieve your symptoms in 1 to 3 days. Nystatin vaginal tablets effectively control troublesome and unpleasant symptoms such as itching, inflammation, and discharge. In most cases, 2 weeks of therapy is sufficient, but prolonged treatment may be necessary. It is important that you continue using this drug during menstruation. This drug has been used to prevent thrush or *Candida* infection in the newborn infant by treating the mother for 3 to 6 weeks before her due date.

Before the development of nystatin pastilles, the vaginal tablet was used as a lozenge to treat *Candida* infections of the mouth.

Cautions and Warnings

Do not take this drug if you know you may be **sensitive** or **allergic** to it. Proper diagnosis is essential for effective treatment. Do not use nystatin without first consulting your doctor.

Possible Side Effects

Nystatin is virtually nontoxic and is generally well tolerated.

Possible Side Effects *(continued)*

Oral Form
▼ Most common: nausea, upset stomach, and diarrhea may occur with large doses.

Vaginal Form
▼ Most common: intravaginal irritation; if this occurs, discontinue the drug and contact your doctor.

Drug and Food Interactions

None known.

Usual Dose

Oral Suspension or Pastilles: 200,000-600,000 units 4 or 5 times a day.

Oral Tablets: 500,000-1,000,000 units 3 times a day.

Vaginal Tablets: 1 tablet inserted high in the vagina daily for 2 weeks.

Overdosage

Nystatin overdose may cause stomach irritation or upset. Call your local poison control center for more information.

Special Information

Do not stop taking nystatin just because you begin to feel better. You must continue taking the medication as prescribed for at least 2 days after the relief of symptoms.

Some nystatin brands require storage in the refrigerator. Ask your pharmacist for specific instructions.

If you forget a dose of nystatin, take it as soon as you remember. If it is almost time for your next dose, skip the one you forgot and continue with your regular schedule. Do not take a double dose.

Special Populations

Pregnancy/Breast-feeding
Pregnant and breast-feeding women may use nystatin without special restriction.

Seniors
Seniors may use nystatin without special restriction.

Generic Name

Olanzapine (oeh-LAN-zuh-pene)

Brand Name

Zyprexa

Type of Drug

Antipsychotic.

Prescribed for

Psychotic behavior and other signs of psychotic disorders. Olanzapine should be prescribed only for people with chronic conditions.

General Information

Olanzapine is a potent antipsychotic that blocks several different chemical receptors in the brain. The exact way in which olanzapine works is not known, but its antipsychotic effect may be produced by its blockage of 2 types of receptors in the brain, those for dopamine and those for serotonin. Olanzapine tablets are well absorbed, but about 40% of each dose is broken down in the liver before it can ever reach the bloodstream. A small portion of each dose of olanzapine is eliminated through the kidneys, but most of it is broken down in the liver by the same systems that break down many other drugs.

Cautions and Warnings

Do not take olanzapine if you are **sensitive** or **allergic** to it.

Women clear olanzapine about 30% more slowly than men, but this effect is not considered a problem. Men and women can generally take the same doses of olanzapine.

Smokers clear olanzapine from their bodies about 40% faster than non-smokers because smoking stimulates systems in the liver that break down this and other drugs. Most people do not require dose adjustments, however.

People with **liver disease** may eliminate this drug more slowly from their bodies. Their drug dosage must be individualized to their needs.

A serious set of side effects known as **neuroleptic malig-**

nant syndrome (NMS) includes a high fever, convulsions, difficult or fast breathing, rapid heartbeat, and rapid pulse. This condition has been associated with antipsychotic medicines. Other symptoms of NMS include muscle rigidity, mental changes, irregular pulse or blood pressure, and increased sweating. NMS can be fatal and requires immediate medical attention.

Tardive dyskinesia (symptoms include lip smacking or puckering, puffing of the cheeks, rapid or worm-like movements of the tongue, uncontrolled chewing motions, and uncontrolled arm or leg movements) can occur and is often considered a reason to stop taking this drug. Report any of these side effects to your doctor.

In a small number of people, olanzapine can cause **dizziness** or **fainting** when rising from a sitting or standing position, especially when people start taking the drug.

Avoid being exposed to **extreme heat**, because antipsychotics can upset your body's temperature-regulating mechanism.

Swallowing problems, and particularly breathing in food intended to be swallowed, have been a problem with antipsychotics, including olanzapine.

Suicide is a danger with all psychotics. People taking this drug should be limited to a 30-day supply of medication at any time to reduce the chances of possible overdose.

Seizures occur in a small number of people taking olanzapine. Olanzapine should be taken with care if you have had seizures or other conditions that can make you more likely to have a seizure.

Possible Side Effects

Olanzapine side effects are not that different from those of an inactive placebo (sugar pill).

▼ Most common: headache, tiredness, agitation, sleeplessness, nervousness, hostility, dizziness, and runny nose.

▼ Less common: fever; abdominal, back, or chest pains; a rigid neck; dizziness or fainting when rising from a sitting or standing position; rapid heartbeat; low blood pressure; constipation,; dry mouth; increased appetite; weight gain; swelling in the arms or legs; joint pain; arm

---

Possible Side Effects *(continued)*

or leg pain; twitching; anxiety; personality changes; restlessness or a feeling that you need to keep moving;
muscle stiffness; tremors; memory loss; difficulty speaking or expressing thoughts; euphoria (feeling high); stuttering; cough; sore throat; double vision or other eye
problems; and symptoms of premenstrual syndrome
(PMS). Other side effects can affect virtually any other
body system or organ. Report anything unusual to your
doctor at once.

Drug Interactions

• Mixing carbamazepine and olanzapine leads to a 50% or
more increase in the rate at which olanzapine is broken down.
This can lead to problems if the olanzapine dose is not
adjusted for this problem.

• Olanzapine may increase the effects of blood-pressure-
lowering drugs and olanzapine's depressant effect on the
nervous system. Dosage adjustments may be needed if you
take one of these combinations.

Food Interactions

None known.

Usual Dose

Adult: starting dose—5–10 mg a day. Maintenance dose—
increase gradually up to 20 mg a day if needed.

Senior: Start with lower doses and increase gradually until
maximum benefit is achieved.

Child (under age 18): not recommended.

Overdosage

The most common overdose symptoms are drowsiness and
slurred speech. Overdose victims should be taken to a hospital emergency room for treatment. ALWAYS bring the
prescription bottle or container with you.

Special Information

Sleepiness occurs in about 25% of people who take olanzapine; this effect may increase with larger doses. Take care
when engaging in activities, such as driving, that require
concentration or coordination.

Avoid alcohol and other nervous-system depressants while taking olanzapine.

Olanzapine can cause dry mouth. See your dentist regularly while you are taking this medication, since dental problems are more likely in these circumstances.

Be sure your doctor knows about all medication you are taking, including over-the-counter products.

If you forget to take a dose of olanzapine, take it as soon as you remember. If it is almost time for your next dose, skip the dose you forgot and continue with your regular schedule. Do not take a double dose of olanzapine. Tell your doctor if you regularly forget doses, since he or she may want to change your dosage schedule to make it easier to remember.

Special Populations

Pregnancy/Breast-feeding

Olanzapine should only be taken by pregnant women if the potential benefits are worth the risks to the fetus. Birth defects and other problems have been seen in women taking olanzapine, but there is no definite link between the drug and these effects.

It is not known if olanzapine passes into human breast milk. Nursing mothers who must take this medication should bottle-feed their babies.

Seniors

Seniors often retain olanzapine in their bodies about 1½ times as long as younger adults. Seniors usually need less olanzapine than a younger adult.

Generic Name

Olopatadine (oe-loe-PAT-uh-dene)

Brand Name

Patanol

Type of Drug

Antihistamine.

Prescribed for

Eye itching due to allergy.

General Information

Olopatadine is an antihistamine that works in the eye to fight histamine released when the eye is irritated because of conjunctivitis (pinkeye). Because little of the drug enters the blood circulation after it is put into the eye, systemic (whole-body) side effects are uncommon.

Cautions and Warnings

Do not use olopatadine if you are **allergic** to it.

Possible Side Effects

▼ Common: headache.

▼ Less common: burning or stinging in the eye, dry eye, sensation that something is in your eye, eye redness, inflammation of the cornea, eyelid swelling, itching, weakness, sore throat, runny nose, common cold symptoms, sinus inflammation, and changes in sense of taste.

Drug Interactions

None known.

Usual Dose

Adult and Child (age 3 and over): 1–2 drops in each eye 2 times a day, 6–8 hours apart.

Child (under age 3): Not recommended.

Overdosage

There is little information about olopatadine overdose. Putting too much of the drug in your eye is likely to be irritating and cause side effects (see "Possible Side Effects"). Accidental ingestion of olopatadine is not likely to be associated with side effects because each bottle contains only 5 mg of the drug. Call your local poison control center or hospital emergency room for more information.

Special Information

If you wear contact lenses, wait at least 15 minutes after using olopatadine before putting in your lenses.

To administer eyedrops, lie down or tilt your head back. Hold the dropper above your eye, gently squeeze your lower lid to form a small pouch, and release the drop or drops of medication inside your lower lid while looking up. Release the lower lid, keeping your eye open. Do not blink for 40 seconds. Press gently on the bridge of your nose at the inside corner of your eye for 1 minute to help circulate the drug in your eye. To avoid infection, do not touch the dropper tip to your finger, eyelid, or any other surface. Wait at least 5 minutes before using another eyedrop or eye ointment.

If you forget a dose of olopatadine, administer it as soon as you remember. If it is almost time for your next dose, skip the one you forgot and continue with your regular schedule. Do not take a double dose.

Special Populations

Pregnancy/Breast-feeding
Antihistamines have not been proven to cause birth defects in humans. Since little olopatadine gets into the circulation, risk of birth defects is low. Do not take any antihistamine without your doctor's knowledge if you are or might be pregnant—especially during the last 3 months of pregnancy, because newborns may have severe reactions to antihistamines. When this drug is considered crucial by your doctor, its potential benefits must be carefully weighed against its risks.

In animal studies, olopatadine passed into breast milk. Nursing mothers using olopatadine should watch their babies for side effects.

Seniors
Seniors may take olopatadine without special precaution.

Generic Name

Olsalazine (ol-SAL-uh-zene)

Brand Name

Dipentum

Type of Drug

Bowel anti-inflammatory.

Prescribed for

Treating and maintaining ulcerative colitis.

General Information

Olsalazine sodium is broken down to an anti-inflammatory compound, mesalamine, after it enters the colon. Mesalamine acts as an anti-inflammatory agent inside the bowel and is effective for ulcerative colitis. The amount of mesalamine absorbed into the blood is 10% to 30%; 70% to 90% of it remains in the colon, where it works on colitis. People who cannot take sulfasalazine may be able to take olsalazine.

Cautions and Warnings

Do not take this product if you are **allergic** to it, to mesalamine, or to aspirin (or aspirin-related compounds) because the active metabolite product of olsalazine is closely related to aspirin.

Possible Side Effects

Many side effects in addition to those listed below have been reported, but their link to olsalazine has not been well established.

▼ Most common: diarrhea and stomach cramps or pain.

▼ Less common: muscle aches, headache, fatigue or drowsiness, depression, nausea, vomiting, upset stomach, bloating, yellowing of the skin or eyes, depression, dizziness, fainting, appetite loss, respiratory infections, and skin rash or itching.

Drug Interactions

None known.

Food Interactions

Take this drug with food to reduce stomach upset.

Usual Dose

1000 mg a day divided into 2 doses.

Overdosage

Overdose symptoms are diarrhea, vomiting, and lethargy. Overdose victims should be made to vomit with ipecac syrup—available at any pharmacy—to remove any remaining medication from the stomach. Call your local poison control center or emergency room before giving the ipecac. Then take the victim to a hospital emergency room for treatment. ALWAYS bring the prescription bottle or container with you.

Special Information

Call your doctor if you develop fever, pale skin, sore throat, unusual bruising or bleeding, unusual tiredness or weakness, yellow eyes or skin, or if your colitis gets worse. Other symptoms, such as diarrhea, abdominal pain, upset stomach, appetite loss, nausea, and vomiting, should be reported if they become particularly bothersome or severe.

If you forget a dose of olsalazine, take it as soon as you remember. If it is almost time for your next dose, take one dose right away and another in 5 or 6 hours, then go back to your regular schedule. Do not take a double dose.

Special Populations

Pregnancy/Breast-feeding
Olsalazine has caused birth defects in lab animals. Olsalazine should not be taken by pregnant women unless its possible benefits have been carefully weighed against its risks.

Olsalazine and mesalamine pass into breast milk, but the importance of this is not known. Nursing mothers should consult their doctors and exercise caution.

Seniors
Seniors may use this drug without special restriction.

Generic Name

Omeprazole (oe-MEP-ruh-zole)

Brand Name

Prilosec

Type of Drug

Proton-pump inhibitor.

Prescribed for

Stomach or duodenal (upper intestinal) ulcers, gastroesophageal reflux disease (GERD), and conditions in which there is an excess of stomach acid; also used to maintain healing of ulcer of the esophagus.

General Information

Omeprazole stops the production of stomach acid by a method that is different from the histamine H_2 antagonists, drugs such as cimetidine and ranitidine that are also used to treat ulcer disease. Omeprazole, like the related drug lansoprazole, interferes with the "proton pump" in the mucous lining of the stomach, at the last stage of acid production. Omeprazole can turn off stomach acid production within 1 hour after it is taken. This drug is also useful in other conditions in which stomach acid plays a key role or in which excess stomach acid is produced.

Omeprazole is accepted for duodenal ulcers. It is prescribed together with amoxicillin or clarithromycin for people with ulcers caused by *Heliobacter pylori* infections. It is also used to treat GERD, a condition in which some stomach contents flow backward into the esophagus (pipe connecting the throat and stomach). This can result in erosion of the esophagus caused by the stomach acid.

Cautions and Warnings

Do not take omeprazole if you have had an **allergic** reaction to it in the past.

Omeprazole should not be taken as maintenance treatment for duodenal ulcers and is not recommended for treatment of GERD beyond 8 to16 weeks.

In animal studies, omeprazole was found to increase the numbers of some **tumors**. These studies have raised questions about the long-term safety of omeprazole and the possible relationship between omeprazole and human tumors. However, there is no current available information that shows a risk for tumors in people taking omeprazole.

Possible Side Effects

Generally, omeprazole causes few side effects. Those that may occur include headache, diarrhea, abdominal pain, nausea, sore throat, upper respiratory infection, fever, vomiting, dizziness, rash, constipation, muscle pain, unusual tiredness, cough, and back pain.

▼ Rare: abdominal swelling, feeling unwell, angina

Possible Side Effects *(continued)*

pain, appetite loss, stool discoloration, irritable bowel, fungal infection in the esophagus, dry mouth, low blood sugar, weight gain, muscle cramps, joint and leg pain, dizziness, fainting, nervousness, sleeplessness, apathy, anxiety, unusual dreams, tingling in the hands or feet, nosebleed, itching and inflammation of the skin, dry skin, hair loss, sweating, frequent urination, and testicle pain.

Drug Interactions

• Omeprazole may increase the effects of diazepam, phenytoin, and warfarin by slowing the breakdown of these drugs by the liver. It may also interact with other drugs broken down by the liver.

• Combining omeprazole and clarithromycin increases the blood levels of both drugs.

• Omeprazole may interfere with the absorption from the stomach of drugs that require stomach acid as part of the process, including iron, ampicillin, and ketoconazole.

• Omeprazole may increase the effects of drugs that reduce the production of blood cells by the bone marrow.

Food Interactions

Omeprazole should be taken immediately before a meal, preferably breakfast.

Usual Dose

20–80 mg a day; up to 120 mg a day has been used for some conditions. Antacids may be taken with omeprazole.

Overdosage

There is limited experience with omeprazole overdose, although people with Zollinger-Ellison syndrome have taken 360 mg a day without problems. Omeprazole overdose symptoms are likely to be similar to side effects. If you suspect an omeprazole overdose, call your local poison control center or hospital emergency room for more information.

Special Information

Call your doctor if you are unusually tired or weak, or if you have a sore throat, fever, sores in the mouth that do not heal, unusual bleeding or bruising, bloody or cloudy urine, urinary difficulties, or if side effects are unusually persistent or bothersome.

Continue taking this drug until your doctor tells you to stop, even though your symptoms may improve after 1 or 2 weeks.

Do not open, crush, or chew the omeprazole capsule; swallow it whole.

If you forget a dose of omeprazole, take it as soon as you remember. If it is almost time for your next dose, skip the one you forgot and continue with your regular schedule. Do not take a double dose.

Special Populations

Pregnancy/Breast-feeding
Omeprazole may be toxic to pregnant animals, but no such problems have been reported in humans. Women who are or might be pregnant should not use omeprazole unless its potential benefits clearly outweigh its risks.

It is not known if omeprazole passes into breast milk; no drug-related problems have been known to occur. Nursing mothers who use this drug should exercise caution and watch their babies for possible side effects.

Seniors
Seniors report the same side effects as younger adults, but older adults could have more drug in the bloodstream. Report any unusual side effects to your doctor.

Generic Name

Ondansetron (on-DANS-eh-tron)

Brand Name

Zofran

The information in this profile also applies to the following drug:

Generic Ingredient: Dolasetron
Anzemet

Type of Drug

Antiemetic.

Prescribed for

Nausea and vomiting due to general anesthetics used during surgery and certain cancer chemotherapy treatments.

General Information

Ondansetron, like granisetron, produces its effect in a unique way. It antagonizes the receptor for a special form of the neurohormone serotonin ($5HT_3$). Receptors of this type are found in both the part of the brain that controls vomiting—the chemoreceptor trigger zone—and in the vagus nerve in the stomach and intestines. Women absorb ondansetron faster than men, and they clear the drug more slowly from their bodies. This means that women will have more ondansetron in the blood than men who take the same dose, but this difference is not reflected in drug response.

Ondansetron and granisetron are extremely effective in preventing nausea and vomiting and work in many situations in which older antiemetics are ineffective.

Cautions and Warnings

Do not take ondansetron if you are **allergic** or **sensitive** to it.

People with **liver failure** must take less ondansetron since the drug accumulates in their bodies and less is needed to produce the same effect. Ondansetron is not intended for **chronic use**: It is meant only for short-term nausea and vomiting prevention.

Possible Side Effects

▼ Most common: headache, not feeling well, and constipation.

▼ Common: anxiety, agitation, dizziness, drowsiness, diarrhea, gynecological problems, itching, urinary difficulty, abnormal heart rhythms, and low blood pressure.

▼ Less common: weakness, fever or chills, dry mouth, liver inflammation, diarrhea, abdominal pains, and rash.

▼ Rare: liver failure, drug allergy, bronchial spasm, excessive tiredness, rapid heart-beat, angina pain, low blood potassium, and grand mal seizures.

Drug Interactions

None known.

Food Interactions

Food increases the amount of ondansetron absorbed but does not affect your ondansetron dose.

Usual Dose

Adult and Child (age 12 and over): 8 mg 3 times a day. People with liver failure should take no more than 8 mg a day.

Child (age 4–11): 4 mg 3 times a day.

Child (under age 4): not recommended.

Overdosage

Doses up to 145 mg have been taken without significant side effects. Call your local poison control center or hospital emergency room for more information. If you go to the emergency room, ALWAYS bring the prescription bottle or container with you.

Special Information

Call your doctor if you begin to have chest tightness, wheezing, breathing difficulties, chest pains, or other unusual or severe side effects.

Ondansetron can cause dry mouth, which can increase your risk of tooth decay or gum disease. Pay special attention to oral hygiene while you are taking this drug.

If you forget to take a dose of ondansetron, take it as soon as you remember. If it is almost time for your next dose, skip the dose you forgot and continue with your regular schedule. Skipping more than 1 dose may increase your chances of vomiting.

Special Populations

Pregnancy/Breast-feeding

Ondansetron studies have revealed no potential for birth defects. Nevertheless, when this drug is considered crucial by your doctor, its potential benefits must be carefully weighed against its risks.

Ondansetron may pass into breast milk. Nursing mothers who take this drug should watch their babies carefully for possible side effects.

Seniors

Seniors may take this drug without restriction.

Ortho-Cept

*see **Contraceptives**, page 246*

Ortho-Novum

see **Contraceptives**, page 246

Generic Name

Oxaprozin (ox-uh-PROE-zin)

Brand Name

Daypro

Type of Drug

Nonsteroidal anti-inflammatory drug (NSAID).

Prescribed for

Rheumatoid arthritis and osteoarthritis.

General Information

Oxaprozin is one of 16 NSAIDs, which are used to relieve pain and inflammation. We do not know exactly how NSAIDs work, but part of their action may be due to their ability to inhibit the body's production of a hormone called prostaglandin as well as the action of other body chemicals, including cyclooxygenase, lipoxygenase, leukotrienes, and lysosomal enzymes. NSAIDs are generally absorbed into the bloodstream quickly. Pain relief comes within 1 hour after taking the first dose of oxaprozin, but its anti-inflammatory effect takes up to 1 week to become apparent and may take a month or more to reach maximum effect. Oxaprozin is broken down in the liver and eliminated through the kidneys.

Cautions and Warnings

People who are **allergic** to oxaprozin or any other NSAID and those with a history of **asthma** attacks brought on by an NSAID, iodides, or aspirin should not take oxaprozin.

Oxaprozin can cause **gastrointestinal (GI) bleeding, ulcers,** and **stomach perforation**. This can occur at any time, with or without warning, in people who take oxaprozin regularly. People with a history of **active GI bleeding** should be cautious about taking any NSAID. People who develop bleeding or ulcers and continue NSAID treatment should be aware of the possibility of developing more serious drug toxicity.

Oxaprozin can affect **platelets and blood clotting** at high doses, and should be avoided by people with clotting problems and by those taking warfarin.

People with **heart problems** who use oxaprozin may experience swelling in their arms, legs, or feet.

Oxaprozin can cause severe toxic effects to the **kidney**. Report any unusual side effects to your doctor, who may need to periodically test your kidney function.

Oxaprozin can make you unusually photosensitive (sensitive to the effects of the sun).

Possible Side Effects

▼ Most common: diarrhea, nausea, vomiting, constipation, stomach gas, stomach upset or irritation, and appetite loss—especially during the first few days of treatment.

▼ Less common: stomach ulcers, GI bleeding, hepatitis, gallbladder attacks, painful urination, poor kidney function, kidney inflammation, blood and protein in the urine, dizziness, fainting, nervousness, depression, hallucinations, confusion, disorientation, tingling in the hands or feet, light-headedness, itching, increased sweating, dry nose and mouth, heart palpitations, chest pain, breathing difficulties, and muscle cramps.

▼ Rare: severe allergic reactions including closing of the throat, fever and chills, changes in liver function, jaundice (yellowing of the skin or whites of the eyes), and kidney failure. People who experience such effects must be promptly treated in a hospital emergency room or doctor's office. NSAIDs have caused severe skin reactions; if this happens to you, see your doctor immediately.

Drug Interactions

• Oxaprozin can increase the effects of oral anticoagulant (blood-thinning) drugs such as warfarin. You may take this combination, but your doctor might have to reduce your anticoagulant dose.

• Taking oxaprozin with cyclosporine may increase the toxic kidney effects of both drugs. Methotrexate toxicity may be increased in people also taking oxaprozin.

• Oxaprozin may reduce the blood-pressure-lowering effect of beta blockers and loop diuretics.

• Oxaprozin may increase phenytoin blood levels, leading to increased side effects. Lithium blood levels may be increased in people taking oxaprozin.

• Oxaprozin blood levels may be affected by cimetidine.

• Probenecid may interfere with the elimination of oxaprozin from the body, increasing the chances for oxaprozin side effects.

• Aspirin and other salicylates may decrease the amount of oxaprozin in your blood. These drugs should never be combined with oxaprozin.

Food Interactions

Take oxaprozin with food or a magnesium/aluminum antacid if it upsets your stomach.

Usual Dose

600–1800 mg taken once a day. Do not exceed 12 mg per lb. of body weight daily.

Overdosage

People have died from NSAID overdoses. The most common signs of overdose are drowsiness, nausea, vomiting, diarrhea, abdominaı pain, rapid breathing, rapid heartbeat, increased sweating, ringing or buzzing in the ears, confusion, disorientation, stupor, and coma. Take the victim to a hospital emergency room at once. ALWAYS bring the prescription bottle or container with you.

Special Information

Take each dose with a full glass of water and do not lie down for 15 to 30 minutes afterward.

Oxaprozin can make you drowsy and/or tired: Be careful when driving or operating hazardous equipment. Do not take any over-the-counter products containing acetaminophen or aspirin while taking oxaprozin. Avoid alcoholic beverages.

Contact your doctor if you develop skin rash or itching, visual disturbances, weight gain, breathing difficulties, fluid retention, hallucinations, black or tarry stools, persistent headache, or any unusual or intolerable side effect.

If you forget to take a dose of oxaprozin, take it as soon as you remember. If you take oxaprozin once a day and it is within 8 hours of your next dose, skip the dose you forgot and continue with your regular schedule. If you take several doses a day and it is within 4 hours of your next dose, skip the one you forgot and continue with your regular schedule. Never take a double dose.

Special Populations

Pregnancy/Breast-feeding

NSAIDs may cross into fetal blood circulation. They have not been found to cause birth defects, but may affect the fetal heart during the second half of pregnancy. Pregnant women should not take oxaprozin without their doctor's approval, particularly during the last 3 months of pregnancy. When the drug is considered crucial by your doctor, its potential benefits must be carefully weighed against its risks.

NSAIDs may pass into breast milk but have caused no problems in breast-fed infants, except for seizures in a baby whose mother was taking the NSAID indomethacin. There is a possibility that a nursing mother taking oxaprozin could affect her baby's heart or cardiovascular system. If you must take oxaprozin, bottle-feed your baby.

Seniors

Seniors may be more susceptible to oxaprozin side effects, especially ulcer disease.

Generic Name

Oxiconazole (ox-ih-KON-uh-zole)

Brand Name

Oxistat

Type of Drug

Antifungal.

Prescribed for

Fungal infections of the skin.

General Information

Oxiconazole nitrate is a general-purpose antifungal drug. It works by interfering with the cell membrane (outer skin) of the fungus. Oxiconazole penetrates the skin after application, but little is absorbed into the bloodstream.

Cautions and Warnings

Do not use oxiconazole if you are **allergic** to it or to any other ingredient in this product.

Large doses of oxiconazole have caused **reduced fertility** in laboratory animals. This should be taken into account when considering the use of this drug, although there is no evidence that oxiconazole reduces fertility in humans.

Possible Side Effects

Oxiconazole side effects are infrequent.
▼ Common: itching and burning.
▼ Rare: stinging, irritation, rash, scaling, tingling, pain, eczema, redness and swelling, and cracked skin.

Drug Interactions

None known.

Usual Dose

Oxiconazole should be applied to affected areas every evening for 2–4 weeks, depending on the fungus type.

Overdosage

People who accidentally swallow this medication should be taken to a hospital emergency room. ALWAYS bring the prescription bottle or container with you.

Special Information

Oxiconazole is meant only for application to the skin. Do not put this drug into your eyes or mouth.

Stop using the drug and call your doctor if skin irritation or redness develops.

If you forget to apply a dose of oxiconazole, apply it as soon as you remember. If it is almost time for your next dose, skip the dose you forgot and continue with your regular schedule.

Special Populations

Pregnancy/Breast-feeding

Oxiconazole is not likely to affect your pregnancy because little is absorbed into the bloodstream. Nevertheless, you should not use this drug without your doctor's knowledge and approval.

Significant amounts of oxiconazole may pass into breast milk. Nursing mothers who use it should watch their infants for possible side effects.

Seniors

Seniors may use oxiconazole without special restriction.

Generic Name

Oxybutynin (ox-ee-BYUE-tih-nin) Ⓖ

Brand Name

Ditropan

Type of Drug

Antispasmodic and anticholinergic.

Prescribed for

Bladder instability including an urgent need to urinate, frequent urination, urinary leakage, and painful urination.

General Information

Oxybutynin directly affects the smooth muscle that controls the opening and closing of the bladder. Oxybutinin is 4 to 10 times more potent than atropine but has only 20% of the anticholinergic effect of that drug and is much less likely to cause side effects.

Cautions and Warnings

Do not take oxybutynin if you are **allergic or sensitive** to it.

Oxybutynin should be used with caution if you have **glaucoma, intestinal obstruction or poor intestinal function, megacolon**, severe or ulcerative **colitis, myasthenia**, or unstable **heart disease** including abnormal heart rhythms, heart failure, or recent heart attack. **Heat prostration** may develop more easily while you are taking this drug because it makes you more sensitive to hot weather or high temperatures.

Oxybutynin should be used with caution if you have **liver or kidney disease**. It may worsen symptoms of an **overactive thyroid gland, coronary heart disease, abnormal heart rhythms,**

rapid heartbeat, high blood pressure, prostate disease, or hiatal hernia.

Possible Side Effects

▼ Most common: dry mouth, decreased sweating, and constipation.

▼ Less common: difficulty urinating, blurred vision, enlarging of the pupils, worsening of glaucoma, palpitations, drowsiness, sleeplessness, weakness, nausea, vomiting, bloating, impotence, reduced production of breast milk, rash, and itching.

Drug Interactions

• Combining oxybutinin and atenolol (a beta blocker) may increase the effect of oxybutynin by increasing the amount of it absorbed by the blood.

• Oxybutynin may reduce the amount of haloperidol in the blood, increasing the risk of worsening of schizophrenic symptoms. Oxybutynin may increase blood levels of digoxin and nitrofurantoin, increasing the risk of side effects.

• Oxybutinin may interfere with the effects of levodopa.

• Amantadine may increase the side effects of oxybutynin.

• Combining oxybutynin with a phenothiazine antipsychotic medication may increase side effects and raise or lower the amount of phenothiazine in the blood.

Food Interactions

Take oxybutynin with food or milk if it upsets your stomach.

Usual Dose

Adult: 10–20 mg a day in divided doses.
Child (age 6 and over): 10–15 mg a day in divided doses.

Overdosage

Oxybutynin overdose symptoms may include restlessness, tremors, irritability, convulsions, hallucinations, flushing, fever, nausea, vomiting, rapid heartbeat, blood-pressure changes, respiratory failure, paralysis, delirium, and coma. Victims should be taken to a hospital emergency room at once. ALWAYS bring the prescription bottle or container with you.

Special Information

Oxybutynin may interfere with your vision and your ability to concentrate. Be careful while driving or doing anything that requires concentration or clear vision.

Your eyes may become more sensitive to bright light while taking oxybutynin; wearing sunglasses or protective lenses should help to alleviate this problem.

Dry mouth may be relieved with sugarless gum, candy, or ice chips. Excessive mouth dryness may lead to tooth decay and should be brought to your dentist's attention if it lasts for more than 2 weeks.

If you forget to take a dose of oxybutynin, take it as soon as you remember. If it is almost time for your next dose, skip the dose you forgot and continue with your regular schedule. Do not take a double dose.

Special Populations

Pregnancy/Breast-feeding
The safety of oxybutynin use by pregnant women is not known. When this drug is considered crucial by your doctor, its potential benefits must be carefully weighed against its risks.

It is not known if oxybutynin passes into breast milk. Nursing mothers should use this drug with caution.

Seniors
Seniors may be more susceptible to the side effects of oxybutynin and should take it with caution.

Generic Name

Paclitaxel (PAK-lih-TAX-ul)

Brand Name

Taxol

Type of Drug

Antineoplastic drug.

Prescribed for

Ovarian and breast cancer; also prescribed for AIDS-related Kaposi's sarcoma.

General Information

Paclitaxel is a natural substance that interferes with the

process of cell division in cancerous cells. Paclitaxel is recommended only after other treatments have failed. People who receive this drug will be premedicated with other drugs such as diphenhydramine, cimetidine, or ranitidine to minimize some side effects.

Studies in ovarian cancer indicate that 22% to 30% of women who receive paclitaxel respond to the drug. Of a total of 92 women studied, there were 6 complete and 18 partial responses. In these studies the average survival for all women taking the drug was between 8 and 16 months. In breast cancer, studies showed response rates ranging from 26% and 30% to 57%; survival averaged almost 1 year.

Paclitaxel is also being studied for cancers of the head and neck, lung, and upper gastrointestinal tract; prostate cancer that does not respond to hormone treatments; and non-Hodgkin's lymphoma.

Cautions and Warnings

Paclitaxel must be prescribed by a physician who is experienced in the use of cancer chemotherapies. Management of drug complications is possible only when adequate treatment facilities are available.

Severe drug sensitivity reactions, including **breathing difficulties; low blood pressure** (symptoms include dizziness and fainting); **swelling of the face, hands, feet, genitals, or internal organs**; and **generalized itching and rash** have occurred in 2% of people taking this drug. People who experience these kinds of reactions should not receive paclitaxel again.

Bone-marrow suppression is the major toxic effect of paclitaxel. Because the bone marrow is where blood cells are manufactured, people with low white-blood-cell counts should not receive paclitaxel.

Fewer than 1% of people who take paclitaxel develop severe **heart problems**; these people may require cardiac therapy while continuing to receive this drug.

Paclitaxel is broken down in the liver and should be used with caution in people with severe **liver disease**.

Possible Side Effects

▼ Most common: reduced blood-cell counts, anemia, infection, drug sensitivity reactions, dizziness or fainting, changes in electrocardiogram (EKG) measurements,

Possible Side Effects *(continued)*

muscle or joint pain, nausea and vomiting, diarrhea, mouth sores, liver inflammation, kidney damage, hair loss, numbness, tingling or burning in the hands or feet, and swelling or retention of fluid.

▼ Less common: bleeding, blood in the urine, bruising, black and tarry stool, severe sensitivity reactions, and slow heartbeat.

▼ Rare: severe heart problems and nail changes.

Drug Interactions

• When paclitaxel is given with cisplatin—another antineoplastic drug—side effects are worse when the paclitaxel is given after the cisplatin.

• Ketoconazole, verapamil, diazepam, quinidine, dexamethasone, cyclosporine, teniposide, etoposide, vincristine, testosterone, estradiol, and retinoic acid may reduce the rate at which paclitaxel is broken down in the body, increasing the possibility of paclitaxel side effects.

• Paclitaxel may increase the amount of doxorubicin in the blood, increasing the possibility of doxorubicin side effects.

Food Interactions

None known.

Usual Dose

Adult: Paclitaxel is given by intravenous injection. Dosage is individualized according to body surface area.
Child: not recommended.

Overdosage

There is little information on paclitaxel overdose, but exaggerated side side effects would be expected. Breathing difficulties, chest pain, burning eyes, sore throat, and nausea have occurred after accidental inhalation of paclitaxel. There is no known antidote for this drug. Overdose victims should be taken to a hospital emergency room for treatment. ALWAYS bring the prescription bottle or container with you.

Special Information

It is important that your care is closely supervised by your doctor while receiving paclitaxel.

Do not receive any immunizations or vaccinations while taking paclitaxel, unless approved by your doctor.

Avoid exposure to people with bacterial or viral infections, especially when your blood counts are likely to be low. Check with your doctor at the first sign of any cold or infection. Do not touch the inside of your mouth or nose unless you have first washed your hands.

Call your doctor if you experience any unusual bleeding or bruising, black or tarry stool, blood in the urine or stool, or pinpoint red spots on the skin.

Be careful about dental hygiene—brushing or flossing—while on this drug because of the possibility of introducing bacteria into your system. Check with your doctor before you have any dental work done and make sure your dentist knows that you are receiving cancer chemotherapy.

Take care to avoid accidental cuts of your skin with a razor, fingernail, or other sharp object. Avoid contact sports or other situations in which bruising or injury could occur.

Special Populations

Pregnancy/Breast-feeding

Paclitaxel can harm the fetus. Women taking this drug must be sure to use an effective contraceptive during treatment. If you are pregnant and must start taking paclitaxel, discuss the possible hazards with your doctor.

It is not known if paclitaxel passes into breast milk, but nursing mothers who must take this drug should bottle-feed their babies because of the possibility of side effects.

Seniors

Seniors may use this drug without special restriction.

Generic Name

Paroxetine (pah-ROX-eh-tene)

Brand Name

Paxil

Type of Drug

Selective serotonin reuptake inhibitor (SSRI).

Prescribed for

Depression; also prescribed for diabetic nerve disease, headache, and premature ejaculation.

General Information

Paroxetine and the other SSRI antidepressants—fluoxetine, fluvoxamine, and sertraline—are chemically unrelated to the older tricyclic and tetracyclic antidepressant drugs. SSRIs work by preventing the movement of the neurohormone serotonin into nerve endings. This forces the serotonin to remain in the spaces surrounding nerve endings, where it works. Paroxetine is effective in treating common symptoms of depression. It can help improve your mood and mental alertness, increase physical activity, and improve sleep patterns. Tolerance to the effects of paroxetine may develop over time. The drug takes between 1 and 4 weeks to start working, although you may start sleeping better within 1 to 2 weeks. Proxetine stays in your body for several weeks after you stop taking it. This fact may be important as your doctor considers when to start or stop treatment. Unlike other SSRIs, paroxetine does not have any weight-reducing effect.

Cautions and Warnings

Do not take paroxetine if you are **allergic** to it. Allergies to non-SSRI antidepressants should not prevent you from taking paroxetine because it is chemically different from other types of antidepressants.

Serious, potentially **fatal reactions may occur if paroxetine and a monoamine oxidase inhibitor (MAOI) are taken together (see "Drug Interactions").**

Paroxetine is broken down in the liver. People with **severe liver or kidney disease** should be cautious about taking this drug and should be treated at lower-than-normal doses.

Studies in animals receiving doses 10 to 20 times the maximum human dose revealed an increase in certain liver **tumors and reduced fertility**. The significance of these results for humans is not known.

A small number of **manic** or **hypomanic** patients may experience an activation of their condition while taking paroxetine.

Paroxetine should be given with caution to people who suffer from **seizures**.

Paroxetine causes low blood levels of uric acid, but has not caused kidney failure.

The possibility of **suicide** exists in severely depressed patients and may be present until the condition is significantly improved. Depressed patients should be allowed to carry only small quantities of paroxetine with them to limit the possibility of overdose.

Possible Side Effects

Paroxetine side effects are generally mild and often related to the size of the dose you are taking; they occur primarily during the first week of treatment. In studies of paroxetine before its release in the U.S., 15% of people taking it had to stop because of side effects. Be sure to report anything unusual to your doctor at once.

▼ Most common: headache, weakness, sleep disturbances, dizziness, and tremors.

▼ Common: nausea, excessive sweating, weakness, dry mouth, constipation, dizziness, decreased sex drive, abnormal ejaculation, blurred vision, dry mouth, and weight gain.

▼ Less common: flushing, pinpoint pupils, increased saliva, cold and clammy skin, dizziness when rising quickly from a sitting or lying position, blood pressure changes, swelling around the eyes and in the arms or legs, coldness in the hands or feet, fainting and dizziness, rapid heart beat, weakness, loss of coordination, unusual walk, changes in the general level of activity, migraines, droopy eyelids, tingling in the hands or feet, acne, hair loss, dry skin, difficulty swallowing, stomach gas, joint pain, muscle pain, cramps and weakness, aggressiveness, abnormal dreaming or thinking, memory loss, apathy, delusions, feelings of detachment, worsened depression, emotional instability, feeling "high," hallucinations, neurosis, paranoia, suicide attempts, teeth grinding, menstrual cramps or pain, bleeding between periods, coughing, bronchospasm, nosebleed, breathing difficulties, conjunctivitis, double vision, difficulty accommodating to bright light, eye pain, ear aches, painful urination, facial swelling, frequent urination, nighttime urination, loss of urinary control, generalized swelling, not feeling well, and lymph swelling.

Possible Side Effects *(continued)*

▼ Rare: Side effects affecting virtually every body system have been reported by people taking paroxetine. They are considered infrequent or rare and affect only a small number of people.

Drug Interactions

• At least 5 weeks should elapse between stopping paroxetine treatment and starting an MAOI antidepressant. Two weeks should elapse between stopping an MAOI and starting paroxetine. Taking these two drugs too close together or at the same time may cause serious, life-threatening reactions.

• People taking warfarin may experience an increase in its effect if they start taking paroxetine. People combining warfarin with paroxetine may experience a bleeding episode. Your doctor should reevaluate your warfarin dosage.

• Paroxetine increases the amount of theophylline in the blood, increasing the possibility of side effects. Report anything unusual to your doctor.

• Paroxetine may reduce the amount of digoxin absorbed into the blood by 15%.

• Cimetidine increases blood levels of paroxetine by about 50% when the drugs are taken together.

• Phenobarbital decreases the amount of paroxetine in the blood and increases the rate at which it is released from the body.

• Paroxetine and phenytoin, which is prescribed for seizure disorders can affect each other. The amount of both drugs in the blood may be decreased and both drugs may be released from the body more quickly than normal. Your doctor should adjust your dosages.

• Alcoholic beverages may increase the tiredness and other depressant effects of paroxetine on the nervous system.

• People who combine l-tryptophan and paroxetine may develop agitation, restlessness, and upset stomach.

• People combining paroxetine with procyclidine, prescribed for Parkinson's disease under the brand name Kemadrin, have experienced increased procyclidine side effects. Your doctor may reduce your procyclidine dosage if necessary.

Food Interactions

None known.

Usual Dose

10–50 mg once a day, morning or night. Seniors, people with kidney or liver disease, and people taking several different drugs should take the lowest effective dosage possible.

Overdosage

In the 18 reported cases of paroxetine overdose, all victims completely recovered. Symptoms of overdose are likely to be the most common side effects. There is no specific antidote for paroxetine overdose. Any person suspected of having taken an overdose should be taken to a hospital emergency room at once, or you may call your local poison control center for information and instructions. If you go to an emergency room, ALWAYS bring the prescription bottle or container with you.

Special Information

Paroxetine can make you dizzy or drowsy. Take care when driving or performing other tasks that require alertness and concentration.

Do not drink alcoholic beverages if you are taking paroxetine.

Be sure your doctor knows if you are pregnant, breast-feeding, or taking other drugs, including over-the-counter drugs, while taking paroxetine. Notify your doctor if you experience any unusual side effects.

If you forget a dose of paroxetine, take it as soon as you remember. If it is almost time for your next dose, skip the dose you forgot and continue with your regular schedule. Do not take a double dose.

Special Populations

Pregnancy/Breast-feeding

There are no conclusive studies of the effects of paroxetine in pregnant women. Do not take this drug if you are or might be pregnant without first weighing its potential benefits against its risks with your doctor.

Paroxetine passes into breast milk in roughly the same concentrations that it enters the bloodstream of nursing mothers. Women taking paroxetine should bottle-feed their babies.

Seniors

Seniors tend to clear paroxetine more slowly from their bodies, although side-effect patterns are essentially unchanged.

Any person with liver or kidney disease—more common among seniors—should receive a lower dose. Be sure to report any unusual side effects to your doctor.

Paxil

see *Paroxetine*, page 831

Brand Name

Pediazole

Generic Ingredients

Erythromycin Ethylsuccinate + Sulfisoxazole Ⓖ

Other Brand Names
Eryzole

Type of Drug

Antibiotic/anti-infective combination.

Prescribed for

Middle-ear and sinus infection in children.

General Information

This combination of the antibiotic erythromycin and the sulfa drug sulfisoxasole was specially formulated for its effect against *Haemophilus influenzae*, an organism responsible for many cases of difficult-to-treat middle-ear infections in children. Pediazole is also useful for a variety of other infections. Each teaspoonful of the medication contains 200 mg of erythromycin and 600 mg of sulfisoxazole. Although the 2 drugs work by completely different mechanisms, they complement each other in the ways in which they attack various organisms. Pediazole is especially valuable in cases of *H. influenzae* middle-ear infection that do not respond to ampicillin, a widely used and generally effective antibiotic.

Cautions and Warnings

Pediazole should not be given to **infants under 2 months** of age because their body systems are not able to break down the sulfisoxazole in this product. Children who are **allergic** to any sulfa drug or to any form of erythromycin should not be given this product.

Possible Side Effects

It is possible for children given this combination product to develop any of the side effects caused by either erythromycin or sulfisoxazole.

▼ Most common: upset stomach, cramps, drug allergy, and rash.

▼ Less common: nausea, vomiting, and diarrhea. Pediazole may make your child more sensitive to sunlight, an effect that can last for many months after the medicine has been discontinued.

Drug Interactions]

• Pediazole may increase the effects of digoxin, tolbutamide, chlorpropamide, methotrexate, theophylline, warfarin, aspirin or other salicylates, phenylbutazone, carbamazepine, phenytoin, and probenecid. Combining Pediazole with any of these drugs may result in an increase in side effects; a dosage adjustment of the interacting drug may be necessary.

Food Interactions

Pediazole is best taken on an empty stomach, at least 1 hour before or 2 hours after meals. However, if it causes stomach upset, have your child take each dose with food. Be sure your child drinks lots of water while using Pediazole.

Usual Dose

The dosage of Pediazole depends on your child's body weight: ½–2 tsp. every 6 hours, usually for 10 days. Follow each dose of Pediazole with a full glass of water.

Overdosage

The strawberry/strawberry-banana flavoring of this product makes it a good candidate for accidental overdose, so be sure it is stored in the area of your refrigerator that is least accessible to your child. Pediazole overdose is most likely to result in blood in the urine, nausea, vomiting, stomach upset and cramps, dizziness, headache, and drowsiness. Overdose victims must be made to vomit as soon as possible with ipecac syrup—available at any pharmacy—to remove any remaining drug from the stomach. Call your child's doctor or a poison control center before doing this. If you must go to a hospital emergency room, ALWAYS bring the prescription bottle or container with you.

Special Information

This product must be stored in the refrigerator and discarded after 2 weeks. Be sure it is labeled with an expiration date when you leave the pharmacy.

Do not stop giving your child this medication when symptoms disappear. It must be taken for the complete course of treatment prescribed by your doctor.

Call your child's doctor if nausea, vomiting, diarrhea, stomach cramps, stomach discomfort when the medication is taken with food, or other symptoms persist. These symptoms may mean that your child is unable to tolerate this antibiotic and will have to receive different treatment. Severe or unusual side effects should be reported to the doctor at once. Especially important are yellow discoloration of the whites of the eyes or skin, darkening of the urine, pale stools, or unusual tiredness, all of which may be signs of liver irritation.

If your child misses a dose of Pediazole, give it as soon as possible. If it is almost time for the next dose, space the missed dose and the next dose by 2 to 4 hours and then continue with the regular dosage schedule.

Generic Name

Pemoline (PEM-oe-lene)

Brand Name

Cylert

Type of Drug

Psychotherapeutic.

Prescribed for

Children with attention-deficit hyperactivity disorder (ADHD); may also be used to treat daytime sleepiness in adults.

General Information

This drug stimulates the central nervous system (CNS), although its exact action in children with ADHD is not known. It should be prescribed only by a qualified physician trained to treat ADHD, and always used as part of a total therapeutic program that includes social, psychological, and educational counseling.

Cautions and Warnings

People who are **allergic or sensitive** to pemoline should not use it. Children under age 6 should not take this drug. The condition of **psychotic** children who take pemoline may get worse. People taking pemoline should have periodic **liver function** tests.

Possible Side Effects

▼ Less common: sleeplessness, appetite loss, stomachache, rash, irritability, depression, nausea, dizziness, headache, drowsiness, and hallucinations.

▼ Rare: drug hypersensitivity, wandering eye, and uncontrolled movements of the lips, face, tongue, and extremities.

Drug Interactions

• Pemoline lowers the seizure threshold; dosages of anticonvulsant drugs may need to be increased.

• Pemoline increases the effects of other nervous-system stimulants, which may cause nervousness, irritability, sleeplessness, and other side effects.

Food Interactions

Take this drug with food if it upsets your stomach.

Usual Dose

37.5–75 mg a day. Do not exceed 112.5 mg a day.

Overdosage

Symptoms of overdose are rapid heartbeat, hallucinations, agitation, uncontrolled muscle movements, and restlessness. Overdose victims must be taken to a hospital emergency room. ALWAYS bring the prescription bottle or container with you.

Special Information

Take your daily dose at the same time each morning. Taking pemoline too late in the day may result in trouble sleeping; call your doctor if this happens.

If you forget a dose of pemoline, take it as soon as you remember. If it is almost time for your next dose, skip the dose you forgot and continue with your regular schedule. Do not take a double dose.

Special Populations

Pregnancy/Breast-feeding

Pemoline crosses into fetal circulation. Animal studies show that large doses of pemoline can cause stillbirths and reduce newborn survival rates. When the drug is considered crucial by your doctor, its potential benefits must be carefully weighed against its risks.

Pemoline passes into breast milk but has caused no problems among breast-fed infants. Nursing mothers who take pemoline should watch their babies for possible side effects from the drug.

Seniors

Seniors are more likely to have reduced kidney or liver function, and should take this drug with caution.

Generic Name

Penbutolol (pen-BUTE-uh-lol)

Brand Name

Levatol

Type of Drug

Beta-adrenergic blocking agent.

Prescribed for

Hypertension (high blood pressure).

General Information

Penbutolol sulfate is one of 15 beta-adrenergic blocking drugs, or beta blockers, that interfere with the action of a specific part of the nervous system. Beta receptors are found all over the body and affect many body functions. This accounts for the usefulness of beta blockers against a wide variety of conditions. The oldest of these drugs, propranolol, affects all types of beta-adrenergic receptors. Newer, more refined beta blockers affect only a portion of that system, making them more useful in treating cardiovascular disorders and less useful for other purposes. Other of the newer beta blockers act as mild stimulants to the heart or have particular characteristics that make them better for specific purposes or certain people.

Cautions and Warnings

You should be cautious about taking penbutolol if you have **asthma, severe heart failure,** a **very slow heart rate,** or **heart block** (disruption of the electrical impulses that control heart rate) because the drug may aggravate these conditions.

People with **angina** who take penbutolol for high blood pressure risk aggravating their angina if they suddenly stop taking this drug. These people should have their drug **dosage reduced gradually** over 1 to 2 weeks.

Penbutolol should be used with caution if you have **liver or kidney disease**, because your ability to eliminate the drug from your body may be impaired.

Penbutolol reduces the amount of blood pumped by the heart with each beat. This reduction in blood flow may aggravate the condition of people with **poor circulation** or **circulatory disease**.

If you are undergoing **major surgery**, your doctor may want you to stop taking penbutolol at least 2 days before surgery to permit the heart to respond more acutely to stresses that can occur during the procedure. This practice is still controversial and may not be appropriate for all surgeries.

Possible Side Effects

Side effects are relatively uncommon and usually mild; normally they develop early in the course of treatment and are rarely a reason to stop taking penbutolol.

▼ Most common: impotence.

▼ Less common: unusual tiredness or weakness, slow heartbeat, heart failure (symptoms include swelling of the legs, ankles, or feet), dizziness, breathing difficulties,

Possible Side Effects *(continued)*

bronchospasm, depression, confusion, anxiety, nervousness, sleeplessness, disorientation, short-term memory loss, emotional instability, cold hands and feet, constipation, diarrhea, nausea, vomiting, upset stomach, increased sweating, urinary difficulties, cramps, blurred vision, skin rash, hair loss, stuffy nose, facial swelling, aggravation of lupus erythematosus (chronic condition affecting the body's connective tissue), itching, chest pain, back or joint pain, colitis, drug allergy (symptoms include fever and sore throat), and liver toxicity.

Drug Interactions

• Penbutolol may interact with surgical anesthetics to increase the risk of heart problems during surgery. Some anesthesiologists recommend having gradually stopped the drug by 2 days before surgery.

• Penbutolol may interfere with the normal signs of low blood sugar and with the action of oral antidiabetes drugs.

• Penbutolol increases the blood-pressure-lowering effects of other blood-pressure-reducing agents, including clonidine, guanabenz, and reserpine; and calcium channel blockers such as nifedipine.

• Aspirin-containing drugs, indomethacin, sulfinpyrazone, and estrogen drugs may interfere with the blood-pressure-lowering effect of penbutolol.

• Cocaine may reduce the effectiveness of all beta blockers.

• Penbutolol may worsen the problem of cold hands and feet associated with ergot alkaloids for migraine headache. People taking both ergot and penbutolol may develop gangrene.

• Penbutolol will counteract thyroid hormone replacement medicines.

• Calcium channel blockers, flecainide, hydralazine, oral contraceptives, propafenone, haloperidol, phenothiazine tranquilizers—molindone and others—quinolone antibacterials, and quinidine may increase the amount of penbutolol in the bloodstream and lead to increased penbutolol effect.

• Penbutolol should not be taken within 2 weeks of taking a monoamine oxidase inhibitor (MAOI) antidepressant.

• Cimetidine increases the amount of penbutolol absorbed into the bloodstream from oral tablets.

• Penbutolol may interfere with the effectiveness of some anti-asthma drugs including theophylline, aminophylline, and especially ephedrine and isoproterenol).

• Combining penbutolol and phenytoin or digitalis drugs may result in excessive slowing of the heart, possibly causing heart block.

• If you stop smoking while taking penbutolol, your dose may have to be reduced because your liver will break down the drug more slowly afterward.

Food Interactions

None known.

Usual Dose

20 mg once a day. Seniors may require more or less medication and must be carefully monitored by their doctors. People with liver problems may require lower doses.

Overdosage

Symptoms of overdose include changes in heartbeat—unusually slow, unusually fast, or irregular—severe dizziness or fainting; breathing difficulties; bluish-colored fingernails or palms; and seizures. The overdose victim should be taken to a hospital emergency room. ALWAYS bring the prescription bottle or container with you.

Special Information

Penbutolol should be taken continuously. When ending penbutolol treatment, dosage should be lowered gradually over a period of about 2 weeks. Do not stop taking this drug unless directed to do so by your doctor: Abrupt withdrawal may cause chest pain, breathing difficulties, increased sweating, and unusually fast or irregular heartbeat.

Call your doctor at once if you develop back or joint pain, breathing difficulties, cold hands or feet, depression, skin rash, or changes in heartbeat. Penbutolol may produce an undesirable lowering of blood pressure, leading to dizziness or fainting; call your doctor if this happens to you. Call your doctor if you experience persistent or bothersome anxiety, diarrhea, constipation, impotence, headache, itching, nausea or vomiting, nightmares or vivid dreams, upset stomach, trouble sleeping, stuffy nose, frequent urination, unusual tiredness, or weakness.

Penbutolol may cause drowsiness, light-headedness, dizziness, or blurred vision. Be careful when driving or performing complex tasks.

It is best to take penbutolol at the same time each day. If you forget a dose, take it as soon as you remember. If it is within 8 hours of your next dose, skip the dose you forgot and continue with your regular schedule. Do not take a double dose.

Special Populations

Pregnancy/Breast-feeding

Infants born to women who took a beta blocker while pregnant had lower birth weights, low blood pressure, and reduced heart rates. Penbutolol should be avoided by women who are or might be pregnant. When the drug is considered crucial by your doctor, its potential benefits must be carefully weighed against its risks.

It is not known if penbutolol passes into breast milk. Nursing mothers taking this drug should bottle-feed their babies.

Seniors

Seniors may absorb and retain more penbutolol in their bodies, and may require less of the drug to achieve results. Your doctor should adjust your dosage to meet your individual needs. Seniors taking penbutolol may be more likely to suffer from cold hands and feet, reduced body temperature, chest pain, general feelings of ill health, sudden breathing difficulties, increased sweating, or changes in heartbeat.

Generic Name

Penciclovir (pen-SYE-kloe-vere)

Brand Name

Denavir

Type of Drug

Antiviral.

Prescribed for

Cold sores.

General Information

Penciclovir works against different types of herpes viruses responsible for common cold sores. Cold sores treated with penciclovir cream go away sooner and are less painful than those that are not treated. Once applied to the skin, penciclovir is converted to its active form and interferes with the production of DNA inside the viral particle; this inhibits the reproductive process of the herpes virus. Drug resistance may develop with repeated use of penciclovir on cold sores. Penciclovir does not pass into the blood and it cannot be found in the urine of people who use it topically.

Cautions and Warnings

Do not use penciclovir if you are **sensitive** or **allergic** to it.

Penciclovir should **be applied only to the face or lips**. Avoid applying it near your eyes because it may be irritating. The effectiveness of penciclovir in people with **compromised immune systems** is not known.

Male animals given massive doses of penciclovir intravenously suffered damage to the testicles. This effect appears to be related to the dose of penciclovir. Men using famciclovir, the oral form of penciclovir, for 8 to 13 weeks experienced no changes in sperm count.

Possible Side Effects

Side effects are generally mild and infrequent. In studies, side effects were similar in type and frequency among people who used penciclovir and those who used an inactive cream.

▼ Common: headache, redness, and swelling.

▼ Less common: skin reactions to the cream.

▼ Rare: loss of skin sensation where the cream has been applied, changes in the sense of taste, and rash.

Drug Interactions

None known.

Usual Dose

Adult: Apply to affected areas every 2 hours, during waking hours, for 4 days.

Child: not recommended.

Overdosage

There is no information on penciclovir overdose or accidental ingestion. Call your poison control center or a hospital emergency room for more information.

Special Information

Begin cold sore treatment as early as possible. Early application of penciclovir cream will help prevent cold sores from appearing and reduce accompanying pain.

It is very important to apply penciclovir cream every 2 hours during the day for the drug to work. If you forget to apply a dose of penciclovir, apply it as soon as you remember. If you realize you forgot a dose within 30 to 45 minutes of your next dose, skip the dose you forgot and continue with your regular schedule.

Special Populations

Pregnancy/Breast-feeding

In animal studies, penciclovir had no effect on the fetus. There is no information on the effect of penciclovir in pregnant women. This drug should be used during pregnancy only if its possible benefits outweigh its risks.

It is not known if penciclovir passes into breast milk, though famciclovir—the oral form of penciclovir—passes into breast milk in concentrations larger than those found in the mother's blood. Nursing mothers who must use penciclovir should bottle-feed their babies until penciclovir treatment has ended.

Seniors

Seniors may use this drug without special precaution.

Type of Drug

Penicillin Antibiotics (pen-ih-SIL-in)

Brand Names

Generic Ingredient: Amoxicillin Ⓖ

Amoxil	Trimox
Biomox	Wymox
Polymox	

Generic Ingredients: Amoxicillin + Potassium Clavulanate
Augmentin

Generic Ingredient: Ampicillin G
D-Amp   Principen
Omnipen   Totacillin
Polycillin

Generic Ingredients: Ampicillin + Probenecid
Polycillin-PRB   Probampacin

Generic Ingredient: Bacampicillin
Spectrobid

Generic Ingredient: Carbenicillin Indanyl Sodium
Geocillin

Generic Ingredient: Cloxacillin Sodium G
Cloxapen   Tegopen

Generic Ingredient: Dicloxacillin Sodium G
Dycill   Pathocil
Dynapen

Generic Ingredient: Nafcillin
Unipen

Generic Ingredient: Oxacillin G
Bactocill   Prostaphlin

Generic Ingredient: Penicillin G G
Pentids

Generic Ingredient: Penicillin V G
Beepen-VK   Pen-Vee K
Betapen-VK   Phenoxymethyl Penicillin
Ledercillin VK   Robicillin VK
Penicillin VK   V-Cillin K
Pen-V   Veetids

Prescribed for

Bacterial and other infections.

General Information

Penicillin antibiotics kill bacteria and other micro-organisms.
While some antibiotics only prevent the invading organisms
from reproducing, penicillin destroys the cell wall of the

invading organisms. Many infections may be treated with almost any kind of penicillin; some may be treated only by a specific penicillin antibiotic.

Penicillin cannot cure a cold, the flu, or any other viral infection and should never be taken unless prescribed by a doctor for a specific illness. Always take penicillin exactly according to your doctor's directions, including the number of pills to take every day and number of days to take the drug. If you do not follow your doctor's directions, you will not get the antibiotic's full benefit.

Cautions and Warnings

Serious and sometimes fatal allergic reactions have occurred with penicillin. Although this is more common following injection of the drug, it has occurred with penicillin taken by mouth and is more common among people with a history of sensitivity to penicillin or those who suffer from multiple allergies. About 5% of people allergic to a penicillin antibiotic are also allergic to the cephalosporin antibiotics.

Some penicillin allergic reactions may be treated with antihistamines or other medications. Sometimes, when an infection is life-threatening and can only be treated with penicillin, minor reactions may be treated with other medication while the penicillin is continued; generally, though, other drugs are substituted to treat the infection.

Cystic fibrosis patients are more likely to suffer from side effects of certain penicillins.

Possible Side Effects

The most important penicillin side effect, seen in up to 10% of people, is allergic reaction. These reactions are more common among people who have had a previous penicillin reaction and those who have had asthma, hay fever, or other allergies. Allergic symptoms include itching, rash, swelling, breathing difficulties, very low blood pressure, blood vessel collapse, peeling skin, chills, fever, muscle aches, arthritis-like pains, and feeling unwell.

About 9% of ampicillin users develop an itchy rash, which is not a true allergic reaction. This rash is more likely to occur when ampicillin is combined with allopurinol.

Possible Side Effects *(continued)*

People who receive injectable penicillin may become lethargic, dizzy, or tired, or experience hallucinations, seizure, anxiety, depression, confusion, agitation, or hyperactivity.

▼ Common: upset stomach, abdominal pain, nausea, vomiting, diarrhea, colitis, sore mouth, coated tongue, anemia, bleeding abnormalities, low platelet and white-blood-cell counts, and oral or rectal fungal infections.

▼ Less common: vaginal irritation, appetite loss, itchy eyes, and feelings of body warmth.

▼ Rare: yellowing of the skin or whites of the eyes.

Drug Interactions

• Penicillin should not be taken with a bacteriostatic antibiotic such as chloramphenicol, erythromycin, tetracycline, or neomycin. Any of these combinations may diminish the effectiveness of penicillin.

• Penicillin may interfere with the effectiveness of oral contraceptive drugs ("the pill").

• Penicillin allergic reaction may be intensified by beta-blocking drugs.

• Ampicillin may reduce the effect of atenolol by interfering with its absorption into the blood.

• Large doses of injectable penicillin may increase the effect of anticoagulant (blood-thinning) drugs.

Food Interactions

Do not take penicillin with fruit juice or carbonated beverages because the acid in these beverages may destroy the drug.

Most penicillins, including bacampicillin suspension, are best absorbed on an empty stomach. These medications may be taken 1 hour before or 2 hours after meals or first thing in the morning and last thing at night with the other doses spaced evenly throughout the day.

Amoxicillin and bacampicillin tablets may be taken without regard to food.

Amoxicillin and potassium clavulanate are best taken right before a meal for optimum drug absorption into the blood and minimum stomach upset.

Usual Dose

Amoxicillin
   Adult: 250–500 mg every 8 hours.
   Child: 10–20 mg per lb. a day divided into 3 doses.

Amoxicillin and Potassium Clavulanate
   Adult: a "250" tablet every 8 hours; a "500" or "875" tablet every 12 hours.
   Child: 10–20 mg per lb. a day divided into 3 doses.

Note: Different strengths of this product are not interchangeable. Take only the exact strength and product your doctor has prescribed.

Ampicillin
   Adult: 1–12 g a day divided into 4–6 doses.
   Child: 25–100 mg per lb. a day divided into 4–6 doses.

Ampicillin with Probenecid
3.5 g of ampicillin and 1 g of probenecid as a single dose for gonorrhea.

Bacampicillin
   Adult: 400–800 mg every 12 hours; 1600 mg plus 1 g of probenecid for gonorrhea.
   Child: 12–25 mg per lb. a day divided into 2 doses.

Carbenicillin Indanyl Sodium
   Adult: 382–764 mg 4 times a day.
   Child: not recommended.

Cloxacillin Sodium
   Adult: 250 mg every 6 hours.
   Child: 25 mg per lb. a day divided into 4 doses.

Dicloxacillin Sodium
   Adult: 125–250 mg every 6 hours.
   Child: 6–12 mg per lb. a day divided into 4 doses.

Nafcillin
   Adult: 250–1000 mg every 4–6 hours.
   Child: 5–25 mg per lb. every 6–8 hours.

Oxacillin
   Adult: 500–1000 mg every 4–6 hours.
   Child: 25–50 mg per lb. a day divided into 4 or 6 doses.

Penicillin G

Adult (age 12 and over): 200,000–800,000 units, or 125–500 mg, every 6–8 hours for 10 days.

Child (under age 12): 12,000–40,000 units per lb. a day divided into 3–6 doses.

Penicillin V

Adult (age 12 and over): 125–500 mg 4 times a day. Persons with severe kidney disease should not take more than 250 mg every 6 hours.

Child (under age 12): 12–25 mg per lb. a day divided into 3 or 4 doses.

Overdosage

Penicillin overdose is unlikely. If it occurs, diarrhea or upset stomach is the primary symptom. Massive overdose may result in seizure or excitability. Call your local poison control center or emergency room for more information. ALWAYS bring the prescription bottle or container with you if you go for treatment.

Special Information

Liquid penicillin should be refrigerated and must be thrown out after 14 days in the refrigerator or 7 days at room temperature.

Call your doctor if you develop black tongue, rash, itching, hives, diarrhea, breathing difficulties, sore throat, nausea, vomiting, fever, swollen joints, unusual bleeding or bruising, or if you are feeling unwell.

Penicillin eradicates most susceptible organisms in 7 to 10 days; be sure to take all the medication prescribed for the full period prescribed. It is best taken at evenly spaced intervals throughout the day.

If you miss a dose of a penicillin antibiotic, take it as soon as possible. If it is almost time for your next dose, space the missed dose and your next dose by 2 to 4 hours and then continue with your regular schedule.

Special Populations

Pregnancy/Breast-feeding

Penicillin has not caused birth defects and is often prescribed for pregnant women. These drugs cross into the fetal circulation and should be used only if absolutely necessary. If you are or might be pregnant, make certain that your doctor knows that you are taking a penicillin antibiotic.

Penicillin is generally safe during breast-feeding; however, small amounts may pass into breast milk and cause upset stomach, diarrhea, allergic reaction, or other problems in the nursing infant.

Seniors

Seniors may take penicillin without special restriction.

Generic Name

Pentostan Polysulfonate Sodium

(PEN-toe-stan pol-ee-SUL-fon-ate)

Brand Name

Elmiron

Type of Drug

Analgesic.

Prescribed for

Bladder pain or discomfort due to cystitis.

General Information

Interstitial cystitis is a painful, long-term infection of the bladder. Pentostan does not affect the infectious process, but it may stick to the membranes of the bladder wall, preventing irritating substances from reaching bladder cells. This drug is related to heparin, an anticoagulant (blood-thinning) drug, and has mild ability to both prevent a blood clot from forming and dissolve one that has already formed. Only 3% of the total dose of pentostan is absorbed into the bloodstream. In studies of pentostan, 29% of people taking it had less pain after 3 months. By 6 months, another 5% reported pain relief.

Cautions and Warnings

Do not take this product if you are **sensitive** or **allergic** to it.

Pentostan is a weak anticoagulant and can cause **black-and-blue marks**, **nosebleeds**, and **bleeding gums**.

People with **liver disease** should use this drug with caution because its breakdown can be reduced in people with liver problems. Also, pentostan can cause mild liver toxicity.

Possible Side Effects

▼ Most common: patchy hair loss beginning within 4 weeks of treatment, diarrhea, and nausea.

▼ Common: headache, emotional upset or depression, dizziness, abdominal pain, and upset stomach.

▼ Rare: sleeplessness, itching, rash, appetite loss, colitis, constipation, esophagus irritation, stomach irritation or gas, bleeding gums, mouth ulcers, vomiting, anemia, black-and-blue marks, allergic reactions, unusual sensitivity to bright light, nosebleeds, breathing difficulties, sore throat, runny nose, double vision, red-eye, bleeding in the eye, ringing or buzzing in the ears, and liver problems.

Drug Interactions

• Aspirin, warfarin, and other blood-thinning drugs should be taken with caution if you are already taking pentostan. There is a chance that pentostan will increase the anticoagulant effect of one of these drugs.

Food Interactions

Take this drug on an empty stomach, at least 1 hour before or 2 hours after a meal.

Usual Dose

Adult: 100 mg 3 times a day.

Overdosage

Overdose symptoms include bleeding, liver problems, and upset stomach. Overdose victims should be taken to a hospital emergency room at once. ALWAYS bring the prescription bottle or container with you.

Special Information

Pentostan has a mild anticoagulant effect. Make sure that your pharmacist, dentist, and all of your doctors know you are taking pentostan. Check with your doctor before combining any drugs, especially aspirin, with pentostan.

Patchy hair loss, usually starting within the first 4 weeks of taking pentostan, occurs in about 4% of people who take this medication.

Pentostan should be taken exactly as directed. If you forget to take a dose, take it as soon as you remember. If it is almost time for your next dose, skip the dose you forgot and continue with your regular schedule. Do not take a double dose.

Special Populations

Pregnancy/Breast-feeding
Animal studies have not revealed any potential problems with pentostan during pregnancy. It is not known if pentostan passes into breast milk. Like all other medications, pentostan should be used by a pregnant woman or nursing mother only when absolutely necessary.

Seniors
Seniors may use this medication without any special precaution.

Generic Name

Pentoxifylline (pen-tox-SIF-uh-lene)

Brand Name

Trental

Type of Drug

Blood-viscosity reducer.

Prescribed for

Blood-vessel spasms and painful leg cramps associated with intermittent claudication. Pentoxifylline has also been used to treat symptoms in people with poor blood flow to the brain and other blood-vessel disease.

General Information

Intermittent claudication is caused by poor blood supply due to arteriosclerotic disease. Pentoxifylline reduces blood viscosity (thickness) and improves the ability of red blood cells to modify their shape. By improving blood flow to the leg muscles, this medication may offer relief to people who experience severe leg pain when they walk. Leg cramps occur when muscles are deprived of oxygen. When blood flow is improved, the cramps are less severe or do not occur at all. Studies of pentoxifylline's effectiveness have yielded mixed results, but the drug may be helpful for people who do not respond to other treatments.

Exercise and physical training are probably more effective than pentoxifylline in the treatment of intermittent claudication. The medication may help people who cannot follow a training program or who are not candidates for surgery, which is another treatment for this condition.

Pentoxifylline has been studied for treating the complications of diabetes, leg ulcers, stroke, sickle-cell disease, high altitude sickness, weak sperm and low sperm count, hearing disorders, and eye circulation disorders.

Cautions and Warnings

People who have had a recent **stroke** or **bleeding** in the eye should not take pentoxifylline because it may worsen their condition. Those who cannot tolerate caffeine, theophylline, or theobromine should not use pentoxifylline since it is chemically related to those products.

The dosage of pentoxifylline should be reduced in people with **kidney disease**. People with poor kidney function may also require less medication than others since pentoxifylline is cleared from the body through the kidneys.

Possible Side Effects

Pentoxifylline side effects are relatively infrequent.

▼ Common: nausea, upset stomach, vomiting, dizziness, and headache.

▼ Less common: chest pains, breathing difficulties, swelling in the arm or leg, low blood pressure, stomach gas, appetite loss, constipation, dry mouth, excessive thirst, tremors, anxiety, confusion, stuffy nose, nosebleeds, flu-like symptoms, sore throat, laryngitis, swollen glands, itching, rash, brittle fingernails, blurred vision, conjunctivitis (pinkeye), earache, a bad taste in the mouth, feeling unwell, and changes in body weight.

▼ Rare: rapid or abnormal heart rhythms, hepatitis (symptoms include yellowing of the skin or whites of the

> **Possible Side Effects** *(continued)*
>
> eyes), reduced white-blood-cell count, and small hemor-
> rhages under the skin.

Drug Interactions

- Pentoxifylline may increase the blood-pressure-lowering
effects of other drugs.
- Your doctor may have to change the dosage of your
blood-pressure medication while you are taking pentoxifylline.
- Pentoxifylline may increase the effects of warfarin.

Food Interactions

Take pentoxifylline with food if it upsets your stomach.

Usual Dose

400 mg 3 times a day.

Overdosage

The severity of overdose symptoms is directly related to the
amount of pentoxifylline taken. Symptoms usually appear 4
to 5 hours after the medication was taken and may last as
long as 12 hours. Pentoxifylline overdose symptoms include
flushing, low blood pressure, fainting, depression, and convulsions. An overdose victim may be made to vomit with
ipecac syrup—available at any pharmacy—to remove any
remaining pentoxifylline from the stomach. Call your doctor
or a poison control center before doing this. If you go to a
hospital emergency room, ALWAYS bring the prescription
bottle or container with you.

Special Information

Call your doctor if any side effects develop. Some people may
have to stop using this medication if side effects become
intolerable. You may feel better within 2 weeks after starting
on pentoxifylline, but treatment should be continued for at
least 2 months to gain maximum benefit.

If you forget a dose of pentoxifylline, take it as soon as you
remember. If it is almost time for your next dose, skip the one
you forgot and continue with your regular schedule. Do not
take a double dose.

Special Populations

Pregnancy/Breast-feeding
Pentoxifylline crosses into fetal circulation but has not been found to cause birth defects. When the drug is considered essential by your doctor, its potential benefits must be carefully weighed against its risks.

Pentoxifylline passes into breast milk and may affect breast-fed infants. Nursing mothers who must take this medication should bottle-feed their babies.

Seniors
Older adults, especially those with kidney disease, are more sensitive to the effects of this drug because they absorb more and eliminate it more slowly than do younger adults. Follow your doctor's directions and report any side effects at once.

Pepcid

see **Famotidine**, page 398

Brand Name

Percocet

Generic Ingredients

Acetaminophen + Oxycodone Hydrochloride G

Other Brand Names
Roxicet   Roxilox
Roxicet 5/500   Tylox

The information in this profile also applies to the following drugs:

Generic Ingredients: Acetaminophen +
Codeine Phosphate G
Aceta with Codeine   Tylenol with Codeine No. 2
Capital with Codeine   Tylenol with Codeine No. 3
Phenaphen with Codeine   Tylenol with Codeine No. 4
  No. 3
Phenaphen with Codeine
  No. 4

Generic Ingredients: Acetaminophen + Hydrocodone Bitartrate

Anexsia 5/500	Lortab
Anexsia 7.5/650	Lortab ASA
Bancap HC	Lortab 2.5/500
Ceta-Plus	Lortab 5/500
Co-Gesic	Lortab 7.5/500
Dolacet	Margesic H
Duocet	Panacet 5/500
Hydrogesic	Stagesic
Hy-Phen	T-Gesic
Lorcet	Vicodin
Lorcet-HD	Vicodin-ES
Lorcet Plus	Zydone
Lorcet 10/650	

Type of Drug

Narcotic-analgesic (pain reliever) combination.

Prescribed for

Mild to moderate pain.

General Information

Percocet is generally prescribed for those who require a greater analgesic effect than acetaminophen alone can deliver or for those who are allergic to or cannot take aspirin.

Percocet is probably not effective for arthritis or other pain caused by inflammation because it does not reduce inflammation.

Cautions and Warnings

Do not take Percocet if you are **allergic or sensitive** to it. Use this drug with extreme caution if you suffer from **asthma or other breathing problems** or if you have **kidney or liver disease** or **viral infection of the liver**. Chronic (long-term) use of Percocet may cause **drug dependence or addiction**.

Oxycodone is a respiratory depressant and affects the central nervous system (CNS), producing sleepiness, tiredness, or inability to concentrate. Be careful if you are driving, operating hazardous or complicated machinery, or performing other functions requiring concentration.

Alcohol may increase the chances of acetaminophen-related liver toxicity and oxycodone-related drowsiness.

Possible Side Effects

▼ Most common: light-headedness, dizziness, sleepiness, nausea, vomiting, appetite loss, and increased sweating. If any of these effects occur, consider asking your doctor to lower your dosage. Most of these side effects will disappear if you lie down. More serious side effects are shallow breathing or breathing difficulties.

▼ Rare: euphoria (feeling high), weakness, headache, agitation, uncoordinated muscle movement, minor hallucinations, disorientation and visual disturbances, dry mouth, constipation, facial flushing, rapid heartbeat, palpitations, faintness, urinary difficulties or hesitancy, reduced sex drive or potency, rash, itching, anemia, lowered blood sugar, and yellowing of the skin or whites of the eyes. Narcotic pain relievers may aggravate convulsions in those who have had convulsions in the past.

Drug Interactions

• Because of its depressant effect and potential effect on breathing, Percocet should be taken with extreme care in combination with alcohol, sleeping medication, tranquilizers, antihistamines, or other drugs producing sedation.

Food Interactions

Percocet is best taken with food or at least half a glass of water to prevent upset stomach.

Usual Dose

Percocet
    Adult: 1 or 2 tablets every 4 hours.
    Child: not recommended.

Tylenol with Codeine
    Adult and Child (age 13 and over): 1–2 tablets every 4 hours.
    Child (age 7–12): equivalent to 5–10 mg of codeine every 4–6 hours; do not exceed 60 mg in 24 hours.
    Child (age 2–6): equivalent to 2.5–5 mg of codeine every 4–6 hours; do not exceed 30 mg in 24 hours.

Vicodin
    Adult: 1 tablet every 6 hours.
    Child: not recommended.

Overdosage

Symptoms include depression of respiration (breathing), extreme tiredness progressing to stupor and then coma, pinpointed pupils, no response to pain stimulation, cold and clammy skin, slowing of heart rate, lowering of blood pressure, yellowing of the skin or whites of the eyes, bluish discoloration of the hands or feet, fever, excitement, delirium, convulsions, cardiac arrest, and liver toxicity (symptoms include nausea, vomiting, pain in the abdomen, and diarrhea). The overdose victim should be made to vomit with ipecac syrup—available at any pharmacy—and be taken to a hospital emergency room immediately. ALWAYS bring the prescription bottle or container with you.

Special Information

Percocet is a respiratory depressant that affects the CNS, producing sleepiness, tiredness, or inability to concentrate. Be careful if you are driving, operating hazardous or complicated machinery, or performing other functions requiring concentration.

If you forget to take a dose of Percocet, take it as soon as you remember. If it is almost time for your next dose, skip the forgotten dose and continue with your regular medication schedule. Do not take a double dose.

Special Populations

Pregnancy/Breast-feeding

High doses of acetaminophen, one of the ingredients in Percocet, have caused problems when taken during pregnancy. The regular use of oxycodone, the other active ingredient in Percocet, during pregnancy may cause the unborn child to become addicted. If used during labor, it may cause breathing problems in the infant. If you are or might be pregnant, do not take Percocet.

The ingredients in Percocet may pass into breast milk. If you must take it, wait 4 to 6 hours after taking the drug before breast-feeding or consider bottle-feeding your baby.

Seniors

Seniors may be sensitive to the depressant effects of the narcotic pain reliever in this combination. Follow your doctor's directions and report any side effects at once.

Brand Name

Percodan

Generic Ingredients

Aspirin + Oxycodone Hydrochloride + Oxycodone Terephthalate Ⓖ

Other Brand Names

Oxycodone with Aspirin   Roxiprin
Percodan-Demi

The information in this profile also applies to the following drugs:

Generic Ingredients: Aspirin + Codeine Phosphate Ⓖ
Empirin with Codeine No. 3   Empirin with Codeine No. 4

Generic Ingredients: Aspirin + Caffeine + Dihydrocodeine Bitartrate
Synalgos-DC

Generic Ingredients: Pentazocine + Acetaminophen
Talacen

Generic Ingredients: Pentazocine + Aspirin
Talwin Compound

Generic Ingredients: Pentazocine + Naloxone
Talwin Nx

Type of Drug

Narcotic-aspirin combination.

Prescribed for

Mild to moderate pain.

General Information

Percodan is one of many combination products containing both a narcotic and a non-narcotic analgesic. It is prescribed for people who need the combination of pain relief and inflammation reduction offered by Percodan.

Cautions and Warnings

Do not take Percodan you are **allergic or sensitive** to it. Use this medication with extreme caution if you suffer from **asthma or any other breathing problems**. Chronic (long-term) use of this drug may cause **drug dependence or addiction**. Percodan is a respiratory depressant and affects the central nervous system (CNS), producing sleepiness, tiredness, or inability to concentrate.

Do not take Percodan if you are **allergic** to any salicylate, including aspirin, or any nonsteroidal anti-inflammatory drug (NSAID). Check with your doctor or pharmacist if you are not sure. This and all other aspirin-containing products should not be taken by **children under age 16**.

People with **liver damage** should avoid Percodan and all products that contain either aspirin or oxycodone.

Alcoholic beverages may aggravate the stomach irritation caused by aspirin. The risk of aspirin-related ulcer is increased by alcohol. Alcohol will also increase the nervous-system depression caused by the oxycodone ingredient in this drug.

Do not use Percodan if you develop **dizziness**, **hearing loss**, or **ringing or buzzing in your ears**.

Percodan may interfere with normal blood coagulation and should be avoided for 1 week before surgery. Ask your surgeon or dentist for a recommendation before taking an aspirin-containing product for pain after surgery.

Possible Side Effects

▼ Most common: light-headedness, dizziness, sleepiness, nausea, vomiting, appetite loss, and increased sweating. If these occur, consider calling your doctor to ask about lowering your dosage. Usually they will go away if you lie down.

▼ Less common: shallow breathing or serious breathing difficulties, euphoria (feeling high), weakness, headache, agitation, uncoordinated muscle movement, minor hallucinations, disorientation, visual disturbances, dry mouth, constipation, facial flushing, rapid heartbeat, palpitations, feeling faint, urinary difficulties or hesitancy, reduced sex drive or potency, rash, itching, anemia, low blood sugar, and yellowing of the skin or whites of the eyes. These drugs may aggravate convulsions in those who have had convulsions.

Drug Interactions

• Interaction with alcohol, tranquilizers, barbiturates, or sleeping pills produces sleepiness or inability to concentrate and seriously increases the depressive effect of Percodan.

• The aspirin component of Percodan may affect anticoagulant (blood-thinning) therapy. Discuss this with your doctor so that the proper dosage adjustment may be made.

• Interaction with adrenal corticosteroids, phenylbutazone, or alcohol may cause severe stomach irritation with possible bleeding.

• The aspirin component of Percodan will counteract the uric-acid-eliminating effect of probenecid and sulfinpyrazone; may counteract the blood-pressure-lowering effect of angiotensin-converting enzyme (ACE) inhibitors and beta-blocking drugs and the effects of diuretics (agents that increase urination) when given to people with severe liver disease; and may increase blood levels of methotrexate and of valproic acid when taken together, leading to increased risk of drug toxicity.

• The aspirin component of Percodan, when taken with nitroglycerin tablets, may lead to an unexpected drop in blood pressure.

• Do not take Percodan with any NSAID. There is no benefit from the combination and the risk of side effects, especially stomach irritation, is significantly increased.

• Large doses of aspirin—2000 mg a day or more—may lower blood sugar, a potentially serious problem in diabetics. Percodan tablets contain 325 mg of aspirin.

Food Interactions

Take with food or half a glass of water to prevent upset stomach.

Usual Dose

Percodan
   Adult: 1 tablet every 6 hours as needed for relief of pain.
   Child: not recommended.

Empirin with Codeine
   Adult: 1–2 tablets 3–4 times a day.
   Child: not recommended.

Synalgos-DC
   Adult: 2 capsules every 4 hours.
   Child: not recommended.

Overdosage

Symptoms of oxycodone—a component of Percodan—overdose include breathing difficulties, extreme tiredness progressing to stupor and then coma, pinpointed pupils, no response to pain stimulation, cold and clammy skin, slowing of heartbeat, dizziness or fainting, convulsions, and cardiac arrest.

Aspirin—a component of Percodan—overdose in severe cases may cause fever, excitement, confusion, convulsions, liver or kidney failure, or bleeding. Symptoms of mild aspirin overdose include rapid and deep breathing, nausea, vomiting, dizziness, ringing or buzzing in the ears, flushing, increased sweating, thirst, headache, drowsiness, diarrhea, and rapid heartbeat.

The overdose victim should be taken to a hospital emergency room immediately. ALWAYS bring the prescription bottle or container with you.

Special Information

Drowsiness may occur: Be careful when driving or operating complicated or hazardous machinery.

Contact your doctor if you develop continuous stomach pain or a ringing or buzzing in the ears.

Do not use an aspirin product such as Percodan if it has a strong odor of vinegar. This is an indication that the product has started to break down in the bottle.

If you forget to take a dose of Percodan, take it as soon as you remember. If it is almost time for your next dose, skip the one you forgot and continue with your regular schedule. Do not take a double dose.

Special Populations

Pregnancy/Breast-feeding

Check with your doctor before taking any aspirin-containing product during pregnancy, including Percodan. Aspirin may cause bleeding problems in the fetus, particularly during the last 2 weeks of pregnancy. Taking aspirin during the last 3 months of pregnancy may lead to a low-birth-weight infant, prolong labor, and extend the duration of pregnancy; it may also cause bleeding in the mother before, during, or after delivery.

Oxycodone, the other ingredient in Percodan, has not been associated with birth defects but taking too much of any other narcotic during pregnancy may lead to the birth of a drug-dependent infant and drug-withdrawal symptoms in the baby. Any narcotic may cause breathing problems in the newborn if taken just before delivery.

The ingredients in Percodan may pass into breast milk. Consider bottle-feeding your baby if you must take this drug.

Seniors

The oxycodone in Percodan may have more of a depressant effect on seniors than on younger adults. Other effects that may be more prominent are dizziness, light-headedness, and fainting, particularly upon rising suddenly from a sitting or lying position.

Generic Name

Pergolide (PER-goe-lide)

Brand Name

Permax

Type of Drug

Antiparkinsonian.

Prescribed for

Parkinson's disease.

General Information

Pergolide mesylate is combined with levodopa or carbidopa to control Parkinson's disease. It works by stimulating a specific nerve ending in the central nervous system that is normally stimulated by the hormone dopamine. Pergolide also inhibits the production of prolactin, a hormone that is involved in the production of breast milk. Pergolide affects growth-hormone levels and the reproductive hormone called luteinizing hormone (LH).

Cautions and Warnings

If you have had a previous **reaction** to pergolide or to other drugs derived from the fungus ergot, do not take this drug.

Pergolide may cause **hallucinations** in about 14% of people who take it. If this happens to you, report it to your doctor at once.

People who are prone to abnormal heart rhythm should be cautious when taking pergolide because of possible cardiac side effects.

Female animals given pergolide develop tumors of the uterus, but there is no information on this effect in humans.

Possible Side Effects

Pergolide can affect virtually any body part or system because of its effect on basic body hormones. In studies of the drug, about 25% of people who started pergolide stopped because of side effects.

▼ Most common: hallucinations, confusion, abnormal twisting body movements, tiredness, difficulty sleeping, nausea, constipation, diarrhea, upset stomach, and runny nose.

▼ Less common: generalized pain; abdominal pain; neck or back pain; migraine headaches; muscle weakness; chest pain; flu-like illness; chills; facial swelling; infections; dizziness when rising from a sitting or lying position; fainting; heart palpitations; changes in blood pressure; abnormal heart rhythm; heart attack; heart failure; changes in appetite; dry mouth; vomiting; stomach gas; yellow discoloration of the skin or eyes; enlarged saliva glands; stomach irritation; intestinal ulcer or obstruction; gum irritation; tooth cavities; colitis; loss of bowel control; blood in the stool; vomiting blood; bursitis; muscle twitching; anxiety; tremors; depression; unusual dreams; personality changes; psychosis; changes in how you walk; loss of coordination; tingling in the hands or feet; speech problems; muscle stiffness; breathing difficulties; hiccups; pneumonia; coughing; sinus irritation; bronchitis; asthma; nosebleed; rash; skin discoloration; skin ulcers; acne; fungal infections; eczema; hair growth or loss; cold sores; increased sweating; visual abnormalities, such as double vision, conjunctivitis, cataracts, retinal detachment, blindness, and eye pain; earaches; middle-ear infection; ringing or buzzing in the ears; deafness; changes in sense of taste; frequent or painful urination; urinary infection; blood in the urine; swelling of the arms or legs; weight gain; anemia; breast

Possible Side Effects *(continued)*

pain; painful menstruation; breast oozing; underactive thyroid; thyroid tumor; diabetes; and muscle, bone, and joint pain.

Drug Interactions

• Many drugs, including the phenothiazines, the thioxanthenes, haloperidol, droperidol, loxapine, methyldopa, molindone, papaverine, reserpine, and metoclopramide will counter the effects of pergolide: They all antagonize the neurohormone dopamine.

• Alcohol, tranquilizers, and other nervous-system depressants will increase the depressant effects of this drug.

• Drugs that cause low blood pressure will exaggerate the blood-pressure-lowering effect of pergolide.

Food Interactions

Take pergolide with food or meals if it upsets your stomach.

Usual Dose

Starting dose—0.05 mg a day. Dosage is increased by 0.1–0.25 mg every third day until an effect is achieved. Maximum dosage is 5 mg a day.

Overdosage

Symptoms of a pergolide overdosage may include nausea, vomiting, agitation, low blood pressure, hallucinations, involuntary bodily and muscular movements, tingling in the arms or legs, heart palpitations, abnormal heart rhythm, and nervous-system stimulation. Overdose victims should be taken to a hospital emergency room for treatment. ALWAYS bring the prescription bottle or container with you.

Special Information

Many people taking pergolide for the first time experience dizziness and fainting caused by low blood pressure. Your doctor will need to increase your pergolide dosage gradually to reduce this effect. However, any dizziness or fainting should be reported to your doctor at once.

Other pergolide side effects to report to the doctor include any nervous-system effects, such as confusion, uncontrolled body movements, or hallucinations; pain or burning on urination; high blood pressure; severe headache; seizure; sudden changes in vision; severe chest pain; fainting; rapid heartbeat; severe nausea; excessive sweating; nervousness; unexplained shortness of breath; and sudden weakness. In addition, make sure your doctor knows about any side effect that is particularly bothersome or persistent.

Do not stop taking pergolide or change your dosage without your doctor's knowledge. It is important to maintain regular contact with your doctor to allow for observation of the drug's effects and side effects.

Be careful while engaging in activities that require concentration and coordination, such as driving: This drug may make you tired, dizzy, or light-headed.

Dry mouth may be relieved by using sugarless gum, candy, ice, or a saliva substitute. Pay special attention to oral hygiene while you are taking pergolide because dry mouth increases the chances of oral infections.

If you take pergolide once a day and forget a dose, take it as soon as you remember. If it is almost time for your next dose, skip the one you forgot and continue with your regular schedule. Do not take a double dose.

If you take pergolide 2 or 3 times a day and forget a dose, take it as soon as you remember. If it is almost time for your next dose, take one dose as soon as you remember and another in 3 or 4 hours, then go back to your regular schedule. Do not take a double dose.

Special Populations

Pregnancy/Breast-feeding
Women who are or might be pregnant should not use pergolide unless its potential benefits have been carefully weighed against its risks.

Pergolide interferes with milk production. Nursing mothers who must take pergolide should bottle-feed their babies.

Seniors
Older adults may take pergolide without special restriction.

Generic Name

Phenelzine (FEH-nel-zine)

Brand Name

Nardil

The information in this profile also applies to the following drug:

Generic Ingredient: Tranylcypromine Sulfate
Parnate

Type of Drug

Monoamine oxidase inhibitor (MAOI).

Prescribed for

Atypical depression and depression that does not respond to other drugs; also prescribed for a variety of conditions including bulimia, cocaine addiction, night terrors, post-traumatic stress disorder, migraine, seasonal affective disorder, and symptoms of multiple sclerosis.

General Information

Monoamine oxidase (MAO) is a complex enzyme system found throughout the body. MAO is responsible for breaking down hormones that make the nervous system work. MAOIs such as phenelzine sulfate interfere with MAO action, causing an increase in the amount of norepinephrine and other monamines stored throughout the nervous system. This increase is what gives phenelzine its therapeutic effect. Phenelzine is well absorbed when taken by mouth. Its effect is long lasting and may continue for up to 2 weeks after you stop taking it.

Cautions and Warnings

Do not take phenelzine if you are **allergic** to it or if you have **pheochromocytoma** (adrenal-gland tumor), **heart failure, liver disease** or **abnormal liver function,** severe **kidney-function loss, heart disease,** or a history of **headaches, stroke, transient ischemic attack (TIA)**—"mini-stroke"—or **high blood pressure**. The most severe reactions to phenelzine, which can be deadly, involve very high blood pressure. Bleeding inside the head has occurred in people with very high blood pressure. Serious, potentially fatal reactions may occur if phenelzine and a selective serotonin reuptake inhibitor (SSRI) antidepressant are taken together (see "Drug Interactions").

Possible Side Effects

▼ Common: dizziness when rising from a sitting or lying position, dizziness, fainting, headache, tremors, muscle twitching, overly reactive reflexes, manic reactions, confusion, memory loss, sleeping difficulties, weakness, uncontrollable muscle movement, fatigue, drowsiness, restlessness, overstimulation, anxiety and agitation, constipation, nausea, diarrhea, abdominal pain, swelling, dry mouth, liver irritation, appetite loss, weight change, and sexual difficulties.

▼ Less common: jitteriness, a need to pace the floor or change positions often, euphoria (feeling high), nerve irritation, chills, a need to repeat words or phrases, convulsions, tingling in the hands or feet, heart palpitations, rapid heartbeat, painful or infrequent urination, blood changes, glaucoma, blurred vision, uncontrolled eyeball movement, sweating, and skin rash.

▼ Rare: poor coordination, coma, hallucinations at high doses, severe anxiety, schizophrenia, delirious reactions, muscle spasm, jerky movements, numbness, and yellowing of the skin or whites of the eyes.

Drug Interactions

• Phenelzine interferes with the blood-pressure-lowering effect of guanethidine. Do not combine these 2 medicines.

• Taking an SSRI antidepressant and phenelzine at the same time or too close together may result in a serious, sometimes fatal reaction characterized by very high fever, rigidity, muscle spasms, mental changes, and changes in blood pressure, pulse, and breathing rate. Two weeks should elapse between stopping phenelzine and taking an SSRI. At least 5 weeks should elapse between stopping an SSRI and taking phenelzine.

• Combining a tricyclic antidepressant and phenelzine can be safe and successful, but it must be done under your doctor's direct supervision. If doses are not strictly controlled, this combination can lead to seizures, sweating, coma, hyperexcitability, high fever, rapid heartbeat, rapid breathing, head-ache, dilated pupils, flushing, confusion, and low blood pressure. When severe, this reaction can be fatal. Generally, 2 weeks must pass between stopping phenelzine and taking a tricyclic antidepressant.

• Phenelzine increases the effects of sulfonylurea-type anti-diabetic drugs, barbiturates, beta blockers, levodopa, meperi-dine, methyldopa, rauwolfia drugs, sulfa drugs, sumatriptan, stimulants, thiazide-type diuretics, and L-tryptophan. The combination of any of these drugs and phenelzine can result in severe reactions.

• Taking dextromethorphan (a cough suppressant found in many over-the-counter [OTC] products) with phenelzine may lead to a high fever and low blood pressure. Avoid this combination.

• Combining phenelzine with another MAOI or methyl-phenidate may lead to excessively high blood pressure.

• Combining tranylcypromine sulfate and disulfiram may lead to delirium, agitation, disorientation, and hallucinations.

Food Interactions

Avoid the following foods while taking phenelzine and for at least 2 weeks after stopping phenelzine:

Alcoholic Beverages: imported beer and ale; red wine, especially Chianti; sherry; vermouth; and distilled spirits.

Cheese and Dairy: processed American cheese, blue cheese, Boursault, natural brick cheese, Brie, Camembert, cheddar, Emmenthaler, Gruyere, mozzarella, Parmesan, Romano, Roquefort, sour cream, Stilton, Swiss cheese, and yo-gurt.

Fruits and Vegetables: avocados, especially when overripe; yeast extracts, including marmite; canned figs; raisins; sauer-kraut; soy sauce; miso soup; and bean curd.

Meat and Fish: beef or chicken liver, meats prepared with a tenderizer, summer sausage, bologna, pepperoni, salami, game, meat extracts, caviar, dried fish, salted herring, pickled and spoiled herring, and shrimp paste.

Other: fava beans, caffeine-containing drinks, chocolate, and ginseng.

Usual Dose

Phenelzine
  Adult and Child (age 17 and over): 15 mg 3 times a day to

start, increased gradually to 90 mg a day. Maintenance dose
may be as low as 15 mg a day.

Senior: 15 mg in the morning. Doses are increased very
gradually.

Child (under age 17): not recommended.

Tranylcypromine Sulfate

Adult and Child (age 17 and over): 10–60 mg a day. Usual
dose is 30 mg a day.

Senior: starting dosage—2½–5 mg a day. Maintenance
dosage—45 mg a day.

Child (under age 17): not recommended.

Overdosage

Early symptoms of phenelzine overdose may include excitement; irritability; hyperactivity; anxiety; low blood pressure;
vascular system collapse; sleeplessness; restlessness; dizziness; fainting; weakness; drowsiness; hallucinations; jaw-
muscle spasms; flushing; sweating; rapid breathing; rapid
heartbeat; movement disorders including grimacing, rigidity,
muscle tremors, and large muscle spasms; and severe headache. Any person suspected of having taken an overdose of
phenelzine must be taken to a hospital emergency room at
once for treatment. ALWAYS bring the prescription bottle or
container with you.

Special Information

Serious side effects of phenelzine include intense headache;
heart palpitations; stiff or sore neck; nausea; vomiting; sweating, sometimes accompanied by fever or cold, clammy skin;
dilated pupils; and sensitivity to bright light. Report these or
any other unusual side effects to your doctor.

Vivid nightmares, agitation, psychosis, and convulsions
occasionally occur 1 to 3 days after phenelzine is abruptly
stopped. Gradually stopping phenelzine should prevent these
problems.

Phenelzine causes drowsiness and blurred vision. Be careful when driving or doing anything that requires concentration, alertness, and coordination. Avoid alcohol.

Diabetics taking phenelzine should be cautious because the
drug may lower blood-sugar readings.

Be sure your surgeon or dentist knows that you are taking
phenelzine before he or she gives you any anesthetic drug.

Do not take any other prescription or OTC drug without first checking with your pharmacist or the doctor who prescribed phenelzine.

If you forget to take a dose of phenelzine, take it as soon as possible up to 2 hours before your next scheduled dose. If it is less than 2 hours until your next dose, skip the dose you forgot and continue with your regular schedule. Do not take a double dose.

Special Populations

Pregnancy/Breast-feeding
Phenelzine should be taken during pregnancy only if the drug's benefits and risks have been considered. Nursing mothers who must take phenelzine should bottle-feed their babies.

Seniors
Seniors are more susceptible to side effects and must be cautious about using phenelzine.

Phenergan

see **Promethazine**, page 923

Generic Name

Phenobarbital (FEEN-oe-BAR-bih-tol)

Brand Name

Solfoton

Type of Drug

Hypnotic, sedative, and anticonvulsant.

Prescribed for

Epileptic and other seizures, convulsions, daytime sedation, sleeplessness, and eclampsia (toxemia in pregnancy).

General Information

Phenobarbital is a sustained-release barbiturate. It takes 30 to 60 minutes to start working and its effect lasts for 10 to 16 hours. Like other barbiturates, phenobarbital appears to act by interfering with nerve impulses to the brain. When used as an anticonvulsant, phenobarbital is not very effective by itself; when used with anticonvulsant agents such as phenytoin, the combined action is dramatic. This combination has been used very successfully to control epileptic seizure.

Cautions and Warnings

Phenobarbital may **dull your physical and mental reflexes**, so you must be extremely careful when driving or doing anything that requires total concentration.

Phenobarbital may be **addicting** if taken for an extended period of time. It may also cause signs of intoxication including **slurred speech, a wobbly walk, rolling of the eyes, confusion, poor judgement, irritability,** and **sleeplessness**. Combining this drug with **alcohol** worsens the situation.

Barbiturates are broken down in the liver and eliminated through the kidneys; people with **liver or kidney disease** should be cautious about taking phenobarbital.

You should not take phenobarbital if you are **sensitive or allergic** to any barbiturate, if you have been **addicted to sedatives or hypnotics**, or if you have a **respiratory condition**.

People with **chronic pain** should be careful about taking this drug because it may mask symptoms or cause stimulation, although using phenobarbital after surgery and in people with cancer has proven effective.

People abruptly stopping this drug may develop seizure. Dosage should be reduced gradually.

Barbiturates may increase your need for vitamin D. A standard vitamin supplement will take care of this problem.

Possible Side Effects

▼ Most common: drowsiness, lethargy, dizziness, drug hangover, breathing difficulties, rash, and general allergic reaction (symptoms include runny nose, watery eyes, sneezing, scratchy throat, and cough).

▼ Less common: nausea, vomiting, constipation and diarrhea, slow heartbeat, low blood pressure, and fainting. Severe adverse reactions may include anemia and yellowing of the skin or whites of the eyes.

Drug Interactions

• Alcohol, monoamine oxidase inhibitor (MAOI) antidepressants, and valproic acid increase the effects of phenobarbital.

• Charcoal, chloramphenicol, and rifampin may counteract the effects of phenobarbital.

• Phenobarbital interferes with the effects of anticoagulant (blood-thinning) drugs, beta-blocker drugs, carbamazepine, chloramphenicol, oral contraceptives ("the pill"), corticosteroids, clonazepam, digitoxin, doxorubicin, doxycycline, felodipine, fenoprofen, griseofulvin, metronidazole, phenylbutazone, quinidine, theophylline, and verapamil.

• Phenobarbital enhances the toxic effects of acetaminophen and methoxyflurane (an anesthetic).

• Phenobarbital has a variable effect on phenytoin and other antiseizure medication and on narcotic drugs. If you are taking one of these drug combinations, your doctor will have to balance your dosages based on the amount of all drugs in the blood.

Food Interactions

Phenobarbital is best taken on an empty stomach but may be taken with food if it upsets your stomach.

Usual Dose

Anticonvulsant
    Adult: 50–100 mg 2–3 times a day.
    Child: 1.3–2.25 mg per lb. of body weight divided into 2 or 3 doses a day.

Sleeplessness
100–320 mg at bedtime.

Daytime Sedation
30–120 mg in 2–3 divided doses.

Overdosage

Severe barbiturate overdose may kill; barbiturates have been used many times in suicide attempts. Overdose symptoms include breathing difficulties, moderate reduction in pupil size, lowered body temperature progressing to fever as time passes, fluid in the lungs, and eventually coma. Anyone suspected of having taken a barbiturate overdose must be taken to a hospital immediately. ALWAYS bring the prescription bottle or container with you.

Special Information

Avoid alcohol and other drugs that depress the nervous system while taking phenobarbital.

Be sure to take this medication exactly as prescribed by your doctor.

This drug causes drowsiness and poor concentration and makes it more difficult to drive a car or perform complicated activities.

Call your doctor at once if you develop fever, sore throat, nosebleeds, mouth sores, unexplainable black-and-blue marks, or easy bruising or bleeding.

If you forget to take a dose of phenobarbital, take it as soon as you remember. If it is almost time for your next dose, skip the one you forgot and continue with your regular schedule. Do not take a double dose.

Special Populations

Pregnancy/Breast-feeding

Barbiturate use during pregnancy may increase the risk of birth defects. However, phenobarbital may be necessary to control major episodes of seizure in certain pregnant women. Regular use of a barbiturate during the last 3 months of pregnancy may cause the baby to be born dependent on the drug. Also, barbiturate use increases the risk of bleeding problems, brain tumor, and breathing difficulties in the newborn. Talk to your doctor about your need to continue phenobarbital during your pregnancy.

Barbiturates pass into breast milk and may cause drowsiness, slow heartbeat, and breathing difficulties in nursing infants. Nursing mothers who must take phenobarbital should bottle-feed their infants.

Seniors

Seniors are more sensitive to the effects of barbiturates and often need less medication than do younger adults. Follow your doctor's directions and report any side effects at once.

Generic Name

Phenytoin (FEN-ih-toin) Ⓖ

Brand Name

Dilantin

The information in this profile also applies to the following drugs:

Generic Ingredient: Ethotoin
Peganone

Generic Ingredient: Fosphenytoin
Cerebyx

Generic Ingredient: Mephenytoin
Mesantoin

Type of Drug

Hydantoin anticonvulsant.

Prescribed for

Epileptic seizure; also prescribed for prevention of seizure following neurosurgery in nonepileptics and for abnormal heart rhythm, especially when caused by digitalis drugs. Phenytoin injection is used to control preeclampsia (a condition in which pregnant women experience severe increases in blood pressure during the second half of pregnancy), trigeminal neuralgia (tic douloureux), and severe skin conditions characterized by the formation of large pustules.

General Information

Phenytoin is one of several hydantoin antiseizure drugs used to control certain seizure disorders. These drugs all inhibit the activity of that area of the brain responsible for grand mal seizures. People may respond to some hydantoins and not others, but the reason for this is not understood. Phenytoin is the most widely prescribed member of this group of drugs.

There are 2 kinds of phenytoin: *prompt*, which must be taken several times a day, and *extended*, which can be taken either once or several times a day. Many people find the extended action more convenient, but the prompt form allows your doctor more flexibility in designing an effective daily dose schedule.

Phenytoin may be used together with other anticonvulsants, such as phenobarbital.

Cautions and Warnings

Do not take phenytoin if you are **allergic** to it or to any other hydantoin anticonvulsant.

If you have been taking phenytoin for a long time and no longer need it, the dosage should be gradually reduced over a period of about a week. Stopping abruptly may bring on severe **epileptic seizures.**

Phenytoin should not be used if you have **low blood pressure, myocardial insufficiency,** a very **slow heart rate,** or certain other **heart problems**. The use of other hydantoins is not limited by these situations.

People with **liver disease** will eliminate phenytoin more slowly from their bodies than others, increasing the chances for drug side effects.

Your doctor will need to take blood tests periodically to be sure that **red- and white-blood-cell counts** have not been affected by phenytoin. Sore throat, feeling unwell, fever, mucous-membrane bleeding, swollen glands, nosebleeds, black-and-blue marks, and easy bruising may be signs of **blood problems**.

Skin rash may be a sign of a serious reaction and may be cause for stopping this medication. Tell your doctor at once if this happens.

Possible Side Effects

▼ Most common: rapid or unusual growth of the gums, slurred speech, mental confusion, nystagmus (rhythmic, uncontrolled movement of the eye), dizziness, insomnia, nervousness, uncontrollable twitching, double vision, tiredness, irritability, depression, tremors, headache. These side effects will generally disappear as therapy continues and the dosage is reduced.

▼ Less common: nausea, vomiting, diarrhea, constipation, fever, rash, balding, weight gain, numbness in the hands or feet, chest pain, water retention, sensitivity to bright light (especially sunlight), conjunctivitis (pinkeye), joint pain and inflammation, and high blood sugar. Phenytoin may cause coarse facial features, lip enlargement and Peyronie's disease (where the penis is permanently deformed or misshapen). Phenytoin skin rash may be accompanied by fever and may be serious or even fatal. Some fatal blood-system side effects have occurred with phenytoin.

▼ Rare: liver damage, including hepatitis, and unusual body-hair growth.

Drug Interactions

• The following drugs may increase the effects of phenytoin, possibly necessitating a decrease in phenytoin dosage: alcoholic beverages in small amounts, allopurinol, amiodarone, aspirin and other salicylate drugs, benzodiazepine tranquilizers and sedatives, chloramphenicol, chlorpheniramine, cimetidine, disulfiram, fluconazole, ibuprofen, isoniazid, metronidazole, miconazole, omeprazole, phenacemide, phenothiazine antipsychotic medicines, phenylbutazone, succinimide antiseizure medicines, sulfa drugs, tricyclic antidepressants, trimethoprim, and valproic acid.

• The following drugs may interfere with the effects of phenytoin, possibly necessitating an increase in phenytoin dosage: alcoholic beverages in alcoholics, antacids, anticancer drugs, barbiturates, carbamazepine, charcoal tablets, diazoxide, folic acid, influenza virus vaccine, loxapine succinate, nitrofurantoin, pyridoxine, rifampin, sucralfate, and theophylline drugs.

• Calcium supplements may slow the absorption of phenytoin.

• Phenytoin may increase the rate at which the following drugs are removed from the body, possibly necessitating an increase in their dosages: amiodarone, carbamazepine, digitalis drugs, corticosteroids, dicumarol, disopyramide, doxycycline, estrogen drugs, haloperidol, methadone, metyrapone, mexiletine, oral contraceptives, quinidine, theophylline drugs, and valproic acid.

• Phenytoin may increase the chances for liver toxicity from acetaminophen, especially if the phenytoin is taken regularly for a seizure disorder.

• Phenytoin may affect certain other drugs in an unpredictable manner. If you take phenytoin and one or more of these drugs, your doctor will have to determine if dosage adjustment is needed: cyclosporine, dopamine, furosemide, levodopa, levonorgestrel, mebendazole, phenothiazine antipsychotic drugs, and oral antidiabetes medicines.

• Combining clonazepam and phenytoin yields unpredictable results: The effect of either drug may be reduced or phenytoin side effects may occur.

• Corticosteroid drugs may mask the effects of phenytoin sensitivity reactions.

• Lithium toxicity may be increased if lithium is taken with phenytoin.

• Phenytoin may decrease meperidine's pain-relieving effects and increase the risk of meperidine side effects. This combination is not recommended.

• Long-term phenytoin therapy may result in extreme folic acid deficiency, or megaloblastic anemia. This imbalance may be corrected with folic acid supplements.

• Warfarin's effects may be increased by adding phenytoin; warfarin dosage must be adjusted accordingly.

Food Interactions

Take phenytoin with food or meals to avoid stomach upset. Calcium can slow phenytoin absorption from the small intestine. Separate your phenytoin dose from high-calcium foods, such as milk, cheese, almonds, hazelnuts, and sesame seeds and calcium supplements, by 1 to 2 hours.

Usual Dose

Adult: starting dose—300 mg a day. Maintenance dose—300–400 mg a day. Dose can be raised gradually to 600 mg a day. Phenytoin extended is taken once a day; phenytoin prompt must be taken throughout the day.

Child: starting dose—2.5 mg per lb. of body weight a day, divided into 2 or 3 equal doses. Maintenance dose—2–4 mg per lb. of body weight a day. Dosage should be adjusted according to the child's needs. Children over age 6 may take the adult dosage, but no child should take more than 300 mg a day.

Overdosage

Overdose symptoms are the same as those listed under "Possible Side Effects." Take the victim to a hospital emergency room at once. ALWAYS bring the prescription bottle or container with you.

Special Information

Call your doctor at once if you feel unwell or if you develop a rash, severe nausea or vomiting, swollen glands, swollen or tender gums, yellowing of the skin or whites of the eyes, joint pain, sore throat, fever, unusual bleeding or bruising, persistent headache, infection, slurred speech, or poor coordination. Tell your doctor if you are pregnant.

Do not stop taking phenytoin or change dosage without your doctor's knowledge.

Phenytoin may cause drowsiness, dizziness, or blurred vision, effects which are increased by alcoholic beverages. Be careful while engaging in any activity that requires concentration and coordination, such as driving.

Phenytoin sometimes produces a pink-brown color in the urine, which is normal and not a cause for concern.

Diabetic patients who take phenytoin must monitor their urine regularly and report any changes to their doctor.

Good oral hygiene—including gum massage, frequent brushing, and flossing—is very important because phenytoin can cause abnormal growth of your gums.

DO NOT SWITCH PHENYTOIN BRANDS without notifying your doctor. Different brands may not be equivalent to each other and may not produce the same effect on your body. Dose adjustment may be required if you do switch.

If you use phenytoin suspension, be sure to shake the bottle vigorously just before you pour the medication out.

Do not use phenytoin capsules that have become discolored. Throw them away.

If you take phenytoin once a day and forget a dose, take it as soon as you remember. If it is almost time for your next dose, skip the one you forgot and continue with your regular schedule. If you take phenytoin several times a day and remember your medicine within 4 hours of your regular time, take it right away. If you do not remember until later, skip the forgotten dose and go back to your regular schedule. Never take a double dose.

Special Populations

Pregnancy/Breast-feeding

Phenytoin crosses into the fetal circulation. The great majority of mothers who take phenytoin deliver healthy babies, but some are born with cleft lip, cleft palate, or heart malformations.

There is a recognized group of deformities, fetal hydantoin syndrome, which affects children of women taking phenytoin, though the drug has not been definitively established as the cause of these deformities. Fetal hydantoin syndrome consists of skull and face abnormalities, a small brain, growth deficiency, deformed fingernails, and mental deficiency. Children born of mothers taking phenytoin are more likely to have a vitamin K deficiency, which can lead to serious, life-threatening bleeding during the first 24 hours of life. Also, mothers taking phenytoin may be deficient in vitamin K, raising the chances for bleeding during delivery.

Phenytoin passes into breast milk and may affect a nursing infant. Nursing mothers taking phenytoin should bottle-feed their babies.

Seniors

Seniors break phenytoin down more slowly and are more sensitive to its side effects. Follow your doctor's directions and report any side effects at once.

Generic Name

Pimozide (PIH-moh-zide)

Brand Name

Orap

Type of Drug

Antipsychotic.

Prescribed for

Tourette's syndrome and chronic schizophrenia in people who have not responded to other drugs.

General Information

Pimozide works on very specific brain cells, those stimulated by the hormone dopamine. This activity allows pimozide to reduce the verbal and physical expressions of Tourette's syndrome, which include inappropriate noises, physical movements, and verbal statements. It should be used only by people with severe symptoms who cannot tolerate or do not respond to haloperidol, the usual treatment for Tourette's syndrome. Pimozide may be prescribed in some cases of chronic schizophrenia, but it should be used only in those that are not marked by agitation, excitement, or hyperactivity.

Cautions and Warnings

Pimozide should be used only for the conditions listed above because of the risk of cardiac and nervous-system side effects. It should not be used in acute schizophrenia or other psychiatric disorders that can be treated with other drugs.

People who are taking pimozide, especially seniors, are at risk for developing **tardive dyskinesia,** a group of severe side effects (symptoms include lip smacking or puckering, puffing of the cheeks, rapid or worm-like tongue movements, uncontrolled chewing motions, and uncontrolled arm and leg movements). There is no treatment for tardive dyskinesia. The chance that these symptoms will occur and become permanent increases as the dose gets larger. If the drug is stopped at the first sign of involuntary movement, tardive dyskinesia may not develop.

People who are **sensitive or allergic** to pimozide or to other antipsychotic drugs should avoid pimozide. Those who are sensitive to haloperidol, loxapine, molindone, and phenothiazine or thioxanthene antipsychotics may also be sensitive to pimozide.

People with **heart disease** or severe **toxic depression** should use this drug with caution because of the possibility that pimozide-related side effects will worsen those conditions.

Sudden **cardiac death** and **seizures** have occurred in Tourette's patients taking pimozide at doses above 20 mg a day. Your doctor should do an electrocardiogram (EKG) before you start on pimozide and periodically throughout treatment to monitor for cardiac warning signs. Pimozide dosage reduction at the first sign of EKG abnormalities can avoid serious problems.

A serious set of side effects known as **neuroleptic malignant syndrome (NMS)** has been associated with pimozide. The symptoms that make up NMS include a high fever, muscle rigidity, mental changes, irregular pulse or blood pressure, increased sweating, and abnormal heart rhythm. NMS is potentially fatal and requires immediate medical attention.

Liver and kidney function are very important because pimozide is removed from the body by these organs. Any loss of organ function demands a corresponding reduction in dosage.

Possible Side Effects

Extrapyramidal effects (unusual body movements, twisting, unusual postures, and restlessness) often develop during the first few days of pimozide treatment; these

---

Possible Side Effects *(continued)*

generally go away if you stop taking the drug. The potential for and severity of these effects increase with increasing drug dosage. Your doctor may prescribe additional medicines to counteract these side effects.

A potentially fatal group of symptoms, neuroleptic malignant syndrome (NMS), has been associated with pimozide (see "Cautions and Warnings" for details).

A condition known as tardive dyskinesia can develop and worsen as treatment continues and the dosage increases (see "Cautions and Warnings" for details).

▼ Less common: dry mouth, constipation or diarrhea, excessive thirst, changes in appetite, belching, salivation, nausea, vomiting, upset stomach, muscle tightness, cramps, changes in posture, rigidity, headache, drowsiness or sedation, sleeplessness, changes in speech and/or handwriting, dizziness, tremors, fainting, depression, excitement, nervousness, behavioral changes, visual or taste disturbances, unusual sensitivity to bright light, cataracts, spots before the eyes, swelling around the eyes, changes in urinary habits, impotence, loss of sex drive, dizziness or fainting when rising suddenly from a sitting or lying position, blood-pressure changes, heart palpitations, chest pain, increased sweating, skin irritation, rash, changes in body weight, menstrual disorders, and breast secretion.

Drug Interactions

• People taking pimozide should exercise caution in taking other antipsychotic drugs because of the possibility of triggering or aggravating tardive dyskinesia (see "Cautions and Warnings").

• Pimozide may increase the medication needs of people with seizure disorders.

• Alcohol, tranquilizers, and other nervous-system depressants can increase pimozide-related drowsiness or sedation.

• Amphetamines, methylphenidate, and pemoline should be stopped before starting pimozide; these drugs can cause abnormal muscle movements that may be confused with Tourette's syndrome.

• Antihistamines and other anticholinergic drugs with a drying effect should not be taken with pimozide; such a combination may produce more severe side effects, such as dry mouth, visual disturbances, and urinary difficulty.

• Tricyclic antidepressants, disopyramide, maprotiline, quinidine, phenothiazines, and procainamide may increase the chance of pimozide cardiac side effects. These drugs and pimozide should be used together only under a doctor's direct care. Phenothiazines may increase pimozide's depressive and anticholinergic effects.

Food Interactions

Low blood-potassium levels may increase the risk of cardiac side effects associated with pimozide. Be sure to eat enough potassium-rich foods, such as bananas and tomatoes.

Usual Dose

Adult and Child (age 12 and over): starting dose—1–2 mg a day. Maintenance dose—10 mg a day.

Child (under age 12): low doses with gradual increases. Children are particularly sensitive to pimozide.

Overdosage

Symptoms of overdose are cardiac abnormalities, severe involuntary movements (see "Possible Side Effects"), low blood pressure, breathing difficulties, and coma. Pimozide overdose victims must be taken to a hospital emergency room at once. ALWAYS bring the prescription bottle or container with you.

Special Information

Pimozide can make you drowsy. Avoid alcohol, tranquilizers, and other drugs that can worsen that effect. Take care when engaging in activities that require concentration, such as driving.

To avoid dizziness, do not rise rapidly from a sitting or lying position.

Dry mouth caused by pimozide may increase the potential for dental cavities, oral infections, and gum disease. Dry mouth may be alleviated by sugarless gum, candy, ice, or a saliva substitute. Blood disorders associated with pimozide may delay healing and cause oral bleeding.

Do not take more pimozide than your doctor has prescribed. Your doctor will need to monitor for cardiac or other drug side effects, so keep regular doctor's appointments. Call your doctor if dry mouth lasts 2 weeks or more, if you develop any unusual side effect—fever, dehydration, heart pain or abnormal rhythm, muscle rigidity, restlessness, involuntary movements, changes in posture, or mood changes—or if other side effects are bothersome or persistent.

If you forget a dose of pimozide, take it as soon as you remember and divide the remaining doses equally throughout the rest of the day. Do not take a double dose.

Special Populations

Pregnancy/Breast-feeding
While some animal studies demonstrated that pimozide affects fetal development, others failed to do so. Regardless, pregnant women should not take pimozide unless its advantages clearly outweigh its risks.

Nursing mothers who must take pimozide should bottle-feed their babies because of possible side effects.

Seniors
Seniors should receive lower doses of pimozide because of increased sensitivity to side effects. Older adults, especially women, are more likely to develop tardive dyskinesia (see "Cautions and Warnings") and Parkinson's disease while taking pimozide.

Generic Name

Pindolol (PIN-doe-lol) Ⓖ

Brand Name

Visken

Type of Drug

Beta-adrenergic blocking agent.

Prescribed for

High blood pressure, abnormal heart rhythms, side effects of antipsychotic drugs, and stage fright and other anxieties.

General Information

Pindolol is one of 15 beta-adrenergic blocking drugs, or beta blockers, that interfere with the action of a specific part of the nervous system. Beta receptors are found all over the body and affect many body functions. This accounts for the usefulness of beta blockers against a wide variety of conditions. The oldest of these drugs, propranolol, affects all types of beta-adrenergic receptors. Newer, more refined beta blockers affect only a portion of that system, making them more useful in treating cardiovascular disorders and less useful for other purposes. Pindolol is a heart stimulant, which makes it better for certain people.

Cautions and Warnings

You should be cautious about taking pindolol if you have **asthma,** severe **heart failure,** a **very slow heart rate,** or **heart block (disruption of the electrical impulses that control heart rate)** because the drug may aggravate these conditions.

People with **angina** who take pindolol for high blood pressure risk aggravating their angina if they suddenly stop taking the drug. These people should have their drug dosage reduced gradually over 1 to 2 weeks.

Pindolol should be used with caution if you have **liver or kidney disease** because your ability to eliminate the drug from your body may be impaired.

Pindolol reduces the amount of blood pumped by the heart with each beat. This reduction in blood flow may aggravate the condition of people with **poor circulation** or **circulatory disease**.

If you are undergoing **major surgery,** your doctor may want you to stop taking pindolol at least 2 days before surgery to permit the heart to respond more acutely to stresses that can occur during the procedure. This practice is still controversial and may not hold true for all surgeries.

Possible Side Effects

Side effects are relatively uncommon and usually mild; normally they develop early in the course of treatment and are rarely a reason to stop taking pindolol.

▼ Most common: impotence.

▼ Less common: unusual tiredness or weakness, slow heartbeat, heart failure (symptoms include swelling of the legs, ankles, or feet), dizziness, breathing difficulties, bronchospasm, depression, confusion, anxiety, nervous-

Possible Side Effects *(continued)*

ness, sleeplessness, disorientation, short-term memory
loss, emotional instability, cold hands and feet, constipation, diarrhea, nausea, vomiting, upset stomach, increased sweating, urinary difficulties, cramps, blurred
vision, skin rash, hair loss, stuffy nose, facial swelling,
aggravation of lupus erythematosus (chronic condition
affecting the body's connective tissues), itching, chest
pain, back or joint pain, colitis, drug allergy (symptoms
include fever and sore throat), and liver toxicity.

Drug Interactions]

• Pindolol may interact with surgical anesthetics to increase the risk of heart problems during surgery. Some
anesthesiologists recommend having gradually stopped the
drug 2 days before surgery.

• Pindolol may interfere with the normal signs of low blood
sugar and with the action of oral antidiabetes drugs.

• Pindolol increases the blood-pressure-lowering effects of
other blood-pressure-reducing agents, including clonidine,
guanabenz, and reserpine; and calcium channel blockers,
(such as nifedipine).

• Aspirin-containing drugs, indomethacin, sulfinpyrazone,
and estrogen drugs may interfere with the blood-pressure-
lowering effect of pindolol.

• Cocaine may reduce the effectiveness of all beta blockers.

• Pindolol may increase the worsen the problem of cold
hands and feet associated with taking ergot alkaloids, used to
treat migraine headache. Gangrene is a possibility in people
taking taking both an ergot and pindolol.

• Pindolol will counteract thyroid hormone replacements.

• Calcium channel blockers, flecainide, hydralazine, oral
contraceptives, propafenone, haloperidol, phenothiazine
tranquilizers—molindone and others—quinolone antibacterials, and quinidine may increase the amount of pindolol in
the bloodstream and lead to increased pindolol effects.

• Pindolol should not be taken within 2 weeks of taking a
monoamine oxidase inhibitor (MAOI) antidepressant.

• Cimetidine increases the amount of pindolol absorbed
into the bloodstream from oral tablets.

• Pindolol may interfere with the effectiveness of some

antiasthma drugs including theophylline and aminophylline, and especially ephedrine and isoproterenol.

• Combining pindolol and phenytoin or digitalis drugs may result in excessive slowing of the heart, possibly causing heart block (a disruption in the electrical impulses that control heart rate).

• If you stop smoking while taking pindolol, your dose may have to be reduced because your liver will break down the drug more slowly afterward.

Food Interactions

None known.

Usual Dose

10–60 mg a day.

Overdosage

Symptoms of overdose include changes in heartbeat—unusually slow, unusually fast, or irregular; severe dizziness or fainting; breathing difficulties; bluish-colored fingernails or palms; and seizures. The victim should be taken to a hospital emergency room. ALWAYS bring the prescription bottle or container with you.

Special Information

Pindolol is meant to be taken continuously. When ending pindolol treatment, dosage should be reduced gradually over a period of about 2 weeks. Do not stop taking this drug unless directed to do so by your doctor: Abrupt withdrawal may cause chest pain, breathing difficulties, increased sweating, and unusually fast or irregular heartbeat

Call your doctor at once if you develop back or joint pain, breathing difficulties, cold hands or feet, depression, skin rash, or changes in heartbeat. Pindolol may produce an undesirable lowering of blood pressure, leading to dizziness or fainting; call your doctor if this happens to you. Call your doctor if you experience persistent or bothersome anxiety, diarrhea, constipation, impotence, headache, itching, nausea or vomiting, nightmares or vivid dreams, upset stomach, trouble sleeping, stuffy nose, frequent urination, unusual tiredness, or weakness.

Pindolol may cause drowsiness, blurred vision, dizziness,

and light-headedness. Be careful when driving or performing complex tasks.

It is best to take pindolol at the same time each day. If you forget a dose, take it as soon as you remember. If you take pindolol once a day and it is within 8 hours of your next dose, skip the dose you forgot and continue with your regular schedule. If you take it twice a day and it is within 4 hours of your next dose, skip the one you forgot and continue with your regular schedule. Never take a double dose.

Special Populations

Pregnancy/Breast-feeding

Infants born to women who took a beta blocker while pregnant had lower birth weights, low blood pressure, and reduced heart rate. Pindolol should be avoided by women who are or might be pregnant while taking it. When the drug is considered crucial by your doctor, its potential benefits must be carefully weighed against its risks.

Pindolol passes into breast milk, but problems are rare. Still, nursing mothers taking it should bottle-feed their babies.

Seniors

Seniors may absorb and retain more pindolol, and may require less of the drug to achieve results. Your doctor should adjust your dosage to meet your individual needs. Seniors taking pindolol may be more likely to suffer from cold hands and feet, reduced body temperature, chest pain, general feelings of ill health, sudden breathing difficulties, increased sweating, or changes in heartbeat.

Generic Name

Pirbuterol (pir-BYUE-ter-ol)

Brand Name

Maxair Inhaler

Type of Drug

Bronchodilator.

Prescribed for

Asthma and bronchospasm.

General Information

Pirbuterol acetate is available only as an inhalant, but it may be taken in combination with other medications to control your asthma. The drug starts working within 5 minutes after it is taken and continues to work for 5 hours. It can be used as necessary to treat asthma attacks or on a regular basis to prevent them.

Cautions and Warnings

Pirbuterol should be used with caution by people with a history of **angina pectoris** (condition characterized by brief attacks of chest pain), **heart disease**, **high blood pressure**, **stroke**, **seizures**, **diabetes**, **prostate disease**, or **glaucoma**.

Using excessive amounts of pirbuterol can lead to **increased breathing difficulties**, rather than relief. In the most extreme cases, people have had **heart attacks** after using excessive amounts of inhalant.

Possible Side Effects

Pirbuterol's side effects are similar to those associated with other bronchodilator drugs.

▼ Most common: shakiness, nervousness and tension, and headache.

▼ Less common: restlessness, weakness, anxiety, confusion, depression, fatigue, fainting, abdominal cramps or pain, low blood pressure, numbness in the hands or feet, weight gain, weakness, fear, tension, tremors, sleeplessness, convulsions, dizziness, headache, flushing, appetite loss, unusual tastes or smells, pallor, sweating, nausea, vomiting, diarrhea, dry mouth, cough, muscle cramps, angina, abnormal heart rhythm, and palpitations.

Drug Interactions

• Pirbuterol's effects may be enhanced by a monoamine oxidase inhibitor (MAOI), antidepressants, thyroid drugs, other bronchodilators, and some antihistamines.

• Pirbuterol may antagonize the effects of blood-pressure-lowering drugs, especially reserpine, methyldopa, and guanethidine.

• The chances of cardiac toxicity may be increased in people taking both pirbuterol and theophylline.

• Pirbuterol is antagonized by beta-blocking drugs such as propranolol.

Food Interactions

None known.

Usual Dose

Adult and Child (over age 12): 1–2 inhalations—0.2 mg each—every 4–6 hours. Do not take more than 12 inhalations a day.

Overdosage

Pirbuterol overdose can result in severe side effects, including heart pain and high blood pressure, although the pressure can drop after a short period of elevation. People who inhale too much pirbuterol should see a doctor, who may prescribe a beta-blocking drug like atenolol or metoprolol to counter the bronchodilator's effects.

Special Information

The drug should be inhaled during the second half of your inward breath. This will allow the medication to reach more deeply into your lungs.

Be sure to follow your doctor's directions for using pirbuterol, and do not take more than 12 inhalations of the drug each day. Using more than is prescribed can lead to drug tolerance and actually worsen your symptoms. If your condition worsens rather than improves after using pirbuterol, stop taking it and call your doctor.

Call your doctor at once if you develop chest pain, rapid heartbeat or heart palpitations, muscle tremors, dizziness, headache, facial flushing, or urinary difficulty, or if you still have trouble breathing after using the pirbuterol.

If you forget to take a dose of pirbuterol, take it as soon as you remember and then continue with your regular schedule. Do not take a double dose.

Special Populations

Pregnancy/Breast-feeding

Pirbuterol should be used by a pregnant woman only when it is absolutely necessary. The potential benefit of using this medication must be carefully weighed against its risks.

It is not known if pirbuterol passes into breast milk. Nursing mothers who take this drug must observe their infants for side effects. You may want to consider bottle-feeding your baby.

Seniors
Seniors are more sensitive to the effects of this drug. Follow your doctor's directions closely and report any side effects at once.

Generic Name

Piroxicam (pih-ROX-ih-kam)

Brand Name
Feldene

Type of Drug
Nonsteroidal anti-inflammatory drug (NSAID).

Prescribed for
Rheumatoid arthritis, juvenile rheumatoid arthritis, osteoarthritis, menstrual pain, and sunburn.

General Information
Piroxicam is one of 16 NSAIDs, which are used to relieve pain and inflammation. We do not know exactly how NSAIDs work, but part of their action may be due to their ability to inhibit the body's production of a hormone called prostaglandin as well as the action of other body chemicals, including cyclooxygenase, lipoxygenase, leukotrienes, and lysosomal enzymes. NSAIDs are generally absorbed into the bloodstream quickly. Pain relief comes within 1 hour after taking the first dose of piroxicam and lasts for 2 to 3 days, but its anti-inflammatory effect takes several days to 2 weeks to become apparent and may take 3 weeks to reach maximum effect. Piroxicam is broken down in the liver and eliminated through the kidneys.

Cautions and Warnings
People who are **allergic** to piroxicam or any other NSAID and those with a history of **asthma** attacks brought on by an NSAID, iodides, or aspirin should not take piroxicam.

Piroxicam can cause **gastrointestinal (GI) bleeding, ulcers, and stomach perforation**. This can occur at any time, with or without warning, in people who take piroxicam regularly. People with a history of **active GI bleeding** should be cautious about taking any NSAID. People who develop bleeding or ulcers and continue NSAID treatment should be aware of the possibility of developing more serious drug toxicity.

Piroxicam can affect **platelets and blood clotting** at high doses, and should be avoided by people with clotting problems and by those taking warfarin.

People with **heart problems** who use piroxicam may experience swelling in their arms, legs, or feet.

Piroxicam can cause severe toxic effects to the **kidney**. Report any unusual side effects to your doctor, who may need to periodically test your kidney function.

Piroxicam can make you unusually photosensitive (sensitive to the effects of the sun).

Possible Side Effects

▼ Most common: diarrhea, nausea, vomiting, constipation, stomach gas, stomach upset or irritation, and appetite loss—especially during the first few days of treatment.

▼ Less common: stomach ulcers, GI bleeding, hepatitis, gallbladder attacks, painful urination, poor kidney function, kidney inflammation, blood and protein in the urine, dizziness, fainting, nervousness, depression, hallucinations, confusion, disorientation, tingling in the hands or feet, light-headedness, itching, increased sweating, dry nose and mouth, heart palpitations, chest pain, difficulty breathing, and muscle cramps.

▼ Rare: severe allergic reactions including closing of the throat, fever and chills, changes in liver function, jaundice (yellowing of the skin or whites of the eyes), and kidney failure. People who experience such effects must be promptly treated in a hospital emergency room or doctor's office. NSAIDs have caused severe skin reactions; if this happens to you, see your doctor immediately.

Drug Interactions

• Piroxicam can increase the effects of oral anticoagulant

(blood-thinning) drugs such as warfarin. You may take this combination, but your doctor might have to change your anticoagulant dose.

• Taking piroxicam with cyclosporine may increase the toxic kidney effects of both drugs. Methotrexate toxicity may be increased in people who are also taking piroxicam.

• Piroxicam may reduce the blood-pressure-lowering effect of beta blockers and loop diuretics.

• Piroxicam may increase phenytoin blood levels, leading to increased side effects. Lithium blood levels may be increased in people taking piroxicam.

• Piroxicam blood levels may be affected by cimetidine.

• Probenecid may interfere with the elimination of piroxicam from the body, increasing the chances for piroxicam side effects.

• Aspirin and other salicylates may decrease the amount of piroxicam in your blood. These drugs should never be combined with piroxicam.

Food Interactions

Take piroxicam with food or a magnesium/aluminum antacid if it upsets your stomach.

Usual Dose

Adult: 20 mg a day.
Child: not recommended.

Overdosage

People have died from NSAID overdoses. The most common signs of overdose are drowsiness, nausea, vomiting, diarrhea, abdominal pain, rapid breathing, rapid heartbeat, increased sweating, ringing or buzzing in the ears, confusion, disorientation, stupor, and coma. Take the victim to a hospital emergency room at once. ALWAYS bring the prescription bottle or container with you.

Special Information

Take each dose with a full glass of water and do not lie down for 15 to 30 minutes afterward.

Piroxicam can make you drowsy and/or tired: Be careful when driving or operating hazardous equipment. Do not take any over-the-counter products containing acetaminophen or aspirin while taking piroxicam. Avoid alcoholic beverages.

Contact your doctor if you develop skin rash or itching, visual disturbances, weight gain, breathing difficulties, fluid retention, hallucinations, black or tarry stools, persistent headache, or any unusual or intolerable side effect.

If you forget to take a dose of piroxicam, take it as soon as you remember. If you take it once a day and it is within 8 hours of your next dose, skip the missed dose and continue with your regular schedule. Do not take a double dose.

Special Populations

Pregnancy/Breast-feeding

NSAIDs may cross into fetal blood circulation. They have not been found to cause birth defects, but animal studies indicate that they may affect the fetal heart during the second half of pregnancy. Pregnant women should not take piroxicam without their doctor's approval, particularly during the last 3 months of pregnancy. When the drug is considered crucial by your doctor, its potential benefits must be carefully weighed against its risks.

NSAIDs may pass into breast milk but have caused no problems in breast-fed infants, except for seizures in a baby whose mother was taking the NSAID indomethacin. Other NSAIDs have caused problems in animal studies. There is a possibility that a nursing mother taking piroxicam could affect her baby's heart or cardiovascular system. If you must take piroxicam, talk with your doctor about bottle-feeding your baby.

Seniors

Seniors may be more susceptible to piroxicam side effects, especially ulcer disease.

Generic Name

Podofilox (poe-DUH-fil-ox)

Brand Name

Condylox

Type of Drug

Antimitotic drug.

Prescribed for

External genital warts or warts around the anal area. Do not use podofilox for any other purpose.

General Information

Podofilox can be either manufactured from chemicals or purified from natural sources. Applying podofilox to warts results in the death of visible wart tissues. The exact way it produces this result is not known. Condylomas or genital warts are caused by the human papillomavirus and can be found in various places including sex organs, anus, and abdomen. The number of warts increases if your immune system is suppressed, as in HIV or AIDS. In women, genital warts have been associated with a risk of cervical cancer. Ask your doctor for more information.

Cautions and Warnings

Do not use podofilox if you are **sensitive or allergic** to it.

Proper diagnosis of genital warts is necessary before you use this product. Be sure to see your doctor before you start using podofilox.

Possible Side Effects

Most common: burning, pain, inflammation, skin erosion, itching, and bleeding.

▼ Common: pain during intercourse, sleeplessness, tingling, bleeding, tenderness, chafing, bad odor, dizziness, scarring, small sores or ulcers, dryness or peeling, difficulty retracting the foreskin, blood in the urine, vomiting, headache, stinging, and redness.

▼ Less common: skin peeling, scabbing, skin discoloration, tenderness, dryness, crusting, skin cracks, soreness, swelling, rash, blisters, and tingling.

Drug Interactions

None known.

Usual Dose

Apply morning and night—every 12 hours—for 3 consecutive days, then apply nothing for 4 days. Repeat this cycle for up to 4 weeks in a row. Use the cotton-tipped applicator supplied with the solution, or your finger if you are using the gel. Try to limit the amount of podofilox that gets on intact skin. Thoroughly wash your hands before and after each application.

Overdosage

Symptoms may include nausea, vomiting, fever, diarrhea, mouth sores, tingling in the hands or feet, mental changes, lethargy, coma, rapid breathing, respiratory failure, blood in the urine, kidney failure, and seizures. Excess podofilox should be washed off the skin as soon as possible. If you get podofilox in your eyes, wash it out at once with cool water and get medical attention.

Victims of overdose or accidental ingestion should be taken to a hospital emergency room. ALWAYS bring the prescription bottle or container with you.

Special Information

Thoroughly wash your hands before and after each podofilox application.

Call your doctor if you develop any unusual side effects. If you do not see any improvement in 4 weeks, stop using the drug and call your doctor.

If you forget a dose of podofilox, apply it as soon as you remember. If it is within 4 hours of your next dose, skip the dose you forgot and continue with your regular schedule.

Special Populations

Pregnancy/Breast-feeding

Podofilox is toxic to animal fetuses at 250 times the maximum human dose. There is no information on the use of podofilox by pregnant women. Talk to your doctor about the possible risks and benefits of podofilox before using it.

It is not known if podofilox passes into breast milk. Nursing mothers who must use this drug should bottle-feed their babies.

Seniors

Seniors may use podofilox without special precaution.

Brand Name

Poly-Vi-Flor

Generic Ingredients

Folic Acid + Sodium Fluoride + Vitamin A + Vitamin B_1 (Thiamine) + Vitamin B_2 (Riboflavin) + Vitamin B_3 (Niacin) + Vitamin B_6 (Pyridoxine) + Vitamin B_{12} (Cyanocobalamin) + Vitamin C + Vitamin D + Vitamin E G

Other Brand Names

Florvite   Soluvite C.T.

Polytabs-F   Vi-Daylin/F*

PolyVitamins Fluoride

Some products in this brand-name group are alcohol or sugar free. Consult your pharmacist.

Type of Drug

Multivitamin supplement with fluoride.

Prescribed for

Vitamin deficiencies and prevention of dental cavities in infants and children.

General Information

Fluoride taken in small daily doses has been effective in preventing cavities in children by strengthening the teeth and making them resistant to cavity formation. Multivitamins with fluoride are also available in preparations with added iron, if iron supplementation is required.

Cautions and Warnings

Too much fluoride can damage teeth. Because of this, Poly-Vi-Flor should not be used where the fluoride content of the water supply exceeds 0.7 parts per million (ppm). Your pediatrician or local water company can tell you the fluoride content of your drinking water.

Possible Side Effects

▼ Common: occasional rash, itching, upset stomach, headache, and weakness.

Food and Drug and Interactions

None known.

Usual Dose

1 tablet or dropperful a day.

Special Information

As with other medications, it is easiest to remember daily doses of Poly-Vi-Flor if they are given at the same time each day.

If you forget to give your child a dose of Poly-Vi-Flor, do so as soon as you remember. If it is almost time for the next dose, skip the dose you forgot and continue with the regular schedule. Do not give a double dose.

Type of Drug

Potassium Replacements

Brand Names

Generic Ingredient: Potassium Chloride, Liquid G

Cena-K $	Kay Ciel $
Kaochlor 10%	Klorvess
Kaochlor S-F $	Potasalan $
Kaon-Cl 20% $	Rum-K

Generic Ingredient: Potassium Gluconate, Liquid G

Kaon $	K-G
Kaylixir	

Generic Ingredient: Potassium Salt Combination, Liquid G

Kolyum $	Twin-K
Tri-K	

Generic Ingredient: Potassium Chloride, Powder G

Gen-K $	Klor-Con $
K+ Care	Klor-Con/25 $
Kato	K-Lyte/Cl
Kay Ciel $	Micro-K LS
K-Lor	

Generic Ingredient: Potassium Salt Combination, Powder G

Klorvess $	Kolyum $

Generic Ingredient: Potassium, Effervescent Tablets Ⓖ

Effer-K	K-Lyte
K+ Care ET	K-Lyte/Cl
Klor-Con/EF Ⓢ	K-Lyte/Cl 50
Klorvess Ⓢ	K-Lyte DS

Generic Ingredient: Potassium Chloride,
Controlled-Release Ⓖ

K+10	K-Lease
Kaon-Cl-10	K-Norm
K-Dur 10	K-Tab
K-Dur 20	Micro-K Extencaps
K-Lease	Micro-K 10 Extencaps
Klor-Con 8	Slow-K
Klor-Con 10	Ten-K
Klotrix	

Generic Ingredient: Potassium Gluconate, Tablets Ⓖ
Available only in generic form.

Prescribed for

Hypokalemia (low blood-potassium levels).

General Information

Potassium is a very important component of body fluids and has a major effect in maintaining the proper tone of all body cells. Potassium is important for the maintenance of normal kidney function and blood pressure; it is required for the passage of electrical impulses throughout the nervous system; and it has a major effect on the heart and all other muscles of the body. Potassium also plays an important role in how the body uses proteins and carbohydrates.

It is important to maintain blood potassium within a specific range to avoid hypokalemia, which is usually caused by extended diuretic treatment, severe diarrhea, vomiting, complications of diabetes, or other medical conditions. Symptoms of hypokalemia are weakness, fatigue, muscle twitching, muscle excitability, severe bowel obstruction caused by greatly reduced movement of intestinal muscles, and abnormal heart rhythms. Low blood potassium also affects electrocardiogram (EKG) readings.

Potassium supplements are available in many forms, each designed to meet specific needs or preferences. Potassium chloride is the form most often prescribed by doctors because it contains the most potassium per unit weight. Another advantage of potassium chloride is that it also gives you chloride ion, another important body-fluid component. Potassium gluconate provides about ⅓ as much potassium as the chloride, so you have to take 3 times as much to get an equal dose of potassium. However, it is preferable to potassium chloride in circumstances when chloride is undesirable.

Foods rich in potassium can provide a natural potassium source and help you avoid the need to take a potassium supplement; they include apricots, acorn squash, avocados, bananas, beans, beef, broccoli, brussels sprouts, butternut squash, cantaloupe, chicken, collard greens, dates, fish, ham, kidney beans, lentils, milk, orange juice, potatoes with the skin, prunes, raisins, shellfish, spinach, split peas, turkey, veal, yogurt, white navy beans, watermelon, and zucchini.

In addition to treating hypokalemia, long-term, moderate-dose potassium supplementation may help reduce blood pressure in people with mild hypertension.

Cautions and Warnings

Potassium replacement therapy should always be monitored and controlled by your physician. Potassium tablets have caused **ulcers** in some patients with compression of the esophagus. Potassium supplements for these patients should be given in liquid form. Potassium tablets have been reported to cause small bowel ulcer, leading to bleeding, obstruction, and/or perforation (formation of a hole through the bowel into the abdomen).

People with **kidney disease** may not be able to efficiently eliminate potassium from their bodies. If people with this problem take a potassium supplement, they may develop **hyperkalemia** (high blood-potassium levels). Hyperkalemia can develop rapidly, without warning or symptoms, and is potentially fatal. Hyperkalemia is often discovered through an EKG, but the following symptoms may also indicate elevated potassium levels: tingling in the hands and feet, feeling of heaviness or weakness in the muscles, listlessness, confusion, low blood pressure, extreme difficulty moving the arms and legs, abnormal heart rhythms, weak pulse, loss of consciousness, pallor, restlessness, and low urine output.

Do not take potassium supplements if you are **dehydrated** or experiencing **muscle cramps** due to excessive sun exposure. Potassium replacements should be used with caution in people with **kidney or heart disease**.

Possible Side Effects

▼ Most common: nausea, vomiting, diarrhea, stomach gas, and abdominal discomfort.

▼ Less common: rash, tingling in hands or feet, weakness and heaviness in the legs, listlessness, mental confusion, decreased blood pressure, and heart-rhythm changes.

Drug Interactions

• Potassium supplements should not be taken with the potassium-sparing diuretics spironolactone or triamterene— diuretics that do not cause the body to lose potassium—or combinations of these drugs. Potassium toxicity may occur.

• Combining potassium supplements with an angiotensin-converting enzyme (ACE) inhibitor may result in hyperkalemia.

• People taking digitalis drugs must be careful to keep their blood-potassium levels within acceptable limits. Too little potassium in the blood may accentuate digitalis side effects and cause toxic reactions.

Food Interactions

Salt substitutes contain large amounts of potassium; do not use them while taking a potassium supplement, unless directed by your doctor. If stomach upset occurs, take potassium supplements with food.

Usual Dose

16–100 milliequivalents (meq) a day.

Overdosage

Potassium overdose is rare, except when accompanied by another condition that interferes with the body's natural processes of maintaining potassium balance. Toxicity may also occur when high doses of potassium supplements are taken in combination with foods high in potassium.

Symptoms of potassium overdose include muscle weakness, tingling in the hands or feet, a feeling of heaviness in the legs, listlessness, confusion, breathing difficulties, low blood pressure, shock, abnormal heart rhythms, and heart attack. Call your doctor, local poison control center, or hospital emergency room for more information. ALWAYS take the prescription bottle or container with you if you go for treatment.

Special Information

Directions for taking and using any potassium supplement must be followed closely. Effervescent tablets, powders, and liquids should be properly and completely dissolved, or diluted in 3 to 8 oz. of cold water or juice and drunk slowly. Noneffervescent tablets or capsules should never be chewed or crushed; they must be swallowed whole.

Many of the controlled-release potassium supplements contain potassium distributed throughout an indigestible wax core or matrix; you may notice the depleted wax matrix in your stool several hours after swallowing a tablet. This is normal and should not be a cause for alarm.

Call your doctor at once if you experience tingling in your hands or feet, a feeling of heaviness in the legs, unusual tiredness or weakness, nausea, vomiting, continued abdominal pain, or black stool.

If you forget to take a dose of potassium, take it right away if you remember within 2 hours of your regular time. If you do not remember until later, skip the dose you forgot and go back to your regular schedule. Do not take a double dose.

Special Populations

Pregnancy/Breast-feeding

Potassium supplements have been found to be safe for use during pregnancy, although you should check with your doctor before taking any drug while pregnant.

Breast-feeding while taking potassium may cause unwanted side effects in your infant. If you must take potassium, consider bottle-feeding your baby. You can resume nursing 1 to 2 days after stopping potassium.

Seniors

Seniors may take potassium supplements without special restriction. Follow your doctor's directions and report any side effects at once.

Generic Name

Pramipexole (pram-ih-PEX-ole)

Brand Name

Mirapex

Type of Drug

Antiparkinsonian.

Prescribed for

Parkinson's disease.

General Information

Pramipexole is thought to relieve symptoms of Parkinson's disease by stimulating dopamine receptors in the brain, but this connection has not been proven. Pramipexole is rapidly absorbed into the blood; although the drug may be found throughout the body, it is useful only when it reaches the brain. Pramipexole is primarily eliminated through the kidneys and is not broken down or changed in the body. Women release the drug about 30% more slowly than men, but this disparity may be due to differences in body weight rather than to a true gender difference. Studies of pramipexole in people with early Parkinson's disease show improvement after 4 weeks of treatment. Similar studies conducted with advanced Parkinson's disease patients show improvement in their conditions after 6 months of treatment.

Cautions and Warnings

Do not take pramipexole if you are **sensitive or allergic** to it. Pramipexole may cause **low blood pressure** and make you **dizzy** or **faint** when rising from a sitting or lying position, especially during the early stages of treatment. About 1 in 10 to 15 people who take pramipexole experience **hallucinations** that may be serious enough to force them to stop taking the medication.

One person taking pramipexole developed a disease in which skeletal muscle is destroyed; report anything unusual to your doctor. Animal studies with pramipexole show that the drug may cause changes in the retina of the eye. Although this effect has not been reported in people, you should nevertheless report any **changes in your vision** to your doctor.

People who stop taking other antiparkinsonians may develop **high fever** and **confusion. Breathing difficulty** caused by lung changes has also been seen with other antiparkinson's disease drugs. These symptoms have not been seen with pramipexole, but are nevertheless considered to be possible consequences of ending pramipexole treatment.

Possible Side Effects

Early Parkinson's Disease
▼ Most common: sleepiness or tiredness and nausea.
▼ Common: sleeplessness, hallucinations, and constipation.
▼ Less common: dizziness, confusion, memory loss, reduced touch sensation, loss of muscle tone, a tendency to frequently change positions or pace the floor, odd thoughts, loss of sex drive or ability to perform sexually, unusual muscle spasms, swelling in the arms or legs, generalized swelling, appetite loss, difficulty swallowing, weight loss, weakness, feeling unwell, fever, and abnormal vision.

Advanced Parkinson's Disease
▼ Most common: dizziness or fainting when rising from a sitting or lying position, abnormal movements, tremors, muscle rigidity, and hallucinations.
▼ Common: sleeplessness.
▼ Less common: accidental injury, weakness, generalized swelling, chest pain, feeling unwell, dizziness, abnormal dreaming, confusion, sleepiness, unusual muscle spasms, unusual walking, muscle stiffness, memory loss, a tendency to frequently change positions or pace the floor, odd thoughts, paranoid reactions, delusions, sleeping problems, frequent urination, urinary infection, loss of urinary control, swelling in the arms or legs, arthritis, twitching, bursitis, muscle weakness, breathing difficulties, runny nose, pneumonia, visual difficulties, difficulty focusing, double vision, constipation, dry mouth, and rash.

Drug Interactions

• Pramipexole may worsen the uncontrolled muscle spasms that are side effects of levodopa because the level of levodopa in your blood is raised by pramipexole. Your doctor may correct this interaction by reducing your levodopa dosage.

• Cimetidine increases the amount of pramipexole absorbed by 50% and lengthens the time it takes for pramipexole to leave your body by 40%. Dose adjustment may be required if you take both drugs.

• Drugs that are eliminated through the kidneys—including cimetidine, ranitine, diltiazem, triamterene, verapamil, quinidine, and quinine—reduce by 20% the ability to clear pramipexole from the body. Your doctor may adjust your dose for this effect.

• Phenothiazine tranquilizers, haloperidol and similar tranquilizers, thioxanthene tranquilizers, metoclopramide, and other drugs that antagonize the effects of dopamine can reduce the effect of pramipexole.

• Pramipexole worsens the sedative effect of tranquilizers, sleeping pills, and other nervous-system depressants.

Food Interactions

Food slows the rate at which pramipexole is absorbed into the blood, though not the total amount absorbed. You may take this drug with food or meals to prevent nausea.

Usual Dose

Adult: starting dose—0.125 mg 3 times a day. Increase gradually to a maximum of 4.5 mg a day. Your dosage depends on your reaction to the medication and how well you tolerate it. Dosage is reduced for people with kidney disease.

Overdosage

Overdose symptoms are likely to be similar to the most common drug side effects, but there has been no experience with pramipexole overdose. Overdose victims should be taken to a hospital emergency room for treatment. ALWAYS bring the prescription bottle or container with you.

Special Information

Pramipexole should be taken only as directed by your doctor. Be sure to tell your doctor if you are pregnant or nursing a baby.

Avoid alcoholic beverages and other nervous-system depressants, especially if you drive a car or do anything else that requires coordination and concentration.

Call your doctor if you develop hallucinations or if anything unusual occurs.

If you forget a dose of pramipexole, take it as soon as you remember. Space any remaining doses evenly throughout the rest of the day. Continue with your regular schedule on the next day. Do not take a double dose.

Special Populations

Pregnancy/Breast-feeding

Pramipexole has not been studied in pregnant women. Women who are or might be pregnant should take this drug only if they have discussed its risks and benefits with their doctors. Nursing mothers should bottle-feed their babies if they are taking pramipexole.

Seniors

Seniors clear pramipexole more slowly than younger adults, most likely due to age-related changes in kidney function.

Pravachol

see *Pravastatin*, page 908

Generic Name

Pravastatin (prah-vuh-STAT-in)

Brand Name

Pravachol

Type of Drug

Cholesterol-lowering agent.

Prescribed for

High blood-cholesterol, LDL-cholesterol, and triglyceride levels, in conjunction with a low-cholesterol diet program; also prescribed to slow the progression of atherosclerosis (hardening of the arteries), reduce the risk of death in people with heart disease, and to treat inherited blood-lipid problems or lipid problems associated with diabetes or kidney disease.

General Information

Pravastatin is one of several cholesterol-lowering drugs that work by inhibiting an enzyme called HMG-CoA reductase. They interfere with the natural process for manufacturing cholesterol in your body, altering that process in order to produce a harmless by-product. Studies have closely related high blood-fat levels—total cholesterol, LDL cholesterol, and triglycerides—to heart and blood-vessel disease. Drugs that reduce levels of any of these blood fats and increase HDL cholesterol—"good" cholesterol—have been assumed for several years to reduce the risk of death and heart attack. Recently, medication in this class has been proven to slow the formation of blood-vessel plaque—associated with atherosclerosis—and reduce the risk of heart attack and death related to heart disease.

Pravastatin reduces total triglyceride, cholesterol, and LDL-cholesterol counts while increasing HDL cholesterol. A very small amount of the drug actually reaches the body's circulation. Most is broken down and eliminated by the liver; 10% to 20% of the drug is released from the body through the kidneys. A significant blood-fat-lowering response is seen after 1 to 2 weeks of treatment. Blood-fat levels are lowest within 4 to 6 weeks after taking pravastatin and remain at or close to that level as long as you continue to take the drug. The effect is known to persist for 4 to 6 weeks after you stop taking it.

Pravastatin generally does not benefit anyone under age 30, so it is not usually recommended for children. It may, under special circumstances, be prescribed for teenagers in the same dose as adults.

Cautions and Warnings

Do not take pravastatin if you are **allergic** to it or to any other HMG-CoA reductase inhibitor.

People with a history of **liver disease** and **those who drink large amounts of alcohol** should avoid drugs in this group because they may aggravate or cause liver disease. Your doctor should take a blood sample to test your liver function every month or so during the first year of treatment.

Pravastatin causes **muscle aches and/or muscle weakness** in a small number of people, which may be a sign of a more serious condition.

At dosages between 50 and 100 or more times the maximum human dose, pravastatin has caused central-nervous-system lesions, liver tumors, and male infertility in laboratory animals. The importance of this information for humans is not known.

Possible Side Effects

Most people who take pravastatin tolerate it quite well.

▼ Common: headache, nausea, vomiting, localized pain, common cold symptoms, and diarrhea.

▼ Less common: constipation, heartburn, upset stomach, muscle aches, dizziness, runny nose, cough, chest pain, itching, rash, heart pains, fatigue, flu symptoms, and urinary changes.

▼ Rare: Effects may occur in virtually any part of the body. Report anything unusual to your doctor.

Drug Interactions

• The cholesterol-lowering effects of pravastatin and colestipol or cholestyramine are additive when the drugs are taken together. Take pravastatin 1 hour before or 4 hours after either of these drugs.

• Pravastatin may increase the effects of warfarin or digoxin. If you take either of these drugs with pravastatin you should be periodically checked by your doctor.

• The combination of cyclosporine, erythromycin, gemfibrozil, or niacin with pravastatin may cause severe muscle aches or degeneration or other muscle problems. These combinations should be avoided.

• Propranolol can interfere with the action of pravastatin, reducing its effectiveness.

• Itraconazole can increase pravastatin levels by 20 times. Avoid this combination by temporarily stopping pravastatin if you take itraconazole.

Food Interactions

None known. Continue your low-cholesterol diet while taking this medication.

Usual Dose

Adult: 10–40 mg at bedtime.
Senior: 10–20 mg at bedtime.

Your daily dosage of pravastatin should be adjusted monthly, based on how well the drug is working to reduce your blood cholesterol.

Overdosage

There are 2 known cases of pravastatin overdose, neither of which caused symptoms or problems. A person suspected of having taken an overdose of pravastatin should be taken to a hospital emergency room. ALWAYS bring the prescription bottle or container with you.

Special Information

Call your doctor if you develop blurred vision or muscle aches, pain, tenderness, or weakness, especially if you are also feverish or feel sick.

Pravastatin is always prescribed in combination with a low-fat diet. Be sure to follow your doctor's dietary instructions precisely, since both diet and medication are necessary to treat your condition. Do not take more cholesterol-lowering medication than your doctor has prescribed, and do not stop taking the medication without your doctor's knowledge.

Pravastatin may cause unusual sensitivity to the sun. Use sunscreen and wear protective clothing while in the sun until you determine whether you are affected.

If you forget to take a dose of pravastatin, take it as soon as you remember. If it is almost time for your next dose, skip the one you forgot and continue with your regular schedule. Do not take a double dose.

Special Populations

Pregnancy/Breast-feeding

Women who are or might be pregnant absolutely must not take pravastatin. Cholesterol is essential to the health and development of a fetus. Anything that interferes with that process will damage the developing brain and nervous system. Since hardening of the arteries is a long-term process, you should be able to stop this medication during pregnancy without developing atherosclerosis. If you become pregnant while taking pravastatin, stop the drug immediately and call your doctor.

A small amount of pravastatin passes into breast milk. Women taking pravastatin should bottle-feed their infants.

Seniors

Seniors may be more sensitive to the effects of pravastatin. Be sure to report any side effects to your doctor.

Generic Name

Prazosin (PRAY-zoe-sin) Ⓖ

Brand Name

Minipress

Combination Products

Generic Ingredients: Prazosin + Polythiazide

Minizide 1   Minizide 5

Minizide 2

Type of Drug

Antihypertensive.

Prescribed for

High blood pressure, benign prostatic hyperplasia (BPH), congestive heart failure, and Raynaud's disease. Prasozin combined with the diuretic polythiazide is used to treat high blood pressure.

General Information

Prazosin hydrochloride is one of several alpha-adrenergic blocking agents, or alpha blockers, that work by opening blood vessels and reducing pressure in them. Other types of blood-pressure-lowering drugs block beta receptors, interfere with the movement of calcium in blood-vessel muscle cells, affect salt and electrolyte balance in the body, or interfere with the production of norepinephrine in the body. Alpha blockers like prazosin block nerve endings known as alpha$_1$ receptors. The maximum blood-pressure-lowering effect of prazosin is seen between 2 and 6 hours after taking a single dose. Prazosin's effect in congestive heart failure is seen within 1 hour of taking the drug. In BPH treatment, prazosin works by relaxing smooth muscles in the prostate and neck of the bladder, which results from the blocking of alpha receptors in the affected muscles. Despite the fact that prazosin reduces the symptoms of BPH, the drug's long-term effect on complications of BPH or the need for urinary surgery is not known. There is no difference in response among different races or between older and younger adults. Prazosin's effect lasts only between 6 and 10 hours. It is broken down in the liver; very little passes out of the body via the kidneys.

Cautions and Warnings

Prazosin may cause **dizziness** and **fainting**, especially the first few doses. This is known as the first-dose effect, which can be minimized by limiting the first dose to 1 mg at bedtime. First-dose effects occur in about 1% of people taking an alpha blocker and may recur if the drug is stopped for a few days and then restarted.

People who are **allergic or sensitive** to any of the alpha blockers should avoid prazosin.

Prazosin may slightly reduce cholesterol levels and increase the high-density-lipoprotein (HDL)/low-density-lipoprotein (LDL) ratio, a positive step for people with a blood-cholesterol problem. People who already have high blood-cholesterol levels should discuss this effect with their doctors.

Possible Side Effects

The incidence of side effects is much lower for prazosin than it is for other alpha blockers.

▼ Most common: dizziness, drowsiness, weakness, nausea, and headache.

▼ Less common: low blood pressure, dizziness when rising from a sitting or lying position, rapid heartbeat, vomiting, dry mouth, diarrhea, constipation, abdominal pain or discomfort, breathing difficulties, stuffy nose, nosebleed, joint or muscle pain, blurred vision, conjunctivitis (pinkeye), ringing or buzzing in the ears, depression, nervousness, tingling in the hands or feet, frequent urination, impotence, poor urinary control, painful erection, itching, sweating, rash, hair loss, fluid retention, and fever.

Drug Interactions

• Prazosin may interact with beta blockers to increase the chance of dizziness or fainting after the first dose of prazosin.

• The blood-pressure-lowering effect of prazosin may be reduced by indomethacin.

• When taken with other blood-pressure-lowering drugs, prazosin produces an exaggerated reduction of blood pressure.

• The blood-pressure-lowering effect of clonidine may be reduced by prazosin.

Food Interactions

None known.

Usual Dose

1 mg 2–3 times a day to start; may be increased to a total daily dose of 20 mg although 40 mg a day has been used in some cases. Dosage must be tailored to individual needs.

Overdosage

Prazosin overdose may produce drowsiness, poor reflexes, and very low blood pressure. Overdose victims should be taken to a hospital emergency room immediately. ALWAYS bring the prescription bottle or container with you.

Special Information

Take prazosin exactly as prescribed. Do not stop taking prazosin unless directed to do so by your doctor. Avoid over-the-counter drugs that contain stimulants because they may increase your blood pressure. Your pharmacist will be able to tell you what you can and cannot take.

Prazosin may cause dizziness, headache, and drowsiness, especially 2 to 6 hours after you take your first dose, although these effects can persist after the first few doses.

Call your doctor if you develop severe dizziness, heart palpitations, or other bothersome or persistent side effects.

Wait 12 to 24 hours after taking your first dose of prazosin before driving or doing anything that requires intense concentration. Take your dose at bedtime to minimize this problem.

Taking your medication at the same time each day will help you remember to take it. If you forget to take a dose of prazosin, take it as soon as you remember. If it is almost time for your next dose, skip the dose you forgot and continue with your regular medication schedule. Do not take a double dose.

Special Populations

Pregnancy/Breast-feeding

There have been no studies of prazosin in pregnant women; its safety for use during pregnancy is not known.

Small amounts of prazosin pass into breast milk. Nursing mothers who must take it should bottle-feed their babies.

Seniors
Seniors, especially those with liver disease, may be more sensitive to the effects and side effects of prazosin. Report any unusual side effects to your doctor.

Premarin

see **Estrogen**, *page 385*

Prempro

see **Estrogen**, *page 385*

Prevacid

see **Lansoprazole**, *page 573*

Prilosec

see **Omeprazole**, *page 815*

Prinivil

see **Lisinopril**, *page 592*

Generic Name

Procainamide (proe-KAY-nuh-mide) Ⓖ

Brand Names

Pronestyl   Procan

Type of Drug

Antiarrhythmic.

Prescribed for

Abnormal heart rhythms.

General Information

Procainamide hydrochloride is often used as treatment for primary arrhythmia (abnormal heart rhythms). It works by slowing the response of heart muscle to nervous-system stimulation. It also slows the rate at which nervous-system impulses are carried through the heart. This drug may be given to patients who do not respond to or cannot tolerate other antiarrhythmic drugs. Procainamide begins working 30 minutes after you take it and continues working for 3 or more hours. As with other antiarrhythmic drugs, studies have not proven that people who take procainamide live longer than people who do not take it.

Short-acting procainamide generic products may be interchanged for one another. However, sustained-release or long-acting products may not be equivalent to each other and should not be interchanged without your doctor's knowledge.

Cautions and Warnings

About 1 of every 200 people taking procainamide in the usual dosage range develops bone marrow depression, a drastic drop in white-blood-cell count, low platelet count, or other **abnormalities of blood components**. Symptoms of such problems include fever, chills, sore throat, mouth sores, bruising, or bleeding: Call your doctor if any of these occur. Because these abnormalities happen most often during the first 3 months of taking procainamide, you should be checked with weekly blood counts during your first 3 months on this drug.

Procainamide should not be taken by people who have complete **heart block** or the arrhythmia called "torsade de pointes," situations which procainamide will worsen rather than improve. Long-term use may cause up to 30% of people taking procainamide to test positive for lupus erythematosus (long-term condition affecting the body's connective tissues) with or without symptoms. Report anything unusual to your doctor.

If you have **myasthenia gravis,** tell your doctor when procainamide is first prescribed; you should be taking a drug other than procainamide. You should also tell your doctor if you are **allergic** to procainamide or to the local anesthetic procaine.

Procainamide may aggravate congestive **heart failure** by reducing the output of an already compromised heart.

This drug is eliminated from the body through the kidney and liver. If you have either **kidney or liver disease**, your dose of procainamide may have to be adjusted.

This drug, like other antiarrhythmics, has not been proven to help people with ventricular arrhythmias live longer.

Possible Side Effects

▼ Common: appetite loss; nausea; itching; symptoms resembling the disease lupus erythematosus (fever and chills, nausea, vomiting, muscle aches, skin lesions, arthritis, and abdominal pains), enlargement of the liver or changes in blood tests, that indicate a change in the liver; soreness of the mouth or throat; unusual bleeding; rash; and fever. If any of these symptoms occur while you are taking procainamide, tell your doctor immediately.

▼ Less common: bitter taste in the mouth, vomiting, diarrhea, weakness, dizziness, mental depression, giddiness, hallucinations, and drug allergy (symptoms include rash, itching, and drug fever).

Drug Interactions

• Procainamide blood levels and the chances of drug side effects are increased by the following: propranolol and other beta blockers; cimetidine, ranitidine, and other H_2 antagonists; lidocaine; quinidine; and trimethoprim.

• Do not take procainamide with other antiarrhythmic drugs unless specifically instructed by your doctor. These combinations can unduly depress heart function.

• The interaction between alcohol and procainamide is variable and may alter the effects of procainamide.

• Avoid over-the-counter (OTC) cough, cold, or allergy remedies containing drugs that have a stimulating effect on the heart. Ask your pharmacist about the ingredients in OTC remedies.

Food Interactions

This medication is best taken on an empty stomach, but you may take it with food if it upsets your stomach.

Usual Dose

Starting dose—1000 mg. Maintenance dose—23 mg a day per lb. of body weight, in doses every 3 hours around the clock, adjusted according to individual needs. Taking a sustained-release product allows doses to be spaced 6 hours apart. Seniors and people with kidney or liver disease are treated with lower doses or given the medication less often.

Overdosage

Procainamide overdose leads to a progressive blockage of nerve impulses within heart muscle, thus slowing the heart rate and causing low blood pressure and other drug side effects. Overdose symptoms, which include abnormal heart rhythms, low blood pressure, tremors, and nervous-system depression, can follow an overdose of 2000 mg; 3000 mg taken in 1 dose can be dangerous. Overdose victims should be taken to an emergency room immediately. ALWAYS bring the prescription bottle or container with you.

Special Information

Call your doctor at once if you develop any sign of infection, including fever, chills, sore throat, or mouth sores, or if you develop any of the following: joint or muscle pain, dark urine, wheezing, weakness, chest or abdominal pains, heart palpitations, nausea, vomiting, diarrhea, appetite loss, dizziness, depression, hallucinations, or unusual bruising or bleeding.

Be sure you discuss with your doctor any drug sensitivity or reaction, especially to procaine or other local anesthetics or to aspirin. Also, be sure your doctor knows if you have heart failure, lupus erythematosus, liver or kidney disease, or myasthenia gravis.

Because procainamide is taken so frequently during the day, it is essential that you follow your doctor's directions about taking your medicine. Taking more medicine will not necessarily help you, and skipping doses or taking them less often than directed may lead to a loss of control over your heart problem.

If you forget to take a dose of procainamide and remember within 2 hours, or within 4 hours if you are taking long-acting procainamide, take it right away. If it is almost time for your next regularly scheduled dose, skip the one you forgot and continue with your regular schedule. Do not take a double dose.

Special Populations

Pregnancy/Breast-feeding

Procainamide passes into the fetal blood circulation, but it has not been found to cause birth defects. If you are or might be pregnant and this drug is considered crucial by your doctor, its potential benefits must be carefully weighed against its risks.

This drug passes into breast milk and may affect a nursing infant. Nursing mothers who must take procainamide should bottle-feed their babies.

Seniors

Seniors are more sensitive to procainamide. Follow your doctor's directions and report any side effects at once.

Procardia XL

see **Nifedipine**, page 781

Generic Name

Prochlorperazine (proe-klor-PER-uh-zene) Ⓖ

Brand Name

Compazine

Type of Drug

Antinauseant and phenothiazine antipsychotic.

Prescribed for

Severe nausea and vomiting; also prescribed for psychotic disorders such as excessive anxiety, tension, and agitation.

General Information

Prochlorperazine is a member of a group of drugs called phenothiazines that act on a portion of the brain called the hypothalamus. These drugs affect areas of the hypothalamus that control metabolism, body temperature, alertness, muscle tone, hormone balance, and vomiting and may be used to treat problems related to any of these functions. The exact way in which phenothiazines work is not completely understood.

Cautions and Warnings

Prochlorperazine may **depress the gag (cough) reflex**. Some people who have taken this drug have accidentally choked to death because the gag reflex failed to protect them. Because of its effect in reducing vomiting, prochlorperazine may obscure symptoms of disease or toxicity due to overdose of other drugs.

Do not take prochlorperazine if you are **allergic** to it or any phenothiazine drug. Do not take prochlorperazine if you have **very low blood pressure; Parkinson's disease;** or **blood, liver, kidney**, or **heart disease**. If you have **glaucoma, epilepsy, ulcers**, or **difficulty passing urine**, prochlorperazine should be used with caution and the under strict supervision of your doctor.

Avoid **extreme heat**, because prochlorperazine can upset your body's normal temperature-control mechanism.

Possible Side Effects

▼ Most common: drowsiness, especially during the first or second week of therapy. If the drowsiness becomes troublesome, call your doctor. Prochlorperazine can cause jaundice (symptoms include yellowing of the skin or whites of the eyes), typically within the first 4 weeks of treatment. The jaundice usually goes away when the drug is discontinued, but there have been cases when it did not. If you notice this effect or if you develop symptoms such as fever or feeling unwell, call your doctor immediately.

▼ Less common: changes in blood components including anemia (a condition characterized by a reduction in the number of red blood cells or amount of hemoglobin or blood), raised or lowered blood pressure, abnormal heart rate, heart attack, feeling faint, and dizziness. Phenothiazines may produce extrapyramidal effects such as spasm of the neck muscles, rolling back of the eyes, convulsions, difficulty swallowing, and symptoms associated with Parkinson's disease. These effects look very serious but disappear after the drug is withdrawn; how-

---

Possible Side Effects *(continued)*

ever, face, tongue, and jaw symptoms may persist for as long as several years, especially in seniors with a history of brain damage. If you experience extrapyramidal effects, contact your doctor immediately.

▼ Rare: Prochlorperazine may cause an increase in psychotic symptoms or may cause paranoid reactions, fatigue, lethargy, restlessness, hyperactivity, confusion at night, bizarre dreams, inability to sleep, depression, euphoria (feeling high), itching, swelling, unusual sensitivity to bright light, red skin or rash, breast enlargement, false-positive pregnancy tests, changes in menstrual flow, impotence, changes in sex drive in males, stuffy nose, headache, nausea, vomiting, appetite loss, changes in body temperature, pallor, excessive salivation or perspiration, constipation, diarrhea, changes in urine and bowel habits, worsening of glaucoma, blurred vision, weakening of eyelid muscles, spasms in bronchial or other muscles, increased appetite, excessive thirst, and skin discoloration, particularly in areas exposed to sunlight.

Drug Interactions

• Be cautious about taking prochlorperazine with barbiturates, sleeping pills, narcotics, other tranquilizers, or any other drug that may produce a depressive effect, including alcohol. Avoid alcoholic beverages.

• Aluminum antacids may interfere with the absorption of prochlorperazine into the bloodstream, reducing its effectiveness. Anticholinergic drugs may reduce the effectiveness of prochlorperazine and increase the risk of side effects.

• Prochlorperazine may reduce the effects of bromocriptine and appetite suppressants. The blood-pressure-lowering effect of guanethidine may be counteracted by this drug.

• Taking lithium together with prochlorperazine or any phenothiazine drug may lead to disorientation, loss of consciousness, and uncontrolled muscle movements. Combining propranolol and prochlorperazine may lead to unusually low blood pressure.

• Blood levels of tricyclic antidepressants may increase if they are taken together with prochlorperazine, which may lead to antidepressant side effects.

Food Interactions

The antipsychotic effectiveness of prochlorperazine may be counteracted by beverages or foods with caffeine such as coffee, tea, cola drinks, or chocolate.

Usual Dose

Adult: 15–150 mg a day, depending on your disease and response. By mouth for nausea and vomiting—15–40 mg a day; rectal suppositories—25 mg twice a day.

Child (40–85 lbs.): 10–15 mg a day. The syrup form contains 5 mg of prochlorperazine per tsp.

Child (30–39 lbs.): 2.5 mg 2–3 times a day.

Child (20–29 lbs.): 2.5 mg 1–2 times a day.

Child (under age 2 or 20 lbs.): not recommended, unless your doctor feels the drug would be life-saving. Usually only 1–2 days of therapy are needed to relieve nausea and vomiting.

For psychosis, doses of 25 mg or more a day may be required.

Overdosage

Symptoms of overdose are depression, extreme weakness, tiredness or a desire to sleep, lowered blood pressure, uncontrolled muscle spasms, agitation, restlessness, convulsions, fever, dry mouth, abnormal heart rhythms, and coma. The victim should be taken to a hospital emergency room immediately. ALWAYS bring the prescription bottle or container with you.

Special Information

Prochlorperazine is a tranquilizer and may have a depressive effect, especially during the first few days of therapy. Care should be taken when performing activities requiring a high degree of concentration, such as driving.

Call your doctor if you develop sore throat, fever, rash, weakness, tremors, visual disturbances, or yellowing of the skin or whites of the eyes.

Prochlorperazine may cause unusual sensitivity to the sun. It may also turn your urine reddish-brown to pink; this is normal and not a cause for concern.

If dizziness occurs, avoid sudden changes in posture and avoid climbing stairs. Use caution in hot weather because this medication may make you more prone to heatstroke.

The liquid form of prochlorperazine may cause skin irritation or rash; do not get liquid prochlorperazine on your skin. Liquid prochlorperazine must be protected from light. Do not take it out of the opaque bottle in which it is dispensed from the pharmacy.

If you miss a dose of prochlorperazine, take it as soon as you remember. If it is almost time for your next dose, skip the dose you forgot and go back to your regular dosage schedule. Do not take a double dose.

Special Populations

Pregnancy/Breast-feeding

Infants born to women who have taken prochlorperazine have experienced side effects—jaundice and nervous-system effects—immediately after birth. Check with your doctor about taking this medication if you are or might be pregnant.

This drug may pass into breast milk and affect a nursing infant. Consider bottle-feeding if you must take this drug.

Seniors

Seniors are more sensitive to the effects of prochlorperazine and usually require lower dosage to achieve the desired results. Some experts feel that they should be treated with ½ to ¼ of the usual adult dosage of this drug.

Generic Name

Promethazine (proe-METH-uh-zeen) Ⓖ

Brand Name

Phenergan

Combination Products

Generic Ingredients: Promethazine + Codeine Phosphate Ⓖ
Pentazine with Codeine Syrup Ⓐ
Phenergan with Codeine Syrup
Pherazine with Codeine Syrup
Prometh with Codeine Syrup Ⓐ

Generic Ingredients: Promethazine + Dextromethorphan Hydrobromide Ⓖ
Phenergan with Dextromethorphan Syrup
Phenameth DM Syrup Ⓐ

Pherazine DM Syrup
Promethazine DM Liquid

Generic Ingredients: Promethazine + Phenylephrine Hydrochloride G
Phenergan VC Syrup
Promethazine VC Plain Syrup
Prometh VC Plain Liquid A

Generic Ingredients: Promethazine + Codeine Phosphate + Phenylephrine Hydrochloride
Para-Hist AT Syrup
Phenergan VC with Codeine Syrup
Pherazine VC with Codeine Syrup
Prometh VC with Codeine Liquid A
Promethist with Codeine Syrup A

Type of Drug

Antihistamine.

Prescribed for

Allergy, motion sickness, nausea, vomiting, nighttime sedation, pain relief when given with a narcotic pain reliever, and postoperative nausea and vomiting.

General Information

Promethazine hydrochloride, one of the older members of the phenothiazine antihistamine group, has been used by millions of people both alone and in combination with cough suppressants and decongestants. Newer antihistamines have replaced promethazine as a routine antihistamine but it is still widely used for its other effects.

Cautions and Warnings

Promethazine should be used with caution if you are **allergic** to it or if you cannot tolerate any other phenothiazine drug such as chlorpromazine and prochlorperazine.

Promethazine should be used with care if you have **very low blood pressure; Parkinson's disease;** or **heart, blood, liver,** or **kidney disease.** This drug should be used with caution and under your doctor's strict supervision if you have an **ulcer, epilepsy, glaucoma,** or **urinary difficulties.**

Children with a history of **sleep apnea (condition characterized by intermittent cessation of breathing during sleep),** a family history of **sudden infant death syndrome**, **liver disease**, or **Reye's syndrome** should not take promethazine.

Possible Side Effects

The suppositories can cause rectal burning or stinging.

▼ Most common: drowsiness, thick mucus, and sedation.

▼ Less common: sore throat and fever; unusual bleeding or bruising; tiredness; weakness; dizziness; feeling faint; clumsiness; unsteadiness; dry mouth, nose, or throat; facial redness; breathing difficulties; hallucinations; confusion; seizure; muscle spasm, especially in the back and neck; restlessness; a shuffling walk; jerky movements of the head and face; shaking and trembling of the hands; blurred vision or other changes in vision; urinary difficulties; rapid heartbeat; sensitivity to the sun; increased sweating; and appetite loss. Children and older adults are more likely to develop difficulty sleeping, excitability, nervousness, restlessness, or irritability.

Drug Interactions

• The sedating effects of promethazine are increased by nervous-system depressants including tranquilizers, alcohol, hypnotics, sedatives, antianxiety drugs, and narcotics. These combinations should be used with extreme caution.

• Use of a monoamine oxidase inhibitor (MAOI) antidepressant together with promethazine may cause low blood pressure and unusual or uncoordinated movements.

• Promethazine will antagonize the effects of amphetamines and other appetite suppressants such as diet pills.

• The combination of promethazine and an oral antithyroid drug may increase the risk of agranulocytosis (condition characterized by a reduction in the number of white blood cells).

• The combination of quinidine and promethazine may increase the cardiac effects of both drugs.

• Increasing the dosage of anticonvulsant medication, bromocriptine, guanadrel, guanethidine, or levodopa may be necessary when any of these drugs are taken with promethazine.

• Riboflavin requirements are increased in people taking promethazine.

• Promethazine may interfere with blood-sugar tests and some home pregnancy tests.

Food Interactions

Take promethazine with food if it upsets your stomach.

Usual Dose

Allergy
   Adult: 12.5 mg before meals and 12.5–25 mg at bedtime.
   Child: 5–12.5 mg 3 times a day and 25 mg at bedtime.

Motion Sickness
   Adult: 25 mg half an hour before travel; repeat in 8–12 hours if needed. Then take 1 dose upon arising and another before dinner.
   Child: 10–25 mg given by mouth or as a suppository.

Nausea and Vomiting
   Adult: 25 mg when needed; repeat up to 6 times a day if necessary.
   Child: 10–25 mg twice a day as needed.

Nighttime Sedation
   Adult: 25–50 mg at bedtime.
   Child: about half the adult dose.

Overdosage

Symptoms of overdose include drowsiness; confusion; clumsiness; dry mouth, nose, or throat; hallucinations; seizure; and other promethazine side effects (see "Possible Side Effects"). Overdose victims should be taken to a hospital emergency room for treatment. ALWAYS bring the prescription bottle or container.

Special Information

People who are taking promethazine must be careful when performing tasks requiring concentration and coordination such as driving because the drug may cause tiredness, dizziness, or light-headedness; avoid alcoholic beverages.

Call your doctor if you develop any of the following: sore throat; dry mouth, nose, or throat; fever; chills; unusual bleeding or bruising; tiredness; weakness; clumsiness; unsteadiness; hallucinations; seizure; sleeping problems; feeling faint; flushing; breathing difficulties; or any other persistent or intolerable side effect.

It is important to maintain good dental hygiene while taking promethazine and to use extra care when using your toothbrush or dental floss because dry mouth may cause you to be more susceptible to oral infections. If the dry mouth caused by promethazine is not eased by gum or hard candy or lasts more than 2 weeks, call your doctor or dentist. Any dental work should be completed prior to starting on this drug.

If you take promethazine twice a day and forget a dose, take it as soon as you remember. If it is almost time for your next dose, take one dose as soon as you remember and another in 5 or 6 hours, then continue with your regular schedule. Do not take a double dose.

If you take promethazine 3 or more times a day and forget a dose, take it as soon as you remember. If it is almost time for your next dose, take one dose as soon as you remember and another in 3 or 4 hours, then continue with your regular schedule. Do not take a double dose.

Special Populations

Pregnancy/Breast-feeding

Antihistamines have not been proven to cause birth defects in humans. Some babies born to women who have taken other phenothiazines have suffered side effects at birth such as yellowing of the skin and whites of the eyes and nervous-system effects. Promethazine taken within 2 weeks before delivery may affect the baby's blood-clotting system. Do not take any antihistamine without your doctor's knowledge if you are or might be pregnant—especially during the last 3 months of pregnancy because newborns may have severe reactions to antihistamines. When promethazine is considered to be crucial by your doctor, its potential benefits must be carefully weighed against its risks.

Nursing mothers who must take promethazine should bottle-feed their infants.

Seniors

Seniors are more sensitive to side effects such as dizziness, sedation, confusion, and low blood pressure and should be careful when taking this drug. Nervous-system side effects including parkinsonism and unusual or uncoordinated movements are also more likely to develop in seniors.

Propacet 100

see. **Propoxyphene Hydrochloride**, *page 934*

Generic Name

Propafenone (proe-puh-FEH-none)

Brand Name

Rythmol

Type of Drug

Antiarrhythmic.

Prescribed for

Life-threatening abnormal heart rhythms.

General Information

Propafenone slows the speed at which nerve impulses travel in the heart and reduces the sensitivity of nerves that are present in heart muscle. It also stabilizes the membranes of heart muscle, making them less sensitive to stimulation by cardiac nerves. Propafenone also has a very mild beta-blocking effect, which helps in stabilizing abnormal rhythms. However, this drug can cause abnormal rhythms of its own and, for that reason, is usually recommended only after other drug treatments have failed.

Cautions and Warnings

Propafenone should not be used by people with severe **heart failure,** very **low blood pressure,** or a very **slow heart rate.** In some cases, propafenone is not recommended for use unless an artificial pacemaker has been implanted to control basic heart function. Cardiac pacemakers may need some programming adjustments because of changes brought about by the drug in the sensitivity of heart muscle to the device.

Propafenone, like certain other antiarrhythmic drugs, can worsen some **abnormal rhythms** or create abnormalities of its own, including severe arrhythmias of the ventricle. Overall, about 5% of people who take this drug will develop abnormal rhythms because of the drug itself.

Most people's bodies break down propafenone relatively quickly and efficiently, but others eliminate it much more slowly. People in the latter group—less than 10% of all users—have 1½ to 2 times as much propafenone in their blood for a given dose and must be treated carefully by their doctors to avoid side effects.

People with **heart failure, chronic bronchitis,** or **emphysema** should probably not use propafenone because the drug's beta-blocking effect may worsen their conditions.

Propafenone should not be the first drug of choice for recent **heart-attack** victims, because it may not help them.

People with **kidney or liver disease** may need lower doses to compensate for reduced drug elimination from the body.

Possible Side Effects

▼ Most common: angina pains, heart failure, heart palpitations, abnormal heart rhythms that may include rhythm changes in the ventricles, dizziness, headache, nausea or vomiting, constipation, changes in senses of taste and smell, upset stomach, blurred vision, and breathing difficulties. Generally, side effects increase as drug dosage is increased.

▼ Less common: weakness, tremors, rash, joint pain, swelling, increased sweating, stomach gas, dry mouth, diarrhea, constipation, cramps, tiredness, headache, sleeplessness, drowsiness, dizziness, fainting, muscle weakness, loss of appetite, anxiety, low blood pressure, low heart rate, and chest pain.

▼ Rare: hair loss, impotence, increased blood sugar, low blood potassium, kidney failure, pain, itching, lupus, unusual dreams, flushing, hot flashes, psychosis, seizures, ringing or buzzing in the ears, gallbladder problems, anemia, bruising, bleeding, and changes in blood components.

Drug Interactions

• The combination of propafenone and some beta blockers, such as metoprolol and propranolol, has been shown to increase beta-blocker concentrations and decrease their rate of release from the body. Beta-blocker dosage reduction is likely to be required.

• Alcohol, tranquilizers, and other nervous-system depressants will increase the depressant effects of this drug.

• Cimetidine and quinidine reduce the rate at which this drug is broken down by the liver and may increase propafenone blood concentrations by 20%; dosage adjustment may be necessary.

• Propafenone increases digoxin levels between 35% and 80%, depending on the drug dosage; the higher the propafenone dose, the greater the effect. Your doctor will need to balance your digoxin dose if you must take both drugs.

• Propafenone may increase the nervous-system side effects of local anesthetics often used during minor surgery or dental work.

• Rifampin may increase the rate at which propafenone is eliminated from the body, resulting in a possible loss of propafenone effect.

• Propafenone will increase the amount of warfarin, an anticoagulant (blood thinner), in the blood by about 40%. Adjusting the warfarin dosage will solve the problem.

Food Interactions

None known.

Usual Dose

Starting dose—150 mg every 8 hours. Dosage may be increased in steps up to 900 mg per day, but the dose may also be reduced. Seniors may need less medication.

Overdosage

Overdose symptoms are usually worst within 3 hours of swallowing propafenone, and may include weakness, tiredness, fever, low blood pressure, and slow heart rate. Overdose victims should be taken to a hospital emergency room immediately. ALWAYS bring the prescription bottle or container with you.

Special Information

See your doctor regularly while you are taking propafenone, and call your doctor if you feel that your rhythm problem is not improving or is worsening, an effect you are most likely to experience at higher drug doses. Other important problems to report to your doctor are chest pain, breathing difficulties, swelling, trembling or shaking, dizziness or fainting, joint pains, a slow heart rate, fever, or chills. Other side effects should be reported if they are persistent or bothersome.

Be careful when driving or performing other complex tasks because of the chance that the drug will make you tired, dizzy, or light-headed; avoid alcoholic beverages.

It is important to take propafenone regularly every day and at evenly spaced times around the clock. Maintaining the drug's effect depends on a steady amount of the drug in your body. If you forget a dose, take it as soon as you remember. If 4 hours or more have passed since the forgotten dose should have been taken, skip it and continue with your regular schedule. Do not take a double dose.

Special Populations

Pregnancy/Breast-feeding

Pregnant animals given 10 to 40 times the maximum prescribed human dose of propafenone have shown that the drug can be toxic to the fetus. Pregnant women should not use this drug unless its advantages have been carefully weighed against its possible risks.

It is not known if this drug passes into breast milk. Nursing mothers who must take it should bottle-feed their babies.

Seniors

Seniors are likely to have age-related loss of kidney and/or liver function and may respond to lower dosages. Propafenone is broken down almost completely by the liver, and its by-products are eliminated by the kidneys; this should be taken into account by your doctor when determining your propafenone dosage.

Generic Name

Propantheline (proe-PAN-thuh-lene) [G]

Brand Name

Pro-Banthine

Type of Drug

Anticholinergic.

Prescribed for

Upset stomach, stomach spasm, and peptic ulcers; also used to treat urinary incontinence.

General Information

Propantheline bromide works by inhibiting the effects of a neurohormone called acetylcholine in the stomach and gastrointestinal (GI) tract. The inhibition of acetylcholine directly reduces the mobility of the GI tract and slows the production of enzymes and other secretions. This helps relieve some of the uncomfortable symptoms associated with peptic ulcer, irritable bowel and/or colon, spastic colon, other GI disorders, and urinary incontinence. Propantheline only relieves symptoms; it does not cure the underlying disease. It may also slow the production of saliva—causing dry mouth; reduce sweating; and cause dilation of the pupil—making it more difficult to adjust to sudden bright light.

Cautions and Warnings

Propantheline should not be used if you are **sensitive or allergic** to it or have **heart disease, Down syndrome, reduced mobility of the stomach and lower esophagus, fever, stomach obstruction, glaucoma, acute bleeding, hiatal hernia, intestinal paralysis, myasthenia gravis (disorder of the muscular system), reduced kidney or liver function, rapid heartbeat, high blood pressure,** or **ulcerative colitis**.

Because propantheline reduces your ability to sweat, its use in hot weather may cause **heat exhaustion**.

Possible Side Effects

▼ Most common: constipation, decreased sweating, and dry skin, eyes, nose, or throat.

▼ Less common: difficulty swallowing and reduced breast-milk flow.

▼ Rare: skin rash; hives or other allergy; confusion, especially in older adults; eye pain; dizziness or fainting when rising from a sitting or lying position; feeling bloated; urinary difficulties; blurred vision or sensitivity to bright light; drowsiness; headache; memory loss; nausea; vomiting; and unusual tiredness or weakness.

Drug Interactions

• Antacids that contain calcium or magnesium, citrates, sodium bicarbonate, and carbonic anhydrase inhibitors may slow the rate at which propantheline is released from the blood, increasing its therapeutic effect and possible side effects.

• Combining propantheline with other anticholinergic drugs, including atropine, belladonna, clidinium, dicyclomine, glycopyrrolate, hyoscyamine, isopropamide, and scopalamine, may lead to intensified side effects.

• Propantheline can reduce stomach acidity and reduce the amount of ketoconazole, an antifungal drug, absorbed into the blood after it is taken by mouth.

• Propantheline may counteract the effect of metoclopramide in reducing nausea and vomiting.

• Taking propantheline together with a narcotic pain reliever may increase the chances of severe constipation.

• Combining propantheline or any other drug that slows the movement of stomach and intestinal muscles with a potassium chloride supplement—especially one that comes in a wax-matrix tablet—may lead to excessive stomach irritation.

Food Interactions

Propantheline is usually taken 30 to 60 minutes before a meal.

Usual Dose

Adult: 7.5–15 mg 3 times a day, and 30 mg at bedtime.
Senior: 7.5 mg 3 times a day.
Child (under age 12): not recommended.

Overdosage

Propantheline overdose may result in blurred vision; clumsiness; confusion; breathing difficulties; dizziness; drowsiness; dry mouth, nose, or throat; rapid heartbeat; fever; hallucinations; weakness; slurred speech; excitement, restlessness or irritability; warmth; and dry or flushed skin. Take the victim to a hospital emergency room for treatment. ALWAYS bring the prescription bottle or container with you.

Special Information

Brush and floss your teeth regularly while taking propantheline. Because the drug can cause dry mouth, you may be more likely to develop cavities or other dental problems while you are taking it. Dry mouth can be relieved by chewing gum or sucking hard candy. Constipation associated with propantheline can be treated by using a stool-softening laxative.

Propantheline may make you drowsy or tired and can cause blurred vision. Take care while driving or performing tasks that require concentration and coordination.

Call your doctor if you develop skin rash or flushing, eye pain, or other side effects—such as dry mouth, urinary difficulties, constipation, or unusual sensitivity to light—that are persistent or bothersome.

If you forget a dose of propantheline, take it as soon as you remember. If it is almost time for your next regularly scheduled dose, skip the one you forgot and continue with your regular schedule. Do not take a double dose.

Special Populations

Pregnancy/Breast-feeding

Propantheline crosses into the circulation of the fetus but has not been found to cause birth defects. Women who are or might be pregnant should not take this drug without their doctor's approval. When propantheline is considered crucial by your doctor, its benefits must be carefully weighed against its risks.

Propantheline passes into breast milk and may reduce the amount of milk you make, but has caused no problems among breast-fed infants. Still, you must consider the potential effect on the nursing infant if you breast-feed while taking this drug.

Seniors

Seniors are more likely to become excited, agitated, confused, or drowsy while taking normal doses of propantheline. Continued use of propantheline may lead to loss of memory because it blocks acetylcholine in the brain, which is responsible for many memory functions.

Generic Name

Propoxyphene Hydrochloride

(proe-POK-sih-fene hye-droe-KLOR-ide)

Brand Names

Darvon	Dolene

Combination Products

Generic Ingredients: Propoxyphene Hydrochloride + Aspirin + Caffeine
Darvon Compound-65

Generic Ingredients: Propoxyphene Hydrochloride + Acetaminophen
E-Lor   Wygesic

The information in this profile also applies to the following drugs:

Generic Ingredient: Propoxyphene Napsylate
Darvon-N

Generic Ingredients: Propoxyphene Napsylate + Aspirin
Darvon-N with ASA

Generic Ingredients: Propoxyphene Napsylate + Acetaminophen
Darvocet-N 100   Propacet 100

Type of Drug

Analgesic.

Prescribed for

Mild to moderate pain relief.

General Information

Propoxyphene hydrochloride is a chemical derivative of methadone, a narcotic pain reliever. Methadone is also used to help detoxify narcotics addicts. It is estimated that propoxyphene hydrochloride is about ½ to ⅔ as strong a pain reliever as codeine and about equally as effective as aspirin. Propoxyphene hydrochloride is widely used for mild pain; it can be addictive when taken for extended periods of time.

Propoxyphene hydrochloride is more effective when combined with aspirin or acetaminophen than when used alone. Propoxyphene hydrochloride is about 30% more potent than propoxyphene napsylate.

Cautions and Warnings

Do not take propoxyphene hydrochloride if you are **allergic** to it or to similar drugs. Psychological or physical **drug dependence (addiction)** may result when propoxyphene hydrochloride is taken in doses larger than those needed for pain relief for long periods of time. The major sign of psychological dependence is anxiety when the drug is suddenly stopped. People may also become physically addicted to propoxyphene hydrochloride; it can be abused to the same degree as codeine.

Never take more of this medication than is prescribed by your doctor.

Propoxyphene hydrochloride should be considered a **dangerous drug**, especially in the hands of anyone who is severely depressed or addiction-prone. Excessive doses of propoxyphene hydrochloride, either by itself or together with alcohol or other nervous-system depressants, are a major cause of **drug-related deaths**. Many of these deaths have occurred in people with a history of emotional disturbances, suicidal ideas or attempts, and misuse of tranquilizers, alcohol, and other nervous-system depressants.

Possible Side Effects

▼ Common: dizziness, sedation, nausea, and vomiting. These effects usually disappear if you lie down and relax for a few moments.

▼ Less common: constipation, stomach pain, skin rashes, light-headedness, headache, weakness, euphoria, and minor visual disturbances. Taking propoxyphene hydrochloride over long periods of time and in very high doses has caused psychotic reactions and convulsions.

Drug Interactions

• Propoxyphene hydrochloride may cause drowsiness when taken with other drugs that cause drowsiness, such as tranquilizers, sedatives, hypnotics, narcotics, alcohol, and possibly antihistamines.

• Carbamazepine levels may be increased by propoxyphene hydrochloride, resulting in dizziness, nausea, and poor coordination.

• Charcoal tablets decrease the absorption of propoxyphene hydrochloride into the bloodstream.

• Cigarette smoking increases the rate at which this drug is broken down in the liver. Heavy smokers may need more propoxyphene hydrochloride to obtain pain relief and will have to take less medicine if they stop smoking.

• Cimetidine may interfere with the breakdown of this drug in the liver, causing confusion, disorientation, breathing difficulties, and seizures.

• Propoxyphene hydrochloride may increase the anticoagulant (blood-thinning) effect of warfarin.

Food Interactions

Take propoxyphene hydrochloride with a full glass of water or with food if it upsets your stomach.

Usual Dose

Propoxyphene Hydrochloride: 65 mg every 4 hours as needed.

Propoxyphene Napsylate: 100 mg every 4 hours as needed. Seniors and people with poor liver or kidney function may need to take the medication less often.

Overdosage

Symptoms resemble those of a narcotic overdose and include the following: decrease in respiratory rate—in some people breathing rate is so low that the heart stops; changes in breathing pattern; pinpointed pupils; convulsions; extreme sleepiness leading to stupor or coma; abnormal heart rhythms; and development of fluid in the lungs. The overdose victim should be taken to a hospital emergency room immediately. ALWAYS bring the prescription bottle or container with you.

Special Information

Use caution while driving or performing any tasks that require you to be awake and alert. Avoid alcohol and other nervous-system depressants.

Call your doctor if you develop serious nausea or vomiting while taking this drug, or if you develop breathing difficulties.

If you forget to take a dose of propoxyphene hydrochloride, take it as soon as you remember. If it is almost time for your next regularly scheduled dose, skip the one you forgot and continue with your regular schedule. Do not take a double dose.

Special Populations

Pregnancy/Breast-feeding

No formal studies of this medication have been done in

pregnant women, but a survey of almost 3,000 pregnant women who took propoxyphene hydrochloride found that 46—1.6%—had infants with birth defects. Animal studies show that high doses of the drug can cause problems in a fetus. Pregnant women who must take propoxyphene hydrochloride should talk to their doctor about the risks of taking this drug.

Small amounts of propoxyphene hydrochloride pass into breast milk, but no problems have been seen in nursing infants.

Seniors

Seniors, especially those with reduced kidney or liver function, are more likely to be sensitive to the effects of this drug, and should be treated with smaller dosages than younger adults.

Generic Name

Propranolol (proe-PRAN-oe-lol) Ⓖ

Brand Name

Inderal

Combination Products

Generic Ingredients: Propranolol + Hydrochlorothiazide Ⓖ
Inderide

Type of Drug

Beta-adrenergic blocking agent.

Prescribed for

High blood pressure, angina pectoris, abnormal heart rhythm, prevention of second heart attack, migraine headache prevention, tremors, aggressive behavior, side effects of antipsychotic drugs, acute panic, stage fright and other anxieties, and schizophrenia; also used to treat bleeding from the stomach or esophagus, and symptoms of hyperthyroidism (overactive thyroid gland). The propranolol-hydrochlorothiazide combination is used only for high blood pressure.

General Information

Propranolol hydrochloride is one of 15 beta-adrenergic blocking drugs, or beta blockers, that interfere with the action of a specific part of the nervous system. Beta receptors are found all over the body and affect many body functions. This accounts for the usefulness of beta blockers against a wide variety of conditions. Propranolol, the oldest beta blocker, was found to affect all types of beta-adrenergic receptors. Newer, more refined beta blockers affect only a portion of that system, making them more useful in treating cardiovascular disorders and less useful for other purposes. Other of the newer beta blockers act as mild stimulants to the heart or have particular characteristics that make them better for specific purposes or certain people.

Cautions and Warnings

You should be cautious about taking propranolol if you have **asthma,** severe **heart failure,** a **very slow heart rate,** or **heart block (disruption of the electrical impulses that control heart rate)** because the drug may aggravate these conditions.

People with **angina** who take propranolol for high blood pressure risk aggravating their angina if they suddenly stop taking the drug. These people should have their drug dosage reduced gradually over 1 to 2 weeks.

Propranolol should be used with caution if you have liver or **kidney disease** because your ability to eliminate this drug from your body may be impaired.

Propranolol reduces the amount of blood pumped by the heart with each beat. This reduction in blood flow may aggravate the condition of people with **poor circulation** or **circulatory disease**.

If you are undergoing **major surgery**, your doctor may want you to stop taking propranolol at least 2 days before surgery to permit the heart to respond more acutely to stresses that can occur during the procedure. This practice is still controversial and may not hold true for all surgeries.

Possible Side Effects

Side effects are relatively uncommon and usually mild; normally they develop early in the course of treatment and are rarely a reason to stop taking propranolol.

▼ Most common: impotence.

▼ Less common: tiredness or weakness, slow heartbeat, heart failure (symptoms include swelling of the

Possible Side Effects *(continued)*

legs, ankles, or feet), dizziness, breathing difficulties, bronchospasm, depression, confusion, anxiety, nervousness, sleeplessness, disorientation, short-term memory loss, emotional instability, cold hands and feet, constipation, diarrhea, nausea, vomiting, upset stomach, increased sweating, urinary difficulties, cramps, blurred vision, skin rash, hair loss, stuffy nose, facial swelling, aggravation of lupus erythematosus (chronic condition affecting the body's connective tissues), itching, chest pain, back or joint pain, colitis, drug allergy (symptoms include fever and sore throat), and liver toxicity.

Drug Interactions

• Propranolol may interact with surgical anesthetics to increase the risk of heart problems during surgery. Some anesthesiologists recommend having gradually stopped the drug 2 days before surgery.

• Propranolol may interfere with the normal signs of low blood sugar and with the action of oral antidiabetes medications.

• Propranolol increases the blood-pressure-lowering effects of other blood-pressure-reducing agents, including clonidine, guanabenz, and reserpine; and calcium channel blockers, such as nifedipine.

• Aspirin-containing drugs, indomethacin, sulfinpyrazone, and estrogen drugs may interfere with the blood-pressure-lowering effect of propranolol.

• Cocaine may reduce the effectiveness of all beta blockers.

• Propranolol may worsen the problem of cold hands and feet associated with ergot alkaloids, used to treat migraine headache. Gangrene is a possibility in people taking both ergot and propranolol.

• The effect of benzodiazepine antianxiety drugs may be increased by propranolol.

• Propranolol will counteract thyroid hormone replacements.

• Calcium channel blockers, flecainide, hydralazine, oral contraceptives, propafenone, haloperidol, phenothiazine tranquilizers—molindone and others—quinolone antibacterials, and quinidine may increase the amount of propranolol in the bloodstream and lead to increased propranolol effects.

- Propranolol should not be taken within 2 weeks of taking a monoamine oxidase inhibitor (MAOI) antidepressant.
- Cimetidine increases the amount of propranolol absorbed into the bloodstream from oral tablets.
- Propranolol may interfere with the effectiveness of some antiasthma medications including theophylline and aminophylline, and especially ephedrine and isoproterenol.
- Combining propranolol and phenytoin or digitalis drugs may result in excessive slowing of the heart, possibly causing heart block.
- Your propranolol dose may have to be reduced if you stop smoking because your liver will break down the drug more slowly after you stop.

Food Interactions

Food increases the amount of propranolol absorbed into the bloodstream. Although it is best to take propranolol without food or on an empty stomach, it is more important to be consistent about taking it with or without food in order to maintain consistent effects.

Usual Dose

30–700 mg a day. Propranolol should be given in the smallest effective dose possible.

Overdosage

Symptoms of overdose include changes in heartbeat—unusually slow, fast, or irregular; severe dizziness or fainting; breathing difficulties; bluish-colored fingernails or palms; and seizures. The victim should be taken to a hospital emergency room. ALWAYS bring the prescription bottle or container with you.

Special Information

Propranolol is meant to be taken continuously. Do not stop taking this drug unless directed to do so by your doctor: Abrupt withdrawal may cause chest pain, breathing difficulties, increased sweating, and unusually fast or irregular heartbeat. When ending propranolol treatment, dosage should be reduced gradually over a period of about 2 weeks.

Call your doctor at once if you develop back or joint pain, breathing difficulties, cold hands or feet, depression, skin rash, or changes in heartbeat. Propranolol may produce an undesirable lowering of blood pressure, leading to dizziness or fainting; call your doctor if this happens to you. Call your doctor if you experience persistent or bothersome anxiety, diarrhea, constipation, impotence, headache, itching, nausea or vomiting, nightmares or vivid dreams, upset stomach, trouble sleeping, stuffy nose, frequent urination, unusual tiredness, or weakness.

Propranolol may cause drowsiness, light-headedness, dizziness, or blurred vision. Be careful when driving or performing complex tasks.

It is best to take propranolol at the same time each day. If you forget a dose of propranolol, take it as soon as you remember. If you take propranolol once a day and it is within 8 hours of your next dose, skip the dose you forgot and continue with your regular schedule. If you take it twice a day and it is within 4 hours of your next dose, skip the dose you forgot and continue with your regular schedule. Never take a double dose.

Special Populations

Pregnancy/Breast-feeding
Infants born to women who took a beta blocker while pregnant had lower birth weights, low blood pressure, and reduced heart rates. Propranolol should be avoided by pregnant women and women who might become pregnant while taking it. When the drug is considered crucial by your doctor, its potential benefits must be carefully weighed against its risks.

Propranolol passes into breast milk in concentrations too small to have any effect.

Seniors
Seniors may absorb and retain more propranolol in their bodies, and require less of the drug to achieve results. Your doctor should adjust your dosage to meet your individual needs. Seniors taking propranolol may be more likely to suffer from cold hands and feet, reduced body temperature, chest pain, general feelings of ill health, sudden breathing difficulties, increased sweating, or changes in heartbeat.

Propulsid

see *Cisapride*, page 204

Proventil

see **Albuterol**, page 25

Provera

see **Medroxyprogesterone Acetate**, page 645

Prozac

see **Fluoxetine**, page 439

Generic Name

Quazepam (QUAH-zuh-pam)

Brand Name

Doral

Type of Drug

Benzodiazepine sedative.

Prescribed for

Short-term treatment of insomnia, difficulty falling asleep, frequent nighttime awakening, and waking too early in the morning.

General Information

Quazepam is a member of the group of drugs known benzo-diazepines. All have some activity as antianxiety agents, as anticonvulsants, or as sedatives. Benzodiazepines work by a direct effect on the brain. They make it easier to go to sleep and decrease the number of times you wake up during the night.

The principal difference among the various benzodiaz-epines lies in how long they work on your body. They all take about 2 hours to reach maximum blood level, but some remain in your body longer, so they work for a longer period of time. Flurazepam and quazepam remain in your body the longest, thus resulting in the greatest incidence of morning "hangover."

Sleeplessness may often signal an underlying disorder that this medication does not treat.

Cautions and Warnings

People with respiratory disease may experience **sleep apnea** (intermittent cessation of breathing during sleep) while taking a benzodiazepine sedative.

People with **kidney or liver disease** should be carefully monitored while taking quazepam. Take the lowest possible dose to help you sleep.

Clinical **depression** may be increased by quazepam and by other drugs that depress the nervous system. Intentional overdose is more common among depressed people who take sleeping pills than among those who do not.

All benzodiazepine drugs can be **addictive** if taken for long periods of time. It is possible for a person taking quazepam to develop drug withdrawal symptoms if the drug is discontinued suddenly. Withdrawal symptoms include tremors, muscle cramps, insomnia, agitation, diarrhea, vomiting, sweating, and convulsions.

Possible Side Effects

▼ Most common: drowsiness, headache, dizziness, talkativeness, nervousness, apprehension, poor muscle coordination, light-headedness, daytime tiredness, muscle weakness, slowness of movement, hangover, and euphoria (feeling high).

▼ Less common: nausea, vomiting, rapid heartbeat and abnormal heart rhythms, confusion, temporary memory loss, upset stomach, stomach cramps and pain, depression, blurred or double vision, constipation, changes in sense of taste, changes in appetite, stuffy nose, nosebleeds, common cold symptoms, asthma, sore throat, cough, breathing difficulties, diarrhea, dry mouth, allergic reaction, fainting, itching, acne, dry skin, sensitivity to bright light or to the sun, rash, nightmares or strange dreams, sleeplessness, tingling in the hands or feet, ringing or buzzing in the ears, ear or eye pain,

---

Possible Side Effects *(continued)*

menstrual cramps, frequent or painful urination, blood in the urine, discharge from the penis or vagina, poor control of urinary function, lower back and joint pain, muscle spasms and pain, fever, swollen breasts, and weight changes.

Drug Interactions

• As with all benzodiazepines, the effects of quazepam are enhanced if the drug is taken with alcohol, antihistamines, tranquilizers, barbiturates, anticonvulsant medications, tricyclic antidepressants, or monoamine oxidase inhibitors (MAOIs). MAOIs are most often prescribed for severe depression.

• Oral contraceptives, cimetidine, disulfiram, and isoniazid may increase the effect of quazepam by interfering with the drug's breakdown in the liver. Probenecid may also increase quazepam's effect.

• Cigarette smoking, rifampin, and theophylline may reduce quazepam's sedating effect.

• The effect of levodopa may be decreased by quazepam.

• Quazepam may increase the amount of zidovudine (an AIDS drug—also known as AZT), phenytoin, or digoxin in your bloodstream, increasing the chances of side effects.

• The combination of clozapine and benzodiazepines has led to respiratory collapse in a few people. Quazepam should be stopped at least 1 week before starting clozapine treatment.

Food Interactions

Quazepam may be taken with food if it upsets your stomach.

Usual Dose

Adult (age 18 and over): 7.5–15 mg at bedtime. Dosage must be individualized for maximum benefit.
Senior: Take the lowest effective dose.
Child (under age 18): not recommended.

Overdosage

The most common symptoms of overdose are confusion, sleepiness, depression, loss of muscle coordination, and slurred speech. Coma may develop if the overdose is particularly large. Overdose symptoms can develop if a single dose of only 4 times the maximum daily dose is taken. Overdose victims must be made to vomit with ipecac syrup—available at any pharmacy—to remove any remaining drug from the stomach: Call your doctor or a poison control center before doing this. If 30 minutes have passed since the overdose was taken or if symptoms have begun to develop, the victim must be taken to a hospital emergency room immediately. ALWAYS bring the prescription bottle or container with you.

Special Information

Never take more of this medication than your doctor has prescribed.

Avoid alcoholic beverages and other nervous system depressants while taking this medication.

Exercise caution while performing tasks that require concentration and coordination: Quazepam may make you tired, dizzy, or light-headed.

If you take quazepam daily for 3 or more weeks, you may experience some withdrawal symptoms after you stop taking it. Talk with your doctor about how best to discontinue the drug.

If you forget to take a dose of quazepam and remember within an hour of your regular time, take it as soon as you remember. If you do not remember until later, skip the dose you forgot and continue with your regular schedule. Do not take a double dose.

Special Populations

Pregnancy/Breast-feeding

Quazepam absolutely must not be used by pregnant women or by women who may become pregnant. Animal studies have shown that this drug passes easily into the fetal circulation and can affect fetal development.

Benzodiazepines pass into breast milk and can affect a nursing infant. Quazepam should not be taken by nursing mothers.

Seniors

Seniors are more susceptible to the effects of quazepam and should take the lowest possible dosage.

Generic Name

Quetiapine (keh-TYE-uh-pene)

Brand Name

Seroquel

Type of Drug

Antipsychotic.

Prescribed for

Psychotic disorders.

General Information

Quetiapine fumarate is a new antipsychotic drug that is effective against a wide variety of symptoms. It may work by antagonizing a number of different types of brain receptors. This means that the drug increases levels of certain neurotransmitters including serotonin, dopamine, and histamine, by preventing them from binding to cell receptors. Quetiapine is rapidly absorbed into the bloodstream and broken down by the liver.

Cautions and Warnings

People who are **sensitive or allergic** to quetiapine should avoid taking it.

A potentially fatal condition called **neuroleptic malignant syndrome** (symptoms include convulsions, breathing difficulties, and back, neck, or leg pain) may occur with some antipsychotic drugs. People who have experienced this syndrome with another antipsychotic drug should be cautious when taking quetiapine.

Antipsychotic drugs are often associated with **involuntary, uncoordinated, and uncontrolled movements**. This reaction is most common among older adults, especially older women. It is impossible to predict if someone will develop this problem when starting a new antipsychotic drug and it is sometimes necessary to continue treatment even when these symptoms are present. Call your doctor if you develop any unusual movements while taking quetiapine.

Quetiapine may make you **dizzy** or cause you to **faint** if you rise suddenly from a sitting or lying position. It should be used with caution if you have a history of **heart disease** including heart attack, angina pains, and abnormal heart rhythms. Take this drug with caution if you have a condition or take any drug that can cause **low blood pressure**.

Animal studies show a tendency to develop **cataracts** while taking quetiapine. People taking this drug for a long period have also developed cataracts, but they have not been directly related to the drug. People taking quetiapine should have an eye exam when they start the drug and every 6 months thereafter to detect any cataract formation.

Quetiapine should be used with caution if you have had a **seizure**, or have a seizure disorder or other condition that may make you more susceptible to seizures, such as Alzheimer's disease.

Quetiapine treatment has been associated with low levels of **thyroid** hormone in the blood. This is usually not a problem, although a small percentage of people taking this drug may need a thyroid supplement.

Quetiapine may cause increases in **blood cholesterol** and **triglyceride levels**.

Quetiapine has caused **liver inflammation** without any symptoms, as measured by increases in enzymes produced by the liver. These enzymes generally return to normal with continued treatment.

The possibility of **suicide** exists in any person with schizophrenia. People at risk of suicide should keep only small amounts of medication at any time.

Possible Side Effects

▼ Most common: dizziness, headache, upset stomach, tiredness, dizziness or fainting when rising from a sitting or lying position, abdominal pain, weight gain, and dry mouth.

▼ Common: swelling in the arms or legs, heart palpitations, spastic movements, difficulty talking, sore throat, runny nose, increased coughing, breathing difficulties, flu symptoms, appetite loss, sweating, and low white-blood-cell counts.

▼ Less common: weight loss, increased blood fats, intolerance to alcohol, dehydration, blood-sugar changes, loss of kidney function, flushing and warmth, electrocardiogram changes, migraine, slow heartbeat, poor blood

Possible Side Effects *(continued)*

flow to the brain, stroke, blood clots, irregular pulse, changes in the electrical impulses in the heart, pneumonia, nosebleed, asthma, abnormal dreaming, uncoordinated or abnormal movement, fainting, uncontrollable or excessive movement, confusion, memory loss, psychosis, hallucination, increased sex drive, urinary difficulties, poor coordination, paranoid feelings, unusual walking, muscle spasm, delusion, manic reactions, apathy, depersonalization, stupor, teeth grinding, catatonic reactions, loss of movement on one side of the body, neck or pelvic pain, suicide attempt, feeling unwell, sun sensitivity, chills, facial swelling, fungal infection, salivation, increased appetite, gum irritation or bleeding, difficulty swallowing, stomach gas, stomach irritation, hemorrhoids, mouth sores, thirst, tooth decay, loss of bowel control, stomach contents coming back up into the throat or mouth, rectal bleeding, tongue swelling, itching, acne, eczema, contact dermatitis, raised rash, seborrhea, skin sores, painful menstruation or menstruation accompanied by unusual pain, vaginal irritation, loss of urinary control, painful urination, impotence, abnormal ejaculation, vaginal infection, vaginal discharge, vaginal bleeding, irritation of the external vagina, testicle inflammation, cystitis, frequent urination, loss of periodic bleeding, oozing of breast milk, eye redness, abnormal vision, dry eyes, ringing or buzzing in the ears, changes in the sense of taste, eyelid inflammation, eye pain, broken bones, muscle weakness, twitching, joint pain, arthritis, leg cramps, bone pain, increased white-blood-cell count, anemia, black-and-blue marks, swollen lymph glands, bluish skin, diabetes, and underactive thyroid gland.

▼ Rare: sugar in the urine, gout, hand swelling, low blood potassium, water intoxication, angina pain, very rapid heartbeat, vein irritation, heart failure, hiccups, rapid and deep breathing, speechlessness, tooth problems, delirium, emotional upset, euphoria (feeling high), reduced sex drive, nerve pain, stuttering, bleeding in the brain, abdominal enlargement, vomiting blood, tongue inflammation, intestinal blockage, blood in the stool, pancreas inflammation, peeling rash, psoriasis, skin color

---

Possible Side Effects *(continued)*

changes, swollen breasts, nighttime urination, kidney failure, abnormal accomodation to changes in light, glaucoma, deafness, loss of red blood cells, very low blood-platelet count, and overactive thyroid gland.

Drug Interactions

• Avoid alcoholic beverages while taking quetiapine; excessive drowsiness may result.

• Quetiapine may antagonize the effects of levodopa and other drugs used to treat Parkinson's disease.

• Combining quetiapine with phenytoin increases the rate at which quetiapine is released from the body by 5 times. You may require an increase in quetiapine dosage to achieve the same effect. Once dosage has been adjusted, special caution should be taken if phenytoin is replaced by another antiseizure drug that does not stimulate the body's breakdown of quetiapine. Other drugs that have a similar effect on quetiapine are thioridazine, carbamazepine, barbiturates, rifampin, and oral corticosteroids.

• Ketoconazole, itraconazole, fluconazole, and erythromycin may affect quetiapine. Caution should be exercised when combining these drugs with quetiapine.

• Quetiapine may reduce the rate at which the body clears lorazepam.

Food Interactions

Taking quetiapine with food increases the amount of drug absorbed by a small amount. This is not likely to change its effect on your body.

Usual Dose

Adult: 150–750 mg a day.

Overdosage

Overdose victims should be taken to a hospital emergency room at once. ALWAYS bring the prescription bottle or container with you.

Special Information

Quetiapine may make you drowsy. Take care while driving or

doing anything that requires alertness, concentration, or coordination.

Antipsychotic drugs may increase your sensitivity to hot weather and your susceptibility to dehydration by interfering with normal temperature-control mechanisms. This problem has not been reported with quetiapine, but be sure to call your doctor if anything unusual develops.

Special Populations

Pregnancy/Breast-feeding

There is no information on the effect of taking quetiapine during pregnancy. It should only be taken during pregnancy if the possible benefits outweigh the risks. Talk to your doctor if you become pregnant or are trying to become pregnant while taking this drug.

Quetiapine passes into breast milk. Nursing mothers who must take quetiapine should bottle-feed their babies.

Seniors

Studies show no differences between seniors' reaction to quetiapine and that of younger adults. Nevertheless, seniors may be more sensitive to some of the side effects of this drug, especially dizziness, fainting, and tiredness because the drug clears the body more slowly in older adults. Call your doctor if anything unusual develops.

Generic Name

Quinapril (QUIN-uh-pril)

Brand Name

Accupril

The information in this profile also applies to the following drug:

Generic Ingredient: Ramipril
Altace

Type of Drug

Angiotensin-converting enzyme (ACE) inhibitor.

Prescribed for

High blood pressure and congestive heart failure.

General Information

ACE inhibitors work by preventing the conversion of a hormone called angiotensin I to another hormone called angiotensin II, a potent blood-vessel constrictor. Preventing this conversion relaxes blood vessels, thus reducing blood pressure and relieving the symptoms of heart failure by making it easier for a failing heart to pump blood through the body. Quinapril also affects the production of other hormones and enzymes that participate in the regulation of blood-vessel dilation; this action probably increases the drug's effectiveness. Quinapril begins working about 1 hour after you take it and lasts for a full 24 hours.

Some people who start taking an ACE inhibitor after they are already on a diuretic (agent that increases urination) experience a rapid blood-pressure drop after their first doses or when the dosage is increased. To prevent this from happening, you may be told to stop taking the diuretic 2 or 3 days before starting the ACE inhibitor or to increase your salt intake during that time. The diuretic may then be restarted gradually. Heart-failure patients generally have been on digoxin and a diuretic before beginning treatment with an ACE inhibitor.

Cautions and Warnings

Do not take quinapril if you have had an **allergic reaction** to it in the past.

Quinapril occasionally causes very **low blood pressure**. Quinapril can affect your kidneys, especially if you have **congestive heart failure**. It is advisable for your doctor to check your urine for changes during the first few months of treatment. Dosage adjustment is necessary if you have **reduced kidney function**.

Rarely, quinapril affects **white-blood-cell count**, possibly increasing your susceptibility to infection. Blood counts should be monitored periodically.

Possible Side Effects

▼ Most common: dizziness, tiredness, headache, and chronic cough. The cough usually goes away a few days after you stop taking the medication.

Possible Side Effects *(continued)*

▼ Less common: nausea, vomiting, and abdominal pain.

▼ Rare: heart palpitations, rapid heartbeat, chest pain, angina, heart attack, stroke, fainting, dizziness when rising from a sitting or lying position, sleepiness, not feeling well, depression, nervousness, constipation, dry mouth, inflammation of the pancreas, sweating, skin rash or peeling, itching, sun sensitivity, kidney failure, reduced white-blood-cell or blood-platelet counts, stomach or intestinal bleeding, high blood pressure, shock, flushing or redness, back pain, visual disturbances, sore throat, and viral infections.

Drug Interactions

• The blood-pressure-lowering effect of quinapril is additive with diuretic drugs and beta blockers. Any other drug that causes a rapid drop in blood pressure should be used with caution if you are taking an ACE inhibitor.

• Quinapril may increase potassium levels in your blood, especially when taken with dyazide or other potassium-sparing diuretics.

• Quinapril may increase the effects of lithium; this combination should be used with caution.

• Antacids may reduce the amount of quinapril absorbed into the blood. Separate doses of these medications by at least 2 hours.

• Quinapril decreases the absorption of tetracycline by about ⅓, possibly because of the high magnesium content of quinapril tablets.

• Quinapril may increase blood levels of digoxin, possibly increasing the chance of digoxin-related side effects.

• Capsaicin may trigger or aggravate the cough associated with quinapril therapy.

• Indomethacin may reduce the blood-pressure-lowering effects of quinapril.

• Phenothiazine tranquilizers and antiemetics may increase the effects of quinapril.

• The combination of allopurinol and quinapril increases the chance of side effects.

Food Interactions

Quinapril is affected by high-fat food in the stomach and

should be taken on an empty stomach, at least 1 hour before or 2 hours after a meal.

Usual Dose

Quinapril

Adult: 10–80 mg once a day. People with kidney disease may require a lower dosage.

Ramipril

Adult: 2.5–20 mg a day. People with moderate to severe kidney disease should begin with 1.25 mg a day; dosage may then be increased up to 5 mg a day.

Overdosage

The principal effect of quinapril overdose is a rapid drop in blood pressure, as evidenced by dizziness or fainting. Take the overdose victim to a hospital emergency room at once. ALWAYS bring the prescription bottle or container with you.

Special Information

ACE inhibitors may cause unexplained swelling of the face, lips, hands, and feet. This swelling can also affect the larynx (throat) and tongue and interfere with breathing. If this happens, go to a hospital emergency room for treatment immediately. Call your doctor if you develop a sore throat, mouth sores, abnormal heartbeat, chest pain, a persistent rash, or loss of taste perception.

You may get dizzy if you rise too quickly from a sitting or lying position.

Avoid strenuous exercise and/or very hot weather because heavy sweating or dehydration can cause a rapid drop in blood pressure.

Avoid over-the-counter diet pills, decongestants, and other stimulants that can raise blood pressure.

If you forget to take a dose of quinapril, take it as soon as you remember. If it is within 8 hours of your next dose, skip the one you forgot and continue with your regular schedule. Do not take a double dose.

Special Populations

Pregnancy/Breast-feeding

ACE inhibitors have caused low blood pressure, kidney failure, slow formation of the skull, and death in fetuses when taken during the last 6 months of pregnancy. Women who are pregnant should not take quinapril. Women who may become pregnant while taking quinapril should use an effective contraceptive method and stop taking the medication if they do become pregnant.

Relatively small amounts of quinapril pass into breast milk, and the effect on a nursing infant is likely to be minimal. However, nursing mothers who must take this drug should consider bottle-feeding: Infants, especially newborns, are more susceptible than adults to the drug's effects.

Seniors

Seniors may be more sensitive to the effects of quinapril than younger adults because of age-related kidney impairment; the starting dose for seniors is 10 mg daily. Your quinapril dosage must be individualized to your needs.

Generic Name

Quinidine (QUIN-ih-dene) G

Brand Names

Cardioquin	Quinidex Extentabs
Quinaglute Dura-Tabs	Quinora
Quinalan	

Type of Drug

Antiarrhythmic.

Prescribed for

Abnormal heart rhythms.

General Information

Derived from the bark of the cinchona tree, which gives us quinine, quinidine works by affecting the flow of potassium into and out of cells of the myocardium (heart muscle). This function helps quinidine affect the flow of nerve impulses throughout the heart muscle. Its basic action is to slow the pulse, which allows control mechanisms in the heart to take over and keep the heart beating at a normal, even rate.

The 3 kinds of quinidine—gluconate, polygalacturonate, and sulfate—provide different amounts of active drug; they cannot be interchanged without dosage adjustments by your doctor. Quinidine sulfate provides the greatest amount of active drug.

Quinidine is available in sustained-release products that require fewer daily doses.

Cautions and Warnings

Do not take quinidine if you are **allergic** to it, to quinine, or to a related drug. Quinidine sensitivity may be masked if you have **asthma, muscle weakness,** or an **infection** when you start taking the medicine.

Liver toxicity related to quinidine sensitivity is rare but has occurred. Unexplained fever or liver inflammation may indicate this effect. People with **kidney or liver disease** should take this medication with caution; lower doses may be necessary.

Like other antiarrhythmic drugs, quinidine can also cause **abnormal heart rhythms**. If this happens you will be told to stop taking the drug; you may also be hospitalized for further evaluation.

People taking quinidine for long periods may experience sudden fainting and/or an abnormal heart rhythm. These may end on their own or respond to medical treatment. Occasionally, these episodes may be fatal.

Possible Side Effects

▼ Most common: nausea, vomiting, abdominal pain, diarrhea, and appetite loss. These may be accompanied by fever.

▼ Less common: Quinidine may cause unusual heart rhythms, but such effects are generally found by your doctor during routine examination or by electrocardiogram. It may also affect components of the blood system and cause irritation of the esophagus, headache, dizziness, feelings of apprehension or excitement, confusion, delirium, muscle ache or joint pain, ringing or buzzing in the ears, mild hearing loss, blurred vision, changes in color perception, sensitivity to bright light, double vision, difficulty seeing at night, flushing of the skin, itching, sensitivity to the sun, cramps, an unusual urge to defecate or urinate, and cold sweat.

▼ Rare: asthma; swelling of the face, hands, and feet; respiratory collapse; and liver problems.

Possible Side Effects *(continued)*

High doses of quinidine may cause rash, hearing loss, dizziness, ringing in the ears, headache, nausea, or disturbed vision. This group of symptoms, called cinchonism, is usually related to taking a large amount of quinidine but may appear after a single dose of the medication. Cinchonism is not necessarily a toxic reaction, but you should immediately report any sign of it to your doctor. Do not stop taking this drug unless instructed to do so by your doctor.

Drug Interactions

• Quinidine increases the effect of warfarin and other oral anticoagulants (blood thinners). Your anticoagulant dose may have to be adjusted.

• Quinidine may increase the effects of metoprolol, procainamide, propafenone, propranolol, and other beta blockers; benztropine, oxybutynin, atropine, trihexyphenidyl, and other anticholinergic drugs; and tricyclic antidepressants.

• The effect of quinidine may be decreased by the following medicines: phenobarbital and other barbiturates, phenytoin and other hydantoins, nifedipine, rifampin, sucralfate, and cholinergic drugs such as bethanechol.

• The effectiveness and side effects of quinidine may be increased by taking amiodarone, some antacids, cimetidine, anything that decreases urine acid levels, and verapamil.

• Quinidine may dramatically increase the amount of digoxin in the blood, causing possible digoxin toxicity. This combination should be monitored closely by your doctor.

• The combination of disopyramide and quinidine may result in increased disopyramide levels and possible side effects; reduced quinidine activity may also result.

• Avoid over-the-counter cough, cold, allergy, or diet preparations. These medications may contain drugs that stimulate the heart and may be dangerous in combination with quinidine. Ask your pharmacist if you have any questions about the contents of a particular cough, cold, or allergy remedy.

Food Interactions

You may take quinidine with food if it upsets your stomach. Quinidine is also available in forms that are less irritating to the stomach. Contact your doctor if upset stomach persists.

Usual Dose

Immediate-release: extremely variable, depending on your disease and response; generally, 600–1200 mg a day.

Sustained-release: generally, 600–1800 mg a day.

Overdosage

Overdose produces depressed mental function, including lethargy, decreased breathing, seizures, and coma. Other symptoms are abdominal pain and diarrhea, abnormal heart rhythms, and symptoms of cinchonism (see "Possible Side Effects"). The victim should be taken to a hospital emergency room. ALWAYS bring the prescription bottle or container with you.

Special Information

Call your doctor if you develop ringing or buzzing in the ears, hearing or visual disturbances, dizziness, headache, nausea, skin rash, breathing difficulties, or any intolerable side effect (see "Possible Side Effects").

Do not crush or chew the sustained-release products.

Some side effects of quinidine may lead to oral discomfort including dry mouth, cavities, periodontal disease, and oral *Candida* infections. See your dentist regularly while taking this drug.

If you forget to take a dose of quinidine and you remember within 2 hours of your regular time, take it right away. If you do not remember until later, skip the dose you forgot and continue your regular schedule. Do not take a double dose.

Special Populations

Pregnancy/Breast-feeding

This drug passes into the fetal blood circulation and may cause birth defects or interfere with fetal development. Check with your doctor before taking it if you are or might be pregnant.

Quinidine passes into breast milk but is considered acceptable for use while breast-feeding. Consult your doctor.

Seniors

Seniors may be more sensitive to the effects of this medication because of the likelihood of decreased kidney function. Follow your doctor's directions and report any side effects at once.

Generic Name

Raloxifene (ral-OX-ih-fene)

Brand Name

Evista

Type of Drug

Selective estrogen receptor modulator (SERM).

Prescribed for

Osteoporosis in post menopausal women.

General Information

After menopause or surgical removal of the ovaries, women commonly experience loss of bone density due to the loss of the body's natural estrogen source. Later, the relative loss is made worse by the fact that cells called osteoblasts, responsible for making new bone tissue, lose their effect; calcium stored in bone is slowly reabsorbed back into the blood to be used for other purposes. At first, bone is lost rapidly because the body's attempt to balance this effect by building new bone rapidly is just not enough to offset the loss. Raloxifene reduces the reabsorption of bone in the bloodstream and slows the overall rate at which bone is broken down and rebuilt. It, like estrogen, works by binding to estrogen receptors in bone. Raloxifene has estrogen-like effects on bone and on blood lipids, reducing the rate at which the body makes cholesterol and other blood fats. It appears that raloxifene does not have estrogen-like effects on uterus and breast tissue.

In clinical studies, raloxifene increased the density of hip bone tissue but those changes were less than the improvement seen in women taking estrogen replacement therapy (ERT). However, studies comparing the effects of raloxifene and estrogen on blood fats showed that raloxifene was better than combined estrogen/progestin hormone replacement therapy (HRT) in improving levels of cholesterol.

Raloxifene is rapidly absorbed into the blood but most of it is broken down in the liver before it circulates throughout the body. As a result, only about 2% of each dose reaches the circulating blood. The raloxifene that does reach the bloodstream is eventually broken down in the liver. Most of the drug leaves the body through the feces. A very small amount passes out through the urine.

Cautions and Warnings

Do not take raloxifene if you are **sensitive or allergic** to it.

People with **cirrhosis** may have about 2½ times as much raloxifene in their blood. People with severe **liver disease** have not been tested on this medication and should not be given it unless they are being closely watched by their doctor.

Women with a past history of **blood clotting problems** such as clots in deep veins, pulmonary embolism (condition characterized by clots in the lungs), or clots in veins supplying the eyes should not take this drug. The greatest risk of blood clotting with raloxifene occurs during the first few months of treatment. Women taking raloxifene should avoid sitting still for long periods of time to protect against unwanted clotting.

There is no reason to take raloxifene **before menopause**. Raloxifene has not been studied in women who have had **breast cancer**.

Possible Side Effects

Most raloxifene side effects are relatively infrequent when compared to placebo (sugar pill). When compared with HRT, raloxifene is less likely to cause breast pain, vaginal bleeding, abdominal pain or stomach gas but more likely to cause hot flashes, chest pain, and infection.

▼ Common: hot flashes and leg cramps.

▼ Less common: infection, flu-like symptoms, weight gain, swelling in the arms or legs, muscle pain, sinus irritation, rash, and sweating.

▼ Rare: chest pain, fever, migraine, nausea, upset stomach, vomiting, stomach gas, stomach irritation, joint pain, arthritis, depression, difficulty sleeping, sore throat, coughing, pneumonia, laryngitis, vaginal irritation, urinary infection, cystitis, and problems with the uterus.

Drug Interactions

• Raloxifene reduces the amount of ampicillin absorbed and the amount of that drug in the blood. Do not combine these drugs.

• The effect of combining raloxifene with ERT is not known. Do not combine these drugs.

• Taking raloxifene with cholestyramine resin reduces the amount of raloxifene absorbed into the blood by 60%. Separate these drugs by at least 1 hour.

• Raloxifene may reduce blood-clotting time if combined with warfarin. If you must take both drugs, your doctor should check your blood from time to time.

• Combining raloxifene with clofibrate, indomethacin, naproxen, ibuprofen, diazepam, or diazoxide may lead to side effects. Be cautious when combining these drugs.

Food Interactions

None known.

Usual Dose

Adult: 60 mg a day. Take extra calcium and vitamin D if you do not get the full daily requirement from the foods you eat.
Child: not recommended.

Overdosage

There is no information on raloxifene overdose in humans. Women taking raloxifene during its study period took as much as 600 mg a day with no problems. Lab animals given a dosage equivalent to 810 times the human dosage also had no problems. Call your local poison control center for more information.

Special Information

Avoid situations in which you will be immobile for an extended period of time. You should avoid sitting in one position or place for several hours without moving. Doing so may lead to the formation of an embolus (blood clot) in a vein.

You should stop taking raloxifene at least 3 days before surgery or any other period where you are going to be immobilized for a long time.

Be sure you are getting sufficient amounts of vitamin D and calcium in your diet. If you think you are not getting enough, consider a calcium and vitamin D supplement.

Regular weight-bearing exercise is helpful because it naturally stimulates the body to build new bone.

Cigarette smoking and alcoholic beverages should be avoided.

If you forget to take a dose of raloxifene, take it as soon as you remember and then continue with your regular dose the next day; it may be taken at any time of the day. If it is almost time for your next dose, skip the dose you forgot. Do not take a double dose.

Special Populations

Pregnancy/Breast-feeding
Raloxifene may not be taken by women who are or might be pregnant because it may damage the fetus.

It is not known if raloxifene passes into breast milk. Raloxifene should be avoided if you are breast-feeding.

Seniors
Seniors may take raloxifene without any special precautions.

Generic Name

Ranitidine (rah-NIT-ih-dene)

Brand Name

Zantac   Zantac 75

Type of Drug

Antiulcer and histamine H_2 antagonist.

Prescribed for

Duodenal (intestinal) and gastric (stomach) ulcers; also prescribed for gastroesophageal reflux disease (GERD), other conditions characterized by the secretions of large amounts of gastric fluids, and to prevent bleeding in the stomach and upper intestines, stress ulcers, and stomach damage caused by nonsteroidal anti-inflammatory drugs (NSAIDs) prescribed for arthritis and pain relief. A surgeon may prescribe ranitidine for a patient under anesthesia when it is desirable for the production of stomach acid to be stopped completely.

General Information

Ranitidine hydrochloride and other H_2 antagonists work by turning off the system that produces stomach acid and other secretions. Ranitidine starts working within 1 hour and reaches its peak effect in 1 to 3 hours. Its effect lasts for up to 15 hours.

Ranitidine is effective in treating ulcer symptoms and preventing complications of the disease. It is prescribed for short-term and maintenance therapy. Since all H_2 antagonists work in the same way, ulcers that do not respond to one will probably not respond to another. The only difference among the H_2 antagonists is their potency. Cimetidine is the least potent, with 1000 mg roughly equal to 300 mg of ranitidine and nizatidine and 40 mg of famotidine. The ulcer-healing rates of all of these drugs are roughly equivalent, as is the risk of side effects.

Cautions and Warnings

Do not take ranitidine if you have had an **allergic reaction** to it or another H_2 antagonist in the past. Caution must be exercised by people with **kidney or liver disease** who take ranitidine because the drug is partly broken down in the liver and passes out of the body through the kidneys. Occasionally, reversible **hepatitis** or other liver abnormality may occur, with or without jaundice (symptoms include yellowing of the skin or whites of the eyes). Reducing acid levels in the stomach of a person with compromised immune functions may lead to a greater chance of some **intestinal worm infections**.

Possible Side Effects

Side effects with ranitidine are rare.

▼ Most common: dizziness, confusion, hallucinations, depression, sleeplessness, hair loss, inflammation of the pancreas, joint pain, and drug reactions.

▼ Less common: headache, blurred vision, agitation or anxiety, nausea, vomiting, constipation, diarrhea, abdominal discomfort, rash, painful breast swelling, impotence, loss of sex drive, and rash.

▼ Rare: reversible reduction in the levels of either white blood cells or blood platelets; hepatitis.

Drug Interactions

• The effects of ranitidine may be reduced if it is taken with antacids. This minor interaction may be avoided by separating doses of these drugs by about 2 to 3 hours.

• Ranitidine may interfere with the absorption of diazepam

tablets into the blood. This interaction is considered of only minor importance and is unlikely to affect most people.

• Ranitidine may increase blood concentrations of glipizide, glyburide, theophylline drugs, and procainamide, increasing the risk of side effects. Interactions between ranitidine and glyburide or a theophylline drug are rare.

• Ranitidine may interact with warfarin, an anticoagulant (blood thinner). Persons taking both drugs may need to have their warfarin dosages adjusted by their doctors.

Food Interactions

You may take ranitidine without regard to food or meals.

Usual Dose

150–300 mg a day. People with severe conditions may require up to 600 mg a day. People with severe kidney disease need less medication.

Overdosage

There is very little experience with ranitidine overdose. Overdose victims may be expected to experience severe side effects, but little else is known. Overdose victims must be made to vomit with ipecac syrup—available at any pharmacy—to remove any remaining drug from the stomach. Call your doctor or a poison control center before doing this. If you must go to the emergency room, ALWAYS bring the prescription bottle or container.

Special Information

It may take several days for ranitidine to begin to relieve stomach pain. You must take this drug exactly as directed and follow your doctor's instructions for diet and other treatments to get the maximum benefit from it.

Call your doctor at once if any unusual side effects develop. Especially important are unusual bleeding or bruising, unusual tiredness, diarrhea, dizziness, rash, or hallucinations. Black, tarry stools or vomiting "coffee-ground"-like material may indicate that your ulcer is bleeding.

If you forget to take a dose of ranitidine, take it as soon as you remember. If it is almost time for your next dose, skip the one you forgot and continue with your regular schedule. Do not take a double dose.

Special Populations

Pregnancy/Breast-feeding
Studies with laboratory animals have revealed no damage to the fetus. However, ranitidine should be avoided by women who are or might be pregnant. When ranitidine use is essential, its possible benefits must be carefully weighed against its risks.

Large amounts of ranitidine pass into breast milk, but no problems have been found in nursing infants. Nursing mothers must consider a possible drug effect while nursing their infants.

Seniors
Older adults respond well to ranitidine but may need less medication than do younger adults to achieve the desired response, because the drug is eliminated through the kidneys and kidney function tends to decline with age. Older adults may be more susceptible to some side effects of this drug, especially confusion.

Generic Name

Ranitidine Bismuth Citrate

(rah-NIT-ih-dene BIZ-muth SIT-rate)

Brand Name
Tritec

Type of Drug
Antibacterial-antiulcer combination.

Prescribed for
Duodenal (upper intestinal) ulcer, in conjunction with clarithromycin.

General Information
Revolutionary research into the causes of ulcer disease and some gastritis has shown that a microorganism known as *Heliobacter pylori* is almost always present. This has led to a major change in the treatment of these diseases. Combination drugs now treat both the ulcer and the infection that may

be the cause of the ulcer. Doctors have developed a variety of approaches to treating ulcers that combine various antibiotic and acid-blocking drugs. Ranitidine bismuth citrate combines two different drugs, and is meant to be used with a third drug, the antibiotic clarithromycin. Other ulcer treatments combine other drugs.

Bismuth works against *H. pylori* by disrupting the bacteria's cell wall. Bismuth is thought to prevent the bacteria from sticking to cells in the stomach lining and may also prevent the bacteria from becoming resistant to certain antibiotics.

Ranitidine turns off the system that produces stomach acid, providing relief from ulcer symptoms.

Cautions and Warnings

Ranitidine bismuth citrate should **not be used alone** for active duodenal ulcers. Active ulcer treatment also requires the antibiotic clarithromycin.

If you have taken clarithromycin for *H. pylori* and your **ulcer symptoms persist,** it is likely that you have a resistant form of the bacteria. A different antibiotic may be needed.

Do not take this drug if you are **sensitive or allergic** to any of its components.

People with **porphyria** should not take ranitidine bismuth citrate and clarithromycin.

People with **kidney disease** should take ranitidine bismuth citrate and clarithromycin with caution. Some people with kidney disease may require lower doses.

Ranitidine may interfere with the **Multistix urine test**. Check with your doctor or pharmacist for more information.

Possible Side Effects

Ranitidine Bismuth Citrate
Side effects can be expected to be minimal. In studies they are approximately equal to those reported with placebo (inactive) pills. For more information, see "Ranitidine."

Ranitidine Bismuth Citrate in Conjunction with Clarithromycin
▼ Most common: diarrhea and changes in sense of taste.

Possible Side Effects *(continued)*

▼ Less common: headache, nausea, vomiting, and gynecological disturbances.

▼ Rare: tremors, abdominal discomfort, stomach pain, rash, and drug reactions.

Drug Interactions

• Combining clarithromycin, ranitidine, and bismuth increases the amount of all three drugs in the blood, as compared with the amounts found when the drugs are taken alone. This interaction is beneficial to people taking the combination.

• High-dose antacids may reduce the amount of ranitidine and bismuth in the blood.

Food Interactions

This drug may be taken with food if it upsets your stomach.

Usual Dose

Adult: 400 mg 2 times a day for 4 weeks; 500 mg of clarithromycin 3 times a day is also taken for the first 2 weeks.

Child: not recommended.

Overdosage

Bismuth overdose may lead to kidney and nervous system toxicity, but this has not been seen with ranitidine bismuth citrate, only with other bismuth products. Ranitidine overdose effects are not usually permanent. Overdose victims should be taken to a hospital emergency room for treatment. ALWAYS bring the prescription bottle or container with you.

Special Information

Bismuth may cause a temporary darkening of your tongue or stool. This is a harmless effect. Darkening of the stool should not be confused with blood in the stool, which turns it black.

If you forget to take a dose of ranitidine bismuth citrate, take it as soon as you remember. If it is almost time for your next dose, skip the dose you forgot and continue with your regular schedule. Do not take a double dose.

Special Populations

Pregnancy/Breast-feeding

Animal studies of ranitidine bismuth citrate do not indicate that the combination affects the fetus. Five women became pregnant while taking ranitidine bismuth citrate. Three had normal babies, 1 had a voluntary abortion, and 1 had a baby with a birth defect, which doctors considered unrelated to the medication.

It is not known if ranitidine bismuth citrate passes into human breast milk; both elements pass into rat breast milk. Nursing mothers taking this medication should watch their babies for any unusual symptoms.

Seniors
Seniors may take this drug without special restriction.

Relafen

see **Nabumetone**, page 748

Retin-A

see **Tretinoin**, page 1117

Generic Name
Rifampin (rih-FAM-pin)

Brand Names

Rifadin   Rimactane

Combination Products

Generic Ingredients: Rifampin + Isonazid + Pyrazinamide
Rifater

Type of Drug
Antitubercular.

Prescribed for
Tuberculosis, meningitis, and other infections.

General Information
Rifampin is an important agent in the treatment of tubercu-

losis. It is not effective alone; rifampin is always used with at least one other tuberculosis drug. Rifampin is also prescribed to eradicate the organism that causes meningitis in carriers, people who are not infected themselves but carry the organism and can spread it to others. Rifampin may also be used to treat staphylococcal infections of the skin, bones, or prostate; legionnaires' disease when erythromycin does not work; and leprosy; and to prevent meningitis caused by *Haemophilus influenzae*, common among children in day care.

Cautions and Warnings

Do not take this drug if you are **allergic** to it or to rifabutin, prescribed for *Mycobacterium avium* complex (an infection associated with advanced cases of AIDS). **Liver damage** and death have been reported in people taking rifabutin; people taking other drugs that may cause liver damage should avoid rifampin. People with liver disease need to be carefully monitored by their doctors and should take a reduced dosage of rifampin.

Bacterial resistance develops very quickly if rifampin is used for meningococcus infection. It should not be used for this purpose.

A few cases of accelerated **lung cancer** growth have been reported, but a link to rifampin use is not established. Rifampin has the potential to **suppress the immune system** in people and animals.

Possible Side Effects

▼ Most common: flu-like symptoms, heartburn, upset stomach, appetite loss, nausea, vomiting, stomach gas, cramps, diarrhea, headache, drowsiness, tiredness, menstrual disturbances, dizziness, fever, pains in the arms and legs, confusion, visual disturbances, numbness, and hypersensitivity to the drug.

▼ Less common: effects on the blood, kidneys, or liver.

Drug Interactions

• Severe liver damage may develop when rifampin is combined with other drugs that cause liver toxicity.

• Rifampin may increase your need for oral anticoagulant (blood-thinning) drugs and may also affect angiotensin-converting enzyme (ACE) inhibitors, especially enalapril; acetaminophen; oral antidiabetes drugs; barbiturates; benzodiazepine tranquilizers; beta blockers; chloramphenicol; clofibrate; corticosteroids; cyclosporine; digitalis drugs; disopyramide; estrogens; phenytoin; methadone; mexiletine; quinidine; sulfa drugs; theophylline drugs; tocainide; and verapamil.

• Women taking birth control pills should use another contraceptive method while taking rifampin.

Food Interactions

Take rifampin 1 hour before or 2 hours after a meal, at the same time every day.

Usual Dose

Adult: 600 mg once a day.
Child: 4.5–9 mg per lb. of body weight, up to 600 mg a day.

Overdosage

Signs of rifampin overdose are nausea, vomiting, and tiredness. Unconsciousness is possible in cases of severe liver damage. Brown-red or orange skin discoloration may also develop. Rifampin overdose victims must be taken to a hospital emergency room at once. ALWAYS take the prescription bottle or container with you.

Special Information

Rifampin may cause a red-brown or orange discoloration of the urine, stool, saliva, sweat, and tears; this is not harmful. Soft contact lenses may become permanently stained.

Call your doctor if you develop flu-like symptoms, fever, chills, muscle pain, headache, tiredness or weakness, appetite loss, nausea, vomiting, sore throat, unusual bleeding or bruising, yellowing of the skin or whites of the eyes, rash, or itching.

If you take rifampin once a day and miss a dose, take it as soon as you remember. If it is almost time for your next dose, skip the dose you forgot and continue with your regular schedule. Do not take a double dose. Regularly missing doses of rifampin increases your chances for side effects.

Special Populations

Pregnancy/Breast-feeding

Animal studies indicate that rifampin may cause cleft palate and spina bifida (birth defect in which bones of the lower spinal column do not form properly, leaving the spinal canal partially exposed) in the fetus. Pregnant women should use this drug only if absolutely necessary.

Nursing mothers taking rifampin should bottle-feed their babies.

Seniors
Seniors with liver disease may be more sensitive to the effects of this drug. Report any side effects at once.

Generic Name

Riluzole (RIL-ue-zole)

Brand Name

Rilutek

Type of Drug

Glutamate-release blocker.

Prescribed for

Amyotrophic lateral sclerosis (ALS), also known as Lou Gehrig's disease.

General Information

ALS is a chronic disease of the nervous system for which there has been no effective drug treatment until now. Riluzole, the first drug ever to have been proven to affect ALS, has a number of different actions, though nobody knows exactly how it works. The drug slows the release of glutamate, which is thought to damage important nerve centers in the brains of people with ALS. Riluzole also protects other aspects of nerve function both inside and outside the nerve cell.

Riluzole extended survival in people with ALS during 18 months of treatment, though muscle strength and nerve function were not improved by the drug. Overall, death rates at the end of the studies were the same whether people took riluzole or not. In one study, the average life extension for people taking riluzole was 60 days.

Taking more than 100 mg a day of riluzole increases drug side effects and is not more effective. About 90% of each riluzole tablet is absorbed into the blood; food interferes with this absorption process.

Riluzole is broken down in the liver and passes out of the body through the kidneys.

Cautions and Warnings

Do not take riluzole if you are **allergic** to it or any of the tablet's ingredients.

Riluzole causes **liver inflammation;** people with severe liver disease should use this drug with caution. Liver function should be checked regularly during treatment with riluzole. People with **kidney disease** should also use riluzole with caution.

People of Japanese descent may eliminate riluzole from their bodies twice as slowly as do Caucasians. The drug may be eliminated more slowly due to genetic factors or because of differences in diet such as decreased use of alcohol, nicotine, and caffeine.

Cigarette smoking is likely to increase the rate at which riluzole is broken down by the liver. The drug may break down more quickly in **women** than in men. There is no indication that either of these factors is important in determining riluzole dosage.

Possible Side Effects

About 14% of people who took riluzole in pre-approval studies stopped taking it because of side effects.

▼ Most common: weakness, nausea, dizziness—twice as common in women than in men—diarrhea, a tingling sensation around the mouth, appetite loss, fainting, and tiredness. These effects increased with increasing dosage.

▼ Common: poor lung function, abdominal pain, pneumonia, and vomiting.

▼ Less common: back pain, headache, upset stomach at high doses, stomach gas, stuffy nose, runny nose, cough, high blood pressure, joint aches, and swelling in the arms and legs. At high doses—urinary infection and painful urination, and dizziness when rising from a lying or sitting position.

▼ Rare: aggravation, feeling unwell, mouth infection, eczema, rapid heartbeat, and vein irritation. Other effects

---

Possible Side Effects *(continued)*

may occur in virtually any body system. Report anything unusual to your doctor at once.

Drug Interactions

• Allopurinol, methyldopa, sulfasalazine, and other drugs that are toxic to the liver may interact with riluzole. Combinations of liver-toxic drugs should be taken with caution.

• Caffeine, theophylline, phenacetin, amitriptyline, and quinolone antibacterials may slow the rate at which riluzole is eliminated from the body.

• Cigarette smoke, charcoal-broiled foods, rifampin, and omeprazole might increase the rate at which riluzole is eliminated from the body.

• Riluzole can accelerate the breakdown of caffeine, theophylline, and tacrine, but these effects have not actually been seen in people.

Food Interactions

Take riluzole on an empty stomach, 1 hour before or 2 hours after meals.

Usual Dose

Adult: 50 mg every 12 hours.
Child: not recommended.

Overdosage

There are no reports of riluzole overdose. Overdose victims should be taken to a hospital emergency room at once. ALWAYS bring the prescription bottle or container with you.

Special Information

Taking more than 50 mg twice a day will not improve your condition and may increase drug side effects.

Call your doctor at once if you become feverish or ill. This could be a sign of a very low white-blood-cell count.

Riluzole should be taken at the same time each day—morning and evening—to get maximum benefit and maintain steady levels of the drug in your blood.

Riluzole can make you dizzy, tired, or faint. Do not drive or do anything that requires concentration until you can judge how riluzole affects you.

People taking riluzole should not drink to excess.

Store riluzole tablets between 68°F and 77°F and protect them from bright light.

If you forget a dose of riluzole, take it as soon as you remember. If it is almost time for your next dose, skip the dose you forgot and continue with your regular schedule.

Special Populations

Pregnancy/Breast-feeding

Riluzole is toxic to pregnant lab animals at doses up to 11 times larger than the maximum human dose. There are no studies of riluzole in pregnant women. It should only be used during pregnancy if the possible benefits outweigh the risks.

It is not known if riluzole passes into breast milk. Nursing mothers who must take riluzole should bottle-feed their babies.

Seniors

Seniors with kidney or liver disease should use riluzole with caution.

Generic Name

Rimantadine (rih-MAN-tuh-dene)

Brand Name

Flumadine

Type of Drug

Antiviral.

Prescribed for

Influenza A viral infection (type A flu).

General Information

Rimantadine hydrochloride is a synthetic antiviral agent that appears to interfere with the reproduction of various strains of the influenza A virus, a common cause of viral infection. Rimantadine is used both to treat and to prevent type A flu. Annual vaccination against the virus is the best way of preventing the flu, but immunity takes 2 to 4 weeks to develop. In the meantime, rimantadine may be taken to prevent viral infection in high-risk people or people who may experience greater exposure to the virus.

Cautions and Warnings

People with **severe liver or kidney disease** clear this drug from their bodies only half as fast as those with normal organ function; they will need to have their dosage adjusted appropriately.

People with a history of **seizures** are likely to suffer another one while taking rimantadine. Call your doctor if this happens to you.

The influenza virus may become **resistant** to rimantadine in up to 30% of people taking the drug. When this happens, the resistant virus can infect people who are not protected by the vaccine.

Possible Side Effects

▼ Most common: sleeplessness, nervousness, loss of concentration, headache, fatigue, weakness, nausea, vomiting, appetite loss, dry mouth, and abdominal pains.

▼ Less common: diarrhea, upset stomach, dizziness, depression, euphoria (feeling high), changes in gait or walk, tremors, hallucinations, convulsions, fainting, ringing or buzzing in the ears, changes in or loss of the senses of taste or smell, breathing difficulties, pallor, rash, heart palpitations, rapid heartbeat, high blood pressure, heart failure, swelling of the ankles or feet, and heart block.

▼ Rare: constipation, swallowing difficulties, mouth sores, agitation, sweating, diminished sense of touch, eye pain or tearing, cough, bronchospasm, increased urination, fever, and fluid oozing from the nipples in women.

Drug Interactions

• The importance of rimantadine's drug interactions is not known because there is no established relationship between the amount of drug in the blood and its antiviral effect.

• Aspirin and acetaminophen may reduce the amount of rimantadine in the blood by about 10%.

• Cimetidine increases the rate at which rimantadine is broken down by the liver.

Food Interactions

Rimantadine is best taken on an empty stomach, or at least 1 hour before or 2 hours after meals. You may take it with food if it upsets your stomach.

Usual Dose

Adult and Child (age 10 and over): 100 mg twice a day. People with severe liver or kidney disease—no more than 100 mg a day.

Child (under age 10): 2.25 mg per lb. of body weight, up to 150 mg, taken once a day.

Overdosage

Symptoms of overdose are likely to be reflected in nervous-system and cardiac side effects. They may include agitation, hallucination, and abnormal heart rhythm. Overdose victims should be made to vomit with ipecac syrup—available at any pharmacy—as soon as possible to remove any remaining drug from the stomach. Call your local poison control center or hospital emergency room before giving ipecac; then follow package directions. Give ipecac only if the victim is conscious. ALWAYS bring the prescription bottle or container with you if you go to a hospital for treatment.

Special Information

Rimantadine may be given to children to prevent influenza infection, but it is not recommended for treatment of their flu symptoms.

Call your doctor if you develop seizures, convulsions, or any other serious or unusual side effects.

If you forget a dose of rimantadine, take it as soon as you remember. If it is almost time for your next dose, skip the dose you forgot and continue with your regular schedule. Do not take a double dose.

Special Populations

Pregnancy/Breast-feeding

In animal studies rimantadine is toxic to fetuses; pregnant animals given 11 times the human dose experience side effects. Pregnant women should take rimantadine only after fully discussing its risks and benefits with their doctors.

Animal studies of rimantadine show breast milk levels

double blood levels within 2 to 3 hours. Nursing mothers taking rimantadine should bottle-feed their babies.

Seniors

Older adults are more likely to suffer from rimantadine side effects of the nervous system, stomach, and intestines. Elderly nursing-home patients should receive no more than 100 mg of rimantadine a day because of the likelihood that they have liver or kidney dysfunction. Otherwise healthy seniors may take this drug without special restriction.

Risperdal

see *Risperidone*, page 977

Generic Name

Risperidone (ris-PER-ih-done)

Brand Name

Risperdal

Type of Drug

Antipsychotic.

Prescribed for

Psychotic disorders and schizophrenia.

General Information

No one knows exactly how risperidone works, but it affects brain receptors for serotonin and dopamine, two important neurohormones. Risperidone is broken down in the liver. Between 6% and 8% of Caucasians and a very small number of Asians have little of the liver enzyme that breaks down risperidone and are considered to be "poor metabolizers" of the drug. Because these people break risperidone down very slowly, the drug takes about 5 days to reach a steady level in their blood. People with normal amounts of the enzyme reach a steady level in about 1 day. People with moderate to severe kidney disease and those with liver disease have trouble releasing risperidone from their bodies and must take a lower daily dose.

Cautions and Warnings

Do not take this drug if you are **sensitive** or **allergic** to it. Because risperidone has not been studied for more than 6- to 8-week periods, people taking it for longer periods must be reevaluated at least every 2 months.

A serious set of side effects known as **neuroleptic malignant syndrome (NMS)** has been associated with some antipsychotic drugs. The symptoms that constitute NMS include high fever, muscle rigidity, mental changes, irregular pulse or blood pressure, sweating, and abnormal heart rhythm. NMS is potentially fatal and requires immediate medical attention.

Risperidone can produce **uncontrolled movements,** including spasm of the neck muscles, rolling back of the eyes, convulsions, difficulty in swallowing, and symptoms associated with Parkinson's disease. These effects look very serious but usually disappear after the drug has been discontinued. Face, tongue, and jaw symptoms may persist, especially in older women, though they can appear at any age. Contact your doctor immediately if you experience any of these symptoms.

Risperidone can cause a life-threatening abnormal heart rhythm called **torsade de pointes.** The drug should therefore be used with caution in people with **heart disease.** Slow heart rate, electrolyte imbalance, and taking other drugs that carry a risk of torsade de pointes may increase the chances of developing this abnormality.

Risperidone, like other dopamine antagonists, raises levels of a hormone called prolactin. Increased prolactin has been associated with **tumors of the pituitary gland, breast, and pancreas**, but no problems have been noted with risperidone specifically.

Possible Side Effects

▼ Most common: sleepiness, sleeplessness, agitation, anxiety, uncontrolled movements, headache, and nasal stuffiness and irritation.

▼ Less common: dizziness, constipation, nausea, vomiting, upset stomach, abdominal pain, increased saliva,

Possible Side Effects *(continued)*

toothache, coughing, upper respiratory infection, sinus infection, sore throat, breathing difficulties, rapid heartbeat, joint or back pain, chest pain, fever, abnormal vision, skin rash, dry skin, and dandruff.

Other side effects have occurred in almost every body system. Be sure to report anything unusual to your doctor.

Drug Interactions

• Risperidone may decrease the effects of levodopa.

• Carbamazepine and clozapine may both increase the rate at which risperidone is released from the body, possibly reducing its effect.

Food Interactions

None known.

Usual Dose

Adult: starting dose—1 mg 2 times a day. Maintenance dose—increase gradually up to 6 mg a day if needed. For long-term treatment, your doctor will prescribe the lowest effective dose of risperidone.

Senior: starting dose—0.5 mg 2 times a day. Increase gradually if needed.

Child: not recommended.

Overdosage

In general, overdose symptoms are exaggerations of risperidone's side effects, including drowsiness, rapid heartbeat, low blood pressure, and abnormal and uncontrolled muscle movements. In 8 reports of overdoses up to 300 mg, no fatalities occurred. Overdose victims should be taken to a hospital emergency room for treatment. ALWAYS bring the prescription bottle or container with you.

Special Information

Risperidone can make you tired and affect your judgment, an effect that increases with increasing dosage. People taking this drug should be careful while driving or engaging in any other activity that requires concentration or clear thinking. Avoid alcoholic beverages.

Some antipsychotic drugs can interfere with the body's temperature-regulating mechanism. Take care to avoid extreme heat while you are taking risperidone.

Some people will develop a rapid heartbeat and may become dizzy or faint when first taking risperidone. This risk can be minimized by starting at a low dose, such as 2 mg a day in adults, or 1 mg in seniors or those with kidney or liver disease.

Risperidone can make you unusually sensitive to the sun. Be sure to wear protective clothes and to apply sunscreen thoroughly before going outside.

Because of the possibility of drug interaction, ensure that your doctor knows about any other prescription or over-the-counter medication you may take. Drugs that affect the liver may interfere with risperidone's breakdown.

If you forget to take a dose of risperidone, take it as soon as you remember. If it is almost time for your next dose, skip the dose you forgot and continue with your regular schedule. Call your doctor if you forget 2 doses in a row.

Special Populations

Pregnancy/Breast-feeding
Studies of risperidone in animals show an increase in birth defects and stillbirth. There are no studies of this drug in pregnant women. There is a report, however, of an infant who was born with an abnormally developed brain after the mother took risperidone. Women of childbearing age who are taking this drug should be extremely careful not to become pregnant. Risperidone should not be taken by women who are already pregnant unless the risk is carefully weighed against the potential benefit.

It is not known if risperidone passes into breast milk. Women who must take this medication should bottle-feed their babies.

Seniors
Seniors often have reduced kidney function and cannot release risperidone as efficiently from their bodies as younger adults do. Your doctor will reduce your daily dose accordingly. Seniors may also be more sensitive to the side effects of risperidone.

Generic Name

Ritonavir (rih-TON-uh-vere)

Brand Name

Norvir

Type of Drug

Protease inhibitor.

Prescribed for

Human immunodeficiency virus (HIV) infection.

General Information

Part of the multidrug cocktail responsible for the most important gains in the fight against acquired immunodeficiency syndrome (AIDS), ritonavir belongs to a group of anti-HIV drugs called protease inhibitors. Triple-drug cocktails are considered responsible for the first overall reduction in the AIDS death rate, recorded in 1996. Protease inhibitors work in a unique way but are not a cure for HIV infection or AIDS. When the HIV virus attacks a cell, it must be converted into viral DNA. Older drugs, known as reverse transcriptase inhibitors, interfere with this step, but they need help in fighting HIV. Protease inhibitors work at the end of the HIV reproduction process, when proteins are "cut" into strands of exactly the right size to duplicate HIV. The protein is cut by a protease enzyme. Protease inhibitors prevent the mature HIV virus from being formed by interfering with this cutting process. Proteins that are cut to the wrong length or that remain uncut are inactive.

Protease inhibitors are always taken with 1 or 2 nucleoside antiviral drugs such as AZT, ddl, ddC, or 3TC. Protease inhibitors revolutionized HIV treatment because when taken in combination, they reduce the amount of HIV virus in the bloodstream to levels that are often undetectable by current methods—CD_4 cell counts (immune system cells) and viral load (amount of virus in the blood) measurements. Multiple-drug therapy has changed the current view of HIV from a fatal disease to a manageable chronic illness.

People taking a protease inhibitor may still develop infections or other conditions associated with HIV disease. Because of this, it is very important for you to remain under the care of a doctor or other health care provider. The long-term effects of ritonavir are not known at this time. You may be able to pass the HIV virus to others even if you are on triple-drug therapy.

Cautions and Warnings

Do not take ritonavir if you are **allergic** to it. People with mild or moderate **liver disease** and **cirrhosis** break down ritonavir more slowly than those with normal liver function and may be more likely to develop side effects. People with cirrhosis should receive a reduced dose of ritonavir.

Ritonavir may raise your blood sugar, worsen your **diabetes**, or bring out latent diabetes. Diabetics who take ritonavir may have to have the dose of their antidiabetes medication adjusted.

Ritonavir interacts with a broad range of other drugs; some of these combinations may be dangerous. Details can be found below in "Drug Interactions."

Ritonavir can affect a wide variety of **blood tests**, including those for triglycerides, liver function, and blood sugar.

Possible Side Effects

▼ Most common: weakness, tiredness, nausea, diarrhea, vomiting, appetite loss, abdominal pains, taste changes, and tingling around the mouth and in the hands or feet.

▼ Rare: drug allergy, back pain, chest pain, chills, facial swelling, worsening diabetes, kidney or neck pain, sunsensitivity, bleeding, low blood pressure, migraines, heart palpitations, bloody diarrhea, abnormal stools, dry mouth, upset stomach, mouth ulcers, anemia, black-and-blue marks, swollen lymph glands, dehydration, arm or leg swelling, muscle cramps, joint pain, abnormal dreaming, changes in gait or walk, agitation, memory loss, anxiety, difficulty swallowing, confusion, convulsions, hallucinations, increased sensitivity to painful or other stimuli, poor coordination, loss of sex drive, impotence, nervousness, nerve pains, personality changes, tremors, fainting, breathing difficulties, worsening asthma, nosebleeds, hiccoughs, coughing, acne, skin rash, dry skin, eczema,

> **Possible Side Effects** *(continued)*
>
> changes in vision, painful urination, blood in the urine, kidney stones, urinary infection, and frequent urination.

Drug Interactions

• The following drugs should not be combined with ritonavir: amiodarone, astemizole, bepridil, bupropion, cisapride, clozapine, encainide, flecainide, meperidine, piroxicam, propafenone, propoxyphene, quinidine, rifabutin, and terfenadine. Ritonavir can be expected to substantially. raise the blood levels of all these drugs, which may cause serious abnormal heart rhythms, blood problems, seizures, and other serious side effects.

• Combining ritonavir with any of the following drugs may cause excessive sedation and breathing difficulties: alprazolam, clorazepate, diazepam, estazolam, flurazepam, midazolam, triazolam, and zolpidem. The effectiveness of other sedative-hypnotics is likely to be reduced by ritonavir. Ritonavir may interact with narcotic pain relievers, but the exact interaction is not predictable.

• Combining rifampin with ritonavir decreases the amount of ritonavir absorbed by about 35%.

• Combining ritonavir with clarithromycin or with zidovudine (AZT) results in more of both drugs in the blood. Mixing ritonavir with isoniazid increases the amount of isoniazid in the blood.

• Combining ritonavir with didanosine (ddI) may reduce the amount of ddI in the blood by about 15%.

• Combining fluconazole or fluoxetine with ritonavir increases the amount of ritonavir in the blood.

• Combining ritonavir with desipramine substantially increases the amount of desipramine in the blood.

• Ritonavir oral solution contains alcohol and will interact with disulfiram or metronidazole. Do not combine these drugs.

• Combining ritonavir with oral contraceptives containing ethinyl estradiol can lower blood hormone levels, possibly reducing their effectiveness. Your doctor may lower the dose of your contraceptive.

• Combining ritonavir with saquinavir, another protease inhibitor, slows the breakdown of saquinavir and increases its blood levels.

• Ritonavir lowers the amount of sulfamethoxazole absorbed into the blood by about 20% and raises trimethoprim by about 20%.

• Combining ritonavir with theophylline reduces the amount of theophylline absorbed by about 40%.

• Taking ritonavir with AZT reduces the amount of AZT in the blood by about 10%.

• Ritonavir is likely to increase the absorption of these drugs into the blood: alpha blockers, antiarrhythmics, anticancer drugs, antidepressants, antiemetics, antifungals, antimalarials, beta blockers, blood-fat reducers, calcium entry blockers, cimetidine, corticosteroids, erythromycin, immunosuppressants, methylphenidate, pentoxifylline, phenothiazines, and warfarin.

• Ritonavir is likely to reduce the amount of these drugs absorbed into the blood: atovaquone, clofibrate, daunorubicin, diphenoxylate, and metoclopramide.

Food Interactions

Ritonavir capsules are best taken with meals because more of the drug is absorbed on a full stomach. Ritonavir oral solution should be taken on an empty stomach, 1 hour before or 2 hours after meals, because food reduces the amount of liquid absorbed. The taste of the oral liquid may be improved by mixing it with chocolate milk, Ensure, or Advera. Do not mix earlier than 1 hour before you take your dose.

Usual Dose

Adult: 600 mg 2 times a day. You may start with a lower dose and increase gradually to avoid stomach upset.

Child: not recommended.

Overdosage

In animal studies, the lethal dose is 10 to 20 times the human dose. People taking 1500 mg a day for 2 days developed tingling in the hands or feet; this symptom went away when the dose was reduced. Take overdose victims to a hospital emergency room at once. ALWAYS bring the prescription bottle or container with you.

Special Information

It is imperative to take your HIV medication exactly as prescribed. Missing doses of ritonavir makes you more likely to become resistant to the drug and to lose the benefits of therapy.

Ritonavir does not cure AIDS. It will not prevent you from transmitting the HIV virus to another person; you must still practice safe sex.

Stay in close touch with your doctor while taking ritonavir and report unusual symptoms.

Ritonavir capsules should be stored in the refrigerator. The liquid may be kept at room temperature, but only for 30 days; refrigeration is recommended.

If you forget a dose of ritonavir, take it as soon as you remember. If it is almost time for your next dose, skip the dose you forgot and continue with your regular schedule. Do not take a double dose.

Special Populations

Pregnancy/Breast-feeding

If you are or become pregnant while taking ritonavir, talk to your doctor. There is little information currently available about the effects of ritonavir on pregnant women and their fetuses.

Nursing mothers who must take ritonavir should bottle-feed their babies. In any case, nursing mothers who are HIV positive should bottle-feed their babies to avoid transmitting the virus through their milk.

Seniors

Seniors may take ritonavir without special restriction.

Generic Name

Ropinirole (roe-PIN-ih-role)

Brand Name

Requip

Type of Drug

Antiparkinsonian.

Prescribed for

Parkinson's disease.

General Information

Ropinirole stimulates dopamine receptors in the brain. This is thought to be how it helps relieve symptoms of Parkinson's disease, though no one actually knows. About half of each dose of ropinirole is rapidly absorbed into the blood and is found throughout the body. Most ropinirole is broken down in the liver; only 1% or 2% leaves the body unchanged. A study of ropinirole in people with early Parkinson's disease showed disease improvement in about 70% of people taking the drug after 10 to 12 weeks of treatment. In the same study, 40% of people taking a placebo (sugar pill) also were considered to have responded to treatment. In another study, 28% of people with advanced Parkinson's disease who received ropinirole for 6 months showed improvement while only 11% of people taking placebo showed improvement.

Cautions and Warnings

Do not take ropinirole if you are **sensitive or allergic** to it. Ropinirole may cause **low blood pressure** and make you **dizzy** or **faint** when rising from a sitting or lying position, especially during the early stages of treatment. About 1 in 10 to 15 people who take ropinirole experience **hallucinations** that may be serious enough to force you to stop taking the drug.

Ropinirole causes **testicular tumors** and **changes to the eye** in lab animals though the meaning of these observations in determining how the drug affects people is not known. People taking this drug should be checked regularly.

People stopping other treatments for Parkinson's disease have developed **high fever** and **confusion**. **Breathing difficulties** caused by lung changes have occurred with the use of other antiparkinsonians. These problems have not been associated with ropinirole but there is a risk that you may experience similar problems if you stop taking ropinirole.

Possible Side Effects

Early Parkinson's Disease
▼ Most common: sleepiness or tiredness, nauseá, dizziness, upset stomach, vomiting, and virus infection.
▼ Common: general pain, sweating, weakness, fainting, abdominal pain, sore throat, and changes in vision.

Possible Side Effects *(continued)*

▼ Less common: dry mouth, flushing, chest pain, feeling unwell, blood-pressure changes, heart palpitations, rapid heart beat, hallucinations, confusion, memory loss, very sensitive reflexes, yawning, unusual movements, difficulty concentrating, appetite loss, stomach gas, swollen arms or legs, runny nose, sinus irritation, bronchitis, breathing difficulties, eye problems, urinary infection, impotence, and poor blood supply to the hands, legs, and feet.

Advanced Parkinson's Disease
▼ Most common: abnormal movements, tremor, muscle rigidity, hallucinations, and urinary infection.
▼ Common: confusion, constipation, pneumonia, sweating, abdominal pain, and twitching.
▼ Less common: dizziness or fainting when rising from a sitting or lying position, unusual dreaming, changes in the way you walk, poor muscle coordination, memory loss, nervousness, tingling in the hands and feet, temporary paralysis, diarrhea, difficulty swallowing, stomach gas, increased salivation, poor urinary control, pus in the urine, arthritis, breathing difficulties, dry mouth, anemia, and weight loss.

Drug Interactions

• Ropinirole may worsen uncontrolled muscle spasm that occurs with levodopa because the level of levodopa in your blood is raised by ropinirole. Your doctor may deal with this interaction by reducing your levodopa dosage.

• Ciprofloxacin, diltiazem, enoxacin, erythromycin, estrogen, fluvoxamine, mexilitene, norfloxacin, and tacrine slow the clearance of ropinirole from the body, increasing its effects. Cigarette smoking has a similar effect on ropinirole.

• Phenothiazine tranquilizers, haloperidol and similar tranquilizers, thioxanthene tranquilizers, and metoclopramide and other drugs that antagonize the effects of dopamine may reduce the effect of ropinirole.

• Ropinirole worsens the sedative effect of tranquilizers, sleeping pills, and other nervous system depressants.

Food Interactions

Food slows the rate at which ropinirole is absorbed into the blood but does not reduce the total amount absorbed. You may take this drug with food or meals to prevent nausea.

Usual Dose

Adult: 0.25 mg 3 times a day to start, gradually increasing to a maximum of 3 mg a day. Your dosage depends on your reaction to the medication and how well you tolerate it. Dosage is reduced for people with kidney disease.

Overdosage

Overdose symptoms are likely to be similar to the most common side effects (see "Possible Side Effects"). There have not been any reported cases of overdose with ropinirole. Overdose victims should be taken to a hospital emergency room for treatment. ALWAYS bring the prescription bottle or container with you.

Special Information

Ropinirole should be taken only as directed by your doctor. Be sure to tell your doctor if you are pregnant or breast-feeding.

Ropinirole causes sedation. Avoid alcoholic beverages and other nervous system depressants, especially if you drive or do anything else that requires coordination and concentration.

Hallucinations may occur with this drug, especially among seniors. Call your doctor if you develop hallucinations or experience any unusual side effects.

If you forget a dose of ropinirole, take it as soon as you remember. Space any remaining doses evenly throughout the rest of the day. Go back to your regular schedule on the next full day. Do not take a double dose.

Special Populations

Pregnancy/Breast-feeding

Ropinirole has not been studied in pregnant women. In animal studies, it has been found to cause birth defects and to damage the fetus. It should be used during pregnancy only if its risks and benefits have been discussed with your doctor.

Nursing mothers who must take this drug should bottle-feed their infants.

Seniors

Hallucinations are more likely in seniors taking ropinirole.

Roxicet

see **Percocet**, page 857

Generic Name

Salmeterol (sal-METE-er-ol)

Brand Name

Serevent

Type of Drug

Bronchodilator.

Prescribed for

Asthma and bronchospasm.

General Information

Salmeterol xinafoate differs from other bronchodilators in that it does not provide immediate symptom relief, but is instead prescribed for long-term prevention. When you first start salmeterol treatment, you may need to continue your other asthma inhalers for symptom relief. After a while, however, you should have less need for the other drugs. Salmeterol works like other bronchodilator drugs, such as albuterol, terbutaline, and metaproterenol, but it has a weaker effect on nerve receptors in the heart and blood vessels; for this reason, it is somewhat safer for people with heart conditions. Still, very large doses of salmeterol may lead to abnormal heart rhythms.

Salmeterol begins working within 20 minutes after a dose and continues for 12 hours. Other drugs in this group work for shorter durations.

Cautions and Warnings

Salmeterol should be used with caution by people with a history of **angina pectoris** (condition characterized by brief attacks of chest pain), **heart disease**, **high blood pressure**, **stroke** or **seizure**, **thyroid disease**, **prostate disease**, or **glaucoma**.

Used in excess, salmeterol can actually lead to more

breathing difficulties, rather than breathing relief. In the most extreme cases, people have had **heart attacks** after using excessive amounts of inhalant bronchodilators.

Long-term use of salmeterol, and related drugs, can lead to increases in certain **ovarian tumors**.

Possible Side Effects

Salmeterol's side effects are similar to those of other bronchodilators, except that its effects on the heart and blood vessels are not as pronounced.

▼ Most common: heart palpitations, rapid heartbeat, tremors, dizziness and fainting, shakiness, nervousness, tension, headache, diarrhea, heartburn or upset stomach, dry or sore and irritated throat, respiratory infections, and nasal or sinus conditions.

▼ Less common: nausea and vomiting, joint or back pain, muscle cramps, muscle soreness, muscle ache or pain, giddiness, viral stomach infections, itching, dental pain, not feeling well, rash, and menstrual irregularity.

Drug Interactions

• Monoamine oxidase inhibitors (MAOIs), tricyclic antidepressants, thyroid drugs, other bronchodilator drugs, and some antihistamines may increase the effects of salmeterol.

• The chances of cardiotoxicity may be increased in people taking both salmeterol and theophylline.

• Salmeterol may antagonize the effects of blood-pressure-lowering drugs, especially reserpine, methyldopa, and guanethidine.

Food Interactions

Do not inhale salmeterol if you have food or anything else in your mouth.

Usual Dose

Adult and Child (age 12 and over): 2 puffs every 12 hours. Each puff delivers 42 mcg of salmeterol.

Child (under age 12): not recommended.

Overdosage

Overdose of salmeterol inhalation usually results in exaggerated side effects, including heart pains and high blood pressure, although blood pressure may drop to a low level after a short period of elevation. People who inhale too much salmeterol should see a doctor. ALWAYS bring the prescription bottle or container with you.

Special Information

Be sure to follow the inhalation instructions that come with the product. Salmeterol should be inhaled during the second half of your inward breath, since this will allow it to reach deeper into your lungs. Wait at least 1 minute between puffs.

Call your doctor immediately if you develop chest pain, palpitations, rapid heartbeat, muscle tremors, dizziness, headache, facial flushing, or urinary difficulty, or if you continue to experience difficulty in breathing after using salmeterol.

If you forget a dose of salmeterol, take it as soon as you remember. If it is almost time for your next dose, skip the one you forgot and go back to your regular schedule. Do not take a double dose.

Special Populations

Pregnancy/Breast-feeding

When used during childbirth, salmeterol may slow or delay natural labor. It can cause rapid heartbeat and high blood sugar in the mother and rapid heartbeat and low blood sugar in the baby.

It is not known whether salmeterol causes birth defects in humans, but it has caused defects in animals. When your doctor considers this drug crucial, its potential benefits must be carefully weighed against its risks.

Salmeterol may pass into breast milk. Nursing mothers who must take this drug should be monitored closely by their doctor, and must observe their infants for side effects.

Seniors

Seniors should use the same dose of salmeterol as younger adults. Follow your doctor's directions closely, and report any side effects at once.

Generic Name

Saquinavir Mesylate

(suh-QUIN-uh-vere MES-uh-late)

Brand Name

Invirase   Fortovase

Type of Drug

Protease inhibitor.

Prescribed for

Advanced human immunodeficiency virus (HIV) infection.

General Information

Part of the multidrug cocktail responsible for important gains in the fight against acquired immunodeficiency syndrome (AIDS), saquinavir is a member of a group of anti-HIV drugs called protease inhibitors. Protease inhibitors work in a unique way. When the HIV virus attacks a cell, it must be converted into viral DNA. Older drugs, known as reverse trascriptase inhibitors, work to prevent this step, but they need help in fighting HIV. Protease inhibitors work at the end of the HIV reproduction process, when proteins are "cut" into strands of exactly the correct size to duplicate HIV. The protein is cut by an enzyme known as protease. Protease inhibitors prevent the mature HIV virus from being formed by inhibiting this cutting process. Proteins that are cut to the wrong length or that remain uncut are inactive.

Protease inhibitors are always taken with 1 or 2 nucleoside antiviral drugs such as AZT, ddI, ddC, or 3TC. They revolutionized HIV treatment because, when taken in combination, they reduce the amount of HIV virus in the bloodstream to levels that are often undetectable by current methods—CD_4 cell counts (immune system cells), and viral load (amount of virus in the blood) measurements. Multiple-drug therapy has changed the current view of HIV from a fatal disease to a manageable chronic illness.

Cautions and Warnings

Do not take this drug if you are **sensitive** or **allergic** to it.

If a serious **toxic reaction** occurs while taking saquinavir, you should stop the drug until your doctor can determine the cause or until the reaction resolves itself. Then treatment can be resumed.

Use caution if you have moderate to severe **liver disease.**

Saquinavir may raise your blood sugar, worsen your **diabetes,** or bring out latent diabetes. Diabetics who take saquinavir may need the dose of their antidiabetes medication adjusted against this effect.

HIV virus may become **resistant** to saquinavir or other protease inhibitors. For this reason it is essential that you **take saquinavir exactly according to your doctor's directions**.

Possible Side Effects

Most saquinavir side effects are mild. Other side effects become more prominent when saquinavir is taken together with antiretroviral drugs; these include weakness, muscle pain, and mouth ulcers.

▼ Most common: diarrhea, nausea, and abdominal discomfort.

▼ Less common: upset stomach, abdominal pain, headache, tingling or numbness in the hands or feet, dizziness, nerve damage, changes in appetite, and rash.

▼ Rare: Saquinavir can affect almost any body system. Report anything unusual to your doctor.

Drug Interactions

• Rifampin and rifabutin increase the rate at which saquinavir is broken down in the liver and reduce the amount of saquinavir in the blood by 80% and 40%, respectively. Do not combine these drugs. Other drugs that can reduce saquinavir blood levels are phenobarbital, phenytoin, carbamazepine, and dexamethasone.

• Blood levels of saquinavir may be elevated by terfenidine, astemizole, ketoconazole, and itraconazole. Other drugs that may elevate saquinavir levels and lead to side effects are calcium channel blockers, clindamycin, dapsone, quinidine, and triazolam.

Food Interactions

Take saquinavir within 2 hours after a full meal. The amount of saquinavir absorbed into the blood is vastly reduced when it is taken on an empty stomach, thus negating its antiviral effects.

Usual Dose

Adult (age 16 and over): 200–400 mg 3 times a day, within 2 hours after a full meal.

Child (under age 16): Saquinavir has been studied in HIV-positive children, but a standard dose has not been established.

Overdosage

One person who took 8,000 mg of saquinavir experienced no acute problems after being made to vomit. In a study of people taking up to 7,200 mg a day for 25 weeks, no unusual effects were seen. Call your local poison control center for more information. Overdose victims should be taken to a hospital emergency room. ALWAYS bring the prescription bottle or container with you.

Special Information

Saquinavir does not cure HIV infection or AIDS. It will not prevent you from transmitting the HIV virus to another person; you must still practice safe sex. You may still develop opportunistic infections or other illnesses associated with advanced HIV disease. The long-term effects of this drug are not known.

It is imperative for you to take this medication exactly according to your doctor's instructions. Missing doses of saquinavir increases the chance that you will become resistant to the drug. It should be taken after meals at the same time as you take your nucleoside antiviral drug. If you forget a dose of saquinavir, take it as soon as you remember. Do not take a double dose of this medication.

Special Populations

Pregnancy/Breast-feeding

Studies with saquinavir in pregnant animals have shown no negative effects on the fetus. There are no studies of saquinavir in pregnant women, but more information is becoming available every day, and a number of HIV-positive pregnant women have been successfully treated with protease inhibitors. When this drug is considered crucial by your doctor, its potential benefits must carefully be weighed against its risks.

It is not known if saquinavir passes into breast milk. Nursing mothers who are HIV-positive and must take saquinavir should bottle-feed their babies.

Seniors
Seniors can take this drug without special precaution.

Generic Name

Selegiline (seh-LEJ-uh-lene)

Brand Names

Atapryl   Eldepryl
Carbex

Type of Drug

Antiparkinsonian; selective monoamine oxidase inhibitor (MAOI).

Prescribed for

Parkinson's disease.

General Information

Selegiline hydrochloride is often combined with levodopa or carbidopa to control Parkinson's disease. Most people who take selegiline find that their doctor can reduce their levodopa or carbidopa dose within a few days.

The exact way in which selegiline works is not known. It is a very strong inhibitor of the form of the enzyme monoamine oxidase (MAO) that is found almost exclusively in the brain. Other MAOIs used as antidepressants work on both forms of MAO and affect the entire body. Selegiline also stimulates dopamine receptors in the brain, possibly by interfering with dopamine's reabsorption into brain nerve endings, thus making it last longer. In order for any drug to work in Parkinson's disease, it must somehow increase the activity of dopamine in the brain.

Some of selegiline's side effects may be caused by methamphetamine and amphetamine, 2 extremely potent stimulants that are products of the body's breakdown of selegiline.

Cautions and Warnings

People who have had a **reaction** to selegiline in the past should be very cautious about using it again.

People already taking sinemet—which contains levodopa and carbidopa—who start on selegiline may experience an increase in **levodopa side effects**. Your doctor can address this problem by reducing your sinemet dosage.

Taking more than 10 mg of selegiline a day may inhibit both kinds of MAO, causing unexpected reactions, including severe and possibly fatal **high blood pressure**.

Selegiline should not be used with meperidine or other **narcotic drugs** because of the chance of severe, possibly fatal, reactions similar to those of other MAOIs.

Possible Side Effects

When selegiline dosage is less than 10 mg per day, most of the side effects experienced are not caused by the drug itself; rather, selegiline increases the side effects of levodopa. That is why it is important for your doctor to reduce your levodopa dosage as much as possible.

▼ Most common: nausea, vomiting, dizziness, lightheadedness or fainting, and abdominal pain.

▼ Less common: tremors or uncontrolled muscle movements, loss of balance, inability to move, increasingly slow movements associated with Parkinson's disease, facial grimacing, falling due to loss of balance, stiff neck, muscle cramps, hallucinations, overstimulation, confusion, anxiety, depression, drowsiness, changes in mood or behavior, nightmares or unusual dreams, tiredness, delusions, disorientation, feeling unwell, apathy, sleep disturbances, restlessness, weakness, irritability, generalized aches and pains, migraine or other headaches, muscle pains in the back or legs, ringing or buzzing in the ears, eye pain, finger or toe numbness, changes in sense of taste, dizziness when rising from a sitting or lying position, blood-pressure changes, abnormal heart rhythm, heart palpitations, chest pain, rapid heartbeat, swelling in the arms or legs, constipation, appetite loss, weight loss, difficulty swallowing, diarrhea, heartburn, rectal bleeding, urinary difficulties, impotence, swelling of the prostate, increased sweating, increased facial hair, hair loss, rash, unusual skin sensitivity to the sun, bruising or black-and-blue marks, asthma, blurred or double vision, shortness of breath, speech problems, and dry mouth.

At doses above 10 mg per day, selegiline may cause muscle twitching or spasms, memory loss, increased energy, transient euphoria (feeling high), grinding of the

Possible Side Effects *(continued)*

teeth, decreased feeling in the penis, and male inability to achieve orgasm.

Drug Interactions

• Selegiline should not be used with meperidine or other narcotics because of the chance of severe, possibly fatal, reactions (see "Cautions and Warnings").

• Combining fluoxetine with MAOIs other than selegiline has been deadly. This effect has not been seen with selegiline, but the combination should be avoided. If you are taking fluoxetine, allow 5 weeks between the time you stop taking it and the time you start on any MAOI. If you are already taking an MAOI, allow at least 2 weeks between the time you stop taking it and the time you start taking selegiline.

Food Interactions

Take selegiline with food to avoid nausea or stomach upset, but avoid the following: Chianti and red wine, vermouth, unpasteurized or imported beer, beef or chicken liver, fermented sausages, tenderized or prepared meats, caviar, dried fish, pickled herring, cheese—American, Brie, cheddar, Camembert, Emmentaler, Boursault, Stilton, and others—avocados, yeast extracts, bananas, figs, raisins, soy sauce, miso soup, bean curd, fava beans, caffeine, and chocolate. These foods and others may cause severe, sudden high blood pressure in people taking selegiline. Your doctor or pharmacist can give you more information on foods to avoid.

Usual Dose

5 mg with breakfast and lunch.

Overdosage

Selegiline overdose symptoms may include excitement, irritability, anxiety, low blood pressure, sleeplessness, restlessness, dizziness, weakness, drowsiness, flushing, sweating, heart palpitations, and unusual movements, including grimacing and muscle twitching. Serious overdoses may lead to convulsions, incoherence or confusion, severe headache, high fever, heart attack, shock, and coma. Overdose victims should be taken to a hospital emergency room for treatment. ALWAYS bring the prescription bottle or container with you.

Special Information

After you have taken selegiline for 2 or 3 days, your doctor will probably reduce your carbidopa or levodopa dose by 10% to 30%. If the disease is still under control, your dosage may be reduced further to the lowest effective dosage that will control your condition.

It is important to maintain regular contact with your doctor while taking selegiline to allow for observation of the drug's effects and side effects. Headache, unusual body movements or muscle spasms, mood changes, or other unusual, persistent, or intolerable side effects should be reported to your doctor at once. Do not stop taking selegiline or change your dosage without your doctor's knowledge.

Selegiline reduces saliva flow in the mouth and may increase the risk of cavities, gum disease, and oral infections. Use candy, ice, sugarless gum, or a saliva substitute to avoid dry mouth.

If you forget to take a dose of selegiline, take it as soon as you remember. If it is almost time for your next dose, take 1 dose right away and another in 5 or 6 hours, then go back to your regular schedule. Do not take a double dose.

Special Populations

Pregnancy/Breast-feeding

Women who are or might be pregnant should not use selegiline unless its potential benefits have been carefully weighed against its risks.

It is not known if selegiline passes into breast milk. Nursing mothers who use this drug should watch their babies for unusual reactions. Report anything unusual to your doctor at once.

Seniors

Seniors may take selegiline without special restriction. Use the lowest effective dose to minimize side effects.

Brand Name

Septra

Generic Ingredients

Sulfamethoxazole + Trimethoprim Ⓖ

Other Brand Names

Bactrim

Bactrim DS

Bactrim Pediatric

Cotrim

Cotrim DS

Cotrim Pediatric

Co-trimoxazole

Septra

Septra Pediatric

Sulfatrim

TMP-SMZ

Type of Drug

Anti-infective.

Prescribed for

A wide variety of infections, including urinary tract infection, bronchitis, and ear infection in children; also prescribed for traveler's diarrhea, pneumocystis carinii pneumonia (PCP) in AIDS and leukemia patients, and prostate infection. Septra may be used to prevent urinary tract infections in women who take the medicine immediately after intercourse. It may also be prescribed for cholera, nocardiosis (lung infection), and *Salmonella* infection.

General Information

Septra is one of many combination products used to treat infections. It is unique because it interferes with the infecting microorganism's normal use of folic acid in two ways, making it more efficient than other antibacterial drugs. It is effective in many situations where other drugs are not. Bacterial resistance to Septra develops more slowly than to either sulfamethoxazole or trimethoprim used alone.

Cautions and Warnings

Do not take Septra if you have a **folic acid deficiency** or are **allergic** to either ingredient or to any sulfa drug, antidiabetes drug, or thiazide-type diuretic. Septra should be used with caution by people with **liver or kidney disease**. Be sure to drink at least 1 full glass of water with each dose of Septra.

Infants under 2 months of age should not be given this combination product.

Symptoms such as unusual bleeding or bruising, extreme tiredness, rash, sore throat, fever, pallor, or yellowing of the skin or eyes may be early indications of a serious **blood disorder**. If any of these effects occur, contact your doctor immediately and stop taking the drug. People taking Septra for **PCP** also have compromised immune function. They may not respond to Septra and are more likely to develop the less common side effects. People taking Septra to prevent PCP experience less severe side effects than people taking Septra to treat PCP.

Septra should not be used for **strep throat,** because of a greater chance of treatment failure than with penicillin.

Possible Side Effects

▼ Most common: nausea, vomiting, upset stomach, loss of appetite, and rash or itching.

▼ Less common: reduced levels of red and white blood cells and platelets, allergic reaction (symptoms include rash, itching, hives, and breathing difficulties), drug fever, swelling around the eyes, arthritis-like pain, diarrhea, coating of the tongue, headache, tingling in the arms or legs, depression, convulsions, hallucinations, ringing in the ears, dizziness, difficulty sleeping, apathy, tiredness, weakness, and nervousness. Septra may also affect your kidneys and cause you to produce less urine.

Drug Interactions

• Septra may prolong the effects of anticoagulant (blood-thinning) agents—such as warfarin—and oral antidiabetes drugs.

• The trimethoprim in Septra may reduce the effectiveness of cyclosporine and increase its toxic effect on the kidney.

• The sulfamethoxazole in Septra can increase the amount of phenytoin and methotrexate in the bloodstream, increasing the chance of side effects. Dosage reduction of phenytoin or methotrexate may be needed to adjust for the presence of Septra.

• Older adults taking a thiazide diuretic with Septra are more likely to develop reduced levels of blood platelets and an increased chance of bleeding under the skin.

• Taking Septra together with dapsone can result in increased blood levels of both drugs. Septra can interfere with the elimination of zidovudine (AZT) through the kidneys, increasing the amount of AZT in the blood.

Food Interactions

Take each dose with a full glass of water. Continue to drink plenty of fluids throughout the day to decrease the risk of kidney-stone formation.

Usual Dose

Adult: 2 regular tablets or 1 Septra DS tablet every 12 hours for 5–14 days, depending on the condition being treated.
Child (67–88 lbs.): 4 tsp. (or 2 tablets) every 12 hours.
Child (45–66 lbs.): 3 tsp. (or 1½ tablets) every 12 hours.
Child (23–44 lbs.): 2 tsp. (or 1 tablet) every 12 hours.
Child (under 22 lbs.): 1 tsp. every 12 hours.
Child (under 2 months): not recommended.

Overdosage

Small overdoses are not likely to cause harm. Larger overdoses can cause exaggerated side effects. Call your local poison control center or emergency room for more information. If you go to the hospital for treatment, ALWAYS bring the prescription bottle or container with you.

Special Information

Take Septra exactly as prescribed for the full length of the prescription. Do not stop taking it just because you are beginning to feel better. Take each dose with a full glass of water, and drink plenty of fluids all day to lower the risk of kidney-stone formation.

Call your doctor if you develop sore throat, skin rash, unusual bleeding or bruising, or any other persistent or intolerable side effect.

You may develop unusual sensitivity to bright light, particularly sunlight. If you have a history of light sensitivity or if you have sensitive skin, avoid prolonged exposure to sunlight while using Septra.

If you miss a dose of Septra, take it as soon as possible. If you take it twice a day and it is almost time for your next dose, take 1 dose as soon as you remember and another in 5 to 6 hours, then go back to your regular schedule. If you take

Septra 3 or more times a day and it is almost time for your next dose, take 1 dose as soon as you remember and another in 2 to 4 hours, then continue with your regular schedule. Never take a double dose.

Special Populations

Pregnancy/Breast-feeding
Septra may affect folic acid in the fetus throughout pregnancy and should be used with caution. It should never be taken near term because of the effects of sulfamethoxazole on the newborn, including yellowing of the skin or eyes. Talk to your doctor about Septra's risks versus its benefits if the drug is to be used during pregnancy.

Premature infants, infants with too much bilirubin in their blood, and those who are deficient in the enzyme known as G-6-PD are more likely to develop problems with Septra. Septra is not recommended for use if you are nursing because of possible effects on the newborn infant.

Seniors
Seniors are more likely to be sensitive to the effects of this drug, especially if they have liver or kidney problems. Severe skin reactions and decreased levels of blood platelets and red and white blood cells are the most common, especially when a thiazide diuretic is also being taken. Your doctor will reduce your Septra dose if you have kidney disease.

Serevent

see *Salmeterol*, page 989

Generic Name

Sertraline (SER-truh-lene)

Brand Name

Zoloft

Type of Drug

Selective serotonin reuptake inhibitor (SSRI).

Prescribed for

Depression; also prescribed for obsessive-compulsive disorder.

General Information

Sertraline and the other SSRI antidepressants—fluoxetine, fluvoxamine, and paroxetine—are chemically unrelated to the older tricyclic and tetracyclic antidepressant drugs. SSRIs work by preventing the movement of the neurohormone serotonin into nerve endings. This forces the serotonin to remain in the spaces surrounding nerve endings, where it works. Sertraline is effective in treating common symptoms of depression. It can help improve your mood and mental alertness, increase physical activity, and improve sleep patterns. Sertraline takes about 4 weeks to work and stays in the body for several weeks after you stop taking it. This fact may be important as your doctor considers when to start or stop treatment.

Significant weight loss is uncommon in people taking sertraline, although the drug may cause a small weight loss of 1 to 2 lbs.

Cautions and Warnings

Do not take sertraline if you are **allergic** to it. Allergies to non-SSRI antidepressants should not prevent you from taking sertraline, because it is chemically different from other types of antidepressants.

Serious, potentially fatal reactions may occur if sertraline and a **monoamine oxidase inhibitor (MAOI)** antidepressant are taken together (see "Drug Interactions").

Sertraline is broken down by your liver; therefore, people with severe **liver disease** should be cautious about taking this drug and should be treated at doses below normal.

People with **reduced kidney function** should take sertraline with caution.

Studies in animals receiving doses 10 to 20 times the maximum human dose revealed an increase in certain **liver tumors** and reduced **fertility**. The significance of these results for humans is not known.

A small number of **manic** or **hypomanic** patients may experience an activation of their condition while taking sertraline.

Sertraline should be used with caution by people who suffer from **seizure** disorders.

SSRIs may affect blood platelets, though their exact effect is not known. Some people have had abnormal **bleeding** while taking these drugs.

Sertraline causes low blood levels of **uric acid**, but has not caused kidney failure.

The possibility of **suicide** exists in severe depression and may be present until the condition is significantly improved. Depressed patients should only be allowed to carry small quantities of sertraline with them to limit the possibility of overdose.

Possible Side Effects

▼ Most common: dry mouth; headache; dizziness; tremors; nausea; diarrhea or loose stools; sleeplessness; tiredness; male sexual dysfunction or abnormal ejaculation, in 15% of men; female sexual dysfunction, in 1.7% of women; and feeling unwell.

▼ Common: excessive sweating, constipation, upset stomach, and agitation.

▼ Less common: heart palpitations, chest pain, nervousness, anxiety, tingling or numbness in the hands or feet, twitching, muscle spasm, confusion, rash, muscle and joint ache, stomach gas, appetite increase or decrease, menstrual disorders, sore throat, runny nose, yawning, changes in vision, ringing or buzzing in the ears, frequent urination, fever, back pain, chills, confusion, reduced skin sensation, rash, nightmares, depersonalization, weight gain, vomiting, and changes in sense of taste.

▼ Rare: urinary disorders, abnormal dreaming or thinking, swelling, weight loss, gastroenteritis, itching, acne, and painful menstruation. Other side effects affecting virtually every body system have been reported by people taking sertraline. They are too numerous to mention here but are considered infrequent or rare and affect only a small number of people. Report anything unusual to your doctor at once.

Drug Interactions

• At least 5 weeks should elapse between stopping sertraline treatment and starting an MAOI antidepressant. Two weeks should elapse between stopping an MAOI and starting sertraline. Taking these 2 drugs too close together or at the same time may cause serious, life-threatening reactions.

• Sertraline may prolong the effects of diazepam and other benzodiazepine-type drugs.

• Cimetidine increases blood levels of sertraline by about 50%.

• People taking warfarin may experience an increase in its effect if they start taking sertraline. Your doctor should re-evaluate your warfarin dosage.

• Sertraline may affect lithium blood levels.

• Sertraline may slow the rate at which tolbutamide, pre-scribed for diabetes, is released from the body. The clinical importance of this interaction is not known.

• Combining alcohol with sertraline is not recommended.

Food Interactions

Food increases the rate at which sertraline is absorbed into the blood—maximum blood concentration is reached 2½ hours sooner when it is taken with food—and may slightly increase the total amount of drug absorbed. To maintain consistent blood levels, sertraline should be taken on an empty stomach, or at least 1 hour before or 2 hours after meals.

Usual Dose

50–200 mg once a day, morning or night. Seniors, people with kidney or liver disease, and people taking several differ-ent drugs should take the lowest effective dose possible.

Overdosage

Three cases of sertraline overdose have been reported and all 3 victims recovered completely. Symptoms of overdose are tiredness, nausea, vomiting, rapid heartbeat, anxiety, dilated pupils, and changes in the heartbeat. There is no specific antidote for sertraline overdose. Overdose victims should be taken to a hospital emergency room for treatment at once. ALWAYS bring the prescription bottle or container with you.

Special Information

Sertraline may make you dizzy or drowsy. Take care when driving or performing other tasks that require alertness and concentration.

Do not drink alcoholic beverages if you are taking sertraline.

Be sure your doctor knows if you are pregnant, breast-feeding, or taking other drugs, including over-the-counter drugs, while taking sertraline. Notify your doctor if you experience any unusual side effects.

If you forget a dose of sertraline take it as soon as you remember. If it is almost time for your next dose, skip the dose you forgot and continue with your regular schedule. Do not take a double dose.

Special Populations

Pregnancy/Breast-feeding
Animal studies at ½ to 4 times the maximum human dose have shown that sertraline has some effect on the fetus. Do not take sertraline if you are or might be pregnant without first weighing its potential benefits against its risks with your doctor.

It is not known if sertraline passes into breast milk. Nursing mothers should be cautious about taking this drug.

Seniors
Seniors tend to clear sertraline more slowly from their bodies, although this does not change side-effect patterns. People with liver or kidney disease—more common among seniors—should take a lower dose. Be sure to report any unusual side effects to your doctor.

Generic Name

Simvastatin (SIM-vah-stat-in)

Brand Name

Zocor

Type of Drug

Cholesterol-lowering agent (HMG-CoA reductase inhibitor).

Prescribed for

High blood-cholesterol, LDL-cholesterol, and triglyceride levels, in conjunction with a low-cholesterol diet program. It is also prescribed to slow the progression of atherosclerosis (hardening of the arteries), reduce the risk of death in people with heart disease, and treat inherited blood-lipid problems or lipid problems associated with diabetes or kidney disease.

General Information

Simvastatin is one of several cholesterol-lowering drugs that work by inhibiting an enzyme called HMG-CoA reductase. They interfere with the natural process for manufacturing cholesterol in your body, altering that process in order to produce a harmless by-product. Studies have closely related high blood-fat levels—total cholesterol, LDL cholesterol, and triglycerides—to heart and blood-vessel disease. Drugs that reduce levels of any of these blood fats and increase HDL cholesterol—"good" cholesterol—have been assumed for several years to reduce the risk of death and heart attack. Recently, medication in this class has been proven to slow the formation of blood-vessel plaque—associated with athero-sclerosis—and reduce the risk of heart attack and death related to heart disease.

Simvastatin reduces total triglyceride, cholesterol, and LDL-cholesterol counts while increasing HDL cholesterol. A very small amount of the drug actually reaches the body's circulation. Most is broken down and eliminated by the liver; 10% to 20% of the drug is released from the body through the kidneys. A significant blood-fat-lowering response is seen after 1 to 2 weeks of treatment. Blood-fat levels are lowest within 4 to 6 weeks after taking simvastatin and remain at or close to that level as long as you continue to take the drug. The effect is known to persist for 4 to 6 weeks after you stop taking it.

Simvastatin generally does not benefit anyone under age 30, so it is not usually recommended for children. It may, under special circumstances, be prescribed for teenagers in the same dose as adults.

Cautions and Warnings

Do not take simvastatin if you are **allergic** to it or to any other HMG-CoA reductase inhibitor.

People with a history of **liver disease** and **those who drink large amounts of alcohol** should avoid drugs in this group because they may aggravate or cause liver disease. Your doctor should take a blood sample to test your liver function monthly during the first year of treatment.

Simvastatin causes **muscle aches and/or muscle weakness** in a small number of people, which may be a sign of a more serious condition.

Simvastatin may cause a mild reduction in vital **sperm count**.

At doses between 50 and more than 100 times the maximum human dose, HMG-CoA reductase inhibitors have caused central nervous system (CNS) lesions, liver tumors, and male infertility in lab animals. The importance of this information for people is not known.

Possible Side Effects

Most people who take simvastatin tolerate it quite well because the drug has fewer side effects than other drugs in this group.

▼ Common: headache.

▼ Less common: nausea, vomiting, diarrhea, abdominal pains, cramps, constipation, stomach gas, upset stomach, weakness, and upper respiratory infection.

▼ Rare: Effects can occur in virtually any body part or system. Report anything unusual to your doctor.

Drug Interactions

• The cholesterol-lowering effects of simvastatin and colestipol or cholestyramine are additive. Take simvastatin 1 hour before or 4 hours after either of these drugs.

• Simvastatin may increase the effects of warfarin or digoxin. If you take either of these drugs with simvastatin, you should be periodically checked by your doctor.

• The combination of cyclosporine, erythromycin, gemfibrozil, or niacin with simvastatin may cause severe muscle aches or degeneration and other muscle problems. These combinations should be avoided.

• Propranolol may interfere with the action of simvastatin, reducing its effectiveness.

• Itraconazole may increase simvastatin levels by 20 times. Avoid this combination by temporarily stopping simvastatin if you take itraconazole.

Food Interactions

None known. Continue your low-cholesterol diet while taking this medicine.

Usual Dose

Adult: 5–40 mg at bedtime.
Senior: 5–20 mg at bedtime.

Your daily dosage of simvastatin may be adjusted monthly, based on your doctor's assessment of how well the drug is working to reduce your blood cholesterol.

Overdosage

There are few reports of simvastatin poisoning; all victims recovered, including one person who took a 450 mg overdose. A person suspected of having taken an overdose of simvastatin should be taken to a hospital emergency room for evaluation and treatment. ALWAYS bring the prescription bottle or container with you.

Special Information

Call your doctor if you develop blurred vision or muscle aches, pain, tenderness, or weakness, especially if you are also feverish or feel sick.

Drugs in this group are always prescribed in combination with a low-fat diet. Be sure to follow your doctor's dietary instructions, since both diet and medication are necessary to treat your condition.

Simvastatin may cause unusual sensitivity to the sun. Use sunscreen and wear protective clothing while in the sun until you determine if you are affected.

Do not take more cholesterol-lowering medication than your doctor has prescribed or stop taking the medication without your doctor's knowledge.

If you forget to take a dose of simvastatin, take it as soon as you remember. If it is almost time for your next dose, skip the one you forgot and continue with your regular schedule. Do not take a double dose.

Special Populations

Pregnancy/Breast-feeding

Pregnant women and those who might be pregnant absolutely must not take simvastatin. Cholesterol is essential to the health and development of a fetus. Anything that interferes with that process will damage the developing brain and nervous system. Since hardening of the arteries is a long-term process, you should be able to stop this medication during pregnancy without developing atherosclerosis. If you become pregnant while taking simvastatin, stop taking the drug immediately and call your doctor.

Simvastatin may pass into breast milk. Women taking simvastatin should bottle-feed their infants to avoid possible interference with the baby's development.

Seniors

Seniors may be more sensitive to the effects of simvastatin and are likely to require less of the drug than do younger adults. Be sure to report any side effects to your doctor.

Brand Name

Sinemet

Generic Ingredients

Carbidopa + Levodopa Ⓖ

Other Brand Names

Sinemet CR

The information in this profile also applies to the following drug:

Generic Ingredient: Carbidopa
Lodosyn

Type of Drug

Antiparkinsonian.

Prescribed for

Parkinson's disease.

General Information

The 2 ingredients in Sinemet—levodopa and carbidopa—work together to produce a beneficial effect in those suffering from Parkinson's disease. Levodopa is the active ingredient that affects Parkinson's disease; carbidopa slows the break-down of levodopa, making more available to the brain.

This combination is so effective that your dose of levodopa may be reduced by about 75%, which results in fewer side effects and, generally, safer drug treatment. Unfortunately, Sinemet is not the ultimate in Parkinson's disease treatment. People still become resistant to the effects of levodopa, even under the improved circumstances offered by this combination.

Carbidopa is sold under the brand name Lodosyn for people who need individual doses of both carbidopa and levodopa. Most people can take one of the available strengths of Sinemet.

Cautions and Warnings

Do not take Sinemet if you are **allergic** to either of its ingredients. If you are switching from levodopa to Sinemet, you should stop taking levodopa 8 hours before your first dose of Sinemet. The sustained-release form of Sinemet has a lesser incidence of nervous-system side effects; the immediate-release version may produce such effects at even lower dosages.

Possible Side Effects

▼ Common: uncontrolled muscle movements, appetite loss, nausea, vomiting, stomach pain, dry mouth, difficulty swallowing, drooling, shaky hands, headache, dizziness, numbness, weakness, feeling faint, grinding of the teeth, confusion, sleeplessness, nightmares, hallucinations, anxiety, agitation, tiredness, feeling unwell, and euphoria (feeling high).

▼ Less common: heart palpitations; dizziness when rising quickly from a sitting or lying position; sudden extreme slowness of movement ("on-off" phenomenon); mental changes, including paranoia, psychosis, depression, and a slowdown of mental functioning; difficulty urinating; muscle twitching; eyelid spasms; lockjaw; burning sensation on the tongue; bitter taste; diarrhea; constipation; stomach gas; flushing of the skin; rash; sweating; unusual breathing; blurred or double vision; pupil dilation; hot flashes; changes in body weight; and darkening of the urine or sweat.

▼ Rare: stomach bleeding or ulcer, high blood pressure, adverse effects on blood components, blood vessel irritation, convulsions, uncontrollable eye-muscle move-

---

Possible Side Effects *(continued)*

---

ments, hiccups, feeling stimulated, body fluid retention, hair loss, vocal hoarseness, and persistent penile erection. The drug may affect blood tests for kidney and liver function; tell your doctor if you are taking it.

Drug Interactions

• Sinemet's effectiveness may be increased by taking anticholinergic drugs, such as trihexyphenidyl.

• Methyldopa, an antihypertensive drug, has the same effect on levodopa as carbidopa. It may increase the amount of levodopa available in the central nervous system and may have a slight effect on Sinemet as well.

• People taking guanethidine or a diuretic to treat high blood pressure may find they need less of either of these medications to control their pressure.

• Reserpine, benzodiazepine tranquilizers, antipsychotic medicines, phenytoin, and papaverine may interfere with the effects of Sinemet. Vitamin B_6 will interfere with levodopa but not with Sinemet.

• People taking Sinemet together with a monoamine oxidase inhibitor (MAOI) may experience a rapid increase in blood pressure. MAOIs should be stopped 2 weeks before starting on Sinemet.

• Sinemet may increase the effects of ephedrine, amphetamines, epinephrine, and isoproterenol. This interaction can result in adverse effects on the heart. This reaction may also occur with some of the antidepressants.

Food Interactions

Immediate-release Sinemet may be taken with food to reduce stomach upset. Sinemet CR, the sustained-release form of this product, should be taken on an empty stomach, because food can increase levodopa levels by 25% to 50%.

Usual Dose

Three different Sinemet strengths are available to allow for individual variation: 10/100, 25/100, and 25/250. The first number represents carbidopa content, the second the levodopa content, in mg.

Dosage must be tailored by your doctor to your individual

needs based on previous drug treatment. Dosage adjustments are made by adding or omitting ½–1 tablet per day. Maximum daily dose is 8 25/250-tablets.

Sinemet CR is started at dosages roughly equal to 10% more levodopa a day than was being taken previously. Dosage adjustments are then tailored to your specific needs.

If extra carbidopa is needed, your doctor may prescribe Lodosyn to be taken together with your Sinemet. Lodosyn is added in steps of no more than 25 mg a day until the desired effect is achieved.

Overdosage

Overdose symptoms are exaggerated side effects. Take the victim to a hospital emergency room. ALWAYS bring the prescription bottle or container with you.

Special Information

Sinemet can cause tiredness or lack of concentration: Take care while driving or operating hazardous machinery.

Call your doctor if you experience dizziness; light-headedness or fainting spells; mood or mental changes; abnormal heart rhythm or heart palpitations; difficulty urinating; persistent nausea, vomiting, or other stomach complaints; or any uncontrollable movements of the face, eyelids, mouth, tongue, neck, arms, hands, or legs. This drug may cause darkening of the urine or sweat. This effect is not harmful, but may interfere with urine tests for diabetes. Make sure all your doctors know you are taking this medication.

Take Sinemet as prescribed and call your doctor before making any adjustments in your treatment.

If you forget to take a dose of Sinemet, take it as soon as you remember. If it is within 2 hours of your next dose, skip the one you forgot and continue with your regular schedule. Do not take a double dose.

Special Populations

Pregnancy/Breast-feeding

Sinemet causes birth defects in laboratory animals, but its effect in humans is not known. Women who are pregnant or breast-feeding should use this drug only if it is absolutely necessary.

Seniors

Older adults may need smaller doses because the enzyme that breaks down levodopa, against which carbidopa pro-

tects, decreases with age, reducing the overall dosage requirement. Seniors, especially those with heart disease, are
more likely to develop abnormal heart rhythm or other
cardiac side effects of this drug.

Seniors who respond to this treatment, especially those
with osteoporosis, should resume activity gradually. Sudden
increases in activity and mobility lead to a greater risk of
broken bones than does a gradual return to physical activity.

Generic Name

Stavudine (STAV-ue-dene)

Brand Name

Zerit

Type of Drug

Antiviral.

Prescribed for

Advanced human immunodeficiency virus (HIV) infection.

General Information

Stavudine is a synthetic nucleoside-type antiviral drug that
inhibits the reproduction of the HIV virus by interfering with
viral DNA duplication. Stavudine can also interfere with DNA
in human cells and may affect the duplication of some body
cells. Stavudine is rapidly absorbed into the blood after it is
swallowed. The drug is eliminated primarily through the
kidneys; people with reduced kidney function should have
their daily dose adjusted. Stavudine is approved only for
adults with AIDS, although the drug has been studied in
children for as long as 3 years. In children who were studied,
stavudine acted similarly to the way it acts in adults.

Cautions and Warnings

Stavudine should be taken only by adults with **advanced HIV
infection** who cannot take or tolerate other AIDS treatments,
or whose disease has progressed despite treatment with
other antiviral drugs. There is no proof that stavudine prolongs lives of people with AIDS. Zidovudine (AZT) does

lengthen lives of people with AIDS and should be used as first-line treatment.

People taking stavudine or any other anti-HIV drug may continue to develop **opportunistic infections** and other complications of the disease, and should remain under the direct care of a doctor.

Peripheral neuropathy is the most common side effect of stavudine (see "Special Information"). People who have had these symptoms before are more likely to have this problem while taking stavudine.

Pancreatic inflammation occurs in 1% of people taking stavudine and has been associated with 14 deaths in people taking this drug.

Possible Side Effects

▼ Most common: peripheral neuropathy, which can produce tingling, burning, numbness, or pain in the hands, arms, feet, or legs; diarrhea; nausea; vomiting; headache; fever; chills; weakness; abdominal pain; back pain; muscle or joint ache; generalized pain; not feeling well; sleeplessness; anxiety; depression; nervousness; breathing difficulties; appetite and weight loss; rash; itching; and sweating.

▼ Common: allergic reactions; flu-like symptoms; swollen lymph glands, usually felt under the arms or in the neck; chest pain; constipation; upset stomach; and dizziness.

▼ Less common: pelvic pain, tumors, high blood pressure, swelling, flushing, stomach ulcers, confusion, migraine headache, sleepiness, tremors, nerve pain, asthma, pneumonia, skin tumors, conjunctivitis, visual disturbances, painful urination, genital pain, painful menstruation, and vaginitis.

▼ Rare: frequent urination, blood in the urine, impotence, fainting, inflammation of the pancreas, nerve pain, and peeling skin.

Food and Drug Interactions

None known.

Usual Dose

Adult: 30–40 mg every 12 hours.

Senior: Dosage reduction may be needed.
Child: not recommended.

Overdosage

Adults given 12 to 14 times the usual daily dose experienced no acute effects. Chronic overdosage, however, can produce peripheral neuropathy (see "Special Information") and liver toxicity. Call your local poison control center for more information. Overdose victims should be taken to a hospital emergency room for treatment. ALWAYS bring the prescription bottle or container with you.

Special Information

Peripheral neuropathy (symptoms include tingling, pain, or numbness in the hands, arms, legs, or feet) occurs in 15% to 20% of people who take stavudine. If the drug is stopped, symptoms may disappear, although they can actually worsen for a time after you stop taking stavudine. If the symptoms do go away, your doctor may restart stavudine treatment at a lower daily dosage.

Your stavudine dosage will be reduced if you develop symptoms of neuropathy or if you have reduced kidney function.

Stavudine does not cure AIDS. It will not prevent you from transmitting the virus to another person; you must still practice safe sex. Stavudine may not prevent some illnesses associated with AIDS from developing. The long-term effects of stavudine are not known.

It is very important to take stavudine according to your doctor's directions. If you forget a dose, take it as soon as you remember. If it is almost time for your next dose, take the dose you forgot, take the next 2 doses 8 hours apart, and then go back to your regular schedule. Do not take a double dose. Call your doctor if you skip more than 2 consecutive doses.

Special Populations

Pregnancy/Breast-feeding

Animal studies showed that stavudine passes to the fetus and causes birth defects, but there is no direct information on what happens in humans. Stavudine should be taken during pregnancy only if it is absolutely necessary.

Animal studies show that stavudine passes into breast milk, but it is not known if this occurs in humans. In any case, mothers who are HIV positive should bottle-feed their babies to avoid transmitting the virus through their milk.

Seniors
Older adults are likely to have reduced kidney function and may need to have their daily dose adjusted accordingly.

Generic Name

Sucralfate (sue-KRAL-fate)

Brand Name

Carafate

Type of Drug

Antiulcer.

Prescribed for

Short-term (less than 8-week) treatment of duodenal (intestinal) ulcer; also used for stomach ulcer, stomach irritation caused by aspirin and nonsteroidal anti-inflammatory drugs (NSAIDs), stomach bleeding, treatment of gastroesophageal reflux disease (GERD), irritation of the esophagus and mouth, throat ulcer caused by radiation and chemotherapy, and prevention of stress ulcer and stomach bleeding.

General Information

Sucralfate works within the gastrointestinal (GI) tract by exerting a soothing local effect on ulcer tissue; very little of the drug is absorbed into the bloodstream. After the drug binds to proteins in the damaged mucous tissue within the ulcer, it forms a barrier to the normal acids and enzymes of the GI tract. This barrier protects the ulcer tissue from further damage, allowing it to heal naturally. Sucralfate is not an antacid and works differently than cimetidine, omeprazole, and other antiulcer drugs, but it is as effective in treating duodenal ulcer disease as these drugs.

Cautions and Warnings

Duodenal ulcer is a chronic disease. Short-term treatments like sucralfate can completely heal an ulcer, but this does not reduce your chances of having another ulcer.

Small amounts of aluminum are absorbed while you take sucralfate. This can be a problem for people with chronic **kidney failure** and for people on dialysis.

Possible Side Effects

Side effects are rarely severe and usually minimal: Only about 5% of people who take sucralfate report them.

▼ Most common: constipation.

▼ Less common: diarrhea, nausea, upset stomach, indigestion, dry mouth, rash, itching, back pain, dizziness, and sleepiness.

Drug Interactions

• Sucralfate may decrease the effects of digoxin, ketoconazole, phenytoin, quinidine, tetracycline, warfarin, and ciprofloxacin, norfloxacin, and other quinolone antibacterials. To avoid this effect, separate doses of these drugs and sucralfate by 2 hours.

• Do not take antacids 30 minutes before or after taking sucralfate.

• Do not take aluminum-containing antacids at all while you are taking sucralfate. This combination increases aluminum absorption into the bloodstream and may lead to aluminum toxicity (symptoms include weakening of the bones and adverse effects on the brain).

Food Interactions

Take each dose on an empty stomach, at least 1 hour before or 2 hours after meals.

Usual Dose

Adult: starting dose—1 tablet 4 times a day for active ulcers. Maintenance dose—1 tablet 2 times a day.
Child: not recommended.

Overdosage

There have been no reports of sucralfate overdose. Animals given the equivalent of 5.5 g per lb. of body weight did not experience any unusual effects. The risk associated with sucralfate overdose is thought to be minimal.

Special Information

Be sure to take the full course of sucralfate treatment prescribed, which usually entails 6 to 8 weeks.

Notify your doctor if you develop constipation, diarrhea, or other GI side effects.

If you forget to take a dose of sucralfate, take it as soon as you remember. If it is almost time for your next dose, skip the one you forgot and continue with your regular schedule. Do not take a double dose.

Special Populations

Pregnancy/Breast-feeding

Sucralfate has not been found to cause birth defects. When the drug is considered crucial by your doctor, its benefits must be carefully weighed against its risks.

It is not known if sucralfate passes into breast milk. Nursing mothers should be cautious when taking sucralfate.

Seniors

Seniors may take sucralfate without special restriction. Follow your doctor's directions and report any side effects at once.

Type of Drug

Sulfa Drugs

Brand Names

Generic Ingredient: Sulfadiazine [G]
Only available in generic form.

Generic Ingredient: Sulfamethizole
Thiosulfil Forte

Generic Ingredient: Sulfamethoxazole [G]
Gantanol

Generic Ingredient: Sulfasalazine [G]
Azulfidine   Azulfidine EN-Tabs

Generic Ingredient: Sulfisoxazole [G]
Gantrisin

Generic Ingredient: Triple Sulfa (Sulfathiazole +
Sulfacetamide + Sulfabenzamide)

Dayto Sulf   Trysul
Gyne-Sulf   V.V.S.
Sultrin

Prescribed for

Infection, particularly infection of the urinary tract. Sulfasalazine may also be prescribed for rheumatoid, juvenile, and
psoriatic arthritis; ulcerative and other forms of colitis;
Crohn's disease; ankylosing spondylitis; and psoriasis.
Sulfisoxazole has also been used to prevent middle ear
infection. Triple sulfa is used only to treat vaginal infection.

General Information

Sulfa drugs have been in use for many years. Before penicillin
was discovered, they were the principal class of drug used to
fight infectious disease. They are prescribed for infections in
various parts of the body but are particularly helpful for
urinary tract infections because sulfas are concentrated in the
urine as they pass out of the body. Sulfa drugs kill bacteria
and some fungi by interfering with the metabolic processes
of these organisms. Some organisms may become resistant
to the effects of sulfa drugs. If possible, your doctor will
screen infected urine, blood, or tissue against a number of
anti-infective drugs in order to pick the one most appropriate
for your infection. Sulfas are usually included in this screening process.

Sulfasalazine is different from the other sulfa drugs in that
only about ⅓ of the drug is absorbed into the bloodstream;
the rest stays in the intestines. Because of its specific anti-
inflammatory and immune system effects, sulfasalazine is
effective against various kinds of colitis and intestinal irritation, and arthritis and other inflammatory problems.

Cautions and Warnings

Do not take a sulfa drug if you are **allergic** to any other sulfa
drug or to a drug chemically related to the sulfas including
thiazide and loop diuretics, carbonic anhydrase inhibitors,
and sulfonylurea-type oral antidiabetes drugs—which do not
include metformin. Do not use any sulfa drug if you are

allergic to PABA-containing sunscreens or local anesthetics, or if you have **porphyria**. Sulfasalazine should not be used by people with **aspirin allergy** or by **children less than 2 years old**.

Sulfa drugs can cause unusual **sensitivity to the sun or bright light**. Use sunscreens and wear protective clothing while taking any of these drugs.

Men taking sulfasalazine may have **low sperm counts** or become **infertile**. This effect reverses when the drug is stopped.

Sulfas should be taken by people with **severe kidney or liver disease** only after a doctor has evaluated their condition and need for the drug. High doses of sulfasalazine were found to cause **liver, bladder, and urinary cancers** in rats.

Deaths in people taking sulfasalazine have been related to a variety of effects on the blood, liver damage, and nervous system changes. **Call your doctor if anything unusual develops while taking a sulfa drug.**

Possible Side Effects

▼ Most common: headache, itching, rash, skin sensitivity to strong sunlight, nausea, vomiting, abdominal or stomach cramps or pain, feeling unwell, hallucination, dizziness, ringing or buzzing in the ears, and chills.

▼ Less common: blood diseases or changes in blood composition, arthritic pain, diarrhea, appetite loss, drowsiness, hearing loss, itchy eyes, fever, hair loss, and yellowing of the skin or whites of the eyes. Sulfasalazine may reduce sperm count.

Drug Interactions

• Sulfa drugs may increase the effects of sulfonylurea-type oral antidiabetes drugs, methotrexate, warfarin, and phenytoin and other hydantoin anti-seizure drugs. Dosages of these drugs may have to be reduced by your doctor.

• The amount of cyclosporine in your blood may be reduced by sulfa drugs, possibly increasing kidney toxicity.

• Sulfa drugs may increase blood levels of indomethacin, probenecid, and aspirin and other salicylates, increasing the possibility of side effects.

• When methenamine and a sulfa drug are taken together, an insoluble substance may form in acid urine. Avoid this combination.

• Erythromycin increases the effect of sulfa drugs against infections caused by *Haemophilus influenzae*, a common cause of middle-ear infections.

• The effects of folic acid and digoxin may be antagonized by sulfasalazine; dosage increases may be needed.

Food Interactions

Sulfa drugs should be taken on an empty stomach with a full glass of water. Sulfasalazine may be taken with food if it upsets your stomach.

Usual Dose

Sulfadiazine
   Adult: 2–4 g a day.
   Child (2 months and over): 34–68 mg per lb. of body weight a day.
   Child (under 2 months): not recommended, except to treat certain infections present at birth. In these cases, dosage is 11.3 mg per lb. of body weight, 4 times a day.

Sulfamethizole
   Adult: 1.5–4 g a day.
   Child (over 2 months): 13–20 mg per lb. of body weight a day, in divided doses.

Sulfamethoxazole
   Adult: 2–3 g a day.
   Child (over 2 months): 23–27 mg per lb. of body weight a day.

Sulfasalazine
   Adult: 1–4 g a day in evenly divided doses.
   Child (age 2 and over): 18–27 mg per lb. of body weight a day, in evenly divided doses.
   Child (under age 2): not recommended.

Sulfisoxazole
   Adult: 2–8 g a day, in 4–6 divided doses.
   Child (over 2 months): 34–68 mg per lb. of body weight a day, in 4–6 divided doses.

Triple Sulfa
  Adult: 1 applicator's worth twice a day for 4–6 days, then
¼–½ applicator's worth twice a day; or 1 intravaginal tablet
morning and evening for 10 days.

Overdosage

Overdose symptoms include appetite loss, nausea, vomiting
and colic, dizziness, headache, drowsiness, unconsciousness,
and high fever. Individuals suspected of having taken a sulfa
drug overdose should be taken to a hospital emergency room
at once. ALWAYS take the prescription bottle or container
with you.

Special Information

Sulfa drugs often cause unusual skin sensitivity to the sun. Be
sure to use adequate sunscreen or wear protective clothing
until you can gauge the degree to which sulfas affect you.
  Sore throat, fever, chills, unusual bleeding or bruising, rash,
and drowsiness are signs of serious blood disorders and
should be reported to your doctor at once. Also call your
doctor if you experience ringing in the ears, blood in the
urine, or breathing difficulties.
  Be sure to take the full course of medication as prescribed,
even if you notice an improvement in your symptoms.
  Sulfasalazine may turn your urine orange-yellow. This is a
harmless reaction. Skin discoloration has also occurred. This
drug may permanently stain soft contact lenses.
  Sulfa drugs may interfere with some tests for sugar in the
urine.
  If you forget to take a dose of a sulfa drug, take it as soon
as you remember. If you take the medicine twice a day and it
is almost time for your next dose, take 1 dose as soon as you
remember, another after 5 to 6 hours, and then go back to
your regular schedule. If you take the medicine 3 or more
times a day and it is almost time for your next dose, take 1
dose as soon as you remember, another after 2 to 4 hours,
and then go back to your regular schedule. Never take a
double dose.

Special Populations

Pregnancy/Breast-feeding
Sulfa drugs pass into the fetal circulation and may affect the

fetus if taken near delivery. Malformations have been seen in animals given these drugs, although not in humans. Pregnant women should not take any sulfa drug unless directed by their doctors. When a sulfa drug is considered crucial by your doctor, its potential benefits should be carefully weighed against its risks.

Small amounts of sulfa drugs pass into breast milk, but this rarely causes problems in healthy, full-term babies. The notable exceptions are premature infants, infants deficient in the enzyme known as G-6-PD, or those with hyperbilirubinemia (condition in which there is too much bilirubin in the blood). A nursing infant may also develop diarrhea, rash, and other problems. Talk to your doctor about taking a sulfa drug while nursing.

Seniors
Seniors who suffer from kidney or liver problems should take sulfa drugs with caution. Follow your doctor's directions and report any side effects at once.

Generic Name

Sulindac (SUH-lin-dak)

Brand Name
Clinoril

Type of Drug
Nonsteroidal anti-inflammatory drug (NSAID).

Prescribed for
Rheumatoid arthritis, juvenile rheumatoid arthritis, osteoarthritis, ankylosing spondylitis, tendinitis, bursitis, painful shoulder, gout, and sunburn.

General Information
Sulindac is one of 16 NSAIDs, which are used to relieve pain and inflammation. We do not know exactly how NSAIDs work, but part of their action may be due to their ability to

inhibit the body's production of a hormone called prostaglandin as well as the action of other body chemicals, including cyclooxygenase, lipoxygenase, leukotrienes, and lysosomal enzymes. NSAIDs are generally absorbed into the bloodstream quickly. Pain relief comes within 1 hour after taking the first dose of sulindac, but its anti-inflammatory effect takes several days to 1 week to become apparent and may take 3 weeks to reach maximum effect. Sulindac must be converted to its active form by the liver before it can have an effect.

Cautions and Warnings

People **allergic** to sulindac or any other NSAID and those with a history of **asthma** attacks brought on by an NSAID, iodides, or aspirin should not take sulindac.

Sulindac can cause **gastrointestinal (GI) bleeding, ulcers,** and **stomach perforation**. This can occur at any time, with or without warning, in people who take sulindac regularly. People with a history of **active GI bleeding** should be cautious about taking any NSAID. People who develop bleeding or ulcers and continue NSAID treatment should be aware of the possibility of developing more serious side effects.

Sulindac can affect **platelets and blood clotting** at high doses, and should be avoided by people with clotting problems and by those taking warfarin.

People with **heart problems** who use sulindac may experience swelling in their arms, legs, or feet.

Sulindac can cause **inflammation of the pancreas**.

People taking sulindac may experience an unusually severe **drug-sensitivity reaction**. Report any unusual symptoms to your doctor at once.

Sulindac can cause severe toxic effects to the **kidney**. Report any unusual side effects to your doctor, who may need to periodically test your kidney function.

Sulindac can make you unusually photosensitive (sensitive to the effects of the sun).

Possible Side Effects

▼ Most common: diarrhea, nausea, vomiting, constipation, stomach gas, stomach upset or irritation, and

Possible Side Effects *(continued)*

appetite loss—especially during the first few days of treatment.

▼ Less common: stomach ulcers, GI bleeding, hepatitis, gallbladder attacks, painful urination, poor kidney function, kidney inflammation, blood and protein in the urine, dizziness, fainting, nervousness, depression, hallucinations, confusion, disorientation, tingling in the hands or feet, light-headedness, itching, increased sweating, dry nose and mouth, heart palpitations, chest pain, breathing difficulties, and muscle cramps.

▼ Rare: severe allergic reactions including closing of the throat, fever, and chills; changes in liver function, jaundice (yellowing of the skin or whites of the eyes), and kidney failure. People who experience such effects must be promptly treated in a hospital emergency room or doctor's office. NSAIDs have caused severe skin reactions; if this happens to you, see your doctor immediately.

Drug Interactions

• Sulindac can increase the effects of oral anticoagulant (blood-thinning) drugs such as warfarin. You may take this combination, but your doctor might have to reduce your anticoagulant dose.

• Taking sulindac with cyclosporine may increase the toxic kidney effects of both drugs. Methotrexate toxicity may be increased in people also taking sulindac.

• Sulindac may reduce the blood-pressure-lowering effect of beta blockers and loop diuretics. Sulindac may increase the effects of thiazide diuretics.

• Sulindac may increase phenytoin blood levels, leading to increased side effects. Lithium blood levels are either decreased or unaffected in people taking sulindac.

• Sulindac blood levels may be affected by cimetidine.

• Probenecid may interfere with the elimination of sulindac from the body, increasing the chances for sulindac side effects.

• Aspirin and other salicylates may decrease the amount of sulindac in your blood. These drugs should never be combined with sulindac.

Food Interactions

Take sulindac with food or a magnesium-aluminum antacid if it upsets your stomach.

Usual Dose

200–300 mg twice a day.

Overdosage

People have died from NSAID overdoses. The most common signs of overdose are drowsiness, nausea, vomiting, diarrhea, abdominal pain, rapid breathing, rapid heartbeat, sweating, ringing or buzzing in the ears, confusion, disorientation, stupor, and coma. Take the victim to a hospital emergency room at once. ALWAYS bring the prescription bottle or container with you.

Special Information

Take each dose with a full glass of water and do not lie down for 15 to 30 minutes afterward. Do not crush or chew any sustained-release NSAID tablet. Check with your pharmacist if you are not sure whether your prescription is immediate- or sustained-release.

Sulindac can make you drowsy and/or tired: Be careful when driving or operating hazardous equipment. Do not take any over-the-counter products containing acetaminophen or aspirin while taking sulindac. Avoid alcoholic beverages.

Contact your doctor if you develop skin rash or itching, visual disturbances, weight gain, breathing difficulties, fluid retention, hallucinations, black or tarry stools, persistent headache, or any unusual or intolerable side effect.

If you forget to take a dose of sulindac, take it as soon as you remember. If you take sulindac once a day and it is within 8 hours of your next dose, skip the dose you forgot and continue with your regular schedule. If you take several doses a day and it is within 4 hours of your next dose, skip the one you forgot and continue with your schedule. Never take a double dose.

Special Populations

Pregnancy/Breast-feeding

NSAIDs may cross into fetal blood circulation. They have not been found to cause birth defects, but animal studies indicate that they may affect a developing fetal heart during the second half of pregnancy. Do not take sulindac without your doctor's approval, particularly during the last 3 months of pregnancy. When the drug is considered crucial by your doctor, its potential benefits must be carefully weighed against its risks.

It is possible that a nursing mother taking sulindac could affect her baby's heart or cardiovascular system. If you must take sulindac, bottle-feed your baby.

Seniors

Seniors may be more susceptible to sulindac side effects, especially ulcer disease.

Generic Name

Sumatriptan (sue-muh-TRIP-tan)

Brand Names

Imitrex

The information in this profile also applies to the following drug:

Generic Ingredient: Naratriptan
Amerge

Type of Drug

Antimigraine.

Prescribed for

Migraine attack.

General Information

Sumatriptan succinate may relieve the pain of a migraine headache by slowing the firing of a specific serotonin receptor (5-HT$_{1D}$). Sumatriptan does not affect other serotonin receptors.

Sumatriptan should not be used until other pain-relieving alternatives such as aspirin, acetaminophen, and other nonsteroidal anti-inflammatory drugs (NSAIDs) have failed. Sumatriptan also relieves the nausea, vomiting, and light and sound sensitivity that generally accompany migraine.

If serious, incapacitating migraine attacks occur more than twice a month, your doctor may recommend that you take medications other than sumatriptan on a regular basis to reduce the number and severity of migraine attacks. These drugs include beta-adrenergic blockers, calcium channel blockers, tricyclic antidepressants, monoamine oxidase inhibitors (MAOIs), methysergide, and, especially for children, cyproheptadine. Other measures that may reduce your need for medication are the identification and avoidance of those factors that trigger headaches, and relaxation or biofeedback techniques.

Only 15% of oral sumatriptan is absorbed but 97% is absorbed after subcutaneous (under the skin) injection. Sumatriptan starts relieving migraine pain within 10 minutes after injection; symptoms such as nausea, vomiting, and light and sound sensitivity begin to resolve within 20 minutes of injection. Sumatriptan's maximum effect occurs in about 2 hours. The drug is broken down by the liver and eliminated from the body through the kidneys. People with liver disease may absorb more medication than those with normal liver function and require lower dosages.

Cautions and Warnings

Do not use this drug if you have had an **allergic** reaction to it in the past.

Sumatriptan should not be used if you have **angina**, poor blood supply to the heart muscle, uncontrolled **high blood pressure**, or a previous **heart attack**. It may be used with caution if you have **abnormal heart rhythms, rapid heartbeat, coronary artery disease, liver or kidney disease**, or **controlled high blood pressure**, or if you have had a previous **stroke**.

Possible Side Effects

▼ Common: Most sumatriptan side effects are mild, last for less than 1 hour after injection, and resolve on their own. Some of these reported side effects, such as nausea, vomiting, dizziness, fainting, a feeling of ill health, drowsiness, and sedation, may also be caused by migraines; it is not clear how much more, if any, sumatriptan adds to the problem.

Possible Side Effects *(continued)*

▼ Less common: abnormal heart rhythms, cardiogram changes, low blood pressure, slow heart rate, fainting, angina pain, chest pressure, flushing and dizziness, painful blood vessel spasms in the legs, kidney failure, seizure, stroke, difficulty swallowing, unusual thirst, dehydration, vomiting, breathing difficulties, skin redness, rash, stomach ulcers, gallstones, swelling of the arms or legs, transient paralysis, loss of muscle control or muscle tone, muscle spasm, hysterical reactions, depression, an intoxicated feeling, painful urination, frequent urination, and kidney stones.

▼ Rare: Coronary artery spasm may be caused by sumatriptan, usually in people with a history of coronary artery disease. Numerous other rare side effects have been reported but their relationship to sumatriptan is not known.

Drug Interactions

• Taking sumatriptan with lithium, MAOIs, and selective serotonin reuptake inhibitor (SSRI) antidepressants may lead to a dangerous condition in which there is too much serotonin in the body. Do not combine these drugs with sumatriptan.

• Ergotamine and dihydroergotamine may add to the effects of sumatriptan. Allow at least 24 hours between taking either of these drugs and taking sumatriptan.

Food Interactions

None known.

Usual Dose

Tablets

Adult (age 18 and over): 1 dose of 25–100 mg as soon as migraine symptoms begin or at any time during an attack. If symptoms do not go away, you may take another dose after checking with your doctor. You should wait at least 2 hours before taking a second dose. Do not take more than 300 mg a day. People with liver disease should take the lowest possible dose.

Child: not recommended.

Nasal Spray

Adult (age 18 and over): 1–2 sprays of 5-mg spray, or 1 20-mg spray into 1 nostril only. The dose may be repeated 2 or more hours later if your headache returns. Do not take more than 40 mg a day. Higher doses may be associated with more frequent side effects.

Injection

Adult (age 18 and over): 6 mg as subcutaneous injection. The dose may be repeated if headache pain returns at the same level or is worse. Do not take more than 12 mg every 1 or 2 days. Single doses larger than 6 mg are no more effective and are not recommended.

Child: not recommended.

Overdosage

Overdose symptoms include convulsions or tremors, tiredness, swelling of the arms or legs, abnormal breathing, bluish discoloration of the skin under the fingernails or lips, weakness, dilated pupils, inflammation, hair loss, and paralysis. The injection may cause scabs and other reactions. Call your local poison control center or hospital emergency room in case of overdose. If you go for treatment, ALWAYS bring the prescription bottle or container with you.

Special Information

Notify your doctor if you have other medical conditions that could make sumatriptan problematic (see "Cautions and Warnings").

Be sure to take sumatriptan at the first sign of a migraine attack, such as pain or aura. You may get a greater effect from the drug if you lie down in a quiet, dark room.

Avoid alcohol because it may worsen your headaches.

Sumatriptan may cause dizziness or drowsiness. Take care if you have to drive or do anything else that requires concentration while taking sumatriptan.

Read and follow the enclosed instructions that come with your prescription.

Call your doctor if your usual dose does not relieve 3 consecutive headaches, if your headaches become worse or more frequent, or if you develop chest pain; difficulty swallowing; chest pressure, tightness, or heaviness; injection site reactions; nausea; vomiting; or other side effects that are particularly bothersome.

If you are taking sumatriptan tablets and develop tightness in the chest or throat; shortness of breath; heart throbbing; swollen eyelids, face, or lips; skin rash; or lumps or hives, contact your doctor. Call your doctor at once if chest pain does not go away.

Sumatriptan causes clouding of the cornea of the eye in dogs; this effect might occur in people taking sumatriptan over a long period, although it has never been reported. People taking this drug regularly should have their eyes checked periodically.

If this medication does not help you, do not continue taking it; your doctor may need to prescribe another drug to relieve your migraine attacks. If you get some relief, you may take a second dose at least 2 hours after the first one.

Special Populations

Pregnancy/Breast-feeding
Animal studies have shown possible toxic effects of sumatriptan on a fetus at varying dosage levels. This medication should be used by pregnant women only after they have fully discussed possible benefits and risks with their doctors.

Sumatriptan may pass into breast milk and should be used with caution by nursing mothers.

Seniors
Most published studies of sumatriptan exclude people over age 65, but small studies in seniors ages 65 to 86 show no special differences in how sumatriptan affects older and younger adults. Nevertheless, seniors may be more likely to experience reduced kidney and/or liver function.

Synthroid

see *Thyroid Hormone Replacements*, page 1079

Generic Name

Tacrine (TAK-rene)

Brand Name
Cognex

Type of Drug

Cholinesterase inhibitor.

Prescribed for

Alzheimer's disease.

General Information

Tacrine is the first and only pill proven to raise levels of acetylcholine in the brain. People with Alzheimer's disease (degenerative condition of the nervous system) develop a shortage of this important neurohormone early in the course of the disease. Low levels of acetylcholine are believed to account for the gradual memory loss and decline in reasoning ability associated with Alzheimer's. Tacrine is not effective in treating problems that develop later as a result of Alzheimer's effect on other brain systems.

Studies of tacrine show that 10% to 25% of people who take it will be helped by the drug. One problem is that not everyone can tolerate it; 12% of people stop taking tacrine because of side effects. Many others who stop because of side effects try again and continue on tacrine. Another problem is that the condition of a person with Alzheimer's disease continues to worsen over time. Evaluating tacrine's effectiveness in a particular Alzheimer's patient is difficult without knowing how the disease would develop in that patient in the absence of the drug. Age and gender do not affect individual response to tacrine.

Larger doses of tacrine are more effective than smaller doses. In a 30-week Alzheimer's study, people who took 120 or 160 mg of tacrine daily, continued to get better for the first 24 weeks. After that, their condition slowly worsened. People taking 80 mg improved for the first 18 weeks, then declined toward their starting point for the rest of the study. Patients who took a placebo (sugar pill) showed minor improvement for a short time, then steadily declined for the rest of the study period.

Cautions and Warnings

People who are **sensitive or allergic** to tacrine or similar drugs and those who have had **liver disease** or **jaundice** (yellow discoloration of the skin or whites of the eyes) should not take this drug.

Tacrine may slow heart rate, adversely affecting some people with heart disease.

Tacrine will increase the amount of stomach acid you make. People with a history of **ulcers** and those **taking nonsteroidal anti-inflammatory drugs (NSAIDs)** should be aware that tacrine may increase the risk of stomach or intestinal bleeding.

People with **asthma, bladder obstruction or other disease, seizure disorders,** or **liver disease** should take this drug with caution because it is likely to worsen or cause a reappearance of these conditions.

Women who take tacrine may be more likely to develop side effects, especially liver inflammation because they have about 1½ times as much of it in their blood as men.

Possible Side Effects

▼ Most common: liver inflammation, headache, nausea or vomiting, diarrhea, dizziness, chills, fever, feelings of ill health, swelling in the legs or feet, blood-pressure changes, broken bones, joint pain and/or inflammation, spasticity, fainting, convulsions, hyperactivity, tingling in the hands or feet, nervousness, sore throat, sinus inflammation, bronchitis, pneumonia, breathing difficulties, sweating, and conjunctivitis (pinkeye).

▼ Less common: facial swelling, dehydration, weight gain, a sickly appearance, swelling, heart failure, heart attack, angina pains, stroke, vein irritation, cardiac insufficiency, heart palpitation, abnormal heart rhythms, migraine headache, slow heart rate, blood clot in the lung, elevated blood cholesterol levels, inflamed tongue, swollen gums, dry mouth or throat, sores in the mouth, upset stomach, increased amount of saliva, difficulty swallowing, irritation of the esophagus or stomach, stomach or intestinal bleeding, ulcers, hemorrhoids, hiatal hernia, bloody stools, diverticulitis, loss of bowel control, impacted colon, gallbladder irritation and/or stones, increased appetite, diabetes, anemia, osteoporosis, tendinitis, bursitis, abnormal dreams, difficulty speaking, memory loss, wandering, muscle twitching, delirium, paralysis, slow muscle movements, nerve inflammation or disease, movement disorders and unusual movements usually associated with Parkinson's disease, apathy, increased sex

Possible Side Effects *(continued)*

drive, paranoid feelings, neurosis, nosebleeds, chest congestion, asthma, rapid breathing, respiratory infection, acne, hair loss, skin rash, eczema, dry skin, herpes zoster (shingles), psoriasis, skin inflammation, cysts, furuncles, cold sores, herpes infections of the skin, blood in the urine, kidney stones, kidney infections, sugar in the urine, painful urination, frequent urination, nighttime urination, puss in the urine, cystitis, urinary urgency, difficulty urinating, vaginal bleeding, genital itching, breast pain, impotence, prostate cancer, cataracts, dry eyes, eye pain, styes, double vision or other visual defects, glaucoma, earache, ringing or buzzing in the ears, deafness, middle or inner ear infections, and unusual taste sensations.

▼ Rare: heat exhaustion; blood infection; severely abnormal heart rhythms; bowel obstruction; duodenal ulcer; changes in thyroid status; reduced white-blood-cell and platelet counts; muscle disease; some sensory loss, especially the sense of touch; tortuous (twisting) movements of the tongue, eyes, or muscles of the face; loss of muscle tone; inflammation of the brain or central nervous system; Bell's palsy; suicidal thoughts; hysteria; psychosis; vomiting blood; fluid in the lungs; lung cancer; sudden choking; peeling skin; oily skin; skin ulcers; skin cancer; melanoma; tumors of the bladder or kidney; kidney failure; urinary obstruction; breast cancer; ovarian cancer; inflammation of the male reproductive tract; blindness; droopy or inflamed eyelids; and inner ear disturbances or inflammation.

Drug Interactions

• Tacrine is likely to increase the effects of some curare-type muscle relaxants used during surgery. Be sure your surgeon knows you are taking it.

• Tacrine increases theophylline concentrations twofold, requiring theophylline dose reduction to avoid side effects.

• Cimetidine increases the absorption of tacrine by 50%. Do not combine these drugs without your doctor's knowledge.

• Tacrine interferes with the effects of all anticholinergic medicines.

• Cigarette smoking speeds the rate at which tacrine is broken down by the liver.

Food Interactions

Food reduces the amount of tacrine absorbed into the blood by 30% to 40%; take it between meals whenever possible. It may be taken with food if it upsets your stomach.

Usual Dose

40–160 mg a day, divided into 4 doses.

Overdosage

Symptoms are salivation, severe nausea or vomiting, increased sweating, slow heartbeat, low blood pressure, collapse, and convulsions. Muscles may become increasingly weak; this can lead to death if the respiratory muscles are involved. Victims should be taken to an emergency room. ALWAYS bring the prescription bottle or container.

Special Information

Call your doctor if you develop very light-colored or black and tarry stools, or if you vomit material that resembles coffee grounds. Report yellowing of the skin or whites of the eyes, rash, or other side effects that are bothersome or persistent. Your doctor may have to stop your treatment if you develop liver inflammation; your doctor will need to take blood samples for at least the first 18 weeks of treatment to watch for signs of this problem.

Abruptly stopping use of tacrine or reducing the dose by 80 mg or more at a time is likely to cause behavioral changes and a noticeable worsening of Alzheimer's symptoms. Do not change doses or stop using tacrine without your doctor's knowledge.

For best results, take tacrine at the same time each day. If you forget a dose, take it as soon as possible. If it is almost time for the next dose, evenly space the remaining doses over the rest of the day and then go back to your regular schedule. Call your doctor if you miss more than one dose.

Special Populations

Pregnancy/Breast-feeding

The effect of tacrine on pregnant women is not known.

Discuss possible risks with your doctor if you are or might be pregnant.

It is not known if tacrine passes into breast milk. Nursing mothers taking tacrine should bottle-feed their infants.

Seniors
Seniors may take this drug without special restriction, except those with liver disease who are more likely to experience toxic side effects.

Generic Name

Tacrolimus (tak-ROE-lim-us)

Brand Name

Prograf

Type of Drug

Immunosuppressant.

Prescribed for

Organ transplantation.

General Information

Formerly known as FK506, tacrolimus is derived from a bacterium and is used to prevent the rejection of transplanted organs. It has been shown to prolong the survival of liver, kidney, heart, bone marrow, small bowel and pancreas, lung and trachea, skin, cornea, and limb transplants in animal studies. In people, the drug is used in liver transplants and has been studied in kidney, bone marrow, heart, pancreas, and small bowel transplants, among others.

Tacrolimus works by inhibiting the activation of T-cells—an essential element of the body's immune response—producing immune-system suppression.

Cautions and Warnings

Transplant patients who are **sensitive or allergic** to tacrolimus should be given another drug. Some people may also be allergic to chemically modified castor oil, which is used in tacrolimus injection.

Tacrolimus may cause **kidney damage**, especially when

taken in high doses. This effect has been noted in 33% to 40% of liver transplant patients. To avoid excess kidney damage, this drug should not be taken with cyclosporine, another organ transplant drug. Administration of these drugs should be separated by at least 24 hours.

Mild elevations of blood potassium were noted in 10% to 44% of liver transplant patients.

Tremors, headaches, muscle function changes, changes in mental state and sense perception, or other nervous system problems occur in about half of the people receiving a liver transplant. **Seizure** has also occurred. In some cases, these side effects may be associated with large amounts of tacrolimus in the blood.

As with other immune suppressants, people taking tacrolimus have an increased risk of developing a **lymphoma or other malignancy**. The risk increases with the degree of immune suppression and the length of time that the drug is taken. A **disorder related to Epstein-Barr virus (EBV) infection** has also been reported.

People with **kidney disease** should receive lower dosages of tacrolimus. People who experience post-transplant reduction in liver function may develop kidney damage.

Mild to moderate **high blood pressure** is a common side effect of tacrolimus and may be a sign of kidney damage. People taking this drug should measure their blood pressure regularly.

Possible Side Effects

▼ Most common: headache, tremors, sleeplessness, tingling in the hands or feet, diarrhea, nausea, constipation, appetite loss, vomiting, liver or kidney abnormalities, high blood pressure, urinary infection, infrequent urination, anemia, increased white-blood-cell counts, reduced blood-platelet counts, changes in blood-potassium level, reduced blood magnesium, high blood sugar, fluid in the lungs and other lung problems, breathing difficulties, itching, rash, abdominal pain, pain, fever, weakness, back pain, abdominal-fluid buildup, and retention of fluid.

▼ Less common: abnormal dreaming, anxiety, confusion, depression, dizziness, instability, hallucination, poor coordination, muscle spasms, psychosis, tiredness, unusual thoughts, double vision or other visual distur-

Possible Side Effects *(continued)*

bances, ringing or buzzing in the ears, upset stomach,
yellowing of the skin or whites of the eyes, difficulty
swallowing, stomach gas, stomach bleeding, fungal infection of the mouth, blood in the urine, chest pain, rapid
heartbeat, low blood pressure, diabetes, black-and-blue
marks, muscle and joint aches, leg cramps, muscle weakness, asthma, bronchitis, coughing, sore throat, pneumonia, stuffy and runny nose, sinus irritation, voice changes,
sweating, and herpes infection.

Drug Interactions

• Tacrolimus should not be taken at the same time as other
immune suppressants so as to avoid excessive suppression
of the immune system.

• Tacrolimus may cause more kidney damage when taken
with other drugs that also cause kidney problems including
aminoglycoside antibiotics, amphotericin B, cisplatin, and
cyclosporine.

• Antifungal drugs, bromocriptine, calcium channel blockers,
cimetidine, clarithromycin, danazol, diltiazem, erythromycin,
methylprednisolone, and metoclopramide may increase tacrolimus blood levels and side effects.

• Carbamazepine, phenobarbital, phenytoin, rifampin, and
rifampicin may reduce the amount of tacrolimus in the blood.

• Vaccination may be less effective during tacrolimus use.
Live vaccines such as those for measles, mumps, rubella, oral
polio, BCG, yellow fever, and TY 21 typhoid should be
avoided.

Food Interactions

Food interferes with the absorption of tacrolimus by the
blood. Take this drug either 1 hour before or 2 hours after
meals.

Usual Dose

Adult and Child: 0.075–0.15 mg per lb. a day divided into 2
doses. Children may require higher dosages than do adults.
Dosing is usually started at the high end of the recommended
dosage and then reduced to the lowest effective level.

Overdosage

Tacrolimus overdose may be expected to produce severe side

effects. Overdose victims should be taken to a hospital emergency room for treatment. ALWAYS bring the prescription bottle or container with you.

Special Information

It is extremely important for you to take this drug exactly as prescribed. If you forget a dose of tacrolimus, take it as soon as you remember. If it is almost time for your next dose, skip the forgotten dose and continue with your regular schedule. Do not take a double dose. Call your doctor if you forget 2 or more doses in a row.

People taking tacrolimus require regular testing to monitor their progress.

Call your doctor at the first sign of fever; sore throat; tiredness; weakness; nervousness; unusual bleeding or bruising; tender or swollen gums; convulsions; irregular heartbeat; confusion; numbness or tingling of your hands, feet, or lips; breathing difficulties; severe stomach pain with nausea; or blood in the urine. Other side effects are less serious but should be brought to your doctor's attention, particularly if they are unusually bothersome or persistent.

It is important to maintain good dental hygiene while taking tacrolimus and to use extra care when using your toothbrush or dental floss because the drug may make you more susceptible to dental infection. Tacrolimus suppresses the normal body systems that fight infection. See your dentist regularly while taking this drug.

Tacrolimus should be continued as long as prescribed by your doctor. Do not stop taking it because of side effects or other problems. If you cannot tolerate the oral form, this drug may be given by injection, though the oral capsules are preferable.

Special Populations

Pregnancy/Breast-feeding

In animal studies using half the human dosage, tacrolimus was lethal to embryos and affected the ability of females to become pregnant. Malformations were seen at higher dosages. The drug passes into the circulation of the fetus and should be used during pregnancy only if absolutely necessary. Babies born to mothers taking this drug have had high blood potassium and poor kidney function.

Tacrolimus passes into breast milk. Nursing mothers who must take tacrolimus should bottle-feed their infants.

Seniors

Seniors may take tacrolimus, but their dosage may have to be reduced to accommodate normal loss of kidney function.

Generic Name

Tamoxifen Citrate (tuh-MOX-ih-fen SYE-trate)

Brand Name

Nolvadex

The information in this profile also applies to the following drug:

Generic Ingredient: Toremifene Citrate
Fareston

Type of Drug

Anti-estrogen.

Prescribed for

Breast cancer and painful breasts in women; swollen or painful breasts and breast cancer in men; pancreatic, endometrial, and liver cell cancer.

General Information

Tamoxifen is effective against estrogen-positive breast cancer in women. It works by competing with the sites in tissues to which estrogenic hormones attach. Once tamoxifen binds to an estrogen receptor, it acts in the same way that estrogen would and prevents the cancer cell from dividing. When used together with chemotherapy after mastectomy surgery, tamoxifen is effective in delaying the recurrence of surgically curable cancers in postmenopausal women and women over age 50. It is used to treat metastatic breast cancer and to prevent breast cancer in high-risk women with no current signs of the disease. Up to 60% of women whose breast cancer has spread to other parts of their bodies may benefit from taking tamoxifen. Another medicine, anastrozole can be given to postmenopausal women with advanced breast cancer who do not respond to tamoxifen.

Cautions and Warnings

Visual difficulties have occurred in patients taking tamoxifen for 1 year or more in doses at least 4 times above the maximum recommended dosage. A few cases of **decreased visual clarity** and other vision problems have been reported at normal doses.

People taking tamoxifen have experienced **liver inflammation** and, rarely, more serious liver abnormalities.

Very high doses of this drug (15 mg per lb. of body weight) may cause liver cancer.

Possible Side Effects

Tamoxifen side effects are generally mild. Severe reactions can sometimes be controlled by lowering dosage.

▼ Most common: hot flashes, weight changes, fluid retention, vaginal discharge, menstrual changes, and nausea. Increased bone and tumor pain sometimes occur shortly after starting tamoxifen. These may be a sign of a good response to the drug and usually decline rapidly.

▼ Less common: vomiting, vaginal bleeding, skin changes, and kidney problems.

▼ Rare: high blood-calcium levels, swelling of the arms or legs, changes in sense of taste, vaginal itching, depression, dizziness, light-headedness, headache, visual difficulties, and reduced white-blood-cell count or platelet count. Ovarian cysts have occurred in premenopausal women with advanced breast cancer who took tamoxifen. Increased tumor pain and incidence of local disease sometimes follow a good response with tamoxifen.

Drug Interactions

• The effects of warfarin and other anticoagulant (blood-thinning) drugs may be increased by tamoxifen. Tamoxifen may increase blood-calcium levels.

• Bromocriptine may increase the amount of tamoxifen in the bloodstream.

Food Interactions

Tamoxifen may be taken with food or milk if it upsets your stomach.

Usual Dose

Tamoxifen: 10–20 mg in the morning and evening.

Toremifene: 60 mg once a day.

Overdosage

Overdose may lead to breathing difficulties or convulsions. Other symptoms are tremors, overactive reflexes, dizziness, and unsteadiness. Overdose victims should be taken to a hospital emergency room for treatment. ALWAYS bring the prescription bottle or container.

Special Information

Take this medication according to your doctor's directions. Inform your doctor if you become very weak or sleepy or if you experience confusion, pain, swelling of the legs, breathing difficulties, blurred vision, bone pain, hot flashes, nausea or vomiting, weight gain, irregular periods, dizziness, headache, or appetite loss while taking this drug. Call your doctor if you vomit shortly after taking a dose of tamoxifen. Your doctor may tell you to take another dose immediately or wait until the next dose.

Women taking tamoxifen should use a condom, diaphragm, or other non-hormonal contraceptive during sexual intercourse until treatment is complete.

If you forget to take a dose of tamoxifen, call your doctor. If you cannot reach your doctor, skip the forgotten dose and continue your regular dosing schedule. Do not take a double dose.

Special Populations

Pregnancy/Breast-feeding

The anti-estrogen effects of tamoxifen can harm a fetus. Although there are no studies of its effects in pregnant women, tamoxifen should be avoided by women who are pregnant. Women taking tamoxifen should use a condom, diaphragm, or other non-hormonal contraceptive during sexual intercourse.

It is not known if tamoxifen passes into breast milk. Nursing mothers taking this drug should bottle-feed their babies.

Seniors

Seniors may take tamoxifen without special restriction.

Generic Name

Tamsulosin (tam-SUE-loe-sin)

Brand Name

Flomax

Type of Drug

Alpha blocker.

Prescribed for

Benign prostatic hyperplasia (BPH).

General Information

Tamsulosin hydrochloride and similar drugs block nerve endings known as alpha$_1$ receptors. In BPH, tamsulosin works by relaxing smooth muscles in the prostate and neck of the bladder. This effect is produced by blocking alpha$_1$ receptors in the affected muscles. Despite the fact that tamsulosin alleviates the urinary symptoms of BPH, the drug's long-term effect on complications of BPH or the need for urinary surgery is not known. Age and race have no effect on response. Symptoms of BPH and prostate cancer may be very similar. Your doctor should be sure to differentiate between them because treatments for each are very different. Alpha blockers are broken down in the liver or pass out of the body through the feces.

Cautions and Warnings

Tamsulosin may cause **dizziness** and **fainting**, especially after the first few doses. This is known as the first-dose effect and may be minimized by limiting the first dose to 1 mg at bedtime. The first-dose effect occurs in about 1% of people taking an alpha blocker and may recur if the drug is stopped for a few days and then restarted.

People who are **allergic or sensitive** to any alpha blocker should avoid the others because of the risk that they will react to them as well.

Tamsulosin, like other alpha blockers, may slightly reduce **cholesterol** levels and increase the high density lipoprotein (HDL)/low density lipoprotein (LDL) ratio, a positive step for people with blood-cholesterol problems. People with high blood-cholesterol levels should discuss this situation with their doctors.

Red- and white-blood-cell counts may be slightly reduced in people taking other alpha blockers. This effect should be monitored in people taking tamsulosin.

Possible Side Effects

▼ Most common: dizziness, weakness, and headache.

▼ Less common: low blood pressure; rapid heartbeat; abnormal heart rhythms; chest pain; flushing in the face, arms, or legs; fainting; vomiting; dry mouth; diarrhea; constipation; abdominal pain or discomfort; stomach gas; breathing difficulties; stuffy nose; sinus inflammation; cold or flu-like symptoms; cough; bronchitis; worsening of asthma; nosebleed; sore throat; runny nose; shoulder, neck, or back pain; pain in the arms or legs; joint pain; arthritis; muscle pain; blurred vision or other visual disturbances; conjunctivitis (pinkeye); eye pain; nervousness; tingling in the hands or feet; tiredness; anxiety; difficulty sleeping; frequent urination; urinary infection; itching; rash; sweating; swelling of the face, arms, or legs; and fever.

▼ Rare: depression, reduced sex drive or abnormal sexual function, fluid retention, and weight gain.

Drug Interactions

• Tamsulosin may interact with beta-blocking drugs to produce a higher rate of dizziness or fainting after taking the first dose of tamsulosin.

• The blood-pressure-lowering effect of tamsulosin may be reduced by indomethacin.

• When taken with blood-pressure-lowering drugs, tamsulosin produces severe reduction of blood pressure.

• The blood-pressure-lowering effect of clonidine may be reduced by tamsulosin.

• This drug does not affect the results of the prostate-specific antigen (PSA) test, often used to monitor the progress of BPH.

Food Interactions

None known.

Usual Dose

Starting dosage—0.4 mg a half hour after the same meal each day. The dosage may be increased by 0.8 mg a day if there has been no response after 2 weeks.

Overdosage

Tamsulosin overdose may produce severe side effects. Overdose victims should be taken to a hospital emergency room at once. ALWAYS bring the prescription bottle or container.

Special Information

Take tamsulosin exactly as prescribed and do not stop taking it unless directed to do so by your doctor. Avoid over-the-counter drugs that contain stimulants because they may increase your blood pressure. Your pharmacist will be able to tell you what you may and may not take.

Tamsulosin may cause dizziness, headache, and drowsiness, especially 2 to 6 hours after you take your first dose, although these effects may persist after the first few doses.

Call your doctor if you develop severe dizziness, heart palpitations, or other bothersome or persistent side effects.

Wait 12 to 24 hours after taking the first dose before driving or doing anything that requires a high level of concentration. You should take it at bedtime to minimize this problem.

If you forget to take a dose of tamsulosin, take it as soon as you remember. If it is almost time for your next dose, skip the forgotten dose and continue with your regular schedule. Taking your medication at the same time each day will help you to remember each dose. If you forget your medication for several days in a row, you will have to begin again at the lower dosage of 0.4 mg a day regardless of the dosage you were taking before.

Special Populations

Pregnancy/Breast-feeding

The effect of tamsulosin in pregnant women is not known. When this drug is considered crucial by your doctor, its potential benefits must be carefully weighed against its risks.

It is not known if tamsulosin passes into breast milk. Nursing mothers who must take this medication should bottle-feed their infants.

Seniors

Seniors may be more sensitive to the actions and side effects of tamsulosin. Report any unusual side effects to your doctor.

Generic Name

Tazarotene (tuh-ZAR-oe-tene)

Brand Name

Tazorac

Type of Drug

Antiacne.

Prescribed for

Mild to moderate acne, and psoriasis.

General Information

Tazarotene is converted to its active form after it is applied to the skin. A retinoid related to vitamin A, tazarotene is in the same family as retinoic acid—the active ingredient in Retin-A antiacne products. Tazarotene remains in or on the skin; very little of it reaches the bloodstream.

Cautions and Warnings

Tazarotene causes **birth defects** in lab animals. Though several women have used this drug and had healthy babies, the exact effect of tazarotene on a fetus is not known. Since there is a possibility that a pregnant woman, especially one who uses tazarotene over as much as 20% of her body to treat psoriasis, might be exposed to unusually large amounts of the drug, it is recommended that women who are or might be pregnant avoid tazarotene.

Tazarotene may cause a temporary **burning** or **stinging** sensation. It may cause severe burning if applied to eczema. Other skin medications and makeup can make the skin very dry and should be avoided while you are using tazarotene. It may also be advisable to "rest" your skin between using other drugs or makeup and starting tazarotene.

Tazarotene can cause **rash, allergy,** or a severe **toxic reaction,** especially if used together with another drug that sensitizes the skin such as a tetracycline antibiotic, a fluoroquinolone, or a phenothiazine tranquilizer.

Possible Side Effects

▼ Most common: peeling skin, a burning or stinging sensation, dry skin, redness, and itching.

▼ Common: irritation, skin pain, cracking, swelling, and skin discoloration.

Drug Interactions

None known.

Usual Dose

Adult: Gently clean your face and apply a thin layer of tazarotene to the affected area every evening.

Overdosage

Applying excessive amounts of tazarotene to your skin can cause redness, peeling skin, or other discomfort. Accidental ingestion of tazarotene may cause symptoms similar to vitamin A overdose. Call your local poison control center for information about what to do in the case of tazarotene ingestion.

Special Information

If skin irritation, redness, itching, or peeling is excessive, stop using tazarotene until your skin is completely healed. Extreme wind or cold may worsen skin irritation.

Special Populations

Pregnancy/Breast-feeding
Women who are or might be pregnant should not use this drug.

It is not known if tazarotene passes into breast milk. Nursing mothers should be aware when using this drug that some may be passed on to their babies.

Seniors
Seniors may use this drug without special restriction.

Tegretol

---

*see **Carbamazepine**, page 153*

Generic Name

Terazosin (ter-AY-zoe-sin)

Brand Name

Hytrin

Type of Drug

Alpha blocker.

Prescribed for

High blood pressure and benign prostatic hyperplasia (BPH).

General Information

Terazosin lowers blood pressure by dilating (widening) blood vessels and reducing pressure within them. Terazosin and similar drugs block nerve endings known as alpha$_1$ receptors. Other blood-pressure-lowering drugs block beta receptors, interfere with the movement of calcium in blood-vessel muscle cells, affect salt and electrolyte (body-fluid) balance, or interfere with the process for manufacturing norepinephrine. The maximum blood-pressure-lowering effect of terazosin is seen between 2 and 6 hours after taking a single dose. Terazosin's effect lasts for 24 hours.

In BPH, terazosin works by relaxing smooth muscles in the prostate and neck of the bladder. This effect is produced by blockage of alpha$_1$ receptors in the affected muscles. Despite the fact that terazosin alleviates the urinary symptoms of BPH, the drug's long-term effect on complications of BPH or the need for urinary surgery is not known. Age and race have no effect on response. Alpha blockers are broken down in the liver or pass out of the body through the feces. About 40% of terazosin passes out of the body via the kidneys.

Cautions and Warnings

Terazosin may cause **dizziness** and **fainting**, especially after the first few doses. This is known as the first-dose effect. This effect may be minimized by limiting the first dose to 1 mg at bedtime. The first-dose effect occurs in about 1% of people taking an alpha blocker and may recur if the drug is stopped for a few days and then restarted.

People who are **allergic or sensitive** to any alpha blocker should avoid the others because of the risk that they will react to them as well.

Terazosin may slightly reduce **cholesterol** levels and increase the high density lipoprotein (HDL)/low density lipoprotein (LDL) ratio, a positive step for people with a blood-cholesterol problems. People with high blood-cholesterol levels should discuss this situation with their doctors.

Red- and white-blood-cell counts may be slightly reduced in people taking terazosin.

People taking terazosin may experience a weight gain of about 2 lbs.

Possible Side Effects

▼ Most common: dizziness, weakness, and headache.

▼ Less common: low blood pressure; rapid heartbeat; abnormal heart rhythms; chest pain; flushing in the face, arms, or legs; fainting; vomiting; dry mouth; diarrhea; constipation; abdominal pain or discomfort; stomach gas; breathing difficulties; stuffy nose; sinus inflammation; cold or flu-like symptoms; cough; bronchitis; worsening of asthma; nosebleed; sore throat; runny nose; shoulder, neck, or back pain; pain in the arms or legs; joint pain; arthritis; muscle pain; blurred vision or other visual disturbances; conjunctivitis ("pinkeye"); eye pain; nervousness; tingling in the hands or feet; tiredness; anxiety; difficulty sleeping; frequent urination; urinary infection; itching; rash; sweating; swelling of the face, arms, or legs; and fever.

▼ Rare: depression, reduced sex drive or abnormal sexual function, fluid retention, and weight gain.

Drug Interactions

• Terazosin may interact with beta-blocking drugs to produce a higher rate of dizziness or fainting after taking the first dose of terazosin.

• The blood-pressure-lowering effect of terazosin may be reduced by indomethacin.

• When taken with other blood-pressure-lowering drugs, terazosin produces severe reduction of blood pressure.

• The blood-pressure-lowering effect of clonidine may be reduced by terazosin.

• This drug does not affect the results of the prostate-specific antigen (PSA) test, often used to monitor the progress of BPH.

Food Interactions

None known.

Usual Dose

Starting dosage—1 mg at bedtime. The dosage may be increased in increments of 1–5 mg to a total of 20–40 mg a day. Terazosin may be taken once or twice a day. Dosages of 10 mg a day are generally needed to control the symptoms of BPH.

Overdosage

Terazosin overdose may produce drowsiness, poor reflexes, and very low blood pressure. Overdose victims should be taken to a hospital emergency room at once. ALWAYS bring the prescription bottle or container.

Special Information

Take terazosin exactly as prescribed and do not stop taking it unless directed to do so by your doctor. Avoid over-the-counter drugs that contain stimulants because they may increase your blood pressure. Your pharmacist will be able to tell you what you may and may not take.

Terazosin may cause dizziness, headache, and drowsiness, especially 2 to 6 hours after you take your first dose, although these effects may persist after the first few doses.

Call your doctor if you develop severe dizziness, heart palpitations, or other bothersome or persistent side effects.

Wait 12 to 24 hours after taking the first dose before driving or doing anything that requires a high level of concentration. You should take it at bedtime to minimize this problem.

If you forget to take a dose of terazosin and you take it once a day, take it as soon as you remember. If you take it twice a day and it is almost time for your next dose, skip the forgotten dose and continue with your regular schedule. Never take a double dose. Taking your medication at the same time every day will help you to remember each dose.

Special Populations

Pregnancy/Breast-feeding

Large doses of terazosin in animals damage the fetus but its effect on pregnant women is not known. When this drug is considered crucial by your doctor, its potential benefits must be carefully weighed against its risks.

It is not known if terazosin passes into breast milk. Nursing mothers who must take this medication should bottle-feed their infants.

Seniors

Seniors may be more sensitive to the action and side effects of terazosin. Report any unusual side effects to your doctor.

Generic Name

Terbinafine (ter-BIN-uh-fene)

Brand Name

Lamisil

Type of Drug

Antifungal.

Prescribed for

Fungal infections of the skin, fingernails, or toenails.

General Information

Terbinafine hydrochloride is a general-purpose antifungal product. It can cure common athlete's foot, jock itch, and ringworm due to a variety of different fungi faster than other medicines of this type. It is also effective against *Candida* and other fungal infections of the skin. Terbinafine is unique because it accumulates in the skin after application and continues to kill fungus organisms even after you stop using it. Most other antifungals do not kill the fungus; they only stop it from growing. Because of its strength, terbinafine may be prescribed for fungal infections of the skin that do not respond to over-the-counter products.

Cautions and Warnings

Do not take this product if you are **allergic** to terbinafine or to any other ingredient in the product. Kidney or liver disease can increase the amount of terbinafine in your blood by 50%.

Terbinafine cream is only meant to be applied to the skin. Do not put it into your eyes, or use for a vaginal infection. Do not swallow terbinafine cream. Only the capsules are meant for oral use.

Laboratory animals fed almost 400 times the daily human dose of terbinafine for 2 years developed tumors. Terbinafine should be used only for specific fungal infections and only as prescribed by your doctor. Rarely, people taking terbinafine have experienced severe eyesight changes or a severe drop in white-blood-cell count, leading to serious infection and fever. Call your doctor if anything unusual develops.

Possible Side Effects

Cream
▼ Most common: itching and irritation of the skin immediately after application.
▼ Less common: burning, irritation, and dryness of the skin.

Tablets
▼ Most common: headache.
▼ Common: diarrhea and rash.
▼ Less common: upset stomach, abdominal pain, nausea, stomach gas, itching, liver irritation, taste changes, and temporary eyesight changes.
▼ Rare: severe reactions of liver or skin, low white-blood-cell count, and allergic reactions.

Drug Interactions

• Cimetidine and terfenadine increase the amount of terbinafine in the blood.
• Rifampin doubles the rate at which terbinafine is released through the kidney. Do not mix these medications.
• Terbinfine increases the rate at which cyclosporine is released from the body, possibly reducing its effect.
• Terbinafine may increase the effect of caffeine on your body.

Food Interactions

Up to 20% more terbinafine may be absorbed when taken with food. Take this medication 1 hour before or 2 hours after eating.

Usual Dose

Cream: Apply to affected areas morning and night for 1–4 weeks. Use exactly as prescribed.

Tablets: 250 mg a day for 6 or 12 weeks, depending on condition being treated.

Overdosage

Terbinafine overdose may lead to tiredness, poor muscle coordination, breathing difficulties, and bulging of the eyes. Overdose victims should be taken to a hospital emergency room. ALWAYS bring the prescription bottle or container with you.

Special Information

Do not put terbinafine cream in contact with your eyes, nose, mouth, or any other mucous membrane tissues.

Do not stop using terbinafine before your prescription is complete, even if your rash clears up. The full prescription may be necessary to eliminate the offending fungus.

Do not cover the cream with plastic wrap or anything else that restricts ventilation unless so instructed by your doctor.

Call your doctor if your skin becomes red, burns, itches, blisters, swells, or if oozing develops.

If you forget a dose, take it as soon as you remember. If it is almost time for your next dose, skip the dose you forgot and continue with your regular schedule.

Special Populations

Pregnancy/Breast-feeding

There is no information on the effect of terbinafine on the fetus. Women who are or might be pregnant should not use terbinafine.

Terbinafine passes into breast milk. Nursing mothers should not use terbinafine.

Seniors

Seniors may use terbinafine without special restriction.

Generic Name

Terbutaline (ter-BUE-tuh-lene)

Brand Names

Brethaire   Bricanyl
Brethine

Type of Drug

Bronchodilator.

Prescribed for

Asthma, bronchospasm, and premature labor.

General Information

Terbutaline sulfate is similar to other bronchodilator drugs, such as metaproterenol and isoetharine, but it has a weaker effect on nerve receptors in the heart and blood vessels. For this reason, it is somewhat safer for people with heart conditions.

Terbutaline tablets begin to work within 30 minutes and continue working for 4 to 8 hours. Terbutaline inhalation begins working in 5 to 30 minutes and continues for 3 to 6 hours. Terbutaline injection starts working in 5 to 15 minutes and lasts for 1½ to 4 hours.

Cautions and Warnings

Terbutaline should be used with caution by people with a history of **angina pectoris** (condition characterized by brief attacks of chest pain), **heart disease, high blood pressure, stroke, seizure, thyroid disease, prostate disease,** or **glaucoma.**

Using excessive amounts of terbutaline can lead to increased difficulty breathing rather than relief. In the most extreme cases, people have had heart attacks after using excessive amounts of inhalant.

Animal studies with terbutaline have revealed a significant increase in certain kinds of tumors.

Possible Side Effects

Terbutaline's side effects are similar to those of other bronchodilators, except that its effects on the heart and blood vessels are not as pronounced.

▼ Most common: heart palpitations, abnormal heart rhythm, tremors, dizziness and fainting, shakiness, nervousness, tension, drowsiness, headache, nausea and vomiting, and heartburn or upset stomach.

▼ Less common: rapid heartbeat, chest pain and discomfort, angina, weakness, sleeplessness, wheezing, bron-

---

Possible Side Effects *(continued)*

chial spasms and difficulty breathing, dry throat, sore or irritated throat, flushing, sweating, and changes in senses of smell and taste.

Drug Interactions

• Terbutaline's effects may be increased by monoamine oxidase inhibitors (MAOIs), tricyclic antidepressants, thyroid drugs, other bronchodilator drugs, and some antihistamines.

• The chances of cardiac toxicity may be increased in people taking both terbutaline and theophylline.

• Terbutaline is antagonized by beta-blocking drugs such as propranolol.

• Terbutaline may antagonize the effects of blood-pressure-lowering drugs, especially reserpine, methyldopa, and guanethidine.

Food Interactions

Terbutaline tablets are more effective taken on an empty stomach—1 hour before or 2 hours after meals—but can be taken with food if they upset your stomach. Do not inhale terbutaline if you have food or anything else in your mouth.

Usual Dose

Inhaler

Adult and Child (age 12 and over): 1 or 2 puffs every 4–6 hours. Each puff delivers 0.2 mg of terbutaline.

Tablets

Adult and Child (age 15 and over): 2.5–5 mg every 6 hours, 3 times a day. Do not take more than 15 mg a day.

Child (age 12–14): 2.5 mg 3 times a day. Do not take more than 7.5 mg a day.

Child (under age 12): not recommended.

Overdosage

Overdose of terbutaline inhalation usually results in exaggerated side effects, including heart pains and high blood pressure, although blood pressure may drop to a low level after a short period of elevation. People who inhale too much terbutaline should see a doctor, who may prescribe a beta-blocking drug such as metoprolol or atenolol to counteract the overdose effect.

Overdose of terbutaline tablets is more likely to trigger changes in heart rate, palpitations, unusual heart rhythms, heart pains, high blood pressure, fever, chills, cold sweats, nausea, vomiting, and dilation of the pupils. Convulsions, sleeplessness, anxiety, and tremors may also develop, and the victim may collapse.

If the overdose was taken within the past 30 minutes, give the victim ipecac syrup—available at any pharmacy—to induce vomiting and to remove any remaining medication from the stomach. DO NOT GIVE IPECAC SYRUP IF THE VICTIM IS UNCONSCIOUS OR CONVULSING. If symptoms have already begun to develop, the victim should be taken to a hospital emergency room. ALWAYS bring the prescription bottle or container with you.

Special Information

If you are inhaling terbutaline, be sure to follow the inhalation instructions that come with the product. The drug should be inhaled during the second half of your inward breath, since this will allow it to reach deeper into your lungs. Wait at least 1 minute between puffs if you use more than 1 puff per dose.

Do not take more terbutaline than your doctor prescribes. Taking more than you need could actually worsen your symptoms. If your condition worsens rather than improves after taking terbutaline, stop taking it and call your doctor.

Call your doctor immediately if you develop chest pains, palpitations, rapid heartbeat, muscle tremors, dizziness, headache, facial flushing, or urinary difficulty, or if you continue to experience difficulty in breathing after using the medication.

If you forget a dose of terbutaline, take it as soon as you remember. If it is almost time for your next dose, skip the one you forgot and return to your regular schedule. Do not take a double dose.

Special Populations

Pregnancy/Breast-feeding

When used during childbirth, terbutaline can slow or delay natural labor. Terbutaline should not be taken after the first 3 months of pregnancy: It can cause rapid heartbeat and high blood sugar in the mother, and rapid heartbeat and low blood sugar in the fetus.

It is not known if terbutaline causes birth defects in humans, but it has caused defects in pregnant animals. When your doctor considers this drug crucial, its potential benefits must be carefully weighed against its risks.

Terbutaline passes into breast milk. Nursing mothers who are taking terbutaline must observe their infants for side effects. You may want to consider bottle-feeding your baby.

Seniors

Seniors are more sensitive to the effects of terbutaline. Follow your doctor's directions closely and report any side effects at once.

Generic Name

Terconazole (ter-KON-uh-zole)

Brand Names

Terazol 3   Terazol 7

Type of Drug

Antifungal.

Prescribed for

Fungal infections of the vagina.

General Information

Terconazole is available as a vaginal cream and as vaginal suppositories. It may also be applied to the skin to treat common fungal infections. The exact mechanism by which terconazole exerts its effect is not known.

Cautions and Warnings

Do not use terconazole if you are **allergic** to it. Proper diagnosis is essential for effective treatment. Do not use this product without first consulting your doctor.

Possible Side Effects

▼ Most common: headache, which affects 1 in 4 women who use it.

Possible Side Effects *(continued)*

▼ Rare: painful menstruation, genital pain, body pain, abdominal pain, fever, chills, vaginal burning or irritation, and itching. Application of terconazole cream to the skin can cause unusual sensitivity to the sun.

Food and Drug Interactions
None known.

Usual Dose
Vaginal Suppositories or Cream: 1 applicator's worth or 1 suppository into the vagina at bedtime for 3 or 7 days, depending on formulation.

Topical: Apply to affected areas of skin twice a day for up to 1 month.

Overdosage
Terconazole overdose may cause irritation or, if swallowed, upset stomach. Call your local poison control center or hospital emergency room for more information.

Special Information
When using the vaginal cream, insert the whole applicatorful of cream high into the vagina. Be sure to complete the full course of treatment prescribed. Call your doctor if you develop burning or itching.

Refrain from sexual intercourse or use a condom to avoid reinfection while using this product. Using sanitary napkins may keep terconazole from staining your clothing.

If you forget to take a dose of terconazole, take it as soon as you remember. If it is almost time for your next dose, skip the dose you forgot and continue with your regular schedule. Do not take a double dose.

Special Populations
Pregnancy/Breast-feeding
Pregnant women should avoid using the vaginal cream during the first 3 months of pregnancy; during the last 6 months, it should be used only if absolutely necessary.

Terconazole may cause problems in breast-fed infants. Women who must use it should bottle-feed their babies.

Seniors
Seniors may take this medication without special restriction. Follow your doctor's directions and report any side effects at once.

Generic Name

Testosterone (tes-TOS-ter-one)

Brand Names

Androderm Transdermal
  System

Testoderm Transdermal
  System

The information in this profile also applies to the following drugs:

Generic Ingredient: Methyltestosterone

Android-10

Android-25

Oreton Methyl

Testred

Virilon

Type of Drug

Hormone replacement.

Prescribed for

Male impotence due to hormone deficiency. Testosterone replacement in men who have lost their testicle function or those who have low blood levels of testosterone. Androgen may be prescribed for boys before they reach puberty to maintain secondary sex characteristics if testosterone is lacking or if puberty is delayed. In women, testosterone may be used to treat metastatic cancer (cancer that has spread from one part of the body to another) and breast enlargement or pain in women who have just given birth.

General Information

Testosterone is the principal androgen (male hormone). In men, testosterone is produced in specific cells in the testicle. Women make small amounts of testosterone in their ovaries and in the adrenal gland, located near the kidney. Testosterone is responsible for the normal growth and development of male sex organs and secondary sex characteristics. These include the prostate, penis, and scrotum; beard, pubic, chest, and underarm hair; vocal cord thickening, which lowers the voice; and body muscle and fat distribution. Androgens are responsible for the adolescent growth spurt. A man using a scrotal testosterone patch may transfer some hormone to his sexual partner, which may result in unwanted changes in the partner's secondary sex characteristics.

Taking testosterone from an outside source causes natural body feedback systems to reduce any remaining natural testosterone production.

Weekly testosterone injection of 200 mg, for up to 1 year, have been studied as a reversible male contraceptive.

Testosterone must be used with caution in children. They should be treated only by specialists who are experienced with testosterone and understand its effects on children's bone development.

Cautions and Warnings

The following people should avoid taking testosterone: **pregnant women**, **men with breast or prostate cancer**, those who are **allergic** to it, and people with **heart or kidney disease**, who may respond to the drug by retaining fluid.

Some athletes have taken testosterone in order to improve performance, but such use is unsafe and ineffective. Male hormones may cause very high blood calcium levels in women with breast cancer and in people who are immobilized; these groups should avoid taking testosterone. Continuous use of high doses of male hormones may cause life-threatening **liver problems**. Taking male hormones for an extended period of time causes **reduced sperm count and semen volume**.

Men taking testosterone as hormone replacement may develop **enlarged breasts**. Sometimes, people taking male hormones develop a condition called **acute intermittent porphyria** (symptoms include abdominal pain, nausea and vomiting, constipation, neurotic or psychotic behavior, and nerve irritation).

Blood **cholesterol may rise** while you are taking testosterone. People with heart disease, those who have had a stroke or transient ischemic attack (TIA)—"mini-stroke"—or who have blood vessel disease, such as claudication, should be cautious about taking a male hormone.

Possible Side Effects

▼ Most common: women—menstrual irregularities, a deepening voice, hairiness, acne, and enlargement of the clitoris. Men—breast soreness or enlargement and excessive erections.

▼ Common: men and women—swelling of the feet or lower legs, rapid weight gain, dizziness, headache, tiredness, flushing or redness of the skin, bleeding, nausea, vomiting, yellow discoloration of the eyes or skin, confusion, depression, thirst, increased urination, and constipation. Men—chills, pain in the scrotum or groin, prostate cancer, and difficult urination.

▼ Less common: men and women—mild acne, diarrhea, increased pubic hair and difficulty sleeping. Men—impotence, irritation or infection of the skin of the scrotum, and decreased testicle size.

▼ Rare: men and women—male pattern baldness, oily skin, jaundice, and changes in liver function tests.

Drug Interactions

• Testosterone may increase the effects of anticoagulants (blood thinners) such as warfarin.

• Taking testosterone with imipramine (an antidepressant) may lead to a paranoid reaction.

• Testosterone may interfere with laboratory tests of thyroid function; it does not affect the thyroid gland or normal thyroid function.

Food Interactions

You may take this drug with food if it upsets your stomach. Food does not interfere with testosterone skin patches.

Usual Dose

Oral Tablets
  Men: 10–30 mg a day.
  Women: 50–200 mg a day.

Skin Patches
Apply nightly. Testoderm patches should be placed on clean dry skin of the scrotum. Androderm System is applied to clean dry skin on your back, abdomen, upper arm, or thigh. Androderm dosage starts at 2 patches a night. Dosage may be adjusted to 1 or 3 patches nightly.

Overdosage

Symptoms of overdose are similar to testosterone side effects. Call your local poison control center or hospital emergency room for more information.

Special Information

If you are using a testosterone skin patch, apply it as directed by your doctor.

Take this medicine exactly according to directions. If you forget a dose, take it as soon as possible. If it is almost time for your next dose, skip the dose you forgot and continue with your regular schedule. Do not take a double dose.

Special Populations

Pregnancy/Breast-feeding

Testosterone and other male hormones must not be used by women who are or might become pregnant. Taking this drug during pregnancy, especially during the first 3 months, results in excessive masculinization of the fetus.

It is not known if testosterone passes into breast milk. Nursing mothers who take testosterone risk side effects in their babies.

Seniors

Older men who take testosterone may have an increased chance of developing prostate disease, including cancer. A marked increase in sex drive may also develop.

Type of Drug

Tetracycline Antibiotics

(TEH-tra-SIKE-lene)

Brand Names

Generic Ingredient: Demeclocycline
Declomycin

Generic Ingredient: Doxycycline Hydrochloride [G]

Doryx	Monodox
Doxy Caps	Vibramycin
Doxychel Hyclate	Vibra-Tabs

Generic Ingredient: Meclocycline Sulfosalicylate
Meclan

Generic Ingredient: Minocycline Hydrochloride
Minocin

Generic Ingredient: Oxytetracycline Ⓖ

E.P. Mycin	Urobiotic-250
Terramycin	Uri-Tet

Generic Ingredient: Tetracycline Hydrochloride Ⓖ

Achromycin V	Teline
Ala-Tet	Teline-500
Nor-Tet	Tetracap
Panmycin	Tetralan 250
Robitet Robicaps	Tetralan-500
Sumycin	Tetram
Sumycin 500	Topicycline

Prescribed for

Infection caused by microorganisms susceptible to these drugs.

General Information

Tetracycline antibiotics are effective against a wide variety of bacterial infection including gonorrhea; infection of the mouth, gums, and teeth; Rocky Mountain spotted fever and other types of fever caused by ticks and lice including Lyme disease; urinary tract infection; and respiratory system infection such as pneumonia or bronchitis. Doxycycline has been prescribed to treat and prevent traveler's diarrhea. Tetracycline hydrochloride has also been used with other drugs to treat amebic infection of the intestinal tract known as amebic dysentery.

Tetracycline antibiotics work by interfering with the normal growth cycle of the invading bacteria, preventing reproduction. This allows the body's normal defenses to fight off the infection. This process is described as bacteriostatic (inhibiting bacterial growth).

Tetracycline antibiotics may be substituted for penicillin in people who are allergic to it. They have also been successfully used to treat skin infection but are not considered the first-choice antibiotic for these applications.

Tetracycline hydrochloride and meclocycline have been used successfully in the treatment of adolescent acne, in low dosages over a long period of time. Adverse effects and toxicity in this type of therapy are almost unheard of.

Cautions and Warnings

Tetracycline antibiotics should not be given to people with **liver disease** or **kidney or urinary problems**.

If the **antibiotic that your doctor has prescribed does not work**, a number of things may have happened. You may not have taken the drug for a long enough period of time. You may be the victim of a superinfection, in which another organism—usually a fungus—unaffected by the tetracycline antibiotic begins to grow in the same area as the bacteria being treated. If this happens, it may seem like a relapse or a new infection. Only your doctor can determine which drug to take for it.

Avoid **prolonged exposure to the sun** if you are taking high dosages of a tetracycline antibiotic, especially demeclocycline, because these antibiotics may interfere with your body's normal sun-screening mechanism, making you more prone to severe sunburn.

If you are **allergic** to any tetracycline antibiotic or any other drug in this category, you are probably allergic to them all. Do not use tetracycline antibiotics if you are allergic to them.

Tetracycline antibiotics should not be used by **children under age 8** because they have been shown to interfere with the development of the long bones and may retard growth. Permanent tooth discoloration may also result.

People taking demeclocycline may experience **diabetes insipidus syndrome** (symptoms include **excessive thirst, urination,** and **weakness**). The severity of this condition depends on the amount of drug taken and is reversible when the drug is withdrawn.

Minocycline may cause **light-headedness, dizziness, or fainting**. People taking this drug must be careful when driving or performing tasks requiring concentration.

Tetracycline antibiotics have been associated with **pseudotumor cerebri** (condition characterized by increased pressure in the brain—symptoms include **headache** and **blurred vision**).

Possible Side Effects

▼ Most common: upset stomach, nausea, vomiting, diarrhea, and rash.

Possible Side Effects *(continued)*

▼ Less common: hairy tongue and itching and irritation of the anal or vaginal region. If these symptoms appear, call your doctor immediately. Periodic physical examinations and laboratory tests should be given to those who are on long-term tetracycline antibiotic treatment.

▼ Rare: appetite loss, peeling skin, sensitivity to the sun, fever, chills, anemia, brown spotting of the skin, reduced kidney function, and liver damage.

Drug Interactions

• Tetracycline antibiotics may interfere with the action of bactericidal (bacteria-killing) agents such as penicillin. You should not take both kinds of antibiotics for the same infection.

• Antacids, mineral supplements, and multivitamins containing bismuth, calcium, zinc, magnesium, or iron may reduce the effectiveness of tetracycline antibiotics—with the exception of doxycycline and minocycline—by interfering with their absorption into the bloodstream. Sodium bicarbonate powder may also be a problem if used as an antacid. Separate doses of an antacid, mineral supplement, vitamin with minerals, or sodium bicarbonate and a tetracycline antibiotic by at least 2 hours.

• Tetracycline antibiotics may increase the effect of anticoagulant (blood-thinning) drugs such as warfarin. Consult your doctor because an adjustment in the anticoagulant dosage may be required.

• Barbiturates, carbamazepine, and hydantoin antiseizure drugs may increase the rate at which doxycycline is broken down by the liver, reducing its effectiveness. More doxycycline or a different antibiotic may be required.

• Cimetidine, ranitidine, and other H_2 antagonists may reduce the amount of tetracycline antibiotic absorbed into the bloodstream, decreasing its effectiveness.

• Tetracycline antibiotics may increase blood levels of digoxin in a small number of people, possibly leading to digoxin side effects. In susceptible people, this effect may last for months after the tetracycline antibiotic has been withdrawn. If you are taking this combination, be vigilant for the appearance of digoxin side effects; call your doctor if they develop.

• Tetracycline antibiotics may reduce insulin requirements for diabetics. If you are using this combination, be sure to carefully monitor your blood-sugar level.

• Tetracycline antibiotics may increase or decrease blood-lithium levels. These drugs may reduce the effectiveness of oral contraceptives ("the Pill"). Breakthrough bleeding or pregnancy is possible; you should use another method of contraception in addition to an oral contraceptive while you are taking one of these antibiotics.

Food Interactions

Take all tetracycline antibiotics, except for doxycycline and minocycline, on an empty stomach, 1 hour before or 2 hours after meals and with 8 oz. of water. The antibacterial effect of these antibiotics may be neutralized when they are taken with food, dairy products such as milk or cheese, or antacids.

Doxycycline and minocycline may be taken with food or milk.

Usual Dose

Demeclocycline
  Adult: 600 mg a day.
  Child (age 9 and over): 3–6 mg per lb. of body weight a day.
  Child (under age 9): not recommended.

Doxycycline Hydrochloride
  Adult and Child (age 9 and over, and over 100 lbs.): starting dosage—200 mg in 2 doses of 100 mg given 12 hours apart. Maintenance dosage—100 mg a day in 1 or 2 doses. For gonorrhea take 300 mg in 1 dose and then a second 300-mg dose in 1 hour; for syphilis, 300 mg a day for not less than 10 days.
  Child (age 9 and over, but under 100 lbs.): starting dosage—2 mg per lb. of body weight divided into 2 doses. Maintenance dosage—1 mg per lb. of body weight as a single daily dose.

Your doctor may double the maintenance dosage for severe infection. An increased incidence of side effects is observed with dosages over 200 mg a day.

Meclocycline Sulfosalicylate
Apply to affected area morning and night.

Minocycline Hydrochloride
  Adult: starting dosage—200 mg. Maintenance dosage—100 mg every 12 hours. Alternate dosage: starting dosage—100–200 mg. Maintenance dosage—50 mg 4 times a day.
  Child (age 9 and over): starting dosage—2 mg per lb. of body weight. Maintenance dosage—1 mg per lb. every 12 hours.
  Child (under age 9): not recommended.

Oxytetracycline and Oral Tetracycline Hydrochloride
  Adult: 250–500 mg 4 times a day.
  Child (age 9 and over): 10–20 mg per lb. of body weight a day in 4 equal doses.
  Child (under age 9): not recommended.

Tetracycline Hydrochloride Ointment and Solution
Apply to affected area morning and night.

Overdosage

Overdose is most likely to affect the stomach and digestive system. Call your local poison control center or hospital emergency room for more information. ALWAYS bring the prescription bottle or container with you if you go for treatment.

Special Information

Do not take any antibiotic after the expiration date on the label. Decomposed tetracycline antibiotics produce a highly toxic substance that may cause serious kidney damage.
  Since the action of a tetracycline antibiotic depends on its concentration within the invading bacteria, it is imperative that you completely follow the doctor's directions and complete the full course of treatment prescribed by your doctor.
  Call your doctor if you develop excessive thirst, urination, weakness, unusual discoloration of the skin or mucous membranes—with minocycline, appetite loss, headache, vomiting, changes in vision, abdominal pain with nausea and vomiting, yellowing of the skin or whites of the eyes, or any other persistent or intolerable side effect including dizziness, light-headedness, or unsteadiness; burning or cramps in the stomach; diarrhea with nausea and vomiting; or itching of the mouth, rectal, or vaginal areas—this may indicate the presence of a superinfection. Call your doctor if your child develops tooth discoloration.

Avoid excessive exposure to the sun while taking tetracycline antibiotics, especially demeclocycline, because these drugs may cause susceptibility to sunburn.

Tetracycline antibiotics may cause dizziness, light-headedness, or fainting. Be careful when doing anything requiring concentration.

If you are using tetracycline hydrochloride topical solution or meclocycline sulfosalicylate for acne, apply the product generously to your skin until the area to be treated is completely wet. Stinging or burning may occur but this will last only for a few minutes. Tetracycline hydrochloride solution may stain your skin yellow but the stain usually washes away. Do not apply the solution or cream inside your eyes, nose, or mouth.

If you miss a dose of a tetracycline antibiotic, take it as soon as possible. If you take the drug once a day and it is almost time for your next dose, space the missed dose and your next dose 10 to 12 hours apart, then go back to your regular schedule. If you take a tetracycline antibiotic twice a day and it is almost time for your next dose, space the missed dose and your next dose by 5 to 6 hours, then go back to your regular schedule. If you take the drug 3 or more times a day and it is almost time for your next dose, space the missed dose and your next dose by 2 to 4 hours, then go back to your regular schedule. Never take a double dose.

Special Populations

Pregnancy/Breast-feeding

Tetracycline antibiotics should not be taken if you are pregnant, especially during the last 5 months of pregnancy. They interfere with the formation of normal skull and bone structures in the fetus.

Tetracycline antibiotics pass into breast milk. They should never be taken if you are breast-feeding because they interfere with the development of your child's skull, bones, and teeth.

Seniors

Seniors, especially those with poor kidney function, are more likely to suffer from less common side effects.

Type of Drug

Thiazide Diuretics

(THYE-uh-zide dye-ue-RET-iks)

Brand Names

Generic Ingredient: Bendroflumethiazide
Naturetin

Generic Ingredient: Benzthiazide
Exna

Generic Ingredient: Chlorothiazide G
Diurigen   Diuril

Generic Ingredient: Chlorthalidone G
Hygroton   Thalitone

Generic Ingredient: Hydrochlorothiazide G
Esidrix   Hydro-Par
Ezide   Oretic
HydroDIURIL

Generic Ingredient: Hydroflumethiazide G
Diucardin   Saluron

Generic Ingredient: Indapamide
Lozol

Generic Ingredient: Methyclothiazide G
Aquatensen   Enduron

Generic Ingredient: Metolazone
Mykrox   Zaroxolyn

Generic Ingredient: Polythiazide
Renese

Generic Ingredient: Quinethazone
Hydromox

Generic Ingredient: Trichlormethiazide G
Diurese   Naqua
Metahydrin

Prescribed for

Congestive heart failure (CHF), cirrhosis of the liver, kidney malfunction, hypertension (high blood pressure), and other conditions where it is necessary to rid the body of excess water.

General Information

Thiazide diuretics increase urine production. They do this by affecting the movement of sodium and chloride in the kidney. Thiazide diuretics reduce sodium, magnesium, bicarbonate, chloride, and potassium-ion levels. Calcium elimination is moderated and uric acid is retained as a result of thiazide treatment. Thiazide diuretics may also raise blood sugar. These drugs are used in the treatment of any disease where it is desirable to eliminate large quantities of water. Thiazide diuretics are often taken with other drugs to treat high blood pressure and other conditions. The exact way in which they reduce blood pressure is not known; sodium elimination is of primary importance. These diuretics begin to work within 2 hours and produce their effect in 2 to 6 hours. The differences between thiazide diuretic drugs lie in duration of effect—6 to 12 hours for some and as long as 48 to 72 hours for others—and quantity of drug absorbed. Thiazide diuretic dosages must be adjusted until maximum therapeutic response at minimum effective dosage is reached. Some of these drugs also may be given by injection.

Cautions and Warnings

Do not take a thiazide diuretic if you are **allergic or sensitive** to any drugs in this group or to **sulfa drugs**. If you have a history of **allergy** or **bronchial asthma**, you may also have a sensitivity or allergy to thiazide diuretics. Thiazide diuretics may aggravate **lupus erythematosus** (chronic condition affecting the body's connective tissue).

Thiazides may raise **total cholesterol, LDL cholesterol**, and **total triglyceride levels**. They should be used with caution by people with moderate to high blood-cholesterol or triglyceride levels. Thiazides should be used with caution if you have severe **kidney disease** because they may precipitate kidney failure; only metolazone and indapamide may be safely given in this group. People with severe **liver disease** should be treated carefully with diuretics because minor changes in electrolyte (body-fluid) balance may cause hepatic coma.

Switching between brands of metolazone is not recommended. They are not equivalent and may not have the same effects on you.

Possible Side Effects

▼ Most common: Thiazide diuretics cause loss of body potassium. Symptoms of low potassium include dry mouth, thirst, weakness, lethargy, drowsiness, restlessness, muscle pain or cramp, muscular tiredness, low blood pressure, decreased frequency of urination and decreased urine production, abnormal heart rate, and upset stomach including nausea and vomiting. Potassium supplements are given to prevent this problem in tablet, liquid, or powder form—or you may eat high-potassium foods such as bananas, citrus fruits, melons, and tomatoes.

▼ Less common: appetite loss, abdominal pain, bloating, diarrhea, constipation, dizziness, yellowing of the skin or whites of the eyes, headache, tingling of the toes and fingers, restlessness, changes in blood composition, unusual sensitivity to the sun, rash, itching, fever, breathing difficulties, allergic reaction, dizziness when rising quickly from a sitting or lying position, muscle spasm, impotence and reduced sex drive, weakness, and blurred vision.

Drug Interactions

• Thiazide diuretics increase the action of other blood-pressure-lowering drugs. Consequently, people with high blood pressure often take more than one drug.

• The possibility of developing imbalances in electrolytes is increased if you take medications such as digitalis drugs, amphotericin B, and adrenal corticosteroids while you are taking a thiazide diuretic.

• If you are taking insulin or an oral antidiabetic drug and begin taking a thiazide diuretic, the insulin or antidiabetic dosage may have to be modified.

• Combining a thiazide diuretic and allopurinol may increase the risk of allopurinol side effects.

• Thiazide diuretics may decrease the effects of oral anticoagulant (blood-thinning) drugs.

• Antigout drug dosage may have to be modified since thiazide diuretics raise blood uric-acid levels.

• Thiazide diuretics may prolong the white-blood-cell-reducing effects of chemotherapy drugs.

• Thiazide diuretics may increase the effects of diazoxide, leading to symptoms of diabetes.

• Thiazide diuretics should not be taken with loop diuretics because the combination may lead to an extreme diuretic effect and extreme effect on blood-electrolyte levels.

• Thiazide diuretics may increase the biological actions of vitamin D, possibly leading to high blood-calcium levels.

• Propantheline or another anticholinergic taken with a thiazide diuretic may increase the diuretic's effect by increasing the amount of drug absorbed.

• There is an increased risk of lithium side effects when combining lithium carbonate with a thiazide diuretic.

• Cholestyramine and colestipol bind thiazide diuretics and prevent them from being absorbed by the blood. Thiazide diuretics should be taken more than 2 hours before cholestyramine or colestipol.

• Methenamine and other urinary agents may reduce the effect of thiazide diuretics by reducing urinary acidity.

• Certain nonsteroidal anti-inflammatory drugs (NSAIDs), particularly indomethacin, may reduce the effectiveness of thiazide diuretics. Sulindac, another NSAID, may increase the effect of thiazide diuretics.

Food Interactions

Thiazide diuretics may be taken with food if they upset your stomach. Your doctor may recommend high-potassium foods like bananas and orange juice to offset the potassium-lowering effect of these drugs.

Usual Dose

Bendroflumethiazide
Starting dosage—not more than 20 mg 1–2 times a day. Maintenance dosage—2.5–5 mg a day.

Benzthiazide
Starting dosage—50–200 mg a day. Daily dosages over 100 mg should be divided into 2 doses. Maintenance dosage—50–150 mg a day.

Chlorothiazide
    Adult: 0.5–1 g 1–2 times a day. Often people respond to intermittent therapy, that is, taking the drug on alternate days or 3–5 days a week. This reduces side effects.

Child (age 6 months and over): 10 mg per lb. of body weight a day in 2 equal doses.

Child (under age 6 months): not more than 15 mg per lb. of body weight a day in 2 equal doses.

Chlorthalidone

50–100 mg a day or 100 mg on alternate days or 3 days a week. 150 or 200 mg a day is sometimes required; dosages of more than 200 mg a day generally do not produce greater response.

Hydrochlorothiazide

Adult: 25–200 mg a day depending on the condition being treated. Maintenance dosage—25–100 mg a day. 200 mg a day is sometimes required.

Child (6 months and over): 1 mg per lb. of body weight a day in 2 doses.

Child (under age 6 months): 1.5 mg per lb. of body weight a day in 2 doses.

Hydroflumethiazide

Starting dosage—50 mg 1–2 times a day. Maintenance dosage—25–200 mg a day. Daily dosages of more than 100 mg should be divided into separate doses.

Indapamide

1.25–2.5 mg every morning. Dosage may be increased to 5 mg a day.

Methyclothiazide

2.5–10 mg a day.

Metolazone

Dosage is individualized to personal need. Zaroxolyn—2.5–20 mg once a day, depending on the condition being treated. Mykrox—0.5 mg once a day, in the morning. Dosage may be increased to 1 mg a day.

Polythiazide

1–4 mg a day.

Quinethazone

50–100 mg a day. Occasionally, dosages of 100 mg are divided into 2 doses. 150–200 mg a day is sometimes required.

Trichlormethiazide

2–4 mg a day.

Overdosage

Symptoms of overdose include tingling in the arms or legs, weakness, fatigue, fainting, dizziness, changes in heartbeat, feeling unwell, dry mouth, restlessness, muscle pain or cramp, urinary difficulties, nausea, and vomiting. Take the victim to a hospital emergency room for treatment at once. ALWAYS bring the prescription bottle or container and any remaining medication with you.

Special Information

Ordinarily, diuretics are prescribed early in the day to prevent excessive nighttime urination from interfering with sleep.

Thiazide diuretics will cause excess urination at first but it will subside after several weeks.

Call your doctor if you develop muscle pain, sudden joint pain, weakness, cramps, nausea, vomiting, restlessness, excessive thirst, tiredness, drowsiness, increased heart or pulse rate, diarrhea, or dizziness. Diabetic patients may experience increased blood-sugar levels and need dosage adjustments of their antidiabetic medication.

Avoid alcohol and other medications while taking a thiazide diuretic, unless directed by your doctor.

Avoid over-the-counter medications for the treatment of coughs, colds, and allergy if you are taking a thiazide diuretic for the treatment of hypertension or congestive heart failure because such medication may contain stimulants. If you are unsure, ask your pharmacist.

If you forget to take a dose of a thiazide diuretic, take it as soon as you remember. If it is almost time for your next dose, skip the one you forgot and continue with your regular schedule. Do not take a double dose.

Special Populations

Pregnancy/Breast-feeding

Diuretics are used to treat specific medical conditions during pregnancy but their routine use during a normal pregnancy is improper. Unsupervised use by pregnant women should be avoided. Thiazide diuretics cross the placenta and may cause side effects in the newborn infant such as jaundice, blood problems, and low potassium levels. Birth defects have not been seen in animal studies.

Thiazide diuretics pass into breast milk. Though no problems have been reported in nursing infants, nursing mothers who must take diuretics should bottle-feed their infants.

Seniors

Seniors are more sensitive to the side effects of thiazide diuretics, especially to dizziness. They should closely follow their doctor's directions and report any side effects at once.

Generic Name

Thiothixene (thee-oe-THIX-ene)

Brand Names

Navane   Thiothixene HCl Intensol

Type of Drug

Thioxanthene antipsychotic.

Prescribed for

Psychotic disorder.

General Information

Thiothixene acts on a portion of the brain called the hypothalamus, which controls metabolism, body temperature, alertness, muscle tone, hormone balance, and vomiting. This drug may be used to treat problems related to any of these functions. Thiothixene is available in liquid form for those who have trouble swallowing tablets.

Cautions and Warnings

Do not take thiothixene if you are **allergic** to it or to chlorprothixene. Avoid using this drug if you have very **low blood pressure, Parkinson's disease,** or **blood, liver, kidney, or heart disease**. If you have **glaucoma, epilepsy, ulcer,** or **difficulty passing urine**, thiothixene should be used with caution and under strict supervision of your doctor.

Avoid exposure to **extreme heat** because this drug may upset your body's normal temperature-control mechanism.

Possible Side Effects

▼ Most common: drowsiness, especially during the first or second week of therapy. If the drowsiness becomes troublesome, call your doctor. Do not allow the

Possible Side Effects *(continued)*

liquid form of this medication to come in contact with your skin because it may cause a contact reaction. Thiothixene may cause jaundice (symptoms include yellowing of the skin or whites of the eyes), usually within the first 2 to 4 weeks. The jaundice usually goes away when the drug is discontinued but there have been cases in which it did not. If you notice this effect or if you develop symptoms such as fever and feeling unwell, call your doctor immediately.

▼ Less common: changes in blood components, including anemia, raised or lowered blood pressure, abnormal heart rate, heart attack, and feeling faint or dizziness.

▼ Rare: Thiothixene may produce extrapyramidal effects, such as spasm of the neck muscles, rolling back of the eyes, convulsions, swallowing difficulties, and symptoms associated with Parkinson's disease. These effects seem very serious but usually disappear after the drug has been withdrawn; however, symptoms affecting the face, tongue, or jaw may persist for as long as several years, especially in older adults with a history of brain damage. If you experience extrapyramidal effects, call your doctor immediately. Thiothixene may cause an unusual increase in psychotic symptoms or may cause paranoid reactions, tiredness, lethargy, restlessness, hyperactivity, confusion at night, bizarre dreams, inability to sleep, depression, and euphoria (feeling high). Other reactions include itching, swelling, unusual sensitivity to bright light, red skin or rash, stuffy nose, headache, nausea, vomiting, appetite loss, change in body temperature, loss of facial color, excessive salivation or perspiration, constipation, diarrhea, changes in urine and stool habits, worsening of glaucoma, blurred vision, weakening of eyelid muscles, spasm in bronchial or other muscles, increased appetite, excessive thirst, and skin discoloration—particularly in exposed areas. There have also been cases of breast enlargement, false-positive pregnancy tests, changes in menstrual flow, impotence, and changes in sex drive in men.

Drug Interactions

• Be cautious about taking thiothixene with barbiturates,

sleeping pills, narcotics or tranquilizers, alcohol, or any other medication that may produce a depressive effect.

• Aluminum antacids may interfere with the absorption of thioxanthene drugs into the bloodstream, reducing their effectiveness.

• Thiothixene may reduce the effects of bromocriptine and appetite suppressants.

• Anticholinergic drugs may reduce the effectiveness of thiothixene and increase the risk of side effects.

• The blood-pressure-lowering effect of guanethidine may be counteracted by thiothixene.

• Taking lithium with thiothixene may lead to disorientation, loss of consciousness, and uncontrolled muscle movement.

• Combining propranolol and thiothixene may lead to unusually low blood pressure.

• Blood concentrations of tricyclic antidepressant drugs may increase if they are taken with thiothixene. This may lead to antidepressant side effects.

Food Interactions

You may take this drug with food if it upsets your stomach.

Usual Dose

Adult and Child (age 12 and over): starting dosage—2 mg 3 times a day. Your doctor may increase the dosage up to 60 mg a day depending on your requirements and response.

Child (under age 12): not recommended.

Overdosage

Symptoms of overdose include depression, extreme weakness, tiredness, coma, lowered blood pressure, uncontrolled muscle spasm, agitation, restlessness, convulsions, fever, dry mouth, and abnormal heart rhythms. The victim should be taken to a hospital emergency room immediately. ALWAYS bring the prescription bottle or container with you.

Special Information

This medication may cause drowsiness. Use caution when driving or operating hazardous equipment and avoid alcoholic beverages.

The drug may also cause unusual sensitivity to the sun and may turn your urine reddish-brown to pink.

If dizziness occurs, avoid sudden changes in posture and climbing stairs. Use caution in hot weather because this drug may make you more prone to heatstroke.

If you forget to take a dose of thiothixene, take it as soon as you remember. If you take 1 dose a day and forget to take a dose, skip the missed dose and continue your regular schedule the next day. If you take more than 1 dose a day, skip the missed dose and continue with your regular schedule. Never take a double dose.

Special Populations

Pregnancy/Breast-feeding
Infants born to women taking this medication have experienced side effects such as jaundice and nervous system effects just after birth. Check with your doctor about taking this medication if you are or might be pregnant.

This drug may pass into breast milk and affect a nursing infant. Nursing mothers who must take this drug should bottle-feed their infants.

Seniors
Seniors are more sensitive to thiothixene's effects and usually require a lower dosage to achieve the desired results. Seniors are also more likely to develop side effects. Some experts feel they should be treated with ¼ to ½ the usual adult dosage.

Type of Drug
Thyroid Hormone Replacements

Brand Names

Generic Ingredient: Levothyroxine Sodium G
Eltroxin   Levoxyl
Levo-T   L-Thyroxin
Levothroid   Synthroid
Levoxine

Generic Ingredient: Liothyronine Sodium G
Cytomel

Generic Ingredient: Liotrix G
Euthroid   Thyrolar

Generic Ingredient: Thyroglobulin
Proloid

Generic Ingredient: Thyroid Hormone 🅖
Armour Thyroid   Thyroid USP
S-P-T   Thyrar
Thyroid Strong

Prescribed for

Hypothyroidism (underactive thyroid gland).

General Information

The major differences between thyroid hormone replacement drugs are their sources and hormone content. The first thyroid hormone replacement drug, thyroid hormone, was and still is, made from beef and pork thyroid. It was effective but lacked standardization, which made it difficult for doctors to control their patients' thyroid conditions. Synthetic thyroid-hormone-replacement drugs are more desirable because their tablet-to-tablet content is easily standardized, ensuring that you are receiving the amount you and your doctor think you are getting. Basically, there are two important thyroid hormones: levothyroxine and liothyronine. Levothyroxine is converted in the blood to liothyronine by the removal of an iodine atom. This process slows the absorption of levothyroxine and lowers the risk of side effects. Liothyronine's potency and its potential for side effects make it less desirable for older adults. Thyroglobulin contains both liothyronine and levothyroxine in a proportion of about 2.5:1—they are normally found in the body in a ratio of 4:1. Because thyroglobulin is a natural product—more difficult to standardize—and levothyroxine is converted naturally to liothyronine, there is no advantage in taking thyroglobulin. Liotrix contains both levothyroxine and liothyronine in the same proportions in which they are found in the body. Since levothyroxine is converted naturally to liothyronine, there is no advantage in taking both hormones. These considerations make levothyroxine the treatment of choice for thyroid hormone replacement.

Although generic versions of virtually all thyroid hormone replacement drugs are sold, the bioequivalence of these drugs has not been established; you should not switch between brands of thyroid hormone replacement drugs—

this applies especially to levothyroxine—without your doctor's knowledge.

Cautions and Warnings

If you have **hyperthyroid disease** (symptoms include headache, nervousness, sweating, rapid heartbeat, chest pain, and other signs of central nervous system [CNS] stimulation) or **high output of thyroid hormone**, you should not use a thyroid hormone replacement drug.

If you have **heart disease** or **hypertension** (high blood pressure), thyroid hormone replacement therapy should not be used unless it is clearly indicated and supervised by your doctor. If you develop **chest pain or other signs of heart disease** while taking this drug, call your doctor immediately.

Thyroid hormone replacement therapy should not be used to treat **infertility** unless the person also has hypothyroidism.

Thyroid hormone replacements have been prescribed for **weight loss**. Thyroid treatments do not work in people with a normal thyroid status unless large dosages are used. Large dosages of thyroid hormone replacement drugs may produce serious or fatal side effects, especially when taken with appetite-suppressing drugs.

Thyroid hormone replacement therapy increases metabolism and may worsen the symptoms of other endocrine system—hormone-related—diseases including **diabetes** and **Addison's disease**. Adjustments in the levels of treatment for these other diseases may be needed when you begin treatment with a thyroid hormone replacement drug.

Possible Side Effects

Side effects are rare except during the initial treatment period when the proper dosage is being established or at a time when your dosage is being adjusted.

▼ Most common: heart palpitations, rapid heartbeat, abnormal heart rhythms, weight loss, chest pain, hand tremor, headache, diarrhea, nervousness, menstrual irregularity, inability to sleep, sweating, and intolerance to heat. These symptoms may be controlled by adjusting the hormone dosage. If you develop any side effects, call your doctor at once so that your dosage may be adjusted.

Drug Interactions

- Colestipol and cholestyramine may reduce the effect of

thyroid hormone replacements by preventing their passage into the bloodstream. Take your thyroid hormone replacement and either colestipol or cholestryamine 4 to 5 hours apart.

• The combination of maprotiline and a thyroid hormone replacement may increase the risk of for abnormal heart rhythms. Your doctor may have to adjust the dosage of your thyroid hormone replacement.

• Aspirin and other salicylate drugs may increase the effectiveness of your thyroid hormone replacement by releasing more drug into the blood from body storage sites.

• Estrogen drugs may increase your need for thyroid hormone replacement therapy.

• Avoid taking over-the-counter drugs that contain stimulants—such as many of the products used to treat cough, cold, or allergy—which affect the heart and may cause symptoms of overdose.

• Thyroid hormone replacement therapy may increase the effect of anticoagulant (blood-thinning) drugs like warfarin. Be sure your doctor knows if you are taking an anticoagulant; to avoid hemorrhage, your anticoagulant dosage will have to be reduced by about ⅓ when you begin thyroid hormone replacement therapy. More adjustments may be made after your doctor reviews your blood tests.

• Diabetics may need to have their doctors increase their insulin or oral antidiabetic drug dosages when they start taking a thyroid hormone replacement.

• Thyroid hormone replacement therapy may reduce the effectiveness of certain beta-blocking drugs when people with hypothyroidism are converted to normal thyroid status. The beta-blocker dosage may need to be increased.

• Theophylline drugs are eliminated from the body more slowly in people with hypothyroidism. Taking a thyroid hormone replacement increases your body's metabolism, including the way in which it processes theophylline drugs. Dosage adjustment of the theophylline drug may be required after your thyroid function is normalized.

Food Interactions

Thyroid hormone replacements should be taken as a single dose, preferably before breakfast. More levothyroxine is absorbed into the bloodstream when it is taken on an empty stomach. It is essential to take levothyroxine at the same time each day.

Usual Dose

Levothyroxine
Starting dosage—as little as 25 mcg a day, which is then increased in steps of 25 mcg once every 3–4 weeks depending upon response. Maintenance dosage—100–400 mcg a day.

Liothyronine
   Adult: 5–100 mcg a day depending on the condition being treated and response to therapy.
   Senior and Child: Begin at the low end of the dosage range and increase slowly until the desired effect has been achieved.

Liotrix
   Adult: a single "¼"–"2" tablet a day, depending on the condition being treated and your response to therapy. Liotrix tablets are rated according to their approximate equivalent to thyroid hormone. A "½" tablet is roughly equal to 30 mg of thyroid hormone, a "1" tablet to 60 mg, a "2" tablet to 120 mg, and so on.
   Senior and Child: Begin at the low end of the dosage range and increase slowly until the desired effect has been achieved.

Thyroglobulin and Thyroid Hormone
Starting dosage—15–30 mg, or ¼–½ grain a day, which is then increased in 15-mg steps every 1–2 weeks until response is satisfactory. Maintenance dosage—30–180 mg a day.

Overdosage

Symptoms of overdose are headache, irritability, nervousness, sweating, rapid heartbeat with unusual stomach rumbling—with or without cramps, chest pain, heart failure, and shock. The patient should be taken to a hospital emergency room immediately. ALWAYS bring the prescription bottle or container with you.

Special Information

Thyroid hormone replacement therapy is usually a lifelong treatment. Be sure you always have a fresh supply of medication on hand and remember to follow your doctor's directions. Do not stop taking the medication unless instructed to do so by your doctor.

Do not switch brands of your thyroid hormone replacement product, especially in the case of levothyroxine, without your doctor's or pharmacist's knowledge. Different brands of the same thyroid hormone replacement are not always equivalent to each other.

Call your doctor if you develop nervousness, diarrhea, excessive sweating, chest pain, increased pulse rate, heart palpitations, intolerance to heat, or any other unusual side effect.

Children beginning thyroid hormone replacement therapy may lose some hair during the first few months but this is only temporary and the hair generally grows back.

If you forget to take a dose of thyroid hormone replacement, take it as soon as you remember. If it is almost time for your next dose, skip the one you forgot and continue with your regular schedule. Do not take a double dose. Call your doctor if you miss 2 or more consecutive doses.

Special Populations

Pregnancy/Breast-feeding

A very small amount of a thyroid hormone replacement enters the fetal bloodstream. These medications have not been associated with any problems when used to maintain normal thyroid function in the mother. Pregnant women who have been taking a thyroid hormone replacement should continue their treatment under medical supervision.

Small amounts of a thyroid hormone replacement pass into breast milk but these medications have not been associated with problems in nursing infants. Nursing mothers should observe their infants for possible thyroid-associated side effects.

Seniors

Seniors may be more sensitive to the effects of thyroid hormone replacements. Thyroid hormone replacement needs are generally about 25% less in people over age 60.

Generic Name

Tiagabine (tee-UH-gah-bene)

Brand Name

Gabitril

Type of Drug

Anticonvulsant.

Prescribed for

Partial seizure.

General Information

The exact way in which tiagabine hydrochloride works is not known, but its action is believed to be related to its ability to improve the activity of GABA, the major inhibitor of nerve transmission in the brain and central nervous system (CNS). This means that tiagabine probably slows GABA-related nerve impulses that lead to a seizure. The medication is well absorbed into the blood after each capsule is swallowed, with the amount of medication in the bloodstream reaching a maximum level in 45 minutes. Tiagabine is broken down in the liver.

Cautions and Warnings

Do not take this medication if you are **sensitive** or **allergic** to it. Several people taking tiagabine have developed a severe **rash**. Report rash or skin changes to your doctor.

People with **liver disease** should take this drug with caution because they eliminate it much more slowly from their bodies. Even moderate liver disease reduces the rate at which tiagabine is eliminated by 60%. Lower dosages are needed to take this effect into account.

A feeling of **severe weakness** has developed in a small number of people taking tiagabine. The weakness goes away when the medication is reduced or stopped.

Tiagabine may bind to parts of the eye. There is no evidence that this produces a long-term effect on the eye; be sure to tell your doctor if you experience any **changes in vision**.

Possible Side Effects

▼ Most common: dizziness, weakness, nervousness, and nausea.

▼ Common: poor concentration, speech or language problems, abdominal or other pain, tremor, sleeplessness, confusion, tiredness, diarrhea, vomiting, sore throat, and rash.

▼ Less common: forgetfulness, tingling in the hands or feet, depression, emotional upset, walking unusually, hostility, rolling of the eyeballs, agitation, hunger, mouth sores, cough, itching, and flushing.

Drug Interactions

• Taking tiagabine with other medications for seizure control, including carbamazepine, phenytoin, phenobarbital, and valproate may affect the amount of each in the blood. This interaction may be handled by your doctor by adjusting dosage.

Food Interactions

Take this drug with food or meals. High-fat meals slow the absorption of tiagabine into the blood but do not reduce the total amount of drug absorbed.

Usual Dose

Adult (age 19 and over): starting dosage—4 mg once a day. Dosage may be increased in steps of 4 or 8 mg to 56 mg a day. Higher amounts should be divided into 2 or 4 doses a day.

Child (age 12–18): starting dosage—4 mg once a day. Dosage may be increased in steps of 4 or 8 mg to 32 mg a day. Higher amounts should be divided into 2 doses a day.

Overdosage

The most common overdose symptoms are tiredness, passing out, agitation, confusion, difficulty talking, hostility, depression, weakness, and muscle spasm. All people who overdosed on tiagabine or accidentally swallowed 1 or 2 pills fully recovered after a day of treatment. People who overdose on tiagabine should be taken to a hospital emergency room for treatment. ALWAYS bring the prescription bottle or container with you.

Special Information

This drug may make you dizzy or tired, or interfere with your concentration. When taking tiagabine be extremely careful while driving or doing anything that requires concentration. Avoid alcoholic beverages or other nervous system depressants.

Be sure to tell your doctor if you experience changes in vision, rash, or anything else unusual.

If you forget to take a dose of tiagabine, take it as soon as you remember. If it is almost time for your next dose, take the dose you forgot and then spread your remaining daily dosage over the hours remaining in the day. Do not take a double dose.

Special Populations

Pregnancy/Breast-feeding

Tiagabine causes birth defects in lab animals. There is no information about the effect of tiagabine in pregnant women. Since seizure disorder itself has been associated with a higher than usual risk of birth defects; discuss with your doctor the need to control seizure. Any medication taken during pregnancy should be taken with caution.

Tiagabine may pass into breast milk. Nursing mothers should only take this medication if its possible benefits clearly outweigh its risks. Bottle-feeding should be considered.

Seniors

Seniors may take this medication without special precautions.

Generic Name

Ticlopidine (tih-KLOE-pih-dene)

Brand Name

Ticlid

Type of Drug

Anticoagulant.

Prescribed for

Reducing risk of stroke; also used to treat intermittent claudication and chronic circulatory occlusion, and to reduce the damage caused by stroke. It is used before open heart surgery to reduce the expected drop in platelet count, during coronary artery bypass surgery to improve the chance of the graft taking, in some forms of kidney disease to help improve the kidney function, and in sickle cell disease to reduce the number and severity of sickle cell attacks.

General Information

Ticlopidine hydrochloride makes blood platelets less "sticky," reducing the risk of blood clotting and the possible consequences of clot formation. It interferes with the functioning of the platelet cell membrane, changing platelet cells irreversibly until they are replaced by new ones. Maximum effect (60% to 70% reduction in platelet function) is seen 8 to 11 days after administration of 250 mg of ticlopidine twice a day. In clinical studies of the drug, patients taking ticlopidine regularly for 2 to 5 years experienced a 24% reduction in incidence of stroke. Ticlopidine reduces stroke risk in people who have already had a stroke or who are considered at high risk for one. People at high risk for stroke include those who have never had a stroke but who have had a heart attack or arterial disease.

Cautions and Warnings

Ticlopidine can cause severe reductions in **white-blood-cell counts**, making you much more susceptible to infection. Some cases have been fatal. Your doctor should take white-blood-cell counts 2 weeks after you begin taking ticlopidine and continue testing every 2 weeks for the first 3 months of treatment. Only people showing signs of infection need to be tested after that period. Blood counts usually return to normal 1 to 3 weeks after you stop taking the drug.

Blood-platelet counts can also be depressed, leading to spontaneous **bruising** or **bleeding. Gastrointestinal bleeding** can also worsen during use of ticlopidine.

Do not take this medication if you are **allergic** to it or if you have an **active bleeding site such as an ulcer**, **reduced blood-cell counts**, or **severe liver disease**.

Ticlopidine causes an 8% to 10% increase in blood **cholesterol** within a month after you start taking the drug.

Patients being switched from an anticoagulant or thrombolytic to ticlopidine should stop the former drug and allow it to clear the system before starting ticlopidine.

People with **severe kidney disease** may need less ticlopidine.

Possible Side Effects

Side effects occur in 60% of all patients who take ticlopidine. About 13% of ticlopidine patients stop taking the drug because of stomach side effects.

▼ Most common: diarrhea, nausea, upset stomach, rash, and stomach pain.

▼ Less common: reduced white-blood-cell counts, vomiting, bruising, stomach gas, itching, dizziness, appetite loss, and liver function changes.

Drug Interactions

• Antacids reduce the amount of ticlopidine absorbed into the blood by 20% when the drugs are taken together; to avoid this, separate doses by at least 1 hour.

• Taking cimetidine on a regular basis can reduce the clearance of ticlopidine from the body by 50%, increasing the risk of drug toxicity and side effects.

• Aspirin has an effect on platelets similar to ticlopidine and may increase the risk of bleeding due to loss of platelet function when taken with ticlopidine. Do not combine these drugs.

• Ticlopidine may slightly reduce blood levels of digoxin. This is not a problem for most people but should be monitored by your doctor in case dosage adjustment is needed.

• Ticlopidine reduces the body's clearance of theophylline; your doctor may need to reduce your theophylline dosage.

Food Interactions

Ticlopidine should be taken with meals to reduce possible stomach upset and maximize the absorption of the drug. To gain maximum benefit from ticlopidine, do not vary the way in which you take it.

Usual Dose

250 mg taken twice a day with food.

Overdosage

Ticlopidine overdose may lead to increased bleeding and liver inflammation. Other possible effects include stomach bleeding, convulsions, breathing difficulties, and low body temperature. Take the victim to a hospital emergency room. ALWAYS bring the prescription bottle or container with you.

Special Information

Call your doctor if you have fever, chills, sore throat, or other indication of infection; severe or persistent diarrhea; skin rashes or bleeding under the skin; yellowing of the skin or whites of the eyes; dark urine; light-colored stools; or other unusual, persistent, or severe side effects.

Bleeding may be more difficult to stop if you are taking ticlopidine. Be sure your doctor, dentist, and other health care professionals know that you are taking this medication.

If you miss a dose of ticlopidine, take it as soon as you can. If it is 4 hours or less until your next regular dose, skip the missed dose and continue your regular dose schedule. Do not take a double dose.

Special Populations

Pregnancy/Breast-feeding

The effect of ticlopidine on a fetus is not known. When the drug is considered crucial by your doctor, its potential benefits must be carefully weighed against its risks.

Ticlopidine may pass into breast milk. Nursing mothers taking ticlopidine should bottle-feed their infants.

Seniors

Seniors may be more sensitive to the effects of ticlopidine because it clears the body more slowly as you age. Follow your doctor's directions and report any side effects at once.

Generic Name

Tiludronate (til-UE-droe-nate)

Brand Name

Skelid

Type of Drug

Biphosphonate.

Prescribed for

Paget's disease of bone. Tiludronate may have the same uses

as other biphosphonate drugs, but it is not yet approved for anything else.

General Information

Tiludronate is one of several drugs that have been used for many years to treat a variety of conditions in which bone mass (mostly calcium) is reabsorbed by the body. Tiludronate is not approved specifically for osteoporosis, but other biphosphonates have been used for this purpose for some time.

Cautions and Warnings

Do not use tiludronate if you are **sensitive** or **allergic** to it.

People with **severe kidney disease** should not take tiludronate.

Possible Side Effects

Tiludronate side effects are generally mild and not usually reason to stop taking the drug.

▼ Most common: nausea and diarrhea.

▼ Common: sinus inflammation, fluid in the lungs, runny nose, upper respiratory infection, upset stomach, vomiting, dizziness, and tingling in the hands or feet.

▼ Less common: coughing, sore throat, stomach gas, aches and pains, cataracts, red-eye, glaucoma, rash, skin disorders, tooth problems, swelling, infection, vitamin D deficiency, and muscle aches.

▼ Rare: tiredness, high blood pressure, fainting, appetite loss, constipation, abdominal pains, and sleeplessness.

Drug Interactions

• Antacids, calcium supplements, and some other oral medicines may interfere with the absorption of tiludronate into the blood. Do not take tiludronate within one hour of any other medicines, or ½ hour of antacids containing aluminum.

• Aspirin may reduce the amount of tiludronate absorbed into the blood by up to ½ when taken within 2 hours afterward.

• Indomethacin causes 2 to 4 times more tiludronate to be absorbed by the body. Separate indomethacin from tiludronate by at least 2 hours. Other nonsteroidal anti-inflammatory drugs (NSAIDs) do not affect tiludronate in this way.

Food Interactions

Food and drink interfere with the absorption of tiludronate into the blood. Do not take the drug within 2 hours of a meal or drink. Tiludronate should be taken only with plain water. Other beverages may interfere with its absorption.

Usual Dose

   Adult: 400 mg a day.
   Child: not recommended.

Overdosage

No specific information is available on tiludronate overdose, but very low blood calcium is likely to result. Overdose victims should be taken to a hospital emergency room. ALWAYS bring the prescription bottle or container with you.

Special Information

Take tiludronate with 6 to 8 oz. of plain water in the morning before any food, drink, or other medication and avoid lying down after you have taken it. You must wait at least 30 minutes between taking tiludronate and anything else for the drug to be absorbed. The longer you wait, the more drug will be absorbed into the blood.

   Exercise, calcium, and vitamin D contribute to the health of your bones. Your doctor will provide a treatment plan.

   If you forget a dose of tiludronate, take it as soon as you remember. If it is almost time for your next dose, skip the dose you forgot and continue with your regular schedule. If you forget your morning dose and take one later in the day, you must have an empty stomach: Wait at least 2 hours after eating and then at least 30 minutes after tiludronate before taking any other medication or food.

Special Populations

Pregnancy/Breast-feeding

Tiludronate is not likely to be used by women who are pregnant or nursing, because osteoporosis is common only after menopause. Tiludronate affects bone formation and can be expected to cause scoliosis (malformation of the spinal cord) in the fetus. In animal studies, very high doses of tiludronate were toxic to the mother. Pregnant women should take tiludronate only if the possible benefits outweigh the risks.

It is not known if tiludronate passes into breast milk. Because tiludronate affects bone formation, nursing mothers who must take this drug should bottle-feed their babies.

Seniors
Seniors may take this drug without special precaution.

Generic Name

Timolol (TIM-oe-lol) G

Brand Names

Blocadren	Timoptic Ocudose
Timoptic	Timoptic-XE

The information in this profile also applies to the following drugs:

Generic Ingredient: Nadolol
Corgard

Generic Ingredient: Sotalol
Betapace

Type of Drug

Beta-adrenergic blocking agent.

Prescribed for

High blood pressure, abnormal heart rhythms, prevention of second heart attack, migraine headache prevention, tremors, stage fright and other anxieties, and glaucoma.

General Information

Timolol is one of 15 beta-adrenergic blocking drugs, or beta blockers, that interfere with the action of a specific part of the nervous system. Beta receptors are found all over the body and affect many body functions. This accounts for the usefulness of beta blockers against a wide variety of conditions. The oldest of these drugs, propranolol, affects beta-adrenergic receptors. Newer, more refined beta blockers affect only a portion of that system, making them more useful in treating cardiovascular disorders and less useful for other purposes. Other of the newer beta blockers act as mild stimulants to the heart or have particular characteristics that make them better for a specific purpose or certain people.

When applied as eyedrops, timolol reduces ocular pressure (pressure inside the eye) by reducing the production of eye fluids and by slightly increasing the rate at which these fluids flow through and leave the eye. People who cannot tolerate timolol eyedrops because of their effect on the heart may be prescribed betaxolol, another beta-blocker eyedrop. Beta blockers produce a greater drop in ocular pressure than either pilocarpine or epinephrine—other glaucoma drugs—and may be combined with these or other drugs to produce a more pronounced drop in pressure.

Cautions and Warnings

You should be cautious about taking timolol if you have **asthma**, severe **heart failure**, a very **slow heart rate**, or **heart block** (disruption of the electrical impulses that control heart rate) because the drug may aggravate these conditions.

People with **angina** who take timolol for high blood pressure risk aggravating their angina if they suddenly stop taking the drug. These people should have their drug dosage reduced gradually over 1 to 2 weeks.

Timolol should be used with caution if you have **liver or kidney disease** because your ability to eliminate the drug from your body may be impaired.

Timolol reduces the amount of blood pumped by the heart with each beat. This reduction in blood flow may aggravate the condition of people with **poor circulation** or **circulatory disease**.

If you are undergoing **major surgery**, your doctor may want you to stop taking timolol at least 2 days before surgery to permit the heart to respond more acutely to stresses that can occur during the procedure. This practice is still controversial and may not hold true for all surgeries.

Timolol eyedrops should not be used by people who cannot tolerate oral beta-blocking drugs, such as propranolol.

Possible Side Effects

Side effects are relatively uncommon and usually mild; normally they develop early in the course of treatment and are rarely a reason to stop taking timolol.

▼ Most common: impotence.

Possible Side Effects *(continued)*

▼ Less common: unusual tiredness or weakness, slow heartbeat, heart failure (symptoms include swelling of the legs, ankles, or feet), dizziness, breathing difficulties, bronchospasm, depression, confusion, anxiety, nervousness, sleeplessness, disorientation, short-term memory loss, emotional instability, cold hands and feet, constipation, diarrhea, nausea, vomiting, upset stomach, increased sweating, urinary difficulties, cramps, blurred vision, skin rash, hair loss, stuffy nose, facial swelling, aggravation of lupus erythematosus (chronic condition affecting the body's connective tissues), itching, chest pain, back or joint pain, colitis, drug allergy (symptoms include fever and sore throat), and liver toxicity.

Drug Interactions

• Timolol may interact with surgical anesthetics to increase the risk of heart problems during surgery. Some anesthesiologists recommend having gradually stopped the drug by 2 days before surgery.

• Timolol may interfere with the signs of low blood sugar and with the action of oral antidiabetes drugs.

• Timolol increases the blood-pressure-lowering effects of other blood-pressure-reducing agents, including clonidine, guanabenz, and reserpine; and calcium channel blockers such as nifedipine.

• Aspirin-containing drugs, indomethacin, sulfinpyrazone, and estrogen drugs may interfere with the blood-pressure-lowering effect of timolol.

• Cocaine may reduce the effectiveness of all beta blockers.

• Timolol may worsen the problem of cold hands and feet associated with ergot alkaloids, used to treat migraine headache. Gangrene is a possibility in people taking both an ergot and timolol.

• Timolol will counteract thyroid hormone replacements.

• Calcium channel blockers, flecainide, hydralazine, oral contraceptives, propafenone, haloperidol, phenothiazine tranquilizers—molindone and others—quinolone antibacterials, and quinidine may increase the amount of timolol in the bloodstream and lead to increased timolol effects.

• Timolol should not be taken within 2 weeks of taking a monoamine oxidase inhibitor (MAOI) antidepressant.

• Cimetidine increases the amount of timolol absorbed into the bloodstream from oral tablets.

• Timolol may interfere with the effectiveness of some antiasthma drugs including theophylline and aminophylline, and especially ephedrine and isoproterenol.

• Combining timolol and phenytoin or digitalis drugs may result in excessive slowing of the heart, possibly causing heart block.

• If you stop smoking while taking timolol, your dose may have to be reduced because your liver will break down the drug more slowly afterward.

• If you use other glaucoma eye medications, separate them to avoid physically mixing them.

• Small amounts of timolol eyedrops are absorbed into the bloodstream and may interact with other drugs in the same way as oral beta blockers, although this is unlikely.

Food Interactions

None known.

Usual Dose

Tablets: 10–60 mg a day divided into 2 doses.

Eyedrops: 1 drop twice a day.

Overdosage

Symptoms of overdose include changes in heartbeat—unusually slow, unusually fast, or irregular—severe dizziness or fainting, breathing difficulties, bluish-colored fingernails or palms, and seizures. The victim should be taken to a hospital emergency room. ALWAYS bring the prescription bottle or container with you.

Special Information

Timolol is meant to be taken continuously. Do not stop taking this drug unless directed to do so by your doctor: Abrupt withdrawal may cause chest pain, breathing difficulties, increased sweating, and unusually fast or irregular heartbeat. When ending timolol treatment, dosage should be reduced gradually over a period of about 2 weeks.

Call your doctor at once if you develop back or joint pain, breathing difficulties, cold hands or feet, depression, skin rash, or changes in heartbeat. Timolol may produce an undesirable lowering of blood pressure, leading to dizziness or fainting; call your doctor if this happens to you. Call your doctor if you experience persistent or bothersome anxiety, diarrhea, constipation, impotence, headache, itching, nausea or vomiting, nightmares or vivid dreams, upset stomach, trouble sleeping, stuffy nose, frequent urination, unusual tiredness, or weakness.

Timolol can cause drowsiness, dizziness, light-headedness, or blurred vision. Be careful when driving or performing complex tasks.

It is best to take timolol at the same time each day. If you forget a dose, take it as soon as you remember. If you take timolol twice a day and it is within 4 hours of your next dose, skip the dose you forgot and continue with your regular schedule. Do not take a double dose.

To administer eyedrops, lie down or tilt your head back. Hold the dropper above your eye, gently squeeze your lower lid to form a small pouch, and release the drop or drops of medication inside your lower lid while looking up. Release the lower lid, keeping your eye open. Do not blink for 40 seconds. Press gently on the bridge of your nose at the inside corner of your eye for 1 minute to help circulate the drug in your eye. To avoid infection, do not touch the dropper tip to your finger, eyelid, or any other surface. Wait at least 5 minutes before using another eyedrop or eye ointment.

If you forget a dose of timolol eyedrops, administer it it as soon as you remember. If it is almost time for your next dose, skip the dose you forgot and continue with your regular schedule. Do not take a double dose.

Special Populations

Pregnancy/Breast-feeding
Infants born to women who took a beta blocker while pregnant had lower birth weights, low blood pressure, and reduced heart rates. Timolol should be avoided by pregnant women and women who might become pregnant while taking it. When the drug is considered crucial by your doctor, its potential benefits must be carefully weighed against its risks.

Timolol passes into breast milk, but problems are rare. Still, nursing mothers taking timolol should bottle-feed their babies.

Seniors
Seniors may absorb and retain more timolol in their bodies, and require less of the drug to achieve results. Your doctor

should adjust your dosage to meet your individual needs. Seniors taking timolol may be more likely to suffer from cold hands and feet, reduced body temperature, chest pain, general feelings of ill health, sudden breathing difficulties, sweating, or changes in heartbeat.

Generic Name

Tizanidine (tih-ZAN-ih-dene)

Brand Name

Zanaflex

Type of Drug

Skeletal muscle relaxant.

Prescribed for

Spastic muscle movements.

General Information

Tizanidine hydrochloride is prescribed for people who suffer from uncontrolled muscle spasms usually associated with a nervous system condition. It is presumed to work on the central nervous system by affecting nerves that control major muscle systems; it has no direct effect on skeletal muscles. Tizanidine begins working between 1 to 2 hours after it is taken, and lasts for 3 to 6 hours.

Tizanidine is a chemical cousin of clonidine, which is prescribed for high blood pressure; however, tizanidine has a very minor effect in lowering blood pressure.

Cautions and Warnings

Do not take tizanidine if you are sensitive or **allergic** to it.

Tizanidine can cause **low blood pressure**. This effect usually begins within 1 hour after taking the drug and reaches its height after 2 to 3 hours. Low blood pressure triggered by tizanidine is associated with **slow heart rate**, **light-headedness**, and **dizziness** when rising from a sitting or lying position.

About 50% of people taking tizanidine experience some **sedation**, which may interfere with everyday activities. Sedation usually begins 30 minutes after taking the drug and continues to get worse for about 1 hour. If a person does not experience sedative effects from tizanidine in the first week of treatment, he or she probably will not experience them at all.

Tizanidine may cause **liver injury**. About 1 of every 20 people who take this drug experience some liver inflammation, although most cases resolve once the drug is stopped. Several people have died from liver failure after taking tizanidine; it should be avoided by people with liver disease.

People taking tizanidine have experienced **hallucinations, delusion**, and **psychotic symptoms**.

Tizanidine should be used with caution by people who have **reduced kidney function**. These people need smaller-than-normal doses to accommodate for the fact that the body cannot clear the drug as efficiently as people with full kidney function.

Possible Side Effects

▼ Most common: dry mouth, sleepiness, tiredness, and weakness.

▼ Common: dizziness.

▼ Less common: uncontrolled muscle movement, nervousness, constipation, sore throat, vomiting, frequent urination, urinary infection, liver inflammation, double vision, flu symptoms, runny nose, speech disorders, fever, depression, anxiety, tingling in the hands or feet, rash, sweating, skin sores, diarrhea, abdominal pain, and upset stomach,

▼ Rare: A variety of rare side effects affecting virtually every body system have been associated with this medication. Call your doctor if anything unusual develops.

Drug Interactions

• Alcoholic beverages add substantially to the sedative effects of tizanidine; they also increase the amount of drug in the blood by about 20%. Avoid this combination.

• Oral contraceptives reduce the amount of tizanidine eliminated from the body by about 50%. This can lead to side effects. People who must combine these drugs should take significantly lower doses of tizanidine than normal.

• Tizanidine may increase the effects of blood-pressure-lowering drugs. Caution must be exercised when tizanidine is combined with these drugs.

• When combined with acetaminophen, tizanidine modestly lengthens the time to reach maximum blood concentrations of acetaminophen, possibly delaying its effect.

Food Interactions

Food increases the speed at which tizanidine is absorbed into the blood, but does not increase the overall amount of the drug that enters the bloodstream. It may be taken without regard to food or meals.

Usual Dose

Adults: 8 mg every 6–8 hours as needed, up to 3 doses a day. Do not exceed 36 mg a day.

Child: not recommended.

Overdosage

One person with multiple sclerosis (MS) attempted suicide by taking 400 mg of tizanidine. This person experienced changes in respiratory rate and very slow breathing, but recovered after hospital treatment. Overdose victims should be taken to a hospital emergency room. ALWAYS bring the prescription bottle or container with you.

Special Information

People taking tizanidine should be careful not to exceed the prescribed dosage. Experience with doses above 24 mg a day over an extended period is limited.

Be careful when driving, operating complex machinery, or doing anything that requires alertness and concentration.

Tizanidine is often prescribed for muscle spasms only as needed. If you take it on a regular basis and forget a dose, take it as soon as you remember. If it is almost time for your next dose, skip the one you forgot and continue with your regular schedule. Do not take a double dose.

Special Populations

Pregnancy/Breast-feeding

Tizanidine has not been studied in pregnant women. It should only be taken if absolutely necessary and after its risks and possible benefits have been carefully weighed.

Tizanidine may pass into breast milk. Nursing mothers who must take this drug should consider bottle-feeding their babies.

Seniors

Seniors clear this drug from their bodies 4 times slower than younger people and should use tizanidine with caution.

Generic Name

Tocainide (toe-KAY-nide)

Brand Name

Tonocard

Type of Drug

Antiarrhythmic.

Prescribed for

Abnormal heart rhythms; also prescribed for muscular dystrophy and trigeminal neuralgia (tic douloureux).

General Information

Tocainide hydrochloride works in the same way as lidocaine, one of the most widely used injectable antiarrhythmic drugs. Tocainide slows the speed at which nerve impulses are carried through the heart's ventricle, helping the heart to maintain a stable rhythm by making heart muscle cells less easily excited. Tocainide affects different areas of the heart than do other widely used oral antiarrhythmic drugs. Tocainide is usually prescribed as a follow-up to intravenous lidocaine for people with life-threatening arrhythmias.

Cautions and Warnings

People taking tocainide may develop **bone-marrow depression**, a drastic **drop in white-blood-cell count**, **low platelet count**, or other **abnormalities of blood components**. Physically, these can be represented by fever, chills, sore throat, mouth sores, bruising, or bleeding. Call your doctor if any of these symptoms occur. Because these abnormalities happen most often during the first 3 months on tocainide, you should have weekly blood counts throughout that period.

This drug should not be used by people who are **allergic** to it, to lidocaine, or to local anesthetics.

Some people using tocainide may develop **respiratory difficulties**, including fluid buildup in the lungs, pneumonia, and irritation of the lungs. Immediately report any cough, wheezing, shortness of breath, or breathing difficulties to your doctor. Tocainide should not be used by people with **heart failure** because the drug can actually worsen that condition.

Like other antiarrhythmic drugs, tocainide may occasionally worsen heart rhythm problems. It has not actually been proven to help people live longer.

Possible Side Effects

▼ Most common: nausea, dizziness, fainting, tingling in the hands or feet, and tremors. These reactions are generally mild and short-lived, and usually go away when dosage is reduced or when you take tocainide with food.

▼ Less common: vomiting, reduced appetite, lightheadedness, confusion, disorientation, hallucinations, nervousness, mood or self-awareness changes, poor muscle coordination, blurred or double vision, increased sweating, giddiness, restlessness, anxiety, low blood pressure, slowing of the heart rate, heart palpitations, chest pains, cold sweats, headache, drowsiness, lethargy, ringing or buzzing in the ears, visual disturbances, rolling of the eyes, diarrhea, unusual feelings of heat or cold, joint inflammation and pain, and muscle aches.

▼ Rare: seizures, depression, psychosis, changes in mental state, changes in sense of taste—which may include a metallic taste—changes in sense of smell, agitation, slurred speech, difficulty concentrating, memory loss, sleeplessness, nightmares, unusual thirst, weakness, upset stomach, abdominal pain and discomfort, difficulty swallowing, breathing difficulties (see "Cautions and Warnings"), changes in white-blood-cell count, anemia, urinary difficulty, hair loss, cold hands or feet, leg pain after minor exercise, dry mouth, earache, fever, hiccups, aches, not feeling well, muscle twitches or spasms, neck or shoulder pain, facial flushing or pallor, and yawning.

Drug Interactions

• Tocainide taken with metoprolol or other beta-blocking drugs may cause too rapid a drop in blood pressure and slow the heart.

• Tocainide may produce additive cardiac side effects if taken with other antiarrhythmic drugs.

• Tocainide may increase the effects of other drugs that depress bone-marrow function, leading to reduced levels of white blood cells and blood platelets.

• Cimetidine and rifampin reduce the amount of tocainide absorbed into the bloodstream. Ranitidine, which can be used instead of cimetidine, does not have this effect.

Food Interactions

None known.

Usual Dose

Adult: 1200–1800 mg a day, in 2–3 doses. Seniors and people with kidney or liver disease usually require lower doses.

Overdosage

The first symptoms of tocainide overdose are usually tremors or other nervous system effects. Other, more serious, side effects may follow. At least 1 person has died of a tocainide overdose. Victims should be taken to an emergency room for treatment. ALWAYS bring the prescription bottle or container with you.

Special Information

Be sure to report any side effects to your doctor, particularly breathing difficulties after exertion, cough, wheezing, tremors, palpitations, rash, easy bruising or bleeding, fever, chills, sore throat or mouth, or mouth sores. Most of these side effects are minor and will respond to minimal dosage adjustments.

Tocainide can make you dizzy or drowsy. Be careful while driving or performing other complex tasks.

Do not take more or less of this drug than prescribed. If you forget to take a dose of tocainide and remember within 4 hours of your regular time, take it right away. If you do not remember until later, skip the dose you forgot and go back to your regular schedule. Do not take a double dose.

Special Populations

Pregnancy/Breast-feeding

Animal studies of tocainide in doses 1 to 4 times larger than the human equivalent revealed an increase in spontaneous abortions and stillbirths. When tocainide is considered essential by your doctor, its potential benefits must be carefully weighed against its risks.

This drug passes into breast milk in amounts as high as or higher than those in the blood, increasing the risk of possible side effects in the nursing infant. Nursing mothers who must take this drug should bottle-feed their babies.

Seniors
Seniors are more sensitive to the side effects of this drug, especially dizziness and low blood pressure. Follow your doctor's directions, and report any side effects at once.

Generic Name

Topiramate (toe-PYE-ruh-mate)

Brand Name

Topamax

Type of Drug

Anticonvulsant.

Prescribed for

Partial onset seizure in adults.

General Information

Topiramate has a broad spectrum of antiepileptic activity. The exact way in which it affects seizures is not known, but possible modes of action are suspected. Topiramate is absorbed well, with blood levels reaching a peak within 2 hours of each dose and about 80% of the medication in each tablet absorbed into the blood. Topiramate passes out of your body through the urine, mostly unchanged. Children appear to clear the drug from their bodies faster than adults.

Cautions and Warnings

Do not take topiramate if you are **sensitive** or **allergic** to it. People who suddenly stop taking this or other anticonvulsant medicines may **worsen their seizures**. Anticonvulsant medicines should be reduced gradually to avoid this effect.

People with moderate to severe **kidney disease** should be treated with half the usual dose; other dosage adjustments may be needed. People with **liver disease** may clear topiramate from their bodies more slowly than others do, but the reasons for this are not well understood. About 1.5% of people taking topiramate develop **kidney stones**. This effect may be avoided by drinking several glasses of water a day during treatment.

Possible Side Effects

Topiramate side effects usually affect the central nervous system.

▼ Most common: slow reflexes; slow thought processes; difficulty concentrating; speech or language problems, especially word-finding; tiredness; dizziness; weakness; poor muscle coordination; tingling in the hands or feet; tremors; depression; nausea; respiratory infections; and visual disturbances, including double vision.

▼ Less common: back or chest pain, leg pain, hot flushes, body odor, swelling, abnormal coordination, agitation, mood changes, aggressive reactions, reduced touch sensation, apathy, emotional instability, depersonalization, itching, rash, upset stomach, appetite loss, abdominal pain, constipation, dry mouth, breast pain, menstrual disorders, painful menstruation, sore throat, sinus inflammation, breathing difficulties, eye pain, weight loss, loss of white blood cells, muscle ache, and hearing loss.

▼ Rare: chills, sweating, gum irritation, blood in the urine, and nosebleeds. Other side effects of topiramate can affect almost any part of the body. Report anything unusual to your doctor.

Drug Interactions

• Certain other anticonvulsant drugs—phenytoin, carbamazepine and valproic acid—reduce the amount of topiramate in your blood.

• Topiramate increases the depressive effect of alcohol and other nervous system depressants. Avoid these combinations.

• Combining topiramate with a carbonic anhydrase inhibitor drug may increase your chances of developing kidney stones.

• Topiramate reduces the effect of oral contraceptive pills

and digoxin. Combining topiramate with one of these drugs may reduce that drug's effectiveness.

Food Interactions

None known.

Usual Dose

Adult: starting dose—50 mg a day. Increase gradually to 200 mg twice a day. People with moderate to severe kidney failure should begin with ½ the usual dose.

Child: not recommended.

Overdosage

Topiramate overdose is likely to cause nervous system depression. People suspected of having taken a topiramate overdose must be taken to a hospital emergency room immediately to remove the drug from the stomach. ALWAYS bring the prescription bottle or container with you.

Special Information

If you forget a dose of topiramate, take it as soon as you remember. If it is almost time for your next dose, skip the dose you forgot and continue with your regular schedule. Do not take a double dose.

Drink several glasses of water or other fluids every day to avoid developing kidney stones.

Be careful when engaging in any activity that requires concentration and coordination, such as driving.

Do not break topiramate tablets; they have a bitter taste.

Special Populations

Pregnancy/Breast-feeding

Animal studies indicate that topiramate may cause birth defects. There are no studies of topiramate in pregnant women; it should only be taken during pregnancy if the risks and potential benefits have been fully discussed with your doctor.

Topiramate passes into the breast milk of lab animals. Nursing mothers who must take topiramate should consider bottle-feeding their babies to avoid topiramate side effects in their infants.

Seniors

Studies of topiramate in seniors show no difference in side effects. Lower dosage may be needed because of age-related kidney impairment.

Toprol XL

see **Metoprolol**, page 695

Generic Name

Tramadol (TRAM-uh-dol)

Brand Name

Ultram

Type of Drug

Non-narcotic pain reliever.

Prescribed for

Mild to moderate pain.

General Information

Tramadol hydrochloride is a synthetic compound that works in the central nervous system (CNS) to relieve pain. The exact way in which this drug works is unknown, but it binds to natural opioid receptors and reduces the uptake of two important neurohormones, serotonin and norepinephrine, into nerves. Pain relief begins about an hour after you take a dose and reaches its maximum effect in 2 to 3 hours. Like the narcotic pain relievers, tramadol can cause dizziness, tiredness, nausea, constipation, sweating, and itching. Unlike the narcotics, this drug causes little interference with breathing and does not cause histamine reactions. It has no effect on heart function.

Cautions and Warnings

Do not take this drug if you are **sensitive or allergic** to it or if you are intoxicated with drugs, alcohol, or narcotics. People who must take **tranquilizers**, **sedatives**, or other **nervous**

system depressants should take reduced doses of tramadol.

Large doses of tramadol may interfere with your **ability to breathe**, especially if you take alcohol at the same time.

Tramadol use should be avoided in people who have had **abdominal conditions** or a **head injury** because the drug may interfere with diagnosing the injury or understanding its severity.

This drug causes **seizure** in test animals; similar reactions have been seen in people taking excessive oral doses of 700 mg or large intravenous doses of 300 mg.

People who are **dependent on narcotics** and who take tramadol may experience withdrawal symptoms.

People with **reduced kidney function** or **liver disease** should receive reduced doses of tramadol because excessive quantities will remain in the blood if usual doses are taken.

Possible Side Effects

▼ Most common: dizziness or fainting, nausea, constipation, headache, tiredness, vomiting, itching, weakness, sweating, upset stomach, dry mouth, and diarrhea.

▼ Less common: feeling unwell, warmth and flushing, nervousness, anxiety, agitation, euphoria (feeling high), emotional instability, trouble sleeping, abdominal pain, appetite loss, stomach gas, rash, visual disturbances, urinary difficulties, and symptoms of menopause.

▼ Rare: allergies, accidents, weight loss, suicidal thoughts, dizziness when rising from a sitting or lying position, rapid heartbeat, heart palpitations, heart pain, seizure, tingling in the hands or feet, difficulty learning or understanding, tremors, hallucinations, memory loss, difficulty concentrating, migraine, unusual walk, stomach bleeding, hepatitis (symptoms include yellowing of the skin or whites of the eyes), mouth lesions, itching, changes in sense of taste, cataracts, deafness, ringing or buzzing in the ears, painful urination, and menstrual difficulties.

Drug Interactions

• Taking carbamazepine at the same time as tramadol increases the rate at which tramadol is broken down in the body, reducing its effectiveness. People taking this combination may need twice the usual dose of tramadol.

• The combination of tramadol with a monoamine oxidase

inhibitor (MAOI) antidepressant may cause severe reactions and should be used with caution.

• Quinidine may slow the breakdown of tramadol because it affects the liver enzyme that breaks down tramadol. The full impact of this interaction is not known.

Food Interactions

None known.

Usual Dose

Adult and Child (age 16 and over): 50–100 mg every 4–6 hours; do not exceed 400 mg a day. People with cirrhosis should receive 50 mg every 12 hours. People with severe kidney disease should receive no more than 100 mg every 12 hours.

Senior: Do not exceed 300 mg a day.

Child (under age 16): not recommended.

Overdosage

The most serious effects of tramadol overdose are breathing difficulties and seizure. Some people have died from tramadol overdose; it is estimated that they took between 3000 and 5000 mg—3 to 5 g—of the drug. The lowest fatal dose was thought to be between 500 and 1000 mg in an 88-lb. woman. Tramadol overdose victims should be taken to a hospital emergency room for treatment at once. ALWAYS bring the prescription bottle or container with you.

Special Information

Drowsiness may occur: Be careful when driving or operating complicated or hazardous machinery.

Do not drink alcoholic beverages while taking tramadol. Hypnotics, opioids, and psychotropic drugs will interact adversely with tramadol.

If you forget a dose of tramadol, take it as soon as you remember. If it is almost time for your next dose, skip the one you forgot and continue with your regular schedule. Do not take a double dose.

Special Populations

Pregnancy/Breast-feeding

Tramadol is toxic to an animal fetus at doses only 3 to 15 times the maximum adult dose. In people, tramadol passes into the circulation of the fetus. When this drug is considered crucial by your doctor, its potential benefits must be carefully weighed against its risks.

Tramadol should not be taken by nursing mothers.

Seniors

In people age 75 and older, blood concentrations of tramadol are somewhat higher than in younger adults. Seniors may also be more sensitive to the side effects of this drug. Seniors should not take more than 300 mg a day.

Generic Name

Trandolapril (tran-DOE-luh-pril)

Brand Name

Mavik

Combination Products

Generic Ingredients: Trandolapril + Verapamil
Tarka

Type of Drug

Angiotensin-converting enzyme (ACE) inhibitor.

Prescribed for

High blood pressure.

General Information

ACE inhibitors work by preventing the conversion of a hormone called angiotensin I to another hormone called angiotensin II, a potent blood vessel constrictor. Preventing this conversion relaxes blood vessels, thus reducing blood pressure and relieving symptoms of heart failure by making it easier for a failing heart to pump blood through the body. Trandolapril also affects the production of other hormones and enzymes that participate in the regulation of blood-vessel dilation; this action probably increases the effectiveness of the medication.

Some people who start taking trandolapril after they are already on a diuretic (agent that increases urination) experience a rapid drop in blood pressure after their first doses or when their dosage is increased. To prevent this from happening, your doctor may tell you to stop taking your diuretic 2 or 3 days before starting trandolapril or to increase your salt intake during that time. The diuretic may then be restarted gradually.

Trandolapril is prescribed for high blood pressure alone or with hydrochlorthiazide or another blood-pressure-lowering drug. The brand-name product Tarka contains trandolapril and verapamil, a calcium channel blocker (see "Verapamil" profile for cautions, side effects, and drug interactions).

Cautions and Warnings

Do not take trandolapril if you are **allergic** to it. Trandolapril causes very **low blood pressure**.

Trandolapril may affect **kidney function**, especially if you have **congestive heart failure**. Your doctor should check your urine for protein content during the first few months of treatment. Dosage adjustment of trandolapril is necessary if you have **reduced kidney function** or **liver cirrhosis**.

Trandolapril may affect **white-blood-cell count**, possibly increasing your susceptibility to infection. Your doctor should periodically monitor your blood counts.

Possible Side Effects

▼ Most common: dizziness, fatigue, headache, nausea, and chronic cough. The cough usually goes away a few days after you stop taking the medication.

▼ Less common: chest tightness or pain, dizziness when rising from a sitting or lying position, fainting, abdominal pain, nausea, vomiting, diarrhea, bronchitis, urinary tract infection, breathing difficulties, weakness, and rash.

▼ Rare: itching; fever; heart attack; stroke; abdominal pain; abnormal heart rhythm; heart palpitations; difficulty sleeping; tingling in the hands or feet; appetite loss; odd taste perception; hepatitis and jaundice; blood in the stool; hair loss; unusual sensitivity to the sun; flushing; anxiety; nervousness; reduced sex drive; impotence; muscle cramps or weakness; muscle aches; arthritis; asthma; respiratory infections; sinus irritation; depression; feeling unwell; sweating; kidney problems; anemia; blurred vision; swelling of the arms, legs, lips, tongue,

Possible Side Effects *(continued)*

face, and throat; upset stomach; and inflammation of the pancreas.

Drug Interactions

• The blood-pressure-lowering effect of trandolapril is additive with diuretic drugs and beta blockers. Any other drug that causes a rapid drop in blood pressure should be used with caution if you are taking trandolapril.

• Trandolapril may increase blood-potassium levels, especially when taken with Dyazide or other potassium-sparing diuretics.

• Trandolapril may increase the effects of lithium; this combination should be used with caution.

• Antacids may reduce the amount of trandolapril absorbed into the blood. Separate these medications by at least 2 hours.

• Capsaicin may trigger or aggravate the cough associated with trandolapril therapy.

• Indomethacin may reduce the blood-pressure-lowering effects of trandolapril.

• Phenothiazine tranquilizers and antiemetics may increase the effects of trandolapril.

• The combination of allopurinol and trandolapril increases the chance of side effects. Avoid this combination.

• Trandolapril increases blood levels of digoxin, which may increase the chance of digoxin-related side effects.

Food Interactions

You may take trandolapril with food if it upsets your stomach.

Usual Dose

Trandolapril
1 mg a day; 2 mg a day in African Americans. Daily dosage may be adjusted up to 6 mg a day. Daily dosages greater than 4 mg may be taken in 2 doses a day.

Trandolapril-Verapamil Combination
   Adult (age 18 and over): 1 tablet a day. This sustained-release combination is available in a variety of strengths.

Overdosage

The principal effect of trandolapril overdose is a rapid drop in blood pressure, as evidenced by dizziness or fainting. Take the overdose victim to a hospital emergency room immediately. ALWAYS bring the prescription bottle or container with you.

Special Information

Trandolapril may cause swelling of the face, lips, hands, or feet. This swelling may also affect the larynx (throat) or tongue and interfere with breathing. If this happens, go to a hospital emergency room at once. Call your doctor if you develop sore throat, mouth sores, abnormal heartbeat, chest pain, persistent rash, or loss of taste perception.

You may get dizzy if you rise too quickly from a sitting or lying position. Avoid strenuous exercise and/or very hot weather because heavy sweating or dehydration can cause a rapid drop in blood pressure.

While taking trandolapril, avoid over-the-counter diet pills, decongestants, and other stimulants that can raise blood pressure.

If you take trandolapril once a day and forget to take a dose, take it a soon as you remember. If it is within 8 hours of your next dose, skip the one you forgot and continue with your regular schedule. If you take trandolapril twice a day and miss a dose, take it right away. If it is within 4 hours of your next dose, take 1 dose immediately and another in 5 or 6 hours, then go back to your regular schedule. Never take a double dose.

Special Populations

Pregnancy/Breast-feeding

When taken during the last 6 months of pregnancy, ACE inhibitors have caused low blood pressure, kidney failure, slow skull formation, and death in fetuses. Women who are or might be pregnant should not take any ACE inhibitors. Sexually active women of childbearing age who must take trandolapril must use an effective contraceptive method to prevent pregnancy. If you become pregnant, stop taking this drug and call your doctor immediately.

Relatively small amounts of trandolapril pass into breast milk, and the effect on a nursing infant is likely to be minimal. However, nursing mothers who must take this drug should consider bottle-feeding: Infants, especially newborns, are more susceptible than adults to the trandolapril side effects.

Seniors

Seniors may be more sensitive to the effects of this drug because of age-related losses in kidney or liver function. Dosage must be individualized to your needs.

Generic Name

Trazodone (TRAE-zoe-done) [G]

Brand Names

Desyrel   Desyrel Dividose

Type of Drug

Antidepressant.

Prescribed for

Depression with or without anxiety, cocaine withdrawal, panic disorder, agoraphobia (fear of open spaces), and aggressive behaviors.

General Information

Trazodone hydrochloride is chemically different from the other types of antidepressant drugs, but is as effective in treating the symptoms of depression. Trazodone may also be less likely to cause side effects than other antidepressants.

In many cases, symptoms will be relieved as early as 2 weeks after starting trazodone treatment; however, 4 or more weeks may be required to achieve trazodone's maximum benefit.

Cautions and Warnings

Do not use trazodone if you are **allergic** to it. Do not use trazodone if you are recovering from a **heart attack**. People with a previous history of **heart disease** should not use trazodone because it may cause abnormal heart rhythms.

Although it is rare, **painful and sustained erections** have occurred in men taking trazodone. If this happens, stop taking the drug and call your doctor. One-third of these cases may require surgery or may lead to a permanent inability to reach erection.

Possible Side Effects

▼ Most common: upset stomach; constipation; abdominal pains; a bad taste in the mouth; nausea; vomiting; diarrhea; palpitations; rapid heartbeat; rash; swelling of the arms or legs; blood pressure changes; breathing difficulties; dizziness; anger; hostility; nightmares; vivid dreams; confusion; disorientation; loss of memory or concentration; drowsiness; fatigue; light-headedness; difficulty sleeping; nervousness; excitement; headache; loss of coordination; tingling in the hands or feet; tremor of the hands or arms; ringing or buzzing in the ears; blurred vision; red, tired, and itchy eyes; stuffy nose or sinuses; loss of sex drive; muscle ache and pain; appetite loss; weight gain or loss; increased sweating; clamminess; and feeling unwell.

▼ Less common: drug allergy, chest pain, heart attack, delusions, hallucinations, agitation, difficulty speaking, restlessness, numbness, weakness, seizures, increased sex drive, reverse ejaculation, impotence, missed or early menstrual periods, stomach gas, increased salivation, anemia, reduced levels of some white blood cells, muscle twitches, blood in the urine, reduced urine flow, increased urinary frequency, and increased appetite. Trazodone may cause elevations in levels of body enzymes, which are used to measure liver function.

Drug Interactions

• Combining trazodone with digoxin or phenytoin may increase the amount of digoxin or phenytoin in your blood, leading to a greater possibility of side effects.

• Trazodone may make you more sensitive to drugs that work by depressing the nervous system, including sedatives, tranquilizers, and alcohol.

• Trazodone may cause a slight reduction in blood pressure. If you are taking medication for high blood pressure and begin to take trazodone, you may find that a minor reduction in the dosage of your blood pressure medication is required. At the same time, the action of clonidine, a drug used to treat high blood pressure, may be inhibited by trazodone. All these interactions must be evaluated by your doctor. Do not make any changes in your blood pressure medication on your own.

• Little is known about the potential interaction between

trazodone and monoamine oxidase inhibitor (MAOI) antidepressants. It is most often recommended that one antidepressant be discontinued 2 weeks before another is begun. If
trazodone and an MAOI are taken together, caution should be
used.

Food Interactions

Take trazodone with food to increase the amount of drug
absorbed into the bloodstream and to reduce the chances of
upset stomach, dizziness, and light-headedness.

Usual Dose

Adult: 150 mg a day with food, to start. This dose may be
increased by 50 mg a day every 3 to 4 days, to a maximum of
400 mg a day. Severely depressed people may be prescribed
as much as 600 mg a day.

Overdosage

Drowsiness and vomiting are the most frequent signs of
trazodone overdose. Other signs are very severe side effects,
especially those affecting mood and heart function. Fever
may be present at first, but as time passes body temperature
will drop below normal. All victims of antidepressant overdosage, especially children, must be taken to an emergency
room immediately. ALWAYS bring the prescription bottle or
container with you.

Special Information

Use care when driving or doing anything that requires concentration and alertness. Avoid alcohol or any other depressant drug while taking trazodone.

Call your doctor if you develop any side effects, especially
blood in the urine, dizziness, or light-headedness. Trazodone
may cause dry mouth, irregular heartbeat, nausea, vomiting,
or breathing difficulties; call your doctor if these symptoms
become severe.

If you forget to take a dose of trazodone, take it as soon as
possible. However, if it is within 4 hours of your next dose,
skip the dose you forgot and go back to your regular schedule. Do not take a double dose.

Special Populations

Pregnancy/Breast-feeding

Trazodone may damage the fetus and generally should not be

taken by women who are or might be pregnant. When the drug is deemed crucial, the risks must be carefully weighed against potential benefits.

Trazodone passes into breast milk. Nursing mothers who must take this drug should consider bottle-feeding their babies.

Seniors

Seniors are likely to be more sensitive to trazodone than younger adults and should start with lower doses, before slowly increasing their trazodone dosage.

Trental

see **Pentoxifylline**, page 854

Generic Name

Tretinoin (TRET-in-oin)

Brand Names

Avita   Retin-A
Renova

Type of Drug

Antiacne.

Prescribed for

Acne and other skin conditions and several forms of skin cancer. Vesanoid capsules are prescribed for acute promyelocytic leukemia (APL), a blood cancer.

General Information

Tretinoin, also known as retinoic acid or vitamin A acid, works against acne by decreasing the cohesiveness of skin cells, causing the skin to peel. Because it irritates skin, other irritants including extreme weather or wind, cosmetics, and some soaps can cause severe irritation. Excessive application of tretinoin will cause more peeling and irritation but will not give better results. Tretinoin is usually not effective in treating severe acne.

Medical research shows that regular application of tretinoin cream to aging skin prevents wrinkling and may even reverse the wrinkling process for some people. Tretinoin causes a temporary "plumping" of the skin when it is applied, peeling the outer layer. This gives the appearance of improved skin and reduced wrinkling. Some tretinoin—about 5%—is absorbed through the skin.

When used to treat APL, tretinoin causes the leukemia cells to mature and reduces the spread of APL cells; the exact way it works is not known.

There is limited information on children's use of tretinoin, though children ages 1 to 16 have used this medication.

Cautions and Warnings

Do not use tretinoin if you are **allergic** to it or any of its components.

This drug may increase the **skin-cancer-causing effects** of ultraviolet light. If you apply this drug to your skin you should allow a "rest period" between uses of tretinoin and other skin irritants or peeling agents. You must also limit sun exposure to treated areas and avoid sunlamps. If you cannot avoid sun exposure, use sunscreen and protective covering.

Do not apply tretinoin close to your eyes, the sides of the nose, or to mucous membrane tissue.

People with APL are at high risk for severe side effects. Oral tretinoin should only be prescribed by a doctor who is experienced in its use and the treatment of APL, and has facilities for laboratory and other services necessary to monitor your progress and response to the drug. About 25% of people with APL treated with tretinoin develop a group of symptoms called retinoic acid-APL syndrome. These symptoms include fever, breathing difficulties, weight gain, and fluid in the lungs. Low blood pressure and loss of heart function may also occur.

Forty percent of people who take oral tretinoin develop a rapid increase in **white-blood-cell count**, which is associated with greater risk of life-threatening complications. Sixty percent of people taking tretinoin develop **high blood-cholesterol or triglyceride levels**.

Retinoids such as tretinoin have been associated with **pseudotumor cerebri** (increased pressure in the brain), especially in children. Early signs of this problem include swelling in the eyes, headache, nausea, vomiting, and visual difficulties.

Possible Side Effects

Skin Products

▼ Common: redness, swelling, or blistering of the skin, or formation of crusts on the skin near the application site. Temporary skin discoloration and greater sun sensitivity may also occur. All side effects disappear after the drug has been stopped.

Capsules

▼ Most common: headache, fever, weakness, and fatigue. These generally go away with time.

▼ Common: skin changes, dry skin and membranes, bone pain and inflammation, itching, sweating, visual disturbances and other eye problems, hair loss, earache or a feeling of fullness in the ears, not feeling well, shivering, bleeding, infection, swelling in the arms or legs, pain, chest discomfort, weight gain, breathing difficulties, pneumonia, wheezing, abdominal pain, diarrhea, constipation, upset stomach, abnormal heart rhythms, blood-pressure changes, vein irritation, dizziness, tingling in the hands or feet, sleeplessness, depression, confusion, and bleeding in the brain.

▼ Less common: muscle aches, pain in the side, skin irritation, facial swelling, loss of color, lymph system problems, asthma, swollen larynx, stomach gas, swollen liver, hepatitis, ulcer, heart failure, heart attack, heart inflammation, kidney problems including kidney failure, painful urination, frequent urination, enlarged prostate, agitation, hallucination, an unusual walk, convulsions, coma, depression, paralysis of the face, and a variety of nervous system problems.

▼ Rare: hearing loss.

Drug Interactions

Skin Products

• Other skin irritants will cause excessive sensitivity, irritation, and side effects. Among the substances that cause this interaction are medications that contain sulfur in topical form, resorcinol, benzoyl peroxide, or salicylic acid; abrasive soaps or skin cleansers; cosmetics, creams, or ointments with a severe drying effect; and products with a high alcohol, astringent, spice, or lime content.

• Tretinoin increases the absorption of minoxidil through the skin when they are applied together, leading to lower blood pressure.

Capsules

• Combining ketoconazole, and other drugs that affect systems in the liver that break down tretinoin, with tretinoin causes a substantial increase in the amount of tretinoin in the blood.

Food Interactions

Tretinoin capsules are better absorbed when taken with food.

Usual Dose

Skin Products: Wash the affected area thoroughly and apply a small amount of tretinoin at bedtime.

Capsules: Dosage is individualized for each person. Doses are calculated from height and weight.

Overdosage

Applying too much tretinoin will cause skin irritation and peeling. Ingesting tretinoin is like taking vitamin A and can be extremely dangerous for pregnant women, who should not take more vitamin A than is contained in their prenatal vitamins. Infants who swallow tretinoin should be taken to a hospital emergency room for treatment. Symptoms of accidental ingestion include headache, facial flushing, abdominal pain, dizziness, and weakness. These symptoms have resolved without apparent aftereffects.

Special Information

Your acne may worsen during the first few weeks of treatment because the drug is acting on deeper, hidden lesions. This is beneficial and is not a reason to stop using tretinoin. Results should be seen in 2 to 3 weeks but may not reach maximum effect for 6 weeks; normal cosmetics can be used during this time.

Keep this drug away from your eyes, nose, mouth, and mucous membranes. Avoid skin exposure to sunlight or sunlamps.

Use your fingertip, a gauze pad, or a cotton swab when applying tretinoin to acne lesions to reduce the chances of applying too much medication that may run onto unaffected areas and irritate your skin.

You may feel warmth and slight stinging when you apply tretinoin. If you develop a burning sensation, peeling, redness, or are uncomfortable, stop using tretinoin for a short time.

If you forget a dose of tretinoin, do not apply the forgotten dose. Skip it and continue with your regular schedule. Do not apply a double dose.

Special Populations

Pregnancy/Breast-feeding

Tretinoin causes abnormal skull formation and other birth defects in animal fetuses at doses 500 to 1000 times the human dose. A pregnant woman taking tretinoin capsules is likely to deliver a severely deformed infant. When applied to the skin, tretinoin is rapidly broken down. When this drug is considered crucial by your doctor, its potential benefits must be carefully weighed against its risks. Women who need to take tretinoin capsules should be tested for pregnancy before treatment is started. Use two reliable forms of contraception while you are taking tretinoin and for 1 month after treatment has ended.

It is not known if tretinoin passes into breast milk. Nursing mothers who must take tretinoin should bottle-feed their babies.

Seniors

Seniors may use this product without special restriction.

Generic Name

Triazolam (trye-AY-zuh-lam)

Brand Name

Halcion

The information in this profile also applies to the following drug:

Generic Ingredient: Temazepam
Restoril

Type of Drug

Benzodiazepine sedative.

Prescribed for

Short-term treatment of insomnia, difficulty falling asleep, frequent nighttime awakening, and waking too early in the morning.

General Information

Triazolam is a member of the group of drugs known as benzodiazepines. All have some activity as antianxiety agents, anticonvulsants, or sedatives. Benzodiazepines work by a direct effect on the brain. They make it easier to go to sleep and decrease the number of times you wake up during the night.

The principal difference among the various benzodiazepines lies in how long they work in your body. They all take about 2 hours to reach maximum blood level, but some remain in your body longer, so they work for a longer period of time. Triazolam has the shortest action. While this virtually eliminates "hangover," it may also cause some people to wake up earlier than they would like because the drug has stopped working. Temazepam is considered to be an intermediate-acting sedative and generally remains in your body long enough to give you a good night's sleep with minimal "hangover."

Sleeplessness may often signal an underlying disorder that this medication does not treat.

Cautions and Warnings

Triazolam has been associated with **memory loss**, especially when higher doses are taken. This effect, known as traveler's amnesia, is most common among people who take this medication to adjust to time zone changes during travel; it may be linked to the use of alcoholic beverages and to attempts at starting daily activity too soon after waking up.

If you abruptly stop taking triazolam, you may experience **rebound sleeplessness**, where sleeplessness is worse during the first 1 to 3 nights after you stop the drug than it was before you started it.

People with respiratory disease may experience **sleep apnea** (intermittent cessation of breathing during sleep) while taking triazolam.

People with **kidney or liver disease** should be carefully monitored while taking triazolam. Take the lowest possible dose to help you sleep.

Clinical **depression** may be increased by triazolam, which can depress the nervous system. Intentional overdose is more common among depressed people who take sleeping pills than among those who do not.

All benzodiazepines can be **addictive** if taken for long periods of time, and it is possible for a person taking a benzodiazepine to develop drug withdrawal symptoms if the drug is suddenly discontinued. Withdrawal symptoms include tremors, muscle cramps, insomnia, agitation, diarrhea, vomiting, sweating, and convulsions.

Possible Side Effects

▼ Common: drowsiness, headache, dizziness, talkativeness, nervousness, apprehension, poor muscle coordination, light-headedness, daytime tiredness, muscle weakness, slowness of movement, hangover, and euphoria (feeling high).

▼ Rare: nausea, vomiting, rapid heartbeat, confusion, temporary memory loss, upset stomach, stomach cramps and pain, depression, blurred or double vision and other visual disturbances, constipation, changes in sense of taste, appetite changes, stuffy nose, nosebleeds, common cold symptoms, asthma, sore throat, cough, breathing difficulties, diarrhea, dry mouth, allergic reaction, fainting, abnormal heart rhythm, itching, acne, dry skin, sensitivity to the sun, rash, nightmares or strange dreams, sleeplessness, tingling in the hands or feet, ringing or buzzing in the ears, ear or eye pains, menstrual cramps, frequent urination or other urinary difficulties, blood in the urine, discharge from the penis or vagina, lower back and other pain, muscle spasms and pain, fever, swollen breasts, and weight changes.

Drug Interactions

• As with all benzodiazepines, the effects of triazolam are enhanced if it is taken with alcohol, antihistamines, tranquilizers, barbiturates, anticonvulsants, tricyclic antidepressants, or monoamine oxidase inhibitors (MAOIs). MAOIs are most often prescribed for severe depression.

• Oral contraceptives, cimetidine, disulfiram, itraconazole, ketoconazole, nefazadone, and isoniazid may increase the effect of triazolam by interfering with the drug's breakdown in the liver. Probenecid may also increase triazolam's effect.

• Cigarette smoking, rifampin, and theophylline may reduce the effect of triazolam.

• Triazolam decreases the effectiveness of levodopa.

• Triazolam may increase the amount of zidovudine (an AIDS drug—also known as AZT), phenytoin, or digoxin in your blood, increasing the chances of side effects.

• Mixing clozapine and benzodiazepines has led to respiratory collapse in a few people. Triazolam should be stopped at least 1 week before starting clozapine treatment.

• The effects of triazolam may be increased by the macrolide antibiotics—azithromycin, erythromycin, and clarithromycin.

Food Interactions

Triazolam may be taken with food if it upsets your stomach.

Usual Dose

Temazepam
  Adult: 15–30 mg at bedtime. The dose must be individualized for maximum benefit.
  Senior: starting dose—5 mg at bedtime. Dosage may be increased if needed.
  Child (under age 18): not recommended.

Triazolam
  Adult (age 18 and over): 0.125–0.5 mg about 30 minutes before sleep.
  Senior: starting dose—0.125 mg, then increase in 0.125 mg steps until the desired effect is achieved.
  Child (under age 18): not recommended.

Overdosage

The most common symptoms of overdose are confusion, sleepiness, depression, loss of muscle coordination, and slurred speech. Coma may develop if the overdose is particularly large. Overdose symptoms can develop if a single dose of only 4 times the maximum daily dose is taken. Overdose victims must be made to vomit with ipecac syrup—available at any pharmacy—to remove any remaining drug from the stomach: Call your doctor or a poison control center before doing this. If 30 minutes have passed since the overdose was taken or if symptoms have begun to develop, the victim must immediately be taken to a hospital emergency room. ALWAYS bring the prescription bottle or container with you.

Special Information

Never take more triazolam than your doctor has prescribed.

Avoid alcoholic beverages and other nervous system depressants while taking triazolam.

Exercise caution while performing tasks that require concentration and coordination. Triazolam may make you tired, dizzy, or light-headed.

If you take triazolam daily for 3 or more weeks, you may experience some withdrawal symptoms when you stop taking it. Talk with your doctor about how best to discontinue the drug.

Do not take triazolam unless circumstances will allow for a full night's sleep and time for the drug to clear your body after you awaken and before you need to be alert and active. The necessary amount of time varies among people; you may have to determine your own level of tolerance.

If you forget to take a dose of triazolam and remember within 1 hour of your regular time, take it as soon as you remember. If you do not remember until later, skip the dose you forgot and continue your regular schedule. Do not take a double dose.

Special Populations

Pregnancy/Breast-feeding

Triazolam should absolutely not be used by pregnant women or by women who may become pregnant. Animal studies have shown that triazolam passes easily into the fetal blood system and can affect fetal development.

Triazolam passes into breast milk and can affect a nursing infant. The drug should not be taken by nursing mothers.

Seniors

Seniors are more susceptible to the effects of triazolam and should take the lowest possible dosage.

Type Of Drug

Tricyclic Antidepressants

Brand Names

Generic Ingredient: Amitriptyline G
Elavil

Generic Ingredients: Amitriptyline + Perphenazine [G]

Etrafon   Triavil 2-25
Etrafon 2-10   Triavil 4-10
Etrafon Forte   Triavil 4-25
Triavil 2-10   Triavil 4-50

Generic Ingredients: Amitriptyline + Chlordiazepoxide
Limbitrol   Limbitrol DS 10-25

Generic Ingredient: Amoxapine [G]
Asendin

Generic Ingredient: Clomipramine
Anafranil

Generic Ingredient: Desipramine [G]
Norpramin

Generic Ingredient: Doxepin [G]
Sinequan

Generic Ingredient: Imipramine [G]
Tofranil   Tofranil-PM

Generic Ingredient: Nortriptyline [G]
Aventyl   Pamelor
Aventyl Pulvules

Generic Ingredient: Protriptyline [G]
Vivactil

Generic Ingredient: Trimipramine
Surmontil

Prescribed for

Depression, with or without symptoms of anxiety or sleep disturbance; chronic pain including migraine, tension headache, diabetic disease, tic douloureux, cancer, herpes lesions, and arthritis; pathologic laughing or weeping caused by brain disease; bulimia; sleep apnea; peptic ulcer disease; cocaine withdrawal; panic disorder; eating disorder; premenstrual depression; and skin problems. Clomipramine is prescribed only for obsessive compulsive disorder (OCD).

General Information

Tricyclic antidepressants block the movement of certain stimulant chemicals—norepinephrine or serotonin—in and out of nerve endings, producing a sedative effect and counteracting the effects of a hormone called acetylcholine, making them anticholinergic drugs. Recent theory holds that antidepressant drugs work by causing long-term changes in the way nerve endings function. They change the sensitivity and function of nerve endings. Although antidepressants immediately block neurohormones, it takes about 2 to 4 weeks for their clinical effects to come into play. If you are not affected after 6 to 8 weeks of drug treatment, call your doctor. Tricyclic antidepressants may also elevate mood, increase physical activity and mental alertness, and improve appetite and sleep patterns in depressed people. These drugs are mild sedatives and are useful in treating mild forms of depression associated with anxiety. Tricyclic antidepressants have been used in treating nighttime bed-wetting in young children but they do not produce long-lasting relief. The combination of amitriptyline and perphenazine, a tranquilizer, is used to treat anxiety, agitation, and depression associated with chronic physical or psychiatric disease. The combination of amitriptyline and chlordiazepoxide, an antianxiety drug, is used to treat anxiety and depression. Tricyclic antidepressants are broken down in the liver.

Cautions and Warnings

Do not take any of these antidepressants if you are **allergic or sensitive** to it or any tricyclic antidepressant. These drugs should not be used if you are **recovering from a heart attack;** rapid heartbeat and fainting when rising from a sitting or lying position are problems associated with protryptiline.

These antidepressants may be taken with caution if you have a history of **epilepsy or other convulsive disorders; seizure,** which may be a special problem with clomipramine; **difficulty urinating; glaucoma; heart disease; liver disease;** or **hyperthyroidism**. The condition of people who are **schizophrenic** or **paranoid** may worsen if they are given a tricyclic antidepressant. **Manic-depressive** people may switch phase; this may also happen if you are changing antidepressants or stopping them. **Suicide** is always a possibility in severely depressed people, who should be allowed to have only **minimal quantities of medication** in their possession at one time.

Amoxapine may cause **very high fever, muscle rigidity, altered mental states, irregular pulse or blood pressure, sweating, abnormal heart rhythms,** and **rapid heartbeat**. This group of symptoms is associated with neuroleptic malignant syndrome (NMS), which may be fatal. If these symptoms develop, stop your medication at once and call your doctor, who may prescribe another antidepressant. Clomipramine may also cause very high fever, especially when used with other drugs; this may also be a sign of NMS.

Amoxapine may also be associated with the potentially irreversible **involuntary muscle movement** of a condition called tardive dyskinesia (symptoms include lip smacking or puckering, puffing of the cheeks, rapid or worm-like tongue movements, uncontrolled chewing motions, and uncontrolled arm and leg movements). This condition is more common among the elderly, especially women. Call your doctor if this develops.

Possible Side Effects

▼ Most common: sedation and anticholinergic effects including blurred vision; disorientation; confusion; hallucinations; muscle spasm or tremors; seizures or convulsions; dry mouth; constipation, especially in older adults; difficulty urinating; worsening glaucoma; and sensitivity to bright light.

▼ Less common: blood-pressure changes, abnormal heart rate, heart attack, anxiety, restlessness, excitement, numbness and tingling in the extremities, poor coordination, rash, itching, fluid retention, fever, allergy, changes in composition of the blood, nausea, vomiting, appetite loss, upset stomach, diarrhea, enlargement of the breasts in men and women, changes in sex drive, and blood-sugar changes.

▼ Rare: agitation, inability to sleep, nightmares, feeling of panic, a peculiar taste in the mouth, stomach cramp, black discoloration of the tongue, yellowing of the skin or whites of the eyes, hair loss, changes in liver function, weight changes, excessive perspiration, flushing, frequent urination, drowsiness, dizziness, weakness, headache, and feeling unwell.

Drug Interactions

• Combining a tricyclic antidepressant with a monoamine oxidase inhibitor (MAOI) antidepressant may cause high fever, convulsions, and death. Do not take MAOIs until at least

2 weeks after amitriptyline has been discontinued. Those who must take both an MAOI and a tricyclic antidepressant require close medical observation.

• Amitriptyline interacts with guanethidine and clonidine. Be sure to tell your doctor if you are taking any drugs for high blood pressure.

• Amitriptyline increases the effects of barbiturates, tranquilizers and other sedative drugs, and alcohol. Barbiturates may decrease the effectiveness of a tricyclic antidepressant.

• Combining a tricyclic antidepressant and a thyroid drug will enhance the effects of both drugs, possibly causing abnormal heart rhythms. The combination of reserpine and a tricyclic antidepressant may cause overstimulation.

• Oral contraceptives ("the Pill") may reduce the effect of a tricyclic antidepressant, as may smoking. Charcoal tablets may prevent antidepressant absorption by the blood. Estrogen may increase or decrease the effect of a tricyclic antidepressant.

• Drugs such as bicarbonate of soda, acetazolamide, quinidine, and procainamide will increase the effect of a tricyclic antidepressant. Cimetidine, methylphenidate, and phenothiazine drugs such as thorazine and compazine block the breakdown of tricyclic antidepressants in the liver, causing them to stay in the body longer and possibly causing severe side effects.

Food Interactions

You may take a tricyclic antidepressant with food if it upsets your stomach.

Usual Dose

Amitriptyline
  Adult and Child (age 12 and over): 25 mg 3 times a day, increased to 150 mg a day if necessary. Dosage must be tailored to your specific needs.
  Senior: Lower dosages are recommended, generally 30–50 mg a day.
  Child (under age 12): not recommended.

Amoxapine
  Adult and Child (age 17 and over): 100–400 mg a day. Hospitalized patients may need up to 600 mg a day. Your dosage must be tailored to your specific needs.

Senior: Lower dosages are recommended. People over age 60 usually take 50–300 mg a day.

Child (under age 17): not recommended.

Clomipramine

Adult: 25–250 mg a day.

Child: 25–100 mg a day.

After the most effective dosage has been determined, it may be taken at bedtime to minimize daytime sedation.

Desipramine

Adult and Child (age 12 and over): 75–300 mg a day. Dosage must be tailored to your needs. People taking high dosages should have regular heart examinations to check for side effects.

Senior: Lower dosages are recommended, usually 25–150 mg a day.

Child (under age 12): not recommended.

Doxepin and Imipramine

Adult: Start with about 75 mg a day in divided doses, then increase or decrease as needed. The final daily dosage may be less than 75 or up to 200 mg. Long-term patients being treated for depression may be given sustained-release medication daily at bedtime or several times a day.

Senior: Starting dosage—30–40 mg a day. Maintenance dosage—usually less than 100 mg daily.

Child (age 6 and over): 25 mg a day, given 1 hour before bedtime for nighttime bed-wetting. If bed-wetting relief does not occur in a week, the daily dosage is typically increased to 50–75 mg depending on age—more than 75 mg a day increases side effects without increasing effectiveness. Doses are often taken in mid-afternoon and at bedtime. The dosage should be gradually reduced to help prevent bed-wetting from recurring.

Nortriptyline

Adult: 25 mg 3 times a day, increased to 150 mg a day if necessary. Dosage must be tailored to your needs.

Senior: Lower dosages are recommended, generally 30–50 mg a day.

Child (age 6–17): 10–20 mg a day.

Child (under age 6): not recommended.

Protriptyline

Adult: 15–60 mg a day in 3–4 divided doses. Protriptyline must not be taken as a single bedtime dose because of its stimulant effect.

Senior: Lower dosages are recommended, usually up to 20 mg a day. Seniors taking more than 20 mg a day should have regular heart examinations. Dosage must be tailored to your needs.

Child: not recommended.

Trimipramine

Adult: 75 mg a day in divided doses to start, then increased as necessary to 150–200 mg. The entire daily dosage may be taken at bedtime or divided into several doses a day. Hospitalized adults may receive up to 300 mg a day.

Senior: Starting dosage—50 mg a day. Maintenance dosage—up to 100 mg daily.

Child: not recommended.

Overdosage

Symptoms of overdose include confusion, inability to concentrate, hallucinations, drowsiness, lowered body temperature, abnormal heart rate, heart failure, enlarged pupils, convulsions, severely lowered blood pressure, stupor, and coma. The overdose victim should be taken to an emergency room immediately. ALWAYS bring the prescription bottle or container.

Special Information

Avoid alcohol and other depressants while taking any tricyclic antidepressant. Do not stop taking your medication unless your doctor specifically tells you to do so. Abruptly stopping a tricyclic antidepressant may cause nausea, headache, and feelings of general ill health.

Tricyclic antidepressants may cause drowsiness, dizziness, and blurred vision. Be careful when driving or operating hazardous machinery. Avoid prolonged exposure to the sun or sunlamps.

Call your doctor immediately if you develop seizure, breathing difficulties or rapid breathing, fever and sweating, blood-pressure changes, muscle stiffness, loss of bladder control, or unusual tiredness or weakness. Dry mouth may lead to an increase in dental cavities and gum bleeding and disease. You should pay special attention to dental hygiene if you are taking a tricyclic antidepressant.

When used for nighttime bed-wetting, doxepin and imipramine are often ineffective or of questionable value.

If you forget to take a dose of your medication, skip the forgotten dose and go back to your regular schedule. Do not take a double dose.

Special Populations

Pregnancy/Breast-feeding

Tricyclic antidepressants cross into the circulation of the fetus. Birth defects including heart, breathing, and urinary problems have been reported when women took a tricyclic antidepressant during the first 3 months of pregnancy. Avoid taking any of these drugs while pregnant.

Small amounts of a tricyclic antidepressant pass into breast milk and may sedate your baby. Nursing mothers who must take a tricyclic antidepressant should bottle-feed their babies.

Seniors

Seniors are more sensitive to the effects of these drugs, especially abnormal heart rhythms and other heart side effects, and often require a lower dosage than younger adults to achieve the same results. Follow your doctor's directions and report any side effects at once.

Tri-Levlen

see **Contraceptives**, page 246

Trimox

see **Penicillin Antibiotics**, page 846

Triphasil

see **Contraceptives**, page 246

Generic Name

Troglitazone (troe-GLIT-uh-zone)

Brand Name

Rezulin

Type of Drug

Antidiabetes.

Prescribed for

Type II diabetes and polycystic ovary syndrome.

General Information

Troglitazone is the first member of a new group of diabetes drugs that lower blood sugar by helping cells become more responsive to insulin. This drug is effective for people with type II diabetes, who generally have enough insulin but whose body cells do not respond to its presence. Troglitazone is not effective alone for people with type I diabetes, who do not manufacture enough insulin. Troglitazone reduces the amount of sugar produced by the liver and increases the amount of sugar used by muscle, liver, and fat cells. It is thought that troglitazone works by affecting genes responsible for the control of sugar and fat use in the body. Unlike the sulfonylurea-type antidiabetes drugs, troglitazone does not increase the amount of insulin made in the liver.

Cautions and Warnings

Do not take troglitazone if you are **allergic** or **sensitive** to it. Troglitazone is broken down in the liver; it should be taken with caution by people with **hepatitis** or **liver disease**; it may be toxic to the liver in some people.

Troglitazone should be used with caution if you have **heart failure**. Animals given 14 times the maximum human dose of troglitazone developed enlarged hearts, a sign of heart failure. This effect has not been seen in people taking troglitazone, but increased blood volume, another sign of heart failure, did occur in some people taking the drug. Since people with heart failure were not included in studies of troglitazone, caution is advised.

Women who are not ovulating but have not gone through

menopause may be at risk of becoming pregnant because troglitazone can trigger **ovulation**.

Possible Side Effects

In studies of troglitazone, people reported similar side effects with both the inactive placebo and the active drug.

▼ Most common: infections, headaches, and pain.

▼ Common: accidental injury, weakness, dizziness, back pain, nausea, runny nose, diarrhea, urinary infection, swelling, and sore throat.

Drug Interactions

• Combining troglitazone with insulin may lead to very low blood sugar; insulin dosage may have to be reduced if this happens. Combining troglitazone with glyburide, a sulfonylurea-type antidiabetes drug, can also excessively lower blood sugar.

• Troglitazone can stimulate the breakdown of other drugs also metabolized in the liver. Cyclosporine, tacrolimus, terfenadine, and blood-fat reducers may be affected; dosage adjustments may be needed.

• Taking cholestryramine and troglitazone together may reduce the amount of troglitazone absorbed into the blood by 70%. These drugs should be separated by several hours.

• Troglitazone may make some contraceptive pills lose their effect. Taking troglitazone with oral contraceptives containing norethindrone and ethinyl estradiol reduces the amount of both hormones in the blood by about 30%. Higher-dose contraceptives or another contraceptive method may be needed.

Food Interactions

Troglitazone should be taken with meals to increase the amount of drug absorbed.

Usual Dose

Adult: 400–600 mg a day.

Overdosage

No information is available, but symptoms may be similar to side effects. Call your local poison control center or hospital emergency room for more information. If you take the victim to an emergency room, ALWAYS bring the prescription bottle or container with you.

Special Information

If you are also taking insulin, be sure to follow your doctor's directions for dose reduction. Your blood sugar and insulin requirements can change if you have fever, trauma, infection, or surgery.

If you forget to take a dose of troglitazone, take it with your next meal. If it is time for your next dose, skip the forgotten dose and continue with your regular schedule. Do not take a double dose.

Special Populations

Pregnancy/Breast-feeding

Troglitazone does not affect pregnant animals or their fetuses. There is no information about the effect of troglitazone in pregnant women, who should only take this medication if the possible benefit outweighs its risks. Most experts recommend that diabetic women who become pregnant and pregnant women who develop gestational diabetes should be controlled with insulin injections. Abnormal blood sugar during pregnancy can seriously affect the fetus, and may cause birth defects.

Troglitazone passes into animal milk; it is not known if the drug passes into human breast milk. Nursing mothers who must take this medicine should bottle-feed their babies.

Seniors

Seniors may take this drug without special precautions.

Trusopt

see **Dorzolamide**, page 348

Brand Name

Tussionex Pennkinetic Ⓐ

Generic Ingredients

Hydrocodone + Chlorpheniramine

Type of Drug

Cough suppressant and antihistamine.

Prescribed for

Cough and other symptoms of a cold or other respiratory condition.

General Information

Tussionex Pennkinetic is one of many cough suppressant-antihistamine combinations that may be prescribed to treat a cough or congestion that has not responded to other medication. The narcotic cough-suppressant ingredient in this combination—hydrocodone—is more potent than codeine.

Cautions and Warnings

Do not use Tussionex Pennkinetic if you are **allergic** to any of its ingredients. Those allergic to codeine may also be allergic to Tussionex Pennkinetic. Chronic (long-term) use of this or any other narcotic-containing drug may lead to **drug dependence or addiction**. Tussionex Pennkinetic may cause **drowsiness, tiredness,** or **loss of concentration**. Use with caution if you have a history of **convulsions, glaucoma, stomach ulcer, hypertension (high blood pressure), thyroid disease, heart disease,** or **diabetes**.

Possible Side Effects

▼ Most common: light-headedness, dizziness, sleepiness, nausea, vomiting, increased sweating, itching, rash, sensitivity to bright light, chills, and dryness of the mouth, nose, or throat.

▼ Less common: euphoria (feeling high), weakness, agitation, uncoordinated muscle movement, disorientation and visual disturbances, minor hallucinations, appetite loss, constipation, flushing of the face, rapid heartbeat, palpitations, feeling faint, urinary difficulties, reduced sexual potency, low blood sugar, anemia, yellowing of the skin or whites of the eyes, blurred or double vision, ringing or buzzing in the ears, wheezing, and nasal stuffiness.

Drug Interactions

• Do not use alcohol or other depressant drugs because

they will increase the depressant effect of Tussionex Pennkinetic.

• This drug should not be combined with monoamine
oxidase inhibitor (MAOI) antidepressants.

Food Interactions

Take Tussionex Pennkinetic with food if it upsets your stomach.

Usual Dose

1 tsp. every 12 hours.

Overdosage

Symptoms of overdose include depression, slowed breathing, flushing of the skin, and upset stomach. Overdose
victims should be taken to an emergency room for treatment.
ALWAYS bring the prescription bottle or container with you.

Special Information

Because of the sedating effects of Tussionex Pennkinetic, use
caution while driving or operating hazardous equipment.

If you forget to take a dose of Tussionex Pennkinetic, take it
as soon as you remember. If it is almost time for your next
dose, skip the one you forgot and continue with your regular
schedule. Do not take a double dose.

Special Populations

Pregnancy/Breast-feeding

While hydrocodone, one of the ingredients in Tussionex
Pennkinetic, has not been associated with birth defects,
taking too much of any narcotic during pregnancy may lead
to the birth of a drug-dependent infant; the baby may experience drug withdrawal symptoms. All narcotics including
hydrocodone may cause breathing problems in the newborn
if taken just before delivery. Antihistamines may pass into the
circulation of the fetus but have not been a source of birth
defects.

Nursing mothers who must take Tussionex Pennkinetic
should bottle-feed their infants.

Seniors

Seniors are more likely to be sensitive to both ingredients in
Tussionex Pennkinetic and may experience more depressant

effects; dizziness, light-headedness or fainting when rising suddenly from a sitting or lying position; confusion; difficult or painful urination; feeling faint; dry mouth, nose, or throat; nightmares; excitement; nervousness; restlessness; or irritability.

Brand Name

Tussi-Organidin NR ⑤

Generic Ingredients

Codeine Phosphate + Guaifenesin Ⓖ

Other Brand Names

Cheracol Cough	Mytussin AC Cough
Guiatuss AC	Robafen AC Cough
Guiatussin with Codeine	Robitussin A-C ⑤

Type of Drug

Cough suppressant and expectorant.

Prescribed for

Cough due to a cold or other upper respiratory infection.

General Information

The cough-suppressant effect of Tussi-Organidin NR Liquid is due to the codeine present in the mixture. Guaifenesin, an expectorant, increases the production of mucus and other bronchial secretions. Once these thick secretions become diluted, it should be easier for the body to deal with them, thus relieving the cough. Many experts question the effectiveness of guaifenesin, especially for removing the mucus that accumulates during serious respiratory conditions such as bronchitis, bronchial asthma, emphysema, cystic fibrosis, or chronic sinusitis. Drinking plenty of fluid will work as well as any expectorant for the average cold or upper-respiratory cough. Expectorants do not suppress your cough.

Cautions and Warnings

Do not take Tussi-Organidin NR Liquid if you are **allergic or sensitive** to it or its codeine ingredient. Chronic (long-term) use of codeine may lead to **drug dependence or addiction**.

Possible Side Effects

▼ Most common: light-headedness, dizziness, sedation or sleepiness, nausea, vomiting, diarrhea, stomach pain, and sweating.

▼ Less common: euphoria (feeling high), weakness, headache, agitation, uncoordinated muscle movement, minor hallucinations, disorientation and visual disturbances, dry mouth, appetite loss, constipation, facial flushing, rapid heartbeat, palpitations, feeling faint, urinary difficulties or hesitancy, reduced sex drive or potency, itching, rash, anemia, lowered blood sugar, and yellowing of the skin or whites of the eyes. Narcotic analgesics such as codeine may aggravate convulsions in those who have had convulsions in the past.

Drug Interactions

• Codeine has a general depressant effect and may affect breathing. Tussi-Organidin NR Liquid should be taken with extreme care in combination with alcohol, sedatives, tranquilizers, antihistamines, or other depressant drugs.

Food Interactions

Tussi-Organidin NR Liquid should be taken with a full glass of water or other fluid.

Usual Dose

2 tsp. every 4 hours as needed for cough relief.

Overdosage

Symptoms include breathing difficulties, pinpoint pupils, lack of response to pain stimulation, cold or clammy skin, slow heartbeat, low blood pressure, convulsions, heart attack, or extreme tiredness progressing to stupor and then coma. The victim should be taken to an emergency room immediately. ALWAYS bring the prescription bottle or container with you.

Special Information

Codeine is a respiratory depressant and affects the central nervous system (CNS), producing sleepiness, tiredness, or an inability to concentrate. Be careful if you are driving or performing other functions requiring concentration. Report persistent or intolerable side effects to your doctor.

If you take Tussi-Organidin NR Liquid 3 or more times a day and forget to take a dose, take it as soon as you remember. If it is almost time for your next dose, take 1 dose as soon as you remember and another in 3 or 4 hours, then go back to your regular schedule. Do not take a double dose.

Special Populations

Pregnancy/Breast-feeding

Tussi-Organidin NR Liquid should be avoided by pregnant women. Codeine may cause breathing problems in infants during delivery.

Nursing mothers should not take products containing codeine because they pass into breast milk and may affect the infant's breathing and general respiratory function.

Seniors

Seniors are more sensitive to the effects of codeine. Follow your doctor's directions and report side effects at once.

Ultram

see *Tramadol*, page 1107

Generic Name

Valacyclovir (val-ay-SYE-kloe-vere)

Brand Name

Valtrex

Type of Drug

Antiviral.

Prescribed for

Herpes zoster (shingles) and recurrent genital herpes.

General Information

Valacyclovir hydrochloride is rapidly converted to the antiviral acyclovir in the liver and intestine after it is absorbed into the blood. Acyclovir, the form valacyclovir takes in order to work, fights herpes virus by inhibiting and inactivating an enzyme that is key to viral reproduction and by affecting the growing viral DNA chain.

Cautions and Warnings

Do not take valacyclovir if you are **allergic** to it, acyclovir, or any component of the tablet.

Some people with advanced **HIV disease**, or who have had a **bone marrow transplant** or an **organ transplant**, taking valacyclovir developed a potentially fatal condition known as TTP (blood-clotting disorder). This drug should not be taken by anyone with **AIDS** or people with a **compromised immune system**.

High doses of acyclovir (the active drug to which valacyclovir is converted in the intestine) taken over long periods of time have caused **reduced sperm count** in lab animals, but this effect has not yet been reported in humans.

Possible Side Effects

▼ Most common: headache, diarrhea, dizziness, weakness, constipation, abdominal pain, appetite loss, nausea, and vomiting.

▼ Less common: aching joints, tingling in the hands or feet, stomach gas, fatigue, rash, not feeling well, leg pain, sore throat, a bad taste in the mouth, sleeplessness, and fever.

Drug Interactions

• Cimetidine and probenecid slow the rate at which valacyclovir is converted to acyclovir, but this does not change valacyclovir's effectiveness. No adjustments in valacyclovir dosage is necessary.

• Cimetidine and probenecid may decrease acyclovir elimination from your body and increase drug blood levels, raising the chance of side effects.

• Combining acyclovir and zidovudine (an AIDS drugs— also known as AZT) may lead to severe drowsiness or lethargy.

Food Interactions

None known.

Usual Dose

Adult: shingles—1000 mg 3 times a day for 7 days. Genital

herpes—500 mg twice a day for 5 days. Dosage is reduced in people with kidney disease.

Child (age 12 and under): not recommended.

Overdosage

There are no known cases of valacyclovir overdose. Acyclovir has been taken in doses of up to 4800 mg a day for 5 days without serious adverse effects. However, if acyclovir overdose were to occur it would likely lead to kidney damage due to the deposition of drug crystals in the kidney. Call your local poison control center for more information.

Special Information

Treatment with valacyclovir must be started as soon as possible after shingles are diagnosed. All information on the effectiveness of this drug was gathered from cases in which treatment was begun within 72 hours of diagnosis.

Women with genital herpes have an increased risk of cervical cancer. Check with your doctor about the need for an annual Pap smear.

Herpes may be transmitted even if you do not have symptoms of active disease. To avoid giving the condition to a sexual partner, do not have intercourse while visible herpes lesions are present. A condom should protect against transmission of the herpesvirus, but spermicidal products or diaphragms do not. Valacyclovir alone will not prevent herpes transmission.

Call your doctor if valacyclovir does not relieve your symptoms, if side effects become severe or intolerable, or if you become pregnant or want to begin breast-feeding.

Check with your dentist or doctor about how to take care of your teeth if you notice swelling or tenderness of the gums.

If you forget a dose of valacyclovir, take it as soon as you remember. If it is almost time for your next dose, skip the dose you forgot and continue with your regular schedule. Do not take a double dose.

Special Populations

Pregnancy/Breast-feeding

Acyclovir crosses into the circulation of the fetus. Animal studies have shown that large doses of acyclovir—up to 125 times the human dose—causes damage to both mother and fetus. While there is no information that acyclovir affects a human fetus, do not use valacyclovir if you are pregnant unless it is specifically prescribed by your doctor and the possible benefit outweighs the risk of taking it. The drug manufacturer maintains a registry of pregnant women taking this drug to keep track of how it affects birth outcomes.

Nothing is known about valacyclovir in nursing mothers. It is known that acyclovir passes into breast milk at concentrations up to 4 times the concentration in blood, and it has been found in the urine of a nursing infant. No side effects have been observed in nursing babies, but mothers who must take valacyclovir should consider bottle-feeding their infants.

Seniors

Valacyclovir has been studied in healthy seniors age 50 and older. People over 50 with shingles tend to have more severe attacks and respond best to valacyclovir treatment if the drug is started within 48 to 72 hours of the appearance of the first rash. Seniors with reduced kidney function should be given a lower dose of oral valacyclovir than younger adults.

Generic Name

Valproic Acid (val-PROE-ik) G

Brand Names

Depakene   Depakote   Depakote Sprinkle

Type of Drug

Anticonvulsant and antimanic.

Prescribed for

Petit mal seizure, absence seizure, and bipolar (manic-depressive) disorder; also prescribed for grand mal, myoclonic, and other seizures; prevention of fever convulsions in children; migraine headache; and anxiety or panic attacks.

General Information

This information applies to both forms of the drug: valproic acid (Depakene) and its related compound, divalproex sodium (Depakote). Divalproex sodium is made up of equal quantities of valproic acid and sodium valproate. The dosage of divalproex is measured in terms of the equivalent dosage of valproic acid.

Valproic acid is chemically unrelated to other medications used in the treatment of seizure disorders. This drug's activity may be related to its ability to increase the levels of gamma-aminobutyric acid (GABA) and to improve GABA's effects in the brain. Valproic acid also has a stabilizing effect on cell membranes within the brain, which may account for some of valproic acid's other effects.

Valproic acid is rapidly absorbed into the bloodstream after it is swallowed; the absorption of divalproate is delayed for about 1 hour until its protective coating dissolves. Valproic acid is broken down in the liver and passes out of the body in the urine.

Cautions and Warnings

Do not take valproic acid if you are **allergic** to it.

Use this drug with caution if you have a history of **liver problems**, because cases of liver failure, some resulting in death, have occurred in people taking valproic acid products. **Children under 2 years old** are especially sensitive to liver failure associated with valproic acid, especially if they are also taking other anticonvulsants or if they have congenital disorders of metabolism, severe seizure disorders, mental retardation, or organic brain disease. After age 2, the chance of a fatal liver reaction decreases tremendously. Valproic acid can also cause ammonia to be present in the bloodstream, another factor that worsens liver disease.

If it is going to occur, serious liver disease usually develops during the first 6 months of valproic acid treatment and is often preceded by feeling unwell, weakness, tiredness, facial swelling, appetite loss, yellowing of the skin or whites of the eyes, vomiting, and loss of seizure control. Your doctor should check your liver function before beginning valproic acid treatment and periodically thereafter.

Valproic acid can affect **platelet function**, leading to bruising, bleeding, or changes in normal blood-clotting function.

Possible Side Effects

Side effects worsen as your valproic acid dose increases.

▼ Most common: nausea, vomiting, indigestion, sedation or sleepiness, weakness, rash, emotional upset, depression, psychosis, aggression, hyperactive behavior, and changes in various blood components.

Possible Side Effects *(continued)*

▼ Less common: diarrhea, stomach cramps, constipation, increased or decreased appetite, headache, loss of eye-muscle control, drooping eyelids, double vision, spots before the eyes, loss of muscle control or coordination, and tremors.

Drug Interactions

- Valproic acid may increase the depressive effects of alcohol, sleeping pills, tranquilizers, phenobarbital, primidone, and other depressant drugs. It may slightly increase the amount of clozapine or zidovudine (AZT) in the blood.
- Dosages of carbamazepine, clonazepam, ethosuximide, lamotrigine, and phenytoin may have to be adjusted when you begin valproic acid treatment.
- Valproic acid may affect oral anticoagulant (blood-thinning) drugs; your anticoagulant dose may have to be adjusted.
- Aspirin, cimetidine, chlorpromazine, erythromycin, and felbamate may increase the risk of valproic acid side effects.
- Rifampin may reduce the effectiveness of valproic acid.
- Valproic acid may increase the need for levocarnitine.
- Valproic acid may increase the risk of bleeding or bruising if taken together with other drugs that affect platelet stickiness. These include aspirin, which also increases valproic acid side effects, dipyridamole, nonsteroidal anti-inflammatory drugs (NSAIDs), sulfinpyrazone, and ticlopidine.
- Valproic acid may cause false-positive reactions in the urine ketone tests used in diabetes.
- Charcoal tablets interfere with the absorption of valproic acid into the bloodstream.

Food Interactions

Food slightly prolongs the time it takes for valproic acid to be absorbed into the bloodstream. Nevertheless, you may take it with food if it upsets your stomach. Do not take divalproate (Depakote) with milk.

Depakote Sprinkle can be taken whole or mixed with a tsp. of pudding, applesauce, or other soft food. The food/drug mixture should be swallowed without chewing as soon as it is mixed.

Mix valproic acid syrup with food to make it taste better.

Usual Dose

7–27 mg per lb. a day. Valproic acid is best taken in 1 dose at bedtime to minimize any sedative effects. Daily dosages greater than 250 mg should be split into 2 or more doses a day.

Overdosage

Valproic acid overdose may result in restlessness, hallucinations, flapping tremors of the hands, deep coma, and death. Call your doctor or take the victim to a hospital emergency room immediately. ALWAYS bring the prescription bottle or container with you.

Special Information

This medication may cause drowsiness: Be careful while driving or operating hazardous machinery.

Do not chew or crush valproic acid capsules or tablets.

Do not switch brands of valproic acid without your doctor's knowledge. In at least 1 case, seizures resulted when a person was switched to a new product after 3 seizure-free years on another brand of valproic acid.

Valproic acid can cause mouth, gum, and throat irritation or bleeding, and increased risk of mouth infections. People taking this medicine should pay special attention to caring for their mouth and gums. Dental work should be delayed if your blood counts are low.

People with a seizure disorder should carry special identification indicating their condition and the drug being taken.

If you take valproic acid once a day and forget a dose, take it as soon as possible. If you do not remember until the next day, skip the dose you forgot and continue with your regular schedule. If you take valproic acid 2 or more times a day and forget a dose, and you remember within 6 hours of your regular time, take it as soon as possible. Take the rest of that day's doses at regularly spaced intervals. Go back to your regular schedule the next day. Never take a double dose.

Special Populations

Pregnancy/Breast-feeding

The chance of birth defects may be increased in pregnant women who take valproic acid during the first 3 months of pregnancy. However, most mothers who take anticonvulsants, including valproic acid, deliver healthy babies. Anticonvulsants should be used only to control maternal seizures.

Valproic acid passes into breast milk and may affect a nursing infant. Nursing women who must take this drug should consider bottle-feeding their babies.

Seniors

Valproic acid is broken down by the liver and passes out of the body through the kidneys. Because seniors often have reduced kidney and liver function, they may accumulate more valproic acid in their bloodstream and may be more likely to develop side effects. Seniors should be treated with smaller doses of valproic acid.

Generic Name

Valsartan (val-SAR-tan)

Brand Name

Diovan

Type of Drug

Angiotensin II antagonist.

Prescribed for

High blood pressure.

General Information

Valsartan is a member of a class of drugs for high blood pressure called angiotensin receptor antagonists. These medications work by interfering with the special sites in blood vessels and other tissues where angiotensin II, a potent hormone that normally helps to maintain blood pressure, exerts its effect. Do not confuse these drugs with the many angiotensin-converting enzyme (ACE) inhibitors in use today; ACE inhibitors interrupt the body's production of angiotensin II instead of blocking its effect.

Valsartan begins to lower blood pressure within 2 hours of taking a dose. Its maximum effect is experienced within 6 hours and lasts for 24 hours. Maximum blood pressure reduction occurs after approximately 4 weeks of taking valsartan. Your doctor may lower your blood pressure further by either raising your valsartan dose or by adding a thiazide-type diuretic to your medication program.

Cautions and Warnings

Do not take valsartan if you are **sensitive** or **allergic** to it.

People with **liver disease** can have up to twice as much valsartan in their blood, which can worsen some liver and kidney function tests. Dosage adjustment is not usually needed, but people with liver or **kidney disease** should be cautious when taking valsartan.

Valsartan can raise **blood potassium** levels.

Possible Side Effects

Side effects are generally mild and go away after a short time.

▼ Most common: fatigue, sleeplessness, upset stomach, viral infections, and abdominal pain.

▼ Rare: dizziness or fainting when rising from a sitting or lying position, allergic reactions, weakness, heart palpitations, chest pain, itching and rash, constipation, dry mouth, upset stomach and gas, back pain, muscle cramps or pain, anxiety, sleeplessness, tingling in the hands or feet, tiredness, breathing difficulties, dizziness, impotence, appetite loss, vomiting, and temporary swelling of the face, hands, feet, genitalia, or other body parts. Other side effects—headache, dizziness, upper respiratory infections, cough, diarrhea, rhinitis, sore throat, swelling and joint pains—are experienced with about the same frequency by people taking a placebo (sugar pills) as by those taking valsartan.

People taking ACE inhibitors have more dry cough than people taking valsartan.

Drug Interactions

• Valsartan may further lower blood pressure when it is taken with other blood-pressure-lowering medications.

Food Interactions

Food moderately affects the absorption of valsartan, but it may be taken without regard to food or meals.

Usual Dose

Adult: 80–320 mg once a day.
Child: not recommended.

Overdosage

The most likely symptoms of valsartan overdose are low blood pressure, dizziness or fainting, and rapid heartbeat. Overdose victims should be taken to a hospital emergency room at once. ALWAYS bring the prescription bottle or container with you.

Special Information

If you forget to take a dose of valsartan, take it as soon as you remember. If it is almost time for your next dose, skip the dose you forgot and continue with your regular schedule. Do not take a double dose.

Avoid strenuous exercise and/or very hot weather because heavy sweating or dehydration can cause a rapid blood-pressure drop.

Avoid over-the-counter diet pills, decongestants, and stimulants that can raise blood pressure.

Special Populations

Pregnancy/Breast-feeding

Valsartan should not be taken during the last 6 months of pregnancy because it can directly affect the fetus, possibly leading to fetal injury or death. If you are or might be pregnant, you should take a different medication for high blood pressure.

Animal studies show that valsartan passes into breast milk, but it is not known if this happens in humans. Nursing mothers should avoid valsartan or bottle-feed their babies because of the chance that it will affect the nursing child.

Seniors

Seniors may take this drug without special precautions.

Vancenase AQ

*see **Corticosteroids, Nasal**, page 266*

Vasotec

*see **Enalapril**, page 365*

Veetids

*see **Penicillin Antibiotics**, page 846*

Generic Name

Venlafaxine (ven-luh-FAX-ene)

Brand Names

Effexor   Effexor XR

Type of Drug

Antidepressant.

Prescribed for

Depression.

General Information

Venlafaxine is chemically different from other types of anti-depressant drugs. It is believed that venlafaxine works by inhibiting the ability of nerve endings in the brain to absorb serotonin, norepinephrine, and dopamine; this drug does not affect monoamine oxidase (MAO). Venlafaxine is well absorbed into the bloodstream and passes out of the body primarily via the urine.

Cautions and Warnings

People with severe **kidney or liver disease** may require smaller than normal doses of venlafaxine because these conditions may cause blood levels of the drug to increase by 30% to 50%.

Venlafaxine can raise **blood pressure**. If this happens, your dosage of venlafaxine may have to be reduced. Venlafaxine has not been fully studied in people with recent heart attack or unstable heart disease, although a small study of the cardiograms of such patients revealed no unusual changes.

Possible Side Effects

Side effects increase as venlafaxine dosage increases.
▼ Most common: blurred vision, tiredness, dry mouth,

Possible Side Effects (continued)

dizziness, sleeplessness, nervousness, tremors, weakness, sweating, nausea, constipation, appetite loss, vomiting, impotence, and abnormal ejaculation.

▼ Less common: changes in sense of taste, ringing in the ears, dilated pupils, high blood pressure, rapid heartbeat, anxiety, reduced sex drive, agitation, chills, yawning, and inability to experience orgasm.

▼ Rare: dizziness when rising from a sitting or lying position, unusual dreaming, muscle stiffness, tingling in the hands or feet, confusion, abnormal thinking, depression, urinary difficulties, twitching, chest pain, trauma, weight loss, itching, rash, diarrhea, upset stomach, gas, menstrual disturbances, and urinary difficulties. Venlafaxine is associated with a variety of other rare side effects including swelling, weight gain, hangover-type reactions, hernia, unusual sensitivity to the sun, suicide attempts, appendicitis, thyroid changes, migraines, angina pain, heart rhythm changes, increased pulse rate, difficulty swallowing, stomach irritation, irritated or bleeding gums, salivation, soft stools, tongue discoloration, ulcers, reduced blood cell counts, abnormal vision, ear pain, acne, hair loss, brittle nails, dry skin, herpes, and hairiness.

Drug Interactions

• Taking venlafaxine within 2 weeks of taking a monoamine oxidase inhibitor (MAOI) antidepressant may cause severe reactions including high fever, muscle rigidity or spasm, mental changes, and fluctuations in pulse, temperature, or breathing rate. People stopping venlafaxine should wait at least 1 week before starting an MAOI.

• Cimetidine reduces the rate at which venlafaxine is broken down in the body and can increase drug levels in the blood, although the effect on the body may be minimal.

Food Interactions

Take each dose of venlafaxine with food.

Usual Dose

Adult: 75–350 mg a day, divided into 2–3 doses. People with severe kidney or liver disease should receive half the usual daily dose. Those with moderate kidney disease may only need their daily dose reduced by 25%.

Child (under age 18): not recommended.

Overdosage

Most people who took an overdose of venlafaxine reported no symptoms, although some became tired. One person experienced mild convulsions and cardiac effects. Contact your doctor or emergency room for more information. People who have taken an overdose of venlafaxine should be brought to a hospital emergency room for treatment. ALWAYS bring the prescription bottle or container with you.

Special Information

Call your doctor if you develop rash, hives, or any other allergic-type reaction.

Venlafaxine may make you tired; take care when driving, performing complex tasks, or operating equipment. Avoid alcoholic beverages.

Because of the possibility of drug interactions, be sure to tell your doctor or pharmacist if you are taking any other medication.

If you forget to take a dose of venlafaxine, take it as soon as you remember. However, if it is almost time for your next dose, skip the dose you forgot and continue with your regular schedule. Do not take a double dose.

Do not suddenly stop taking this drug. Venlafaxine dosage should be gradually reduced over a 2-week period.

Special Populations

Pregnancy/Breast-feeding

Animal studies of venlafaxine in doses 10 times larger than the maximum human dose indicate that venlafaxine may lead to low birth weights and other problems. No information is available on the effect of venlafaxine on human pregnancy. It should only be taken during pregnancy if it is deemed crucial and if the potential benefits outweigh the risks.

It is not known if venlafaxine or its by-products pass into breast milk. Nursing mothers who must take the drug should consider bottle-feeding their babies.

Seniors

Seniors may be more sensitive to the side effects of venlafaxine.

Ventolin

*see **Albuterol**, page 25*

Generic Name

Verapamil (vuh-RAP-uh-mil) Ⓖ

Brand Names

Calan	Isoptin
Calan SR	Isoptin SR
Covera HS	Verelan

Type of Drug

Calcium channel blocker.

Prescribed for

Angina pectoris and Prinzmetal's angina, high blood pressure, abnormal heart rhythm, asthma, cardiomyopathy, migraine headache, nighttime leg cramps, and bipolar (manic-depressive) disorder.

General Information

Verapamil hydrochloride is one of many calcium channel blockers available in the U.S. These drugs block the passage of calcium, an essential factor in muscle contraction, into the heart and smooth muscles. Such blockage of calcium interferes with the contraction of these muscles, which in turn dilates (widens) the veins and vessels that supply blood to them. This action has several beneficial effects. Because arteries are dilated, they are less likely to spasm. In addition, because blood vessels are dilated, both blood pressure and the amount of oxygen used by the heart muscle is reduced. Verapamil is therefore useful in treating not only high blood pressure but also angina pectoris (brief attacks of chest pain), a condition related to poor oxygen supply to the heart muscle. Other calcium channel blocker are prescribed for abnormal heart rhythm, heart failure, cardiomyopathy (loss of blood-pumping ability due to damaged heart muscle), and diseases that involve blood-vessel spasm, such as migraine headache and Raynaud's syndrome.

Verapamil affects the movement of calcium only into muscle cells; it has no effect on calcium in the blood.

The sustained-release brands of verapamil should be used only for high blood pressure.

Cautions and Warnings

Verapamil may cause **low blood pressure** in some patients.

Patients taking a beta-blocking drug who begin taking verapamil may develop **heart failure**.

Do not take this drug if you have had an **allergic reaction** to it.

Verapamil may cause **angina** when treatment is first started, when dosage is increased, or if the drug is rapidly withdrawn. This can be avoided by reducing dosage gradually.

Studies have shown that people taking calcium channel blockers—usually those taken several times a day, not those taken only once daily—have a greater chance of having a **heart attack** than do people taking beta blockers or other medication for the same purposes. Discuss this with your doctor to be sure you are receiving the best possible treatment.

In small numbers of people, verapamil can interfere with the movement of nervous impulses within the heart, leading to an unusual **slowing of heart rate**.

People with **hypertrophic cardiomyopathy** (progressive weakening and destruction of heart muscle) who are receiving up to 720 mg a day of verapamil are at risk of developing severe cardiac side effects. Most of these effects respond to dosage reduction, and people generally may continue on verapamil at a lower dose.

People with severe **liver disease** break down verapamil much more slowly than do people with mildly diseased or normal livers. Your doctor should take this into account when determining your daily verapamil dosage. Caution is recommended in people with severe **kidney disease**, though dose adjustment may not be needed.

Verapamil may slow the transmission of nerve impulses to muscle in people with **Duchenne's muscular dystrophy**, possibly causing respiratory muscle failure. Reduced verapamil dosage may be needed.

Possible Side Effects

Side effects of calcium channel blockers are generally mild and rarely cause people to stop taking them. Verap-

Possible Side Effects *(continued)*

amil generally causes fewer side effects than other calcium channel blockers.

▼ Most common: skin rash; low blood pressure; slowed
heartbeat; heart failure or lung congestion marked by
coughing, wheezing, or breathing difficulties; tiredness or
weakness; swelling of the ankles, feet, or legs; headache;
dizziness; light-headedness; constipation; and nausea.

▼ Rare: chest pain, rapid or irregular heartbeat, unusual production of breast milk, bleeding or tender gums,
fainting, flushing, and feeling warm. Other rare side
effects have affected a variety of body systems. Report
anything unusual to your doctor.

Some patients taking verapamil have experienced heart
attack and abnormal heart rhythm, but the occurrence of
these effects has not been directly linked to verapamil.

Drug Interactions

• Long-term verapamil use will cause the levels of digoxin
and digitoxin drugs in the blood to increase by 50% to 70%.
The dose of these drugs will have to be lowered drastically if
verapamil is added.

• Disopyramide should not be taken within 48 hours of
taking verapamil because of possible interaction.

• Patients taking verapamil together with quinidine may
experience very low blood pressure, slow heartbeat, and fluid
in the lungs.

• Verapamil's effectiveness and its side effects may be
reversed by taking calcium products, including antacids.

• Verapamil may interact with beta-blocking drugs to cause
heart failure, very low blood pressure, or increased angina.
However, in many cases these drugs have been taken together with no problem. Low blood pressure can also result
from taking verapamil with fentanyl (a narcotic pain reliever).

• Verapamil may cause unexpected blood pressure reduction in patients also taking other medication to control their
high blood pressure.

• Cimetidine and ranitidine increase the amount of verapamil in the blood and may account for a slight increase in its
effect.

• The combination of dantrolene and verapamil may lead

to high blood-calcium levels and heart muscle depression. If you are taking dantrolene, a calcium channel blocker other than verapamil should be prescribed by your doctor.

• Verapamil may increase the effects of carbamazepine, cyclosporine, and theophylline products, increasing the chance of side effects with those drugs.

• Verapamil may decrease the amount of lithium in your body, leading to a possible loss of antimanic control, lithium toxicity, and psychotic symptoms.

• Rifampin, barbiturates, phenytoin and similar antiseizure medicines, vitamin D, and sulfinpyrazone may decrease the amount of verapamil in your blood and its effect on your body.

Food Interactions

Take immediate-release products at least 1 hour before or 2 hours after meals. Take sustained-release products with food if they upset your stomach.

Usual Dose

120–480 mg a day, according to your needs.

Overdosage

Overdose of verapamil can cause low blood pressure. Symptoms are dizziness, weakness, and slowed heartbeat. If you have taken an overdose of verapamil, call your doctor or go to an emergency room. ALWAYS bring the prescription bottle or container with you.

Special Information

Call your doctor if you develop abnormal heart rhythm, swelling in the arms or legs, breathing difficulties, increased heart pain, dizziness, light-headedness, or low blood pressure. Do not stop taking verapamil abruptly.

If you forget to take a dose of verapamil, take it as soon as you remember. If it is almost time for your next dose, skip the one you forgot and continue with your regular schedule. Do not take a double dose.

Special Populations

Pregnancy/Breast-feeding

Verapamil may cause birth defects or interfere with fetal

development. Check with your doctor before taking it if you are or might be pregnant.

Verapamil passes into breast milk. Taking verapamil while nursing may cause problems; nursing mothers should take this drug only if absolutely necessary.

Seniors

Seniors are more sensitive to the side effects of verapamil and are more likely to develop low blood pressure while taking it. Follow your doctor's directions and report any side effects at once.

Generic Name

Warfarin (WOR-far-in) G

Brand Names

Coumadin   Sofarin
Panwarfin

The information in this profile also applies to the following drugs:

Generic Ingredient: Anisindione
Miradon

Generic Ingredient: Dicumarol G
Only available in generic form.

Type of Drug

Oral anticoagulant (blood thinner).

Prescribed for

Blood clots or coagulation; also prescribed for reducing the risk of recurrent heart attack or stroke and recurrent transient ischemic attack (TIA), and small cell carcinoma of the lung.

General Information

Anticoagulation is generally used to prevent the development of blood clots in the arms and legs, pulmonary embolism, heart attack, stroke, and abnormal heart rhythms. Warfarin prevents the formation of blood clots or coagulation by suppressing the body's normal production of vitamin-K-dependent factors essential to the coagulation process. If you are taking warfarin, you must take it exactly as prescribed. Notify your doctor at the earliest sign of unusual bleeding or bruising; blood in your urine or stool; or black, tarry stools. Warfarin may be affected by many other drugs, and its interactions with these drugs may be dangerous (see "Drug Interactions").

Warfarin may also be extremely dangerous if not used properly. Periodic blood tests to monitor clotting time or the time it takes to begin the clotting process are required for proper control of warfarin therapy.

Warfarin may help to prevent recurrent TIA.

Cautions and Warnings

Do not take warfarin if you are **allergic** to it. Anisindione is usually reserved for people allergic to warfarin.

Warfarin must be taken with care if you have any **blood-clotting disease**. Use of warfarin may be dangerous and should be discussed with your doctor if you have: **threatened abortion; past or planned eye or nervous system surgery; protein C deficiency**—a hereditary condition; **liver inflammation or disease; kidney disease; any infection being treated with an antibiotic;** active **tuberculosis;** severe or prolonged **dietary deficiencies; stomach ulcer or bleeding; bleeding from the genital or urinary areas;** moderate to severe uncontrolled **high blood pressure;** severe **diabetes; vein irritation; disease of the large bowel,** such as diverticulitis or ulcerative colitis; and subacute bacterial endocarditis. People with **congestive heart failure** may be more sensitive to dicumarol than to other anticoagulants. Talk to your doctor if you have any of these conditions.

Anisindione can cause **hepatitis** and **agranulocytosis** (condition characterized by a reduction in the number of white blood cells).

Anticoagulant therapy may increase the release of microplaques into the bloodstream. These microplaques may block very small blood vessels, leading to **purple toe syndrome** (condition that occurs when pressure exerted by normal walking leads to bleeding into the skin of your toes). This usually goes away when anticoagulant treatment is stopped but it may be a sign of a more serious problem present in another part of your body.

Women taking anticoagulants may be at risk of **ovarian**

bleeding when they ovulate. Report anything unusual to your doctor.

People taking warfarin must be extremely careful to **avoid cuts, bruises, or other injuries that may cause internal or external bleeding**.

Possible Side Effects

Warfarin and Dicumarol

▼ Most common: bleeding, which may occur with usual dosages and even when the results of blood tests used to monitor anticoagulant therapy are normal. If you bleed abnormally while you are taking anticoagulants and have eliminated the possibility of drug interactions, call your doctor immediately—another problem may be present.

▼ Less common: abdominal cramps, nausea, vomiting, diarrhea, fever, anemia, adverse effects on blood components, hepatitis, jaundice (symptoms include yellowing of the skin or whites of the eyes), itching, rash, hair loss, sore throat or mouth, red or orange urine, painful or persistent erection in males, and purple-toe syndrome.

Anisindione

▼ Common: rash.

▼ Less common: headache, sore throat, blurred vision, hepatitis, liver or kidney damage, jaundice (symptoms include yellowing of the skin or whites of the eyes), red or orange urine, and a variety of effects on blood-system components.

Drug Interactions

• Anticoagulants may have more drug interactions than any other kind of drug. Your doctor and pharmacist should keep records of all medications you take to review for possible negative drug interactions.

• Drugs that may increase the effect of warfarin include the following: acetaminophen; aminoglycoside antibiotics; amiodarone; androgen; aspirin and other salicylate drugs; beta blockers; cephalosporin antibiotics; chloral hydrate; chloramphenicol; chlorpropamide; cimetidine; clofibrate; corticosteroids; cyclophosphamide; dextrothyroxine; diflunisal; disulfiram; erythromycin; fluconazole; gemfibrozil; glucagon;

hydantoin antiseizure drugs—blood levels of the hydantoins may also be increased in this interaction; ifosfamide, an influenza virus vaccine; isoniazid; ketoconazole; loop diuretics; lovastatin; metronidazole; miconazole; mineral oil; moricizine; nalidixic acid; nonsteroidal anti-inflammatory drugs (NSAIDs); omeprazole; penicillin; phenylbutazone; propafenone; propoxyphene; quinidine; quinine; quinolone antibacterials; sulfa drugs; sulfinpyrazone; tamoxifen; tetracycline antibiotics; thioamines; thyroid hormones; and vitamin E.

• Some drugs decrease the effect of warfarin and the interaction may be just as dangerous. Some examples are alcohol, aminoglutethimide, ascorbic acid (vitamin C), barbiturates, carbamazepine, cholestyramine, dicloxacillin, glutethimide, ethchlorvynol, etretinate, meprobamate, griseofulvin, estrogen, oral contraceptives ("the Pill"), chlorthalidone, nafcillin, rifampin, spironolactone, sucralfate, thiazide-type diuretics, trazodone, and vitamin K.

• No matter what the interaction, it is essential that your doctor and pharmacist know about every medication you are taking including over-the-counter (OTC) drugs containing aspirin. Consult your physician or pharmacist before using any OTC drugs.

Food Interactions

Warfarin is best taken on an empty stomach because food slows the rate at which it is absorbed by the blood.

Vitamin K counteracts the effects of warfarin. Avoid eating large quantities of vitamin-K-rich foods, such as spinach and other green, leafy vegetables. Any change in dietary habits or alcohol intake may affect warfarin's action.

Usual Dose

Warfarin: 2–15 mg or more a day; dosage is variable and must be individualized by your doctor.

Anisindione: 300 mg the first day, 200 mg the second day, 100 mg the third day, and 25–250 mg daily thereafter.

Dicumarol: 200–300 mg the first day, then 25–200 mg a day.

Overdosage

The primary symptom of overdose is bleeding. Bleeding may make itself known by appearance of blood in the urine or stool, an unusual number of black-and-blue marks, oozing of blood from minor cuts, or bleeding from the gums after brushing the teeth. If bleeding does not stop within 10 to 15 minutes, call your doctor. Your doctor may tell you to skip a dose of warfarin or go to a hospital or doctor's office for blood evaluations, or he or she may give you a prescription for vitamin K, which antagonizes the effect of warfarin. This approach has some dangers because it may complicate subsequent anticoagulant therapy. Your doctor must make this decision.

Special Information

Do not change warfarin brands without your doctor's knowledge. Different brands of warfarin may not be equivalent to each other and may not produce the same effect on your blood.

Do not stop taking warfarin unless directed to do so by your doctor. Be sure you have enough medication when you travel or at times when you may not have access to your regular pharmacy.

Do not stop or start ANY other medication without your doctor's and/or pharmacist's knowledge. Avoid alcohol, aspirin and other salicylates, and drastic changes in your diet, since all of these may affect your response.

Call your doctor if you develop unusual bleeding or bruising, red or black tarry stool, or red or dark-brown urine.

Warfarin may turn your urine a red or orange color. This is different from blood in the urine—which causes urine to appear red or brownish in color—and generally happens only if your urine has less acid in it than normal.

If you forget to take a dose of warfarin, take it as soon as you remember, then continue with your regular schedule. If you do not remember until the next day, skip the missed dose and continue with your regular schedule. Do not take a double dose, since doubling the dose may cause bleeding. Be sure to call your doctor if you forget a dose.

Special Populations

Pregnancy/Breast-feeding

Warfarin should not be taken by pregnant women. If you are taking warfarin and become pregnant, call your doctor immediately. Warfarin passes into the circulation of the fetus and causes bleeding, brain and other abnormalities, and stillbirth in 30% of fetuses exposed to the drug.

In some pregnant women, the benefits to be gained from taking warfarin may outweigh its risks, but the drug should not be taken during the first 3 months of pregnancy. The decision to use an anticoagulant is an important one that should be made by you and your doctor. Pregnant women who need an anticoagulant are often given heparin—which must be injected—because it does not cross into the fetal bloodstream.

Warfarin and dicumarol pass into breast milk in an inactive form. Full-term babies are not affected by warfarin but dicumarol may affect a nursing child. The effect on premature babies is not known. Nursing mothers who must take dicumarol should bottle-feed their babies.

Seniors
Seniors may be more sensitive to the effects of warfarin. The reason for this is not clear but may involve a reduced ability to clear the drug from the body. Seniors generally require lower doses to achieve the same results.

Xanax

see **Alprazolam**, page 35

Type of Drug
Xanthine Bronchodilators (ZAN-thene)

Brand Names

Generic Ingredient: Aminophylline G
Norphyl   Truphylline
Phyllocontin

Generic Ingredient: Dyphylline G
Dilor   Lufyllin-400
Dilor-400   Neothylline
Lufyllin

Generic Ingredient: Oxtriphylline G
Choledyl   Choledyl SA

Generic Ingredient: Theophylline Ⓖ

Aerolate*	Theo-Dur
Aquaphyllin Ⓐ	Theo-Dur Sprinkle
Asmalix	Theo-Sav
Bronkodyl	Theo-X
Elixomin	Theobid Duracaps
Elixophyllin	Theobid Jr. Duracaps
Lanophyllin Ⓢ	Theochron
Quibron-T Dividose	Theoclear-80 Ⓐ
Quibron-T/SR Dividose	Theoclear L.A.
Respbid	Theolair Ⓐ
Slo-bid Gyrocaps	Theolair-SR
Slo-Phyllin*	Theophylline SR
Slo-Phyllin Gyrocaps	Theospan-SR
Sustaire	Theostat-80
T-Phyl	Theovent
Theo-24	Uniphyl

*Some products in this brand-name group are alcohol or sugar free. Consult your pharmacist.

Prescribed for

Asthma and bronchospasm associated with emphysema, bronchitis, and other diseases; also prescribed for essential tremors and chronic obstructive pulmonary disease (COPD).

General Information

Xanthine bronchodilators are a mainstay of therapy for bronchial asthma and similar diseases. Although the dosage of each of these drugs is different, they all work by relaxing bronchial muscles and helping to reverse spasms. The exact way in which they work is not known, however.

Some xanthine bronchodilators are sustained-release products that act throughout the day. These minimize potential side effects by avoiding the peaks and valleys associated with immediate-release xanthine drugs. They also allow you to reduce the total number of daily doses.

Initial treatment with a xanthine bronchodilator requires your doctor to take blood samples to assess how much of the drug is in your blood. For theophylline, the standard against which all other members of the group are compared, a level of between 10 and 20 mcg per ml—quantity per blood volume—is generally considered desirable. For dyphylline, the minimum effective level is 12 mcg per ml. Dosage adjustments may be required based on these blood tests and on your response to the therapy.

Because dyphylline is not eliminated by the liver, it is not subject to many of the drug interactions or limitations placed on the other xanthine bronchodilators. However, dosage must be altered in the presence of kidney failure.

Cautions and Warnings

Do not use a xanthine bronchodilator if you are **allergic** or **sensitive** to any of these medications. If you have a **stomach ulcer**, congestive **heart failure**, **heart disease**, **liver disease**, **low blood-oxygen levels**, or **high blood pressure**, or are an **alcoholic**, you should use this drug with caution. People with **seizure disorders** should not take a xanthine bronchodilator unless they are receiving appropriate anticonvulsant medicines. Theophylline may cause or worsen preexisting **abnormal heart rhythm**. Any change in heart rate or rhythm warrants your doctor's immediate attention.

Status asthmaticus, a medical condition in which the breathing passages are almost completely closed, does not respond to oral bronchodilators. Victims of this condition must be taken to a hospital emergency room at once for treatment.

Serious side effects, including convulsions, serious arrhythmias, and death, may be among the initial signs of drug toxicity. Periodic monitoring by your physician is mandatory if you are taking one of these drugs.

Possible Side Effects

Side effects are directly related to the amount of drug in your blood. As long as you stay in the proper range—below 20 mcg per ml of blood—you should experience few, if any, problems.

▼ Most common: nausea; vomiting; stomach pain; diarrhea; irritability; restlessness; difficulty sleeping; rectal irritation or bleeding, especially with suppositories; and rapid breathing.

▼ Less common: excitability, high blood sugar, muscle twitching or spasms, heart palpitations, seizures, brain damage, or death. These effects are more likely when drug levels reach 35 mcg per ml or more.

Possible Side Effects *(continued)*

▼ Rare: vomiting blood, regurgitating stomach contents while lying down, fever, headache, rash, hair loss, and dehydration.

Drug Interactions

• Taking two xanthine bronchodilators together may increase side effects.

• Xanthine bronchodilators are often given in combination with a stimulant drug such as ephedrine. Such combinations can cause excessive stimulation and should be used only as your doctor specifically directs.

• Reports have indicated that combining erythromycin, flu vaccine, allopurinol, beta blockers, calcium channel blockers, cimetidine—and, rarely, ranitidine—oral contraceptives, corticosteroids, disulfiram, ephedrine, interferon, mexiletine, quinolone antibacterials, or thiabendazole with a xanthine bronchodilator will increase blood levels of the xanthine bronchodilator. Higher blood levels mean the possibility of more side effects. Tetracycline may also increase the chances for xanthine bronchodilator side effects.

• The following drugs may decrease theophylline levels: aminoglutethimide, barbiturates, charcoal, ketoconazole, rifampin, sulfinpyrazone, sympathomimetic drugs, and phenytoin and other hydantoin anticonvulsants. The hydantoin level may also be reduced.

• Smoking cigarettes or marijuana makes xanthine bronchodilators less effective by increasing the rate at which your liver breaks them down. This does not apply to dyphylline.

• Drugs that may either increase or decrease xanthine bronchodilator levels include carbamazepine, isoniazid, and furosemide and other loop diuretics. Persons combining a xanthine bronchodilator with one of these drugs must be evaluated individually. Again, consult your doctor when combining xanthine bronchodilators with any of these drugs.

• People with an overactive thyroid clear xanthine bronchodilators faster and may require a larger dose. People with an underactive thyroid have the opposite reaction. Correcting thyroid function through medical or surgical treatment will normalize your response to a xanthine bronchodilator.

• A xanthine bronchodilator may counteract the sedative effect of valium and other benzodiazepine tranquilizers.

• Xanthine bronchodilators may interfere with or interact with a number of different drugs used during anesthesia. Your doctor may temporarily alter your bronchodilator dose or change drugs to avoid this problem.

• Blood lithium levels may be lowered by xanthine bronchodilators.

• Probenecid may increase the effects of dyphylline by interfering with its removal from the body through the kidneys.

• Xanthine bronchodilators may counteract the sedative effects of propofol.

Food Interactions

To obtain a consistent effect from your medication, take it at the same time each day on an empty stomach, at least 1 hour before or 2 hours after meals.

Theophylline is eliminated from the body faster if your diet is high in protein and low in carbohydrates. Eating charcoal-broiled beef also aids theophylline elimination. Conversely, the rate at which your body eliminates theophylline is reduced by a high-carbohydrate, low-protein diet. You may take some food with a liquid or immediate-release xanthine bronchodilator if it upsets your stomach. Dyphylline is not affected in this way.

Caffeine—a xanthine derivative—may add to the side effects of the xanthine bronchodilators, except dyphylline. Avoid large amounts of caffeine-containing products, such as coffee, tea, cola, cocoa, and chocolate, while taking one of these drugs.

Usual Dose

Aminophylline
 Adult (age 16 and over): 100–200 mg every 6 hours. Sustained-release—200–500 mg a day in 1–3 doses.
 Child (under age 16): 50–100 mg every 6 hours, or 1–2.5 mg per lb. of body weight every 6 hours.

Each 100 mg of aminophylline is equal in potency to 79 mg of theophylline. Aminophylline dosage is calculated on the basis of theophylline equivalents and must be tailored to your specific condition. The best dose is the lowest that will control your symptoms.

Dyphylline
 Adult: up to 7 mg per lb. of body weight 4 times a day.
 There is no established theophylline equivalent dosage for

dyphylline. Dyphylline dosage must be tailored to your specific condition and must be reduced in the presence of kidney failure. The best dose is the lowest that will control your symptoms.

Oxtriphylline
   Adult: about 2 mg per lb. of body weight, 3 times a day. Sustained-release—400–600 mg every 12 hours.
   Child (age 1–9): 2.8 mg per lb. of body weight 4 times a day.

Each 100 mg of oxtriphylline is roughly equal to 64 mg of theophylline. Oxtriphylline dosage is calculated on the basis of theophylline equivalents and must be tailored to your specific condition.

Theophylline
   Adult: up to 6 mg per lb. of body weight a day, to a maximum daily dose of 900 mg. Sustained-release—same dosage, but taken 1–3 times a day.
   Child (age 12–16): up to 8.1 mg per lb. of body weight a day.
   Child (age 9–11): up to 9 mg per lb. of body weight a day.
   Child (age 1–8): up to 10.9 mg per lb. of body weight a day.
   Infant (6–52 weeks): Your doctor will calculate total daily dosage in mg by a formula that factors in age and weight. Under 6 months, give ⅓ the total daily dosage every 8 hours; age 26 weeks—1 year, give ¼ the total daily dosage every 6 hours.
   Premature Infant (25 days and over): 0.68 mg per lb. of body weight every 12 hours.
   Premature Infant (under 24 days): 0.45 mg per lb. of body weight every 12 hours.

These dosage guidelines may seem backward because children require more drug per lb. of body weight than do adults. This is because children break down xanthine bronchodilators faster than adults do.

Theophylline dosage must be tailored to your specific condition. The best dose is the lowest that will control your symptoms.

Overdosage

The first symptoms of overdose are loss of appetite, nausea, vomiting, nervousness, difficulty sleeping, headache, and restlessness. These symptoms are followed by rapid or abnormal heart rhythm, unusual behavior, extreme thirst, delirium, convulsions, very high temperature, and collapse.

These serious toxic symptoms are rarely experienced after overdose by mouth, which generally produces loss of appetite, nausea, vomiting, and stimulation. The overdose victim should be taken to a hospital emergency room immediately. ALWAYS bring the prescription bottle or container with you.

Special Information

Do not chew or crush coated or sustained-release capsules or tablets. Doing so could result in the immediate release of large amounts of the drug, possibly causing serious side effects.

To ensure consistent effectiveness, take your medication at the same time and in the same way, with or without food, every day.

Call your doctor if you develop nausea, vomiting, heartburn, sleeplessness, jitteriness, restlessness, headache, rash, severe stomach pain, convulsions, or a rapid or irregular heartbeat. Acute drug toxicity may descend abruptly, with little or no warning; serious side effects such as convulsions, life-threatening arrhythmias, and death may result. Periodic monitoring by your physician is mandatory if you are taking a xanthine bronchodilator.

Do not change xanthine bronchodilator brands without notifying your doctor or pharmacist. Different brands of the same bronchodilator may not be identical in their effect on your body.

If you forget to take a dose of your xanthine bronchodilator, take it as soon as you remember. If it is almost time for your next dose, skip the one you forgot and continue with your regular schedule. Do not take a double dose.

Special Populations

Pregnancy/Breast-feeding

Xanthine bronchodilators pass into the fetal circulation. They do not cause birth defects, but they may produce dangerous drug levels in a newborn's bloodstream. Babies born to women who take one of these drugs may be nervous, jittery, and irritable, and may gag or vomit when fed. Pregnant women who must use a xanthine bronchodilator to control asthma or other conditions should talk with their doctors about the risks of this medication.

These drugs pass into breast milk and may cause a nursing infant to be nervous and irritable or to have difficulty sleeping. Nursing mothers who must use one of these drugs should bottle-feed their babies.

Seniors

Seniors, especially men age 55 and over, may take longer to clear the xanthine bronchodilators from their bodies than do younger adults. Seniors with heart failure or other cardiac conditions, chronic lung disease, a viral infection with fever, or reduced liver function may require a lower dosage of this medication to account for the clearance effect.

Generic Name

Zafirlukast (zah-fere-LUE-kast)

Brand Name

Accolate

Type of Drug

Leukotriene receptor antagonist (LTRA).

Prescribed for

Asthma prevention.

General Information

Zafirlukast is the first of a new group of antiasthma drugs, LTRAs. LTRAs counteract the effects of leukotrienes, chemicals that are a part of the body's allergic or reactive response. In asthma, the presence of leukotrienes has been associated directly with swelling of tissues and tightening of muscles in the throat, causing it to close during an attack. Zafirlukast prevents this from happening by preventing leukotriene chemicals from binding to nerve endings in the throat. Zafirlukast is absorbed into the bloodstream after the tablets are swallowed. About 10% of each dose leaves the body through the kidneys; the rest is broken down in the liver.

Cautions and Warnings

Zafirlukast does not treat asthma attacks. It is to be used only as a preventive treatment.

Do not take zafirlukast if you are **allergic** or **sensitive** to it.

People with **liver damage** have 50% to 60% more zafirlukast in their blood and may need to take a lower dose.

Possible Side Effects

▼ Most common: headache.

▼ Less common: nausea, diarrhea, and infections.

▼ Infrequent: dizziness, abdominal pain, vomiting, general pain, weakness, accidental injury, muscle aches, fever, back pain, liver inflammation, and upset stomach.

Drug Interactions

• Aspirin increases the amount of zafirlukast in the blood by almost 50%.

• Zafirlukast interferes with the functioning of some enzyme systems in the liver that are responsible for breaking down certain drugs. The effects of other drugs broken down in the liver may be enhanced if they are taken with zafirlukast.

• Erythromycin, terfenadine, and theophylline reduce the amount of zafirlukast in the blood by 30% to 50%.

• Zafirlukast increases the effect of warfarin, which may lead to dangerous bleeding because the blood cannot clot. People who take both of these medications must have their warfarin dosage adjusted to take this effect into account.

Food Interactions

Food interferes with the absorption of zafirlukast into the blood. Take each dose at least 1 hour before or 2 hours after meals.

Usual Dose

Adult and Child (age 12 and over): 20 mg 2 times a day.
Child (under age 12): not recommended.

Overdosage

Animals given as much zafirlukast as 1000 mg per lb. of body weight have survived. There is little information, however, about the effect of zafirlukast overdose in people. Overdose victims should be taken to a hospital emergency room. ALWAYS bring the prescription bottle or container with you.

Special Information

Zafirlukast must be taken on a regular basis to prevent

asthma attacks. If you stop taking the medication, the chances are that your attacks will become frequent and get worse. You should continue taking zafirlukast even if you are having an asthma attack, unless instructed by your doctor to stop.

If you forget to take a dose of zafirlukast, take it as soon as you remember. If it is almost time for your next dose, skip the dose you forgot and continue with your regular schedule. Do not take a double dose.

Special Populations

Pregnancy/Breast-feeding

Pregnant animals given very high doses of zafirlukast had spontaneous abortions and other problems, but there is no information on its possible effect in pregnant women. When this drug is considered crucial by your doctor, its potential benefits must carefully be weighed against its risks.

Zafirlukast passes into breast milk and can affect a nursing infant. Nursing mothers who must take this medication should bottle-feed their babies.

Seniors

In studies of zafirlukast, people age 55 and older reported more infections—mostly mild or moderate respiratory infections—than did younger people. Report anything unusual to your doctor. Seniors eliminate zafirlukast from their bodies more slowly than younger people and can have 2 to 3 times as much drug in their blood; a dosage adjustment may be required.

Generic Name

Zalcitabine (zal-SYE-tuh-bene)

Brand Name

Hivid

Type of Drug

Antiviral.

Prescribed for

Human immunodeficiency virus (HIV) infection, either alone or in combination with zidovudine (AZT).

General Information

Zalcitabine, also known as ddC or dideoxycytidine, was first approved for use in multiple-drug treatment of acquired immunodeficiency syndrome (AIDS), but it can be used alone in people who cannot tolerate AZT or whose disease has progressed while taking AZT. Zalcitabine interferes with the reproduction of the HIV virus by interrupting its internal DNA manufacturing process. DNA carries the essential genetic messages that direct all life processes; by acting on the DNA of HIV, zalcitabine interferes with the life of the HIV virus. Zalcitabine was originally approved because of its ability to increase blood levels of CD4 cells. CD4 cells represent the level of immune function and are considered important indicators of the severity of an AIDS-related infection.

Zalcitibine has been compared with didanosine (ddI) as a single-drug treatment for HIV infection. In these studies, both drugs were equally effective in prolonging the time to the next AIDS-defining event, but survival comparisons favored zalcitabine. When zalcitibine was given together with AZT to people who had not previously received AZT, the combination was better than AZT alone. People who had been taking AZT and then added zalcitibine did not benefit more than people who took either drug alone.

Cautions and Warnings

Zalcitibine has caused **severe, potentially fatal side effects**. Although it is rare, people taking zalcitibine, AZT, or didanosine can develop lactic acidosis (a potentially fatal metabolic imbalance).

Between 22% and 35% of people taking zalcitibine experience **nervous system inflammation**, which is generally signaled by numbness and burning pain in the hands and feet. These symptoms may be followed by sharp shooting pains or a severe and continuous burning pain. If the drug is continued, these pains may become permanent and require narcotic pain relievers. People who already have signs of this kind of nerve damage should not take zalcitabine. Stop taking zalcitabine if the numbness, burning, and pain become moderately uncomfortable. If the symptoms get better on their own after you stop taking the drug, you may, after consultation with your doctor, start taking zalcitabine again in a smaller dosage.

Fatal inflammation of the pancreas has occurred in less

than 1% of people taking zalcitabine. People with a history of pancreatic inflammation should take this drug only after careful consideration. Symptoms of inflammation of the pancreas include major changes in blood-sugar levels, rising blood levels of triglycerides, a drop in blood calcium, nausea, vomiting, and abdominal pain. People who develop pancreatic inflammation must stop taking zalcitabine.

Mouth ulcers developed in about 3% of people taking zalcitibine during clinical studies. Infrequently, people taking zalcitabine develop **ulcers of the esophagus**.

People taking zalcitabine may develop **heart failure**. People who already have heart failure should take this drug only after careful consideration.

Do not take zalcitabine if you are **allergic** to it or any ingredient in the zalcitabine tablet.

Zalcitibine may worsen the condition of people with **liver disease**. Death from liver failure may also occur with zalcitabine. **Alcohol abuse** aggravates the liver problems associated with zalcitabine.

Possible Side Effects

▼ Most common: mouth sores, nausea and vomiting, appetite loss, abdominal pain, itching, rashes, headache, muscle ache, joint pain, tiredness, sore throat, fever, chest pain, and weight loss.

▼ Less common: swallowing difficulties, constipation, stomach irritation and ulcers, night sweats, and foot pain.

▼ Rare: muscle weakness, pain, not feeling well, high blood pressure, heart palpitations, abnormal heart rhythms, dizziness, dry mouth, ulcers in the esophagus, upset stomach, tongue inflammation or ulcers, hemorrhoids, rectal bleeding, stomach bleeding, enlarged abdomen, gum disease, stomach gas, pancreatic inflammation, enlarged salivary glands, throat pain, rectal ulcers, diabetes, high blood sugar, low blood calcium, impotence, hot flushes, hepatitis, yellowing of the skin and whites of the eyes, abnormal liver function, nosebleeds, arthritis, cold hands or feet, leg cramps, muscle inflammation, seizures, poor muscle control, loss of coordination, Bell's palsy, migraine headache, nerve pain, stupor, fainting, tremors and twitching, confusion, loss of concentration, sleeplessness, agitation, hallucination,

---

Possible Side Effects *(continued)*

emotional instability, depersonalization reactions, anxiety, depression, euphoria (feeling high), abnormal thought patterns, memory loss, cough, breathing difficulties, flu-like symptoms, blue discoloration of the hands or feet, skin reactions, acne, hair loss, sweating, abnormal vision, hearing difficulties, loss of or changes in sense of taste, burning and itching eyes, eye pain, ringing or buzzing in the ears, and arm, wrist, or shoulder pain.

Drug Interactions

• Chloramphenicol, cisplatin, dapsone, didanosine, disulfiram, ethionamide, glutethimide, gold, hydralazine, iodoquinol, isoniazid, metronidazole, nitrofurantoin, phenytoin, ribavirin, vincristine, and other drugs that can cause nervous system inflammation should be avoided while taking zalcitabine.

• Drugs such as probenecid, foscarnet, cimetidine, amphotericin, and aminoglycoside-type antibiotics may interfere with the elimination of zalcitabine from the kidneys, increasing the chance of side effects.

• Drugs that may cause inflammation of the pancreas—including intravenous pentamidine—should not be taken with zalcitabine.

• Taking metoclopramide together with zalcitabine moderately reduces the amount of zalcitabine absorbed into the blood.

Food Interactions

Food interferes with the amount of zalcitabine absorbed and the speed at which it is absorbed into the blood. Take zalcitabine on an empty stomach, or 1 hour before or 2 hours after meals.

Usual Dose

Adult and Child (age 13 and older): 0.75 mg every 8 hours. For people with poor kidney function, dosage may be reduced to 0.75 mg once or twice a day.

Overdosage

Zalcitabine overdose victims generally experience side effects of the drug, especially inflammation of the nervous system. There is little experience with treating zalcitabine overdose. Victims should be taken to a hospital emergency room for testing and monitoring. ALWAYS bring the prescription bottle or container with you.

Special Information

Zalcitabine is not an AIDS cure. It will not prevent you from transmitting the HIV virus to another person; you must still practice safe sex. Patients may still develop AIDS-related opportunistic infections while taking this drug.

Zalcitabine may cause anemia and affect other components of the blood. Your doctor should perform blood tests to check for any changes.

People taking zalcitabine should take good care of their teeth and gums to minimize the possibility of oral infections.

Call your doctor if you develop any of the following symptoms of zalcitabine toxicity: numbness and burning pain in the hands and feet; sharp, shooting pains or a severe and continuous burning pain; nausea; vomiting; or abdominal pain.

If you forget to take a dose of zalcitabine, take it as soon as you remember. If it is almost time for your next dose, allow 2 to 4 hours to pass between the dose your took late and your next dose, and then continue with your regular schedule. Do not take a double dose. Call your doctor for more specific advice if you forget to take several doses.

Special Populations

Pregnancy/Breast-feeding

In animal studies, zalcitabine causes the development of malformed fetuses. There are no studies of pregnant women taking this drug. Women who are or might become pregnant should use effective contraception while taking zalcitibine.

It is not known if zalcitabine passes into breast milk. In any case, mothers who are HIV positive should bottle-feed their babies to avoid transmitting the virus through their milk.

Seniors

People with reduced kidney function, including older adults, should receive smaller doses of zalcitabine than those with normal kidneys.

Zantac

see **Ranitidine**, page 962

Zestril

see **Lisinopril**, page 592

Ziac

see **Bisoprolol**, page 122

Generic Name

Zidovudine (zih-DOE-vuh-dene) G

Brand Name

Retrovir

Type of Drug

Antiviral.

Prescribed for

Human immunodeficiency virus (HIV) infection.

General Information

Zidovudine, also known as azidothymidine, compound S, and AZT—which it is commonly called—was the first drug approved for use in the U.S. under a special government program. Drugs in this program are released to the public before they have been tested completely for safety and effectiveness because of the severity of the specific disease they are designed to treat. AZT inhibits the production of several viruses, including the HIV virus that causes acquired immunodeficiency syndrome (AIDS). It works by interfering with specific enzymes within the virus that are responsible for essential steps in HIV's reproduction process. It has been generally recognized that AZT helps people with AIDS to live longer, although an international study of AIDS patients questions this claim. Treatment recommendations emphasize that AZT should be used to fight the HIV virus only in the later stages of the illness, when symptoms have developed and CD4 cell counts are below 500. CD4 cells are an important part of the immune system. Numbers of such cells in the blood are widely regarded as an indication of the severity of the disease; fewer CD4 cells usually indicate more serious AIDS-related conditions. Early treatment of HIV-positive patients who do not have symptoms are now focused on general health measures and supportive therapies. The true safety and effectiveness of AZT after prolonged use, and in people with less-advanced HIV disease, are not known.

Cautions and Warnings

AZT may cause severe reductions in white- and red-blood-cell counts and should be taken with caution by people with **bone-marrow disease** or those whose bone marrow has already been compromised by other treatments. Your doctor should take a blood count every 2 weeks; if problems develop, the dosage should be reduced.

In rare instances, people taking AZT or other nucleoside-type antivirals have developed **lactic acidosis** (a potentially fatal metabolic imbalance). Symptoms of lactic acidosis may include unexplained rapid breathing, breathing difficulties, and reduced blood-bicarbonate levels—which your doctor can detect with a routine blood test.

People with **impaired kidney or liver function** should use this drug with caution.

Prolonged use of AZT may cause **muscle irritation and abnormalities** similar to those caused by HIV infection.

Possible Side Effects

Adult

▼ Most common: anemia, reduced white-blood-cell counts, headache, nausea, sleeplessness, and muscle aches.

▼ Less common: body odor, chills, flu-like symptoms, greater susceptibility to feeling pain, back pain, chest pain, swelling of the lymph nodes, flushing and warmth,

Possible Side Effects *(continued)*

constipation, swallowing difficulties, swelling of the lips
and tongue, bleeding gums, mouth sores, stomach gas,
flatulence, bleeding from the rectum, joint pain, muscle
spasms, tremors, twitching, anxiety, confusion, depression, emotional flare-ups, dizziness, fainting, loss of mental sharpness, cough, nosebleeds, runny nose, sinus
inflammation, hoarseness, acne, itching, rash, double
vision, sensitivity to bright light, hearing loss, painful or
difficult urination, and frequent urination.

Child
▼ Most common: anemia, reduced white-blood-cell
counts, vomiting, abdominal pains, fever, and sleeplessness.
▼ Less common: headache, blood infection, nervousness, and irritability.
▼ Rare: nausea, diarrhea, weight loss, seizures, heart
failure and other cardiac abnormalities, blood in the
urine, and bladder infections.

Drug Interactions

• Combining AZT with other drugs that can damage your
kidneys, including pentamidine, dapsone, amphotericin B,
flucytosine, vincristine, vinblastine, adriamycin, and alfa- and
beta-interferon, increases the chance of loss of some kidney
function.

• Probenecid may reduce the rate at which your body
eliminates AZT, increasing the amount of the drug in your
blood and the chances for side effects. Other drugs that can
reduce the liver's ability to break down AZT are acetaminophen, aspirin, indomethacin, and trimethoprim; combining
any of these drugs with AZT may lead to increased side
effects.

• Acyclovir is often used in combination with AZT to
combat opportunistic infections in AIDS patients; however,
this combination may cause lethargy or seizures.

• Other drugs that can cause anemia, including ganciclovir
or zalcitabine, should be used carefully in combination with
AZT because of the risk of worsening drug-related anemia.

• Taking AZT together with rifampin or rifampicin may
reduce the amount of AZT absorbed into the blood.

• Taking phenytoin and AZT together may affect the amounts of both drugs in the blood, usually increasing the amount of AZT. The effect on phenytoin blood levels varies. This combination can result in either too much phenytoin—leading to phenytoin side effects—or too little phenytoin—leading to a possible increase in the number of seizures. Your doctor should check your phenytoin levels if you are also taking AZT.

Food Interactions

AZT is best taken on an empty stomach, but you may take it with food if it upsets your stomach.

Usual Dose

Adult: symptomatic AIDS—100 mg every 4 hours around the clock, even if sleep must be interrupted. Dosage may be reduced if side effects develop. Asymptomatic AIDS—100 mg every 4 hours during waking hours. Combination therapy with zalcitabine—200 mg of AZT with 0.8 mg of zalcitabine every 8 hours.

Pregnancy: AZT is used to prevent transmission of HIV infection to the fetus. After 14 weeks of pregnancy—100 mg 5 times a day, until labor starts. During labor and delivery—intravenously, until the umbilical cord is clamped.

Child (age 3 months–12 years): up to 100 mg every 6 hours.

Infant: about 1 mg per lb. of body weight every 6 hours by mouth, starting within 12 hours of birth and continuing through 6 weeks of age. The drug may be given intravenously if necessary.

Overdosage

The most serious effect of AZT overdose is suppression of bone marrow and its ability to make red and white blood cells. Overdose victims should be taken to a hospital emergency room at once. ALWAYS bring the prescription bottle or container with you.

Special Information

AZT does not cure AIDS. It will not decrease the chance of your transmitting the HIV virus to another person; you must still practice safe sex. AZT may not prevent some illnesses associated with AIDS or AIDS-related complex (ARC) from continuing to develop.

See your doctor if any significant change in your health

occurs. Periodic blood counts are very important while taking AZT to detect possibly serious side effects. Avoid acetaminophen, aspirin, and other drugs that may increase AZT toxicity.

Be sure to take this drug exactly as prescribed—around the clock if needed, even though it will interfere with your sleep. Do not take more AZT than your doctor has prescribed.

People taking AZT must take especially good care of their teeth and gums to minimize the chance of developing oral infections.

If you miss a dose of AZT, take it as soon as possible. If it is almost time for your next dose, allow 2 to 4 hours to pass between the dose you took late and your next dose, and then continue with your regular schedule. Do not take a double dose.

Protect AZT capsules and liquid from light.

Special Populations

Pregnancy/Breast-feeding

To avoid conceiving a child that could be born infected with HIV, HIV-positive women should use effective contraception. However, if you are HIV-positive and pregnant, talk to your doctor about taking or continuing your AZT. AZT treatment in HIV-positive women who are pregnant has been shown to sharply reduce the chances of transmitting the HIV virus to babies. Treatment should begin by the 14th week of pregnancy and continue through delivery. The baby should also be given AZT for the first 6 weeks of life. Studies have shown that the risk of birth defects is not increased by taking AZT during pregnancy.

It is not known if AZT passes into breast milk. In any case, mothers who are HIV positive should bottle-feed their babies to avoid transmitting the virus through their milk.

Seniors

Seniors may be at a greater risk of AZT side effects because of reduced kidney function.

Generic Name

Zileuton (zih-LUE-tun)

Brand Name

Zyflo Filmtab

Type of Drug

Leukotriene receptor inhibitor.

Prescribed for

Asthma prevention and long-term treatment.

General Information

Zileuton belongs to a new group of antiasthma drugs which inhibit the formation of leukotrienes, chemicals that are a natural part of the body's allergic or reactive response. In asthma, leukotrienes have been associated directly with swelling of tissues and tightening of muscles in the throat, causing it to close during an attack. Since zileuton interferes with the formation of leukotrienes, people taking it should have fewer and less severe asthma attacks. Zileuton differs from zafirlukast, a leukotriene receptor antagonist, which interferes with the action of leukotrienes in a developing reaction. The drug is absorbed into the bloodstream after the tablets are swallowed, and most of it is broken down in the liver.

Cautions and Warnings

Zileuton does not treat asthma attacks. It is to be used only as prevention and long-term treatment for asthma.

Do not take Zileuton if you are **allergic** or **sensitive** to it or if you have active **liver disease**. Dose adjustments are not needed for people with kidney disease.

Zileuton can cause low **white-blood-cell counts;** these usually return to normal after the drug is stopped.

Possible Side Effects

▼ Most common: headache.

▼ Common: general pain, upset stomach, nausea, and liver inflammation.

▼ Less common: abdominal pain, weakness, accidental injury, and muscle aches.

▼ Rare: joint pain, chest pain, red-eye, constipation, dizziness, fever, stomach gas, muscle stiffness, sleeplessness, swollen lymph glands, not feeling well, neck pain or rigidity, nervousness, itching, tiredness, urinary infections, vaginal inflammation, and vomiting.

Drug Interactions

• Zileuton increases the effects of theophylline, terfenadine, propranolol, and warfarin, leading to an increased drug
effect and possibly dangerous side effects. People who must
combine these drugs should have their doctors adjust their
dosages.

• Zileuton has been tested with digoxin, oral contraceptives, phenytoin, and prednisone; no interaction with these
drugs has been found.

Food Interactions

None known.

Usual Dose

Adult and Child (age 12 and older): 600 mg 4 times a day.
Child (under age 12): not recommended.

Overdosage

Animals given as much zileuton as 1000 mg per lb. of body
weight have survived. There is little information, however,
about the effect of zileuton overdose in people. Overdose
victims should be taken to a hospital emergency room for
treatment. ALWAYS bring the prescription bottle or container
with you.

Special Information

Zileuton must be taken on a regular basis to prevent asthma
attacks. If you stop taking the medication, the chances are
that your attacks will become more frequent and get worse.
You should continue taking zileuton even if you are having an
asthma attack, unless instructed by your doctor to stop.

Liver inflammation is the most serious side effect of zileuton; your doctor should periodically check your liver function
while you are taking this drug. Call your doctor if you develop
any signs of liver damage (symptoms include severe itching,
dark-colored urine, flu, tiredness, appetite loss, yellowing of
the skin or whites of the eyes, abdominal pain, and stomach
or intestinal problems).

Because zileuton can interact with other drugs, be sure to
tell your doctor and pharmacist about all of the medications
you are taking.

Zileuton is only one part of your asthma treatment. Do not

stop taking any of your other asthma medications or change their dosages without your doctor's knowledge.

Taking zileuton with meals and at bedtime will help you remember all of your daily tablets. If you forget a dose of zileuton, take it as soon as you remember. If it is almost time for your next dose, skip the dose you forgot and continue with your regular schedule. Do not take a double dose.

Special Populations

Pregnancy/Breast-feeding
Studies with pregnant rats given zileuton indicated there might be a problem, but there is no information on its possible effect in pregnant women. When this drug is considered crucial by your doctor, its potential benefits must carefully be weighed against its risks.

Zileuton may pass into breast milk and affect a nursing infant. Nursing mothers who must take this medication should consider bottle-feeding their babies.

Seniors
Seniors may take zileuton without special precaution.

Zithromax

see **Azithromycin**, page 90

Zocor

see **Simvastatin**, page 1006

Generic Name

Zolmitriptan (zol-mih-TRIP-tan)

Brand Name
Zomig

Type of Drug
Antimigraine.

Prescribed for

Migraine.

General Information

Zolmitriptan may work by slowing the activity of certain serotonin-controlled nerves in the brain. Specifically, it is thought that zolmitriptan relieves the pain of migraine headache by slowing the firing of the serotonin receptor 5-HT$_{1B/1D}$ in blood vessels in the brain and in nerves that may cause blood vessels in the brain to become constricted. Zolmitriptan does not affect most other serotonin receptors.

Zolmitriptan relieves only your migraine symptoms. It has not been approved for cluster headache. Drugs similar to zolmitriptan are currently used for cluster headache and zolmitriptan is likely to be approved for it in the future. Zolmitriptan does not prevent a migraine from developing and should only be used if you are having an attack. It should not be used until other pain-relieving alternatives have been tried including aspirin, acetaminophen, and other nonsteroidal anti-inflammatory drugs (NSAIDs). Zolmitriptan also relieves the nausea, vomiting, and light and sound sensitivity that generally accompany migraine.

If serious, incapacitating migraine occurs more often than twice a month, your doctor may have you take medication other than zolmitriptan on a regular basis to reduce the number and severity of migraine attacks. Some of the drugs you may be advised to take are beta-adrenergic blockers, calcium channel blockers, tricyclic antidepressants, monoamine oxidase inhibitor (MAOI) antidepressants, methysergide, and cyproheptadine—especially in children. You may be able to reduce your need for medication by avoiding factors that trigger migraine. Relaxation or biofeedback techniques may also help.

Zolmitriptan, unlike sumatriptan (a related antimigraine drug), is well absorbed after you swallow it and reaches maximum blood concentrations in 2 hours. It starts relieving migraine pain within an hour. Zolmitriptan's maximum effect occurs in about 2 hours.

Cautions and Warnings

Do not use this drug if you have had an **allergic reaction** to it in the past.

Zolmitriptan should not be used if you have **angina, poor**

blood supply to the heart muscle, or uncontrolled hypertension (high blood pressure) or have had a **heart attack**.

It is strongly recommended that antimigraine drugs of this type not be taken by people at risk of **heart disease** as indicated by known factors including hypertension, high blood cholesterol, smoking, obesity, diabetes, and a family history of heart disease. In this case, a medical evaluation providing assurance that you are not at risk of heart disease should be done before this drug is prescribed.

Do not take zolmitriptan if your **headache is unusual** in any way. Call your doctor at once.

Strokes and some fatalities have been reported in people taking antimigraine drugs of this type. Death is likely to have occurred because a stroke-related headache was treated with antimigraine medication and was not identified as a symptom of stroke. People with migraine headache are more likely to have a stroke or bleeding in the brain.

Most of this drug is broken down in the liver. About 17% of it is eliminated through the kidneys. People with severe **liver disease** do not break down the drug as efficiently as others and may develop **hypertension** in rare cases. Dosages below 2.5 mg a day are recommended. No special caution is required for people with kidney disease.

Zolmitriptan may accumulate in the eye, possibly leading to chronic (long-term) problems though no problems have been identified in studies. Call your doctor if you experience any **changes in vision**.

Possible Side Effects

Side effects are usually mild or moderate, are not long-lasting, and are the same in men and women regardless of age. Certain side effects get worse as dosage increases, especially tingling in the hands or feet; chest, neck, jaw, or throat tightness or heaviness; dizziness; tiredness; weakness; and nausea.

▼ Most common: chest, jaw, or neck tightness; tingling; warmth or burning; dizziness; and fainting.

▼ Less common: reduced sensation, chest pressure; chest heaviness, chest tightness, dry mouth, upset stomach, difficulty swallowing, nausea, weakness, heart palpitations, muscle ache and weakness, sweating, allergic reaction, chills, facial swelling, fever, feeling unwell, sen-

Possible Side Effects *(continued)*

sitivity to bright light, abnormal heart rhythms, hypertension, fainting, increased appetite, swollen tongue, sores
in the mouth or throat, stomach irritation, liver function
changes, thirst, swelling, back pain, leg cramp, tendon
inflammation, agitation, anxiety, depression, emotional
instability, sleeplessness, bronchitis, bronchial spasm,
nosebleeds, hiccups, laryngitis, yawning, itching, rash,
hives, dry eye, eye pain, unusual sound or smell sensitivity, ear pain, ringing or buzzing in the ears, blood in the
urine, cystitis, frequent urination, and the need to urinate.

▼ Rare: slowing of heartbeat, extra heart contractions,
dizziness and fainting when rising from a sitting or lying
position, rapid heartbeat, vein irritation, black-and-blue
marks, electrocardiogram changes, appetite loss, constipation, vomiting blood, pancreas irritation, blood in the
stool, ulcer, blue discoloration due to poor blood flow,
blood-cell abnormalities, high blood sugar, arthritis, muscle
stiffness, twitching, uncontrolled movement, memory
loss, apathy, euphoria (feeling high), hallucinations, weakness, voice changes, breathing difficulties, double vision,
tearing, painful menstruation, and miscarriage.

Drug Interactions

• MAOIs may drastically increase the effects of zolmitriptan
by slowing its breakdown in the liver. Do not take these drugs
together. If you are taking an MAOI, wait 2 weeks after you
stop taking it before using zolmitriptan.

• Ergotamine and dihydroergotamine may increase the
effects of zolmitriptan. Allow at least 24 hours between taking
either of these drugs and taking zolmitriptan.

• Do not mix zolmitriptan with sumatriptan or any similar
antimigraine drug.

• Cimetidine doubles the length of time that zolmitriptan
remains in the blood. You may need a lower dosage of
zolmitriptan if you are combining these drugs.

• Combining zolmitriptan with selective serotonin reuptake
inhibitor (SSRI) antidepressants including fluoxetine, fluvoxamine, paroxetine, and sertraline may cause weakness, overly
sensitive reflexes, or poor coordination.

Food Interactions

None known.

Usual Dose

Adult (age 18 and over): 1.25–5 mg as soon as migraine symptoms begin or at any time during the attack. If the symptoms do not go away, you may take another tablet in 2 hours; do not take more than 10 mg a day. People with liver disease should take the lowest possible dosage of zolmitriptan.

Child: not recommended.

Overdosage

There are no reports of zolmitriptan overdose. Overdose symptoms are likely to be severe side effects. Overdose victims should be taken to a hospital emergency room for treatment since they need to be watched for at least 15 hours after taking the overdose or while overdose symptoms persist. Always bring the prescription bottle or container with you.

Special Information

Notify your doctor if you have other medical conditions or heart disease risk factors such as hypertension, high cholesterol, diabetes, obesity, or a history of smoking.

People with moderate or severe liver disease should begin with lower dosages of zolmitriptan and have their blood pressure checked regularly.

Be sure to take zolmitriptan at the first sign of a migraine such as pain or aura. You may get a greater effect from the drug if you lie down in a quiet, dark room.

Avoid alcoholic beverages because they may worsen your headache.

Zolmitriptan may make you dizzy or drowsy. Take care if you have to drive or do anything else that requires concentration while taking zolmitriptan.

Read and follow instructions for use that come with the drug.

Call your doctor if the usual dosage does not relieve 3 consecutive migraines, if your migraines become more frequent or worse, if you are pregnant or breast-feeding, or if you experience chest pain; breathing difficulties or difficulty swallowing; hypertension; chest pressure, tightness, or heaviness; nausea; vomiting; or other side effects that are particularly bothersome.

If you are taking zolmitriptan tablets and develop tightness in the chest or throat, shortness of breath, or heart throbbing, call your doctor. Call your doctor at once if chest pain does not go away.

People taking zolmitriptan should have their eyes checked periodically.

Special Populations

Pregnancy/Breast-feeding

There are no studies of zolmitriptan in pregnant women. Animal studies show that it may have toxic effects on the fetus at varying dosage levels. When this drug is considered crucial by your doctor, its potential benefits must be carefully weighed against its risks.

It is not known if zolmitriptan passes into breast milk. In animal studies, the level of zolmitriptan found in breast milk was 4 times that found in the blood. Nursing mothers should take this drug with caution.

Seniors

Studies of zolmitriptan exclude people over age 65 but suggest that it has the same effect on seniors as on younger adults.

Zoloft

see **Sertaline**, *page 1002*

Generic Name

Zolpidem (ZOLE-pih-dem)

Brand Name

Ambien

Type of Drug

Sedative.

Prescribed for

Insomnia.

General Information

Zolpidem is a nonbenzodiazepine sleeping pill that works in the brain in much the same way as do benzodiazepine sleeping pills and tranquilizers. Unlike the benzodiazepines, however, zolpidem has little muscle-relaxing or antiseizure effects. It is meant for short-term use—7 to 10 days—and should not be taken regularly for longer than that without your doctor's knowledge, although it has been studied for longer periods of time. Unlike a benzodiazepine, zolpidem causes little or no hangover, and there are no rebound effects on nights following treatment when you do not take any medication. Zolpidem has only a minimal effect on sleep stages such as the all-important rapid eye movement (REM) stage, in which many important functions are accomplished including dreaming. Zolpidem is broken down in the liver.

Cautions and Warnings

Sleeping problems are often part of a physical or psychological illness. Drugs like zolpidem may treat the symptom—sleeplessness—but do not affect the **underlying reason for not being able to sleep**. They should be taken only with your doctor's knowledge. If you still cannot sleep after 7 to 10 days of taking zolpidem, it may mean that the underlying problem is getting worse and that you should see your doctor for other treatment.

Zolpidem has little effect on memory, unlike some of the short-acting benzodiazepine sleeping pills. It has caused **amnesia (memory loss)** but this happens mostly at dosages larger than 10 mg a night.

Suddenly stopping zolpidem after having taken it for some time may produce **drug withdrawal** (symptoms include fatigue, nausea, flushing, light-headedness, crying, vomiting, stomach cramps, panic, nervousness, and general discomfort). Other serious signs of drug withdrawal such as feeling unwell, sleeplessness, muscle cramp, abdominal cramp, increased sweating, tremor, and convulsions have not been seen after sudden withdrawal from zolpidem. People with a **history of substance abuse** may be more likely to develop drug dependence on zolpidem.

Zolpidem has all the effects of other nervous system depressants and may cause **loss of coordination and concentration**. It should be taken only before bedtime and never if you need to do something that requires concentration. There is a possibility that activities to be performed on the day following a zolpidem dose may also be affected, especially if alcohol was taken with zolpidem.

People with **liver disease** are much more sensitive to the effects of zolpidem and need less medication to produce the same effect than do people with normal liver function. People with severe **kidney disease** should be watched for unusual side effects.

Zolpidem should be avoided in the presence of severe **depression**, severe **lung disease, sleep apnea** (condition characterized by intermittent cessation of breathing during sleep), and drunkenness or you run the risk of increasing the depressive effects of zolpidem or worsening your overall condition.

Possible Side Effects

Short-term Use (10 Days or Less)

▼ Most common: drowsiness, dizziness, and diarrhea.

▼ Less common: chest pain, fatigue, unusual dreams, memory loss, anxiety, nervousness, difficulty sleeping, appetite loss, vomiting, and runny nose.

▼ Rare: Effects may occur in almost any part of the body.

Long-term Use

▼ Most common: drowsiness, a feeling of being drugged.

▼ Common: headache, allergy symptoms, back pain, flu-like symptoms, lethargy, sensitivity to light, depression, upset stomach, constipation, abdominal pain, muscle and joint pain, upper respiratory infection, sinus irritation, sore throat, rash, urinary infection, heart palpitations, and dry mouth.

▼ Rare: Effects may occur in almost any part of the body.

Drug Interactions

• Zolpidem is a central nervous system (CNS) depressant. Avoid alcohol because its effects and those of zolpidem compound each other. Other nervous system depressants including tranquilizers, narcotics, barbiturates, monoamine oxidase inhibitor (MAOI) antidepressants, antihistamines, and antidepressants may have a similar effect. Taking a benzodiazepine such as diazepam with zolpidem may result in excessive depression, tiredness, sleepiness, breathing difficulties, or similar symptoms.

Food Interactions

For the most rapid and complete effect, take zolpidem on an empty stomach at least 2 hours after a meal.

Usual Dose

Adult (age 18 and over): 10 mg immediately before bedtime.
Senior: 5 mg immediately before bedtime.
Child: not recommended.

People with severe liver disease should take 5 mg immediately before bedtime.

Overdosage

Zolpidem overdose results in excessive nervous system depression, from unconsciousness to light coma. Combining zolpidem with alcohol or other nervous system depressants may be fatal or affect other body organs. Zolpidem overdose victims should be taken to a hospital emergency room at once. ALWAYS bring the prescription bottle or container.

Special Information

Zolpidem may cause tiredness, drowsiness, and an inability to concentrate. Be careful if you are driving, operating machinery, or performing other activities that require concentration on the day following a zolpidem dose.

People taking zolpidem on a regular basis may develop drug withdrawal reaction if the medication is stopped suddenly (see "Cautions and Warnings").

If you forget a dose of zolpidem, take it as soon as you remember. If it is almost time for your next dose, skip the forgotten one and continue with your regular schedule. Do not take a double dose.

Special Populations

Pregnancy/Breast-feeding

Animal studies with large dosages show that zolpidem may affect the fetus. Because there is no reliable information about its effect during pregnancy, it should be used only if it is clearly needed.

Small amounts of zolpidem pass into breast milk but its effect on a nursing infant is not known. Nursing mothers who must take this drug should bottle-feed their infants.

Seniors

Seniors are likely to be more sensitive to the action of zolpidem and its side effects. Seniors should take the lowest effective dosage. Report unusual side effects to your doctor.

Zyrtec

*see **Cetirizine**, page 178*

Acetaminophen and Aspirin: Two Frequently Recommended Over-the-Counter Drugs

Generic Name

Acetaminophen (uh-SEE-tuh-MIN-uh-fen)

Brand Names

Acephen	*Mapap
Aceta	Maranox
Apacet	Meda Cap/Tab
Arthritis Foundation Pain	Neopap
Reliever Aspirin Free	Oraphen-PD
Aspirin Free Anacin	*Panadol
Maximum Strength	Redutemp
Aspirin Free Pain Relief	Ridenol
Dapacin	Silapap △
Feverall	Tapanol
*Genapap	*Tempra
Genebs	*Tylenol
Halenol	Uni-Ace △
Liquiprin △	Uniserts

Some products in this brand-name group are alcohol or sugar free. Consult your pharmacist.

Type of Drug

Antipyretic and analgesic.

Prescribed for

Relief of pain and fever for people who cannot or do not want to take aspirin or a nonsteroidal anti-inflammatory drug (NSAID). Acetaminophen may be given to children about to receive a DTP vaccination to reduce the fever and pain that commonly follow the vaccination.

General Information

Acetaminophen is generally used to relieve pain and fever associated with the common cold, flu, viral infections, or other disorders where pain or fever may occur. It is also used to relieve pain in people who are allergic to aspirin, or those who cannot take aspirin because of potential interactions with other drugs such as oral anticoagulants. It can be used to relieve pain from a variety of sources, including arthritis, headache, and tooth and periodontic pain, although it does not reduce inflammation.

Cautions and Warnings

Do not take acetaminophen if you are **allergic** or **sensitive** to it. Do not take acetaminophen for **more than 10 days in a row** unless directed by your doctor. Do not take more than is prescribed or recommended on the package.

Use this drug with extreme caution if you have **kidney or liver disease** or **viral infections of the liver**. Large amounts of alcohol increase the liver toxicity of large doses or overdoses of acetaminophen. **Avoid alcohol** if you regularly take acetaminophen. Some people are more sensitive to this effect than others.

Possible Side Effects

This drug is relatively free from side effects when taken in recommended doses. For this reason it has become extremely popular, especially among those who cannot take aspirin.

▼ Rare: large doses or long-term use may cause liver damage, rash, itching, fever, lowered blood sugar, stimulation, yellowing of the skin or whites of the eyes, and/or a change in the composition of your blood.

Drug Interactions

• Acetaminophen's effects may be reduced by long-term use or large doses of barbiturate drugs, carbamazepine, phenytoin and similar drugs, rifampin, and sulfinpyrazone. These drugs may also increase the chances of liver toxicity if taken with acetaminophen.

• Alcoholic beverages increase the chances for liver toxicity and possible liver failure associated with acetaminophen.

Food Interactions

None known.

Usual Dose

Adult and Child (age 12 and over): 300–600 mg 4 to 6 times a day, or 1000 mg 3 to 4 times a day. Avoid taking more than 2.6 g (8 325-mg tablets) a day for long periods of time.

Child (age 11): 480 mg 4–5 times a day.

Child (age 9–10): 400 mg 4–5 times a day.

Child (age 6–8): 320 mg 4–5 times a day.

Child (age 4–5): 240 mg 4–5 times a day.
Child (age 3): 160 mg 4–5 times a day.
Child (age 1–2): 120 mg 4–5 times a day.
Child (age 4–11 months): 80 mg 4–5 times a day.
Child (under 4 months): 40 mg 4–5 times a day.

Overdosage

Acute acetaminophen overdose may cause nausea, vomiting, sweating, appetite loss, drowsiness, confusion, abdominal tenderness, low blood pressure, abnormal heart rhythms, yellowing of the skin and whites of the eyes, and liver and kidney failure. Liver damage has occurred with 12 extra-strength tablets or 18 regular-strength tablets, but most people need larger doses—20 extra-strength or 30 regular-strength tablets—to damage their livers. Regular use of large doses for long periods—3000 to 4000 mg a day for a year—can also cause liver damage, especially if alcohol is involved. Acetaminophen overdose victims should be made to vomit as soon as possible by using ipecac syrup—available at any pharmacy—or another method recommended by your poison control center. Then take the victim to a hospital emergency room for further evaluation. ALWAYS bring the prescription bottle or container with you.

Special Information

Unless abused, acetaminophen is a beneficial, effective, and relatively nontoxic drug. Follow package directions and call your doctor if acetaminophen does not work in 10 days for adults or 5 days for children.

Alcoholic beverages will worsen the liver damage that acetaminophen can cause. People who take this drug on a regular basis should limit their alcohol intake.

If you forget to take a dose of acetaminophen, take it as soon as you remember. If it is within an hour of your next dose, skip the dose you forgot and continue with your regular schedule. Do not take a double dose.

Special Populations

Pregnancy/Breast-feeding

Acetaminophen is considered safe during pregnancy when taken in usual doses. Taking continuous high doses of the drug may cause birth defects or interfere with fetal development. Three cases of congenital hip dislocation appear to have been associated with acetaminophen. Check with your doctor before taking this drug if you are or might be pregnant.

Small amounts of acetaminophen may pass into breast milk, but the drug is considered harmless to nursing infants.

Seniors

Seniors may take acetaminophen as directed by a doctor.

Generic Names

Aspirin, Buffered Aspirin (AS-prin) G

Brand Names

Alka-Seltzer with Aspirin	Ecotrin
Arthritis Pain Formula	Empirin
Ascriptin	Genprin
Aspergum	Halfprin
Bayer	Magnaprin
Bufferin	Measurin
Buffex	Norwich
Cama Arthritis Pain Reliever	Wesprin
Easprin	ZORprin

Type of Drug

Analgesic and anti-inflammatory agent.

Prescribed for

Mild to moderate pain, fever, arthritis, and inflammation of bones, joints, or other body tissues. People who have had a stroke or transient ischemic attack (TIA)—oxygen shortage to the brain—may have aspirin prescribed to reduce the risk of having another such attack. Aspirin may also be prescribed as an anticoagulant (blood-thinning) drug in people with unstable angina, and to protect against heart attack. Aspirin has a definite beneficial effect if it is taken as soon as possible after having a heart attack.

General Information

Aspirin may be the closest thing we have to a wonder drug. It has been used for more than a century for pain and fever relief and is now used for its effect on the blood as well.

Aspirin is the standard against which all other drugs are

compared for relieving pain and for reducing inflammation. Chemically, aspirin is a member of the group of drugs called *salicylates*. Other salicylates include sodium salicylate, sodium thiosalicylate, choline salicylate, and magnesium salicylate (trilisate). These drugs are no more effective than regular aspirin, although two of them—choline salicylate and magnesium salicylate—may be a little less irritating to the stomach. They are all more expensive than aspirin.

Aspirin reduces fever by causing the blood vessels in the skin to open, allowing heat to leave the body more rapidly. Its effects on pain and inflammation are thought to be related to its ability to prevent the manufacture of complex body hormones called prostaglandins. Of all the salicylates, aspirin has the greatest effect on prostaglandin production.

Many people find that they can take buffered aspirin but not regular aspirin. The addition of antacids to aspirin can be important to patients who must take large doses of aspirin for chronic arthritis or other conditions. In many cases, aspirin is the only effective drug and can be tolerated only with the antacids present.

Cautions and Warnings

People with **liver damage** should avoid aspirin. People who are **allergic** to aspirin may also be allergic to nonsteroidal anti-inflammatory drugs (NSAIDs) such as indomethacin, sulindac, ibuprofen, fenoprofen, naproxen, tolmetin, and meclofenamate sodium or to products containing *tartrazine* (a commonly used orange dye and food coloring). People with **asthma** and/or **nasal polyps** are more likely to be allergic to aspirin.

Alcoholic beverages may worsen the stomach irritation caused by aspirin. Alcohol increases the risk of aspirin-related ulcers.

Stop taking aspirin if you develop **dizziness, hearing loss,** or **ringing or buzzing in your ears**.

Reye's syndrome is a life-threatening condition characterized by vomiting and stupor or dullness and may develop in **children** with influenza (flu) or chickenpox if treated with aspirin or other salicylates. Up to 30% of people who develop Reye's syndrome can die, and permanent brain damage is possible in those who survive. Because of this, authorities advise against giving children under age 16 aspirin or another salicylate, especially those with chickenpox or the flu. Take acetaminophen instead.

Aspirin **interferes with normal blood clotting** and should therefore be avoided for 1 week **before surgery**. Ask for your surgeon or dentist's recommendation before taking aspirin for pain after surgery.

Possible Side Effects

▼ Most common: nausea, upset stomach, heartburn, loss of appetite, and loss of small amounts of blood in the stool.

▼ Less common: hives, rashes, liver damage, fever, thirst, and visual difficulties. Aspirin may contribute to the formation of stomach ulcers and bleeding. People who are allergic to aspirin and those with a history of nasal polyps, asthma, or rhinitis may experience breathing difficulty and a stuffed nose.

Drug Interactions

• People taking anticoagulant (blood-thinning) drugs should avoid aspirin because it increases the effect of the anticoagulant.

• Aspirin may increase the possibility of stomach ulcer when taken together with adrenal corticosteroids, phenylbutazone, or alcoholic beverages.

• Aspirin will counteract the uric-acid-eliminating effect of probenecid and sulfinpyrazone. Aspirin may counteract the blood-pressure-lowering effect of ACE inhibitor and beta-blocking drugs. Aspirin may also counteract the effects of some diuretics in people with severe liver disease.

• Aspirin may increase blood levels of methotrexate and of valproic acid when taken with either of these drugs, leading to increased chances of drug toxicity. Mixing aspirin and nitroglycerin tablets may lead to an unexpected drop in blood pressure.

• Do not take aspirin with an NSAID. There is no benefit to the combination, and the chance of side effects—especially stomach irritation—is vastly increased.

• Large aspirin doses (2000 mg a day or more) can lower blood sugar. This can be a problem in diabetics who take insulin or oral antidiabetes drugs to control their condition.

Food Interactions

Because aspirin can cause upset stomach and bleeding, take each dose with food, milk, or a glass of water.

Usual Dose

Adult: aches, pains, and fever—325–650 mg every 4 hours. Arthritis and rheumatic conditions—up to 5200 mg a day in divided doses. Rheumatic fever, up to 7800 mg a day in divided doses. To prevent heart attack, stroke, or TIA—325 mg every 2 days or 80–160 mg a day.

Child (under age 16): not recommended because of the risk of Reye's syndrome (see "Cautions and Warnings").

Overdosage

Aspirin may be lethal for adults in overdoses of 30 regular-strength tablets—325 mg each—or 20 maximum-strength tablets—500 mg. Aspirin may be lethal for children in overdoses of 12 regular-strength tablets or 8 maximum-strength tablets.

Symptoms of mild overdose are rapid and deep breathing, nausea, vomiting, dizziness, ringing or buzzing in the ears, flushing, sweating, thirst, headache, drowsiness, diarrhea, and rapid heartbeat.

Severe overdose may cause fever, excitement, confusion, convulsions, liver or kidney failure, coma, and bleeding.

The initial treatment of aspirin overdose involves making the patient vomit to remove any drug remaining in the stomach. Further treatment depends on how the situation develops and what must be done to maintain the patient. Do not induce vomiting until you have spoken with your doctor or poison control center. If in doubt, go to a hospital emergency room.

Special Information

Contact your doctor if you develop continuous stomach pain or ringing or buzzing in the ears.

Do not use an aspirin product if it has a strong odor of vinegar. This is an indication that the product has started to break down in the bottle.

If you forget to take a dose of aspirin, take it as soon as you remember. If it is almost time for your next dose, skip the dose you forgot and continue with your regular schedule. Do not take a double dose.

Special Populations

Pregnancy/Breast-feeding

Check with your doctor before taking any aspirin-containing

product during pregnancy. Aspirin may cause bleeding problems in the fetus during the last 2 weeks of pregnancy. Taking aspirin during the last 3 months of pregnancy may extend the length of pregnancy, prolong labor, and lead to a low-birthweight infant. It can also cause bleeding in the mother before, during, or after delivery.

Aspirin has not caused any problems among nursing mothers or their infants.

Seniors

Aspirin, especially in the larger doses that an older adult may take to treat arthritis and rheumatic conditions, may be irritating to the stomach. Seniors with liver disease should not use aspirin.

Twenty Questions to Ask Your Doctor and Pharmacist About Your Prescription

1. What is the name of this medication?

2. What results may be expected from taking it?

3. How long should I wait before reporting if this medication does not help me?

4. How does the medication work?

5. What is the exact dosage of the medication?

6. What time of day should I take it?

7. Do alcoholic beverages have an effect on this medication?

8. Do I have to take special precautions with this medication in combination with other prescription medications I am taking?

9. Do I have to take special precautions with this medication in combination with over-the-counter medications?

10. Does food have any effect on this medication?

11. Are there any special instructions I should have about how to use this medication?

12. How long should I continue to take this medication?

13. Is my prescription renewable?

14. For how long a period may my prescription be renewed?

15. Which side effects should I report, and which ones may I disregard?

16. May I save any unused part of this medication for future use?

17. How should I store this medication?

18. How long may I keep this medication without it losing its strength?

19. What should I do if I miss a dose of this medication?

20. Does this medication come in a less expensive, generic form?

Other Points to Remember
for Safe Drug Use

- Store your medications in a sealed, light-resistant container to maintain maximum potency, and be sure to follow any special storage instructions listed on your prescription bottle or container, such as "refrigerate," "do not freeze," "protect from light," or "keep in a cool place." Protect all medications from excessive humidity.
- Make sure you tell the doctor everything that is wrong. The more information your doctor has, the more effective will be your treatment.
- Make sure each doctor you see knows about all the medications you use regularly, including prescription and over-the-counter (OTC) medications.
- Keep a record of any bad reaction you have had to a medication.
- Fill each prescription you are given. If you do not fill a prescription, make sure your doctor knows you are not taking the medication.
- Do not take extra medication without consulting your doctor or pharmacist.
- Follow the label instructions exactly. If you have any questions, call your doctor or pharmacist.
- Report any unusual symptoms that develop after taking any medication.
- Do not save unused medication for future use unless you

have consulted your doctor. Dispose of unused medication by flushing it down the toilet.

- Never keep medications where children may see or reach them.
- Always read the label before taking your medication. Do not trust your memory.
- Consult your pharmacist for guidance on the use of medications.
- Do not share your medication with anyone. Your prescription was written for you and only you.
- Be sure the label stays on the container until the medication is used or destroyed.
- Keep the label facing up when pouring liquid medication from the bottle.
- Do not use a prescription medication unless it has been specifically prescribed for you. Whenever you travel, carry your prescription in its original container.
- If you move to another city, ask your pharmacist to forward your prescription records to your new pharmacy. Carry important medical facts about yourself in your wallet. Such things as drug allergies, chronic diseases (e.g., diabetes), and special requirements may be very useful.
- Do not hesitate to discuss the cost of medical care with your doctor or pharmacist.
- Exercise your right to make decisions about purchasing medications:
  1. If you suffer from a chronic condition, you will probably save money by buying in larger quantities.
  2. Choose your pharmacist as carefully as you choose your doctor.
  3. Remember, the cost of your prescription includes the professional services offered by your pharmacy. If you want more service, you may have to pay for it.

THE TOP 200 PRESCRIPTION DRUGS IN THE UNITED STATES

RANKED BY NUMBER OF PRESCRIPTIONS DISPENSED FROM JANUARY TO MAY 1997

(Generic products are followed by manufacturer name in parentheses.)

1. Premarin
2. Trimox
3. Synthroid
4. Lanoxin
5. Hydrocodone with APAP (Watson)
6. Prozac
7. Vasotec
8. Zantac
9. Albuterol (Warwick)
10. Coumadin sodium
11. Prilosec
12. Zoloft
13. Procardia XL
14. Norvasc
15. Claritin
16. Zocor
17. Biaxin
18. Cardizem CD
19. Zestril
20. Augmentin
21. Paxil
22. Amoxil
23. Furosemide (Mylan)
24. Triamterene/HCTZ (Geneva)
25. Trimethoprim/ sulfamethoxazole (Teva)
26. Cipro
27. Prempro
28. K-Dur
29. Glucophage
30. Cephalexin (Teva)
31. Acetaminophen wlith codeine (Teva)
32. Amoxicillin trihydrate (Teva)
33. Hytrin
34. Propoxyphen-N with APAP (Mylan)
35. Pravachol
36. Ultram
37. Veetids
38. Dilantin
39. Propacet 100
40. Mevacor
41. Pepcid
42. Zithromax Z-Pak

43. Humulin N
44. Ambien
45. Prinivil
46. Relafen
47. Atrovent
48. Ibuprofen (Par)
49. Pondimin*
50. Alprazolam (Geneva)
51. Accupril
52. Ortho-Novum 7/7/7
53. Levoxyl
54. Claritin-D 12 Hr
55. Lotensin
56. Triphasil 28
57. Glucotrol XL
58. Verapamil SR (Zenith Goldline)
59. Propulsid
60. Lescol
61. Acetaminophen with codeine (Purpac)
62. Cephalexin (Apothecon)
63. Cardura
64. Amitriptyline HCl (Mylan)
65. Proventil inhaler
66. Ibuprofen (Greenstone)
67. Depakote
68. Adalat CC
69. Cefzil
70. Axid
71. Zithromax
72. Hydrochlorothiazide (Zenith Goldline)
73. Atenolol (Mylan)
74. Ceftin
75. Estrace
76. Daypro
77. Diflucan
78. Glyburide (Copley)
79. Nitrostat
80. Prednisone (Schein)
81. Imitrex
82. Medroxyprogesterone (Greenstone)
83. Humulin 70/30
84. Azmacort
85. Provera
86. BuSpar
87. Ery-Tab
88. Atenolol (Lederle)
89. Klonopin
90. Toprol-XL
91. Lotrisone
92. Lodine
93. Lorazepam (Mylan)
94. Imdur
95. Flonase
96. Atenolol (Geneva)
97. Cycrin
98. Methylphenidate (MD)
99. Lorazepam (Purpac)
100. Roxicet
101. Alprazolam (Greenstone)
102. Deltasone
103. Naproxen (Mylan)
104. Albuterol (Zenith Goldline)
105. Zyrtec
106. Calan SR
107. Vancenase AQ
108. Ventolin
109. Trental
110. Desogen
111. Hydrocodone with APAP (Qualitest)
112. Fosamax
113. Redux*
114. Estraderm
115. Prevacid
116. Serevent
117. Risperdal
118. Phentermine HCl (Eon)
119. One Touch
120. Lo/Ovral-28
121. Cozaar
122. Monopril

123. Neomycin/Polymyxin/HC (Schein)
124. Batroban
125. Metoprolol tartrate (Mylan)
126. Gemfibrozil (Warner-Chilcott)
127. Lasix
128. Ortho-Tri-Cyclen 28
129. Potassium chloride (Ethex)
130. Cyclobenzaprine HCl (Mylan)
131. Dyazide
132. Glyburide (Greenstone)
133. Ortho-Cept 28
134. Retin-A
135. Xanax
136. Dilacor XR
137. Ziac
138. Phenergan
139. Trusopt
140. Tri-Levlen 28
141. Macrobid
142. Cimetidine (Mylan)
143. Effexor
144. Humulin R
145. Tegretol
146. Klor-Con 10
147. Carisoprodol (Schein)
148. Metoprolol tartrate (Geneva)
149. Lorabid
150. Glynase PresTab
151. Vanceril
152. Glipizide (Mylan)
153. Nitro-Dur
154. Seldane*
155. Furosemide (Roxane)
156. Ortho-Cyclen-28
157. Lestrin-FE 1.5/30
158. Cefaclor (Mylan)
159. Altace
160. Floxin
161. Darvocet-N 100
162. Methylprednisolone (Duramed)
163. Amoxicillin trihydrate (Warner-Chilcott)
164. Clonazepam (Teva)
165. Diazepam (Mylan)
166. Captopril (Apothecon)
167. Doxycycline hyclate (Zenith Goldline)
168. Lamisil
169. Temazepam (Mylan)
170. Alprazolam (Mylan)
171. Clonidine HCl (Mylan)
172. Elocon
173. Dicyclomine HCl (Rugby)
174. Diclofenac sodium (Geneva)
175. Verelan
176. Zestoretic
177. Guaifenesin/PPA (Duramed)
178. Tobradex
179. Clozaril
180. Albuterol (Dey)
181. Ritalin
182. Timoptic-XE
183. Tamoxifen citrate (Barre-National)
184. Atenolol (Apothecon)
185. Wellbutrin
186. Beconase AQ
187. Suprax
188. Zovirax tablets
189. Contuss-XT
190. Ticlid
191. Hydrochlorothiazide (Lederle)
192. Serzone
193. Oruvail
194. Tenormin
195. Furosemide (Zenith Goldline)

196. Zovirax capsules
197. Sumycin
198. Loestrin-FE 1/20-2

199. Ortho-Novum 1/35 28
200. Promethazine with
     codeine (Barr)

*No longer being sold.

Source: NPA Plus™, IMS America, Ltd., 1997

Index of Generic and Brand-Name Drugs

ABOUT THE EDITOR

Educated at Columbia University, Dr. Harold Silverman has been a hospital pharmacist, author, educator, and pharmaceutical industry consultant. Currently, he is Vice Chairman of *Interscience*, a global health-care communications consultancy. Professionally, Dr. Silverman seeks to help people understand why medicines are prescribed and how to get the most from them. In addition to *THE PILL BOOK*, Dr. Silverman is coauthor of *THE VITAMIN BOOK: A No-Nonsense Consumer Guide* and *The MED FILE Drug Interactions System*. He is also the author of *THE PILL BOOK GUIDE TO SAFE DRUG USE, THE CONSUMER'S GUIDE TO POISON PROTECTION, THE WOMAN'S DRUG STORE,* and *TRAVEL HEALTHY.* Dr. Silverman's contributions to the professional literature include more than 70 articles, research papers, and textbook chapters. He is a member of many professional organizations and has served as an officer for several, including the New York State Council of Hospital Pharmacists, for which he served as president. He has taught pharmacology and clinical pharmacy at several universities and won numerous awards for his work. Dr. Silverman resides in a Washington suburb with his wife, Judith Brown, and their son, Joshua.